# The Year in Hematology
## 1978

# The Year in Hematology

## 1978

Edited by

### Robert Silber, M.D.

*New York University School of Medicine*
*New York, New York*

### Joseph LoBue, Ph.D.

*Graduate School of Arts and Science*
*New York University*
*New York, New York*

and

### Albert S. Gordon, Ph.D.

*Graduate School of Arts and Science*
*New York University*
*New York, New York*

PLENUM MEDICAL BOOK COMPANY
NEW YORK AND LONDON

The Library of Congress cataloged the first volume of this title as follows:

---

The year in hematology, 1977/edited by Albert S. Gordon, Robert Silber,
    and Joseph LoBue — New York: Plenum Medical Book Co., c1977.
    xx. 595 p.: ill.; 24 cm.
    Includes bibliographies and index.
    ISBN 0-306-32401-6

    1. Hematology. 2. Blood — Diseases. I. Gordon, Albert Saul, 1910-
        II. Silber, Robert, 1931-        , III. LoBue, Joseph.
    [DNLM: 1. Hematology — Period. W1YE395]
    RC633.Y4                          616.1'5                          77-8412

---

Library of Congress Catalog Card Number 77-8412
ISBN 0-306-32402-4

# Contributors

**George P. Canellos,** M.D., Chief of Medicine, Sidney Farber Cancer Institute; Professor of Medicine, Harvard Medical School; Senior Associate in Medicine, Peter Bent Brigham Hospital, Boston, Massachusetts

**Jack K. Chamberlain,** M.D., Assistant Professor, Department of Medicine, University of Rochester School of Medicine, Rochester, New York

**Richard A. Cooper,** M.D., Professor of Medicine, Chief, Hematology–Oncology Section, Department of Medicine, and Director, Cancer Center, University of Pennsylvania School of Medicine, Philadelphia, Pennsylvania

**Martha E. Fedorko,** M.D., Associate Professor, Rockefeller University, New York, New York

**Allan L. Goldstein,** Ph.D., Professor and Chairman, Department of Biochemistry, The George Washington University Medical Center, Washington, D.C.

**Robert L. Goodman,** M.D., Sidney Farber Cancer Institute; Harvard Medical School, Boston, Massachusetts. Present Affiliation: Associate Professor and Chairman, Department of Radiation Therapy, University of Pennsylvania, Philadelphia, Pennsylvania

**Brigid G. Leventhal,** M.D., Associate Professor of Oncology and Pediatrics, The Oncology Center, Johns Hopkins Hospital, Johns Hopkins University, Baltimore, Maryland

**Marshall A. Lichtman,** M.D., Professor, Departments of Medicine and of Radiation Biology and Biophysics, University of Rochester School of Medicine, Rochester, New York

**Teresa L. K. Low,** Ph.D., Assistant Professor, Department of Biochemistry, The George Washington University Medical Center, Washington, D.C.

**Malcolm A. S. Moore,** Ph.D., Member, Sloan-Kettering Institute for Cancer Research, New York, New York

**Alexander Nakeff,** Ph.D., Assistant Professor, Section of Cancer Biology, Division of Radiation Oncology, Department of Radiology, Washington University School of Medicine, St. Louis, Missouri

**Arthur W. Nienhuis,** M.D., Chief, Clinical Hematology Branch, National Heart, Lung, and Blood Institute, National Institutes of Health, Bethesda, Maryland

**Robert D. Rosenberg,** M.D., Ph.D., Associate Professor of Medicine, Harvard Medical School; Sidney Farber Cancer Institute; Beth Israel Hospital, Boston, Massachusetts

**Tapio Rytömaa,** M.D., Head, Medical Research Group, Institute of Radiation Protection; Docent, Experimental Cell Research, University of Helsinki, Helsinki, Finland

**Patricia A. Santillo,** B.S., Senior Technologist, Hematology Unit, University of Rochester School of Medicine, Rochester, New York

**Arthur T. Skarin,** M.D., Senior Medical Oncologist, Sidney Farber Cancer Institute; Assistant Professor of Medicine, Harvard Medical School; Associate in Medicine, Peter Bent Brigham Hospital, Boston, Massachusetts

**Frederick Valeriote,** Ph.D., Professor and Head, Section of Cancer Biology, Division of Radiation Oncology, Department of Radiology, Washington University School of Medicine, St. Louis, Missouri

**Michael Weiner,** M.D., The Oncology Center, Johns Hopkins Hospital, Baltimore, Maryland. Present Affiliation: Instructor, Clinical Pediatrics, College of Physicians and Surgeons, Columbia University, New York, New York

**Jacqueline Whang-Peng,** M.D., Medicine Branch, National Cancer Institute, National Institutes of Health, Bethesda, Maryland

**Neal S. Young,** M.D., Visiting Expert, Clinical Hematology Branch, National Heart, Lung, and Blood Institute, National Institutes of Health, Bethesda, Maryland

**Robert C. Young,** M.D., Medicine Branch, National Cancer Institute, National Institutes of Health, Bethesda, Maryland

**Adel A. Yunis,** M.D., Professor, Departments of Medicine and Biochemistry and Director, Division of Hematology, University of Miami School of Medicine; Howard Hughes Laboratories for Hematological Research, Howard Hughes Medical Institute, Miami, Florida

# Preface

A thorough knowledge of the literature is an embarkation point for scientists exploring the unknown, teachers who share the fruit of their reading with students, and clinicians who apply this information to better care for the ill. This blunt justification is offered in appreciation for the work of contributors to this volume as well as to those questioning the need of "yet another review."

The editors believe that no single article by itself can furnish either the entire information or all the concepts that encompass a given field. We have found, however, that each article in the previous and present volume has brought to us the "state of the art" as could best be absorbed by an interested outsider. The skilled writer allows the reader to share in the excitement of unraveling a complex biologic phenomenon.

The response to the previous volume has encouraged the editors in their task of assembling articles that analyze a rapidly developing area and synthesize concepts which hopefully point to new directions. As always, comments and suggestions for future reviews are welcome. This book is dedicated to Maxwell M. Wintrobe, who has done so much for hematology.

Robert Silber, M.D.
Joseph LoBue, Ph.D.
Albert S. Gordon, Ph.D.

# Contents

## Chapter 2

## Culture of Granulocytic Stem Cells and Its Application to Clinical Problems

Malcolm A. S. Moore



## Chapter 3

## Abnormalities of Red Cell Membrane Lipids: Clinical–Biophysical Correlates

Richard A. Cooper

## Chapter 4

# Hemoglobin Switching in Sheep and Man

Neal S. Young and Arthur W. Nienhuis



## Chapter 5

# Mechanisms Underlying Marrow Toxicity from Chloramphenicol and Thiamphenicol

Adel A. Yunis

Chapter 6

# Morphologic and Functional Observations on Bone Marrow Megakaryocytes

Martha E. Fedorko

## Chapter 7

## Mechanisms of Heparin Therapy

Robert D. Rosenberg



## Chapter 8

## Factors Thought to Contribute to the Regulation of Egress of Cells from Marrow

Marshall A. Lichtman, Jack K. Chamberlain, and Patricia A. Santillo

## Chapter 9

## Structure and Function of Thymosin and Other Thymic Factors

Teresa L. K. Low and Allan L. Goldstein



## Chapter 10

## Chalones and Blood Cells

Tapio Rytömaa

## Chapter 11

# Cytogenetic Studies in Leukemia

Jacqueline Whang-Peng and Robert C. Young

## Chapter 12

## Leukemia Antigens

Brigid G. Leventhal and Michael Weiner



## Chapter 13

## Recent Advances in the Treatment of Malignant Lymphomas: Hodgkin's Disease

George P. Canellos, Arthur T. Skarin, and Robert L. Goodman

## Chapter 14

## Recent Advances in the Treatment of Malignant Lymphoma: Non-Hodgkin's Lymphoma

Arthur T. Skarin, George P. Canellos, and Robert L. Goodman

# Effects of Anticancer Agents on Hematopoietic Progenitor Cells

## Frederick Valeriote and Alexander Nakeff

## 1.1. Introduction

The hematopoietic system is a major locus for the toxic effects exerted by anticancer agents. Consequently, the end cells of this system and most importantly the platelets and white blood cells are carefully monitored during chemotherapy and their levels employed to adjust drug dosages accordingly. There has therefore developed an extensive though widely scattered literature on the effects of anticancer agents upon these end cells. Unfortunately, no one has yet drawn this literature together and we do not intend to do so here. Rather, our focus will be on the action of anticancer agents on the earliest cells of the different hematopoietic lines. Unlike the former situation, the literature is quite limited; the assays for these cells have only recently been developed and few initial studies have examined the effects of anticancer agents. However, it is most important

FREDERICK VALERIOTE and ALEXANDER NAKEFF • Section of Cancer Biology, Division of Radiation Oncology, Department of Radiology, Washington University School of Medicine, St. Louis, Missouri 63110.

to understand drug effects at this level since it is the consequence of this interaction both in terms of cytotoxicity and the proliferative and differentiative response of the residual cells which presents itself days to weeks later at the end-cell level. An excellent review of the literature on the effect of anticancer agents on these precursor cells has recently appeared (Marsh, 1976).

## 1.2. Cell Compartments of the Hematopoietic System

This chapter specifically concerns progenitor cells of the hematopoietic system which we define as those clonogenic cells either culturable *in vitro* in a variety of culture systems to give rise to colonies or transferable *in vivo* to give rise to spleen colonies in syngeneic hosts. Whereas the *in vitro* assays usually give rise to morphologically similar cells in a colony, the *in vivo* spleen colony is quite heterogeneous, representing the progeny of the stem cell of the hematopoietic system and giving rise to groups of cells in the spleen ranging from clusters of cells which are usually not counted (such as megakaryocyte colonies) to larger colonies (erythroid) which are enumerated in the assay.

One approach to analyze drug effects on progenitor cells is from a cell kinetic point of view. Figure 1 shows our kinetic representation of the hematopoietic system indicating the compartment name, the designation given by us or other investigators to different specific cellular components

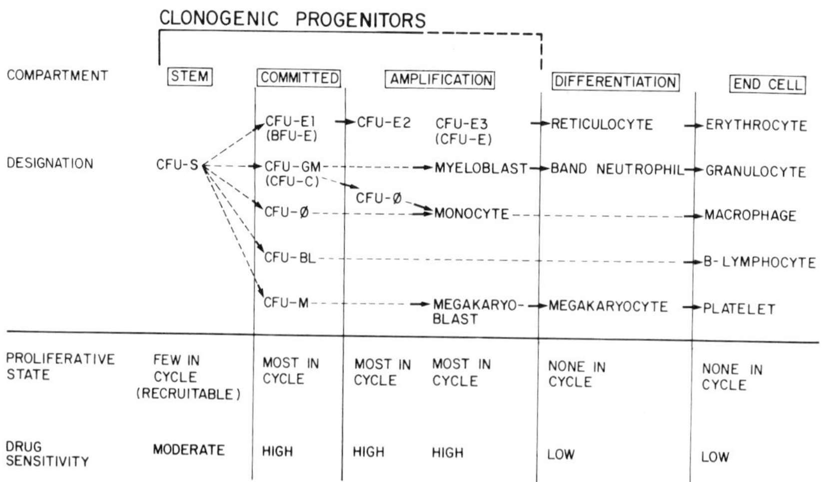


**Fig. 1.** Cell kinetic model of the hematopoietic system.

of the hematopoietic system, the proliferative state of these cells usually determined by their response to specific anticancer agents, and our interpretation of their sensitivity to anticancer agents. We have shown the stem cell to be the basic progenitor cell. Although only a small fraction of these cells are probably in cycle normally, they can be rapidly recruited into cycle when required. From this cell is derived the committed progenitor cells or the "limited stem cells" of Nowell and Wilson (1971). These progenitor cells are in rapid cell cycle and move into an amplification compartment comprised of either mature progenitors or immature but morphologically identifiable cells whose function is to provide a large input of cells into a more differentiating compartment. These first three compartments are considered by us to comprise the *progenitor* cells. The next cellular compartment is the differentiating compartment in which there may be some vestigial proliferative capacity. However, the main function of this compartment is the production of required enzymes or structural proteins to carry out the cellular differentiated function to be required of the functional cell. The final compartment is represented by the end-cell in which there is generally no proliferation. These cells carry out their function and then die or are removed. As we discuss shortly, evidence exists describing the proliferative state of a number of the progenitor cells; further, we attribute much of the drug sensitivity of the hematopoietic system to destruction of cells in the proliferating compartments.

One might expect different agents to yield different quantitative effects following administration not only because of the different proliferative states but also because of different transit times of the precursors in and through their compartments. However, some effects do not seem explainable on this basis. For example, Levin (1972), in reviewing the effects of anticancer agents on thrombopoiesis, points out that while nitrogen mustard has a similar effect on all elements, vincristine demonstrates no thrombocytopenia at doses which produce significant leukopenia.

## 1.3. Action of Anticancer Agents at the Cellular Level

Before discussing the action of anticancer agents on the precursor cell population, it is necessary first to describe the action of anticancer agents from a cellular point of view to provide a firm conceptual basis upon which to develop an understanding of the action of these agents on the hematopoietic system. Anticancer agents fall into two broad categories termed phase-specific and cycle-specific agents (Valeriote and van Putten,

1975; Valeriote and Edelstein, 1977). The phase-specific agents kill cells selectively in one phase of the cell cycle and therefore have little if any effect on nonproliferating cells even at relatively high doses. These drugs are characterized by a limit to the extent of cell killing that can be achieved as a function of dose since after the dose of drug is reached at which all cells in the sensitive phase are killed, the residual insensitive cells define the surviving fraction of the population. Because of this, a number of strategies have been developed for the administration of phase-specific agents such as fractionation or infusion of the drugs so that a large fraction of a tumor cell population can enter the sensitive phase and be killed while cytotoxic levels of the agent are maintained. The rationale and execution of these strategies are discussed in a recent review (Valeriote, 1978). The second category of agents, the cycle-specific agents, will destroy cells in any phase of the cell cycle although they may preferentially kill in one phase compared to another. Generally they are more effective on proliferating (in cycle) than nonproliferating cells (Valeriote and van Putten, 1975).

## 1.4. CFU-S

### 1.4.1. Cytotoxicity of Anticancer Agents to CFU-S

This group of cells must maintain itself as well as respond to appropriate controls forcing it to give rise to a spectrum of differentiated descendants. Till and McCulloch (1961) established an assay system for a class of cells which had these characteristics. This so-called spleen colony assay has since been taken to quantitate hematopoietic stem cells, or colony-forming units, spleen (CFU-S). From extensive modeling of this compartment both in the steady state as well as following radiation insult, it was hypothesized that a fraction of these cells were normally not in cycle but rather in a nonproliferative, $G_0$ state (Lajtha *et al.*, 1962).

This model was provided further support when it was subsequently demonstrated through the use of agents which selectively kill cells in the DNA-synthetic phase of the cell cycle (such as high-specific-activity tritiated thymidine, cytosine arabinoside, or hydroxyurea) that only a small proportion of stem cells were in cycle. However, these techniques have some difficulties with interpretation of the data as indicated by Lord *et al.* (1974); for example, the specific activity of the $[^3H]$-TdR should not be higher than about 24 Ci/mmol. Also, hydroxyurea may not have an immediate effect because endogenous pools of deoxyribonucleotides must first be depleted before cell killing will commence (Byron, 1972). We have summarized in Table I a number of studies in which these agents

**Table I.** Cytotoxic Effect of S-Phase-Specific Agents on Normal CFU-S

| Agent used | Surviving fraction | Mouse strain | Reference |
|---|---|---|---|
| Hydroxyurea | 0.94 | BALB/C | Hodgson *et al.*, 1975 |
| | 0.81–0.84 | $CF_1$ | Monette *et al.*, 1974 |
| | 0.80–0.85 | $CF1_s$ | Rickard *et al.*, 1970 |
| | 0.80[a] | C3H | Vassort *et al.*, 1971 |
| | 0.84 | HSB | Boyum *et al.*, 1974 |
| | 0.90 | NMR1 | Necas *et al.*, 1976 |
| | 1.0[b] | NMR1 | Necas *et al.*, 1976 |
| | 0.80–0.98 | NMR1 | Necas and Neuwirt, 1976 |
| Tritiated thymidine | 0.77[c] | C57BL | Blackett *et al.*, 1974 |
| | 0.96[c] | C57BL | Blackett *et al.*, 1974 |
| | 0.97 | C57BL | Vassort *et al.*, 1973 |
| | 0.93 | C57BL | Guzman and Lajtha, 1970 |
| | 0.75–0.78 | C3H | Croizat *et al.*, 1970 |
| | 0.80 | C3H | Vassort *et al.*, 1973 |
| | 0.89–1.01 | $(C57BL \times C3H)F_1$ | Becker *et al.*, 1965 |
| | 0.97 | $(C57BL \times C3H)F_1$ | Guzman and Lajtha, 1970 |
| | 0.97–0.98 | $(BALB/C \times CBA)F_1$ | Gidali *et al.*, 1974 |
| | 0.85–1.09 | CPB/S | Lahiri, 1973 |
| | 0.72–1.00 | $(C3H \times AKR)F_1$ | Lajtha *et al.*, 1969 |
| | 0.40–0.68[d] | $(C3H \times AKR)F_1$ | Lajtha *et al.*, 1969 |
| | 1.0 | $(C3H \times AKR)F_1$ | Byron, 1975 |
| Cytosine arabinoside | 0.93 | C57BL | Millard and Okell, 1975 |

[a]Same result obtained when $[^3H]$-TdR was used.
[b]Endogenous colonies.
[c]Lower value obtained for *in vivo* suicide.
[d]Autorepopulation assay.

have been employed and the surviving fraction obtained. It is of interest that for one of these studies in which two strains of mice were examined (Vassort *et al.*, 1973), a significant difference in the surviving fraction was obtained; in most cases only a small fraction of cells were killed. Thus, although there is a difference between mouse strains, in the steady state, between 0 and 20% of the CFU-S are in cycle in mouse marrow. We have not referred to results from tissues other than marrow although limited data for spleen (Guzman and Lajtha, 1970) and fetal liver (Becker *et al.*, 1965) exist indicating that a greater proportion of these cells are normally in cycle.

As already indicated, the proliferative state is a most important factor in determining sensitivity of a cell population to the lethal effects of anticancer agents. This factor is relevant in considering CFU-S since these cells are generally out of cycle but can be brought into cycle by a variety of procedures.

The major experimental system employed to study proliferation-dependent cytotoxicity has been proliferating CFU-S obtained following transplantation of bone marrow into irradiated or drug-treated donor mice. The transplanted cells do not seem to become totally proliferating for a number of hours following transplantation as evidenced by the growth of these cells (Valeriote and Bruce, 1967). The initial study of Becker *et al.* (1965) showed that a single exposure to [$^3$H]-TdR could destroy 65% of these cells. Other investigators have repeated this and shown the same effect (e.g., 62% destroyed in CPB/S mice) (Lahiri, 1973). This increase from few to the vast majority of cells being sensitive to this S-phase probe demonstrated the tremendous reserve capability of this population. An identical effect was noted for other phase-specific agents such as vinblastine (Valeriote and Bruce, 1967) where a tenfold difference in sensitivity was noted between CFU-S in the two proliferative states in AKR mice. The effect is also found for cycle-specific agents such as 5-fluorouracil (Bruce and Meeker, 1967), which is very proliferation dependent in its cytotoxicity, and a nontoxic dose may produce a survival difference of over 1000-fold. A comprehensive study in this area has been done by van Putten's group showing that agents varied in their differential response to the two cell populations (van Putten *et al.*, 1972).

Anticancer agents will cause a recruitment of CFU-S in $G_0$ into cycle as a result of destruction of themselves or their progeny. There is ample evidence in experimental systems that significant recruitment can be suprisingly fast; after 6 hr following a single dose of vinblastine (Hanks, 1972; Valeriote and Bruce, 1967), within 12 hr of a single dose of hydroxyurea (Monette *et al.*, 1974), 24 hr following cyclophosphamide (Eaves and Bruce, 1974); or by 48 hr after melphalan (Dunn, 1974). Surprisingly few data are available on the changing sensitivity of CFU-S to anticancer agents with repeated courses of treatment. This recruitment is likely in response to a depletion of proliferating progeny of stem cells since the rapid recruitment occurs even in mice in which only a few percent of the CFU-S are in cycle (Vassort *et al.*, 1973). Sensenbrenner *et al.* (1973) found CFU-S to become fully sensitive to a number of agents (MTX, 6-MP, Act-D, and CY) within 48 hr. BCNU was an anomaly as the sensitivity was maximal initially and then decreased; however, it has been shown repeatedly that BCNU is less effective on proliferating cells (Bhuyan *et al.*, 1977). Much of the work reported in the literature for recruitment of CFU-S by radiation, anticancer agents, or other agents (discussed later) has been summarized in Table II. The treatment used to force the cells into cycle is indicated in the first column. The anticancer agent employed to "probe" the proliferative extent of the stimulated population is listed in the third column, and the cytotoxicity found (usually maximum) is shown in the fourth column to indicate the greater

**Table II.** Recruitment of CFU-S into Cycle by Different Agents

| Proliferative (recruitment) stimulus | Time (or interval) studied | Agent (probe) used | Surviving fraction (minimum) | Mouse strain | Reference |
|---|---|---|---|---|---|
| Radiation (650 R) | 0–54 hr | Hydroxyurea | 0.4 (at 54 hr), 0.2 (at 15 hr)[a] | NMR1 | Necas et al., 1976 |
| Radiation (continuous for 2–3 wks at 40 rads/day) | — | Tritiated thymidine<br>In vivo<br>In vitro | <br>0.58<br>0.53 | C57BL | Blackett et al., 1974 |
| Radiation (continuous for 2–3 wks at 38 rads/day) | — | Cytosine arabinoside<br>In vivo<br>In vitro | <br>0.48<br>0.46 | C57BL | Millard and Okell, 1975 |
| Radiation (150 R) | 0–144 hr | 5-Fluorouracil | $4 \times 10^{-3}$ (at 12 hr) | AKR | Eaves and Bruce, 1974 |
| Radiation (450 R) | 4–46 days | Tritiated thymidine | 0.5 (4–10 days) | (C57BL × C3H)$F_1$ | Guzman and Lajtha, 1970 |
| Hydroxyurea (10 mg/mouse) | 0–48 hr | Hydroxyurea | 0.48 (at 12 hr) 0.62 (at 24 hr) | C3H | Vassort et al., 1971 |
| Hydroxyurea (50 mg/mouse) | 0–48 hr | Hydroxyurea | 0.43 (at 16 hr) | C3H | Vassort et al., 1971 |
| Hydroxyurea (10 mg/mouse) | 1–24 hr | Tritiated thymidine | 0.5 (at 12 hr), 0.65 (at 20 hr) | C3H | Vassort et al., 1973 |
| Hydroxyurea (10 mg/mouse) | 1–15 hr | Tritiated thymidine | 0.55 (at 12 hr) | C57BL | Vassort et al., 1973 |
| Hydroxyurea (900 mg/kg) | 7–27 hr | Hydroxyurea | 0.15 (at 14 hr) | NMR1 | Necas and Neuwirt, 1976 |
| Myleran (35 mg/kg) | 5 days | Cytosine arabinoside | 0.77 | C57BL | Millard and Okell, 1975 |
| Testosterone propionate (0.1 mg/g) | 1–24 hr | Tritiated thymidine | 0.5–0.75 | (C3H × AKR)$F_1$ | Byron, 1972 |
| Testosterone propionate (0.1 mg/g) | 2–3 hr | Hydroxyurea | 0.75 | (C3H × AKR)$F_1$ | Byron, 1972 |
| Tritiated thymidine (1 mCi/mouse) | 1–24 hr | Tritiated thymidine | 0.65 (12 and 20 hr) | C3H | Vassort et al., 1973 |
| Tritiated thymidine (1 mCi/mouse) | 1–15 hr | Tritiated thymidine | 0.60 (at 12 hr) | C57BL | Vassort et al., 1973 |
| Endotoxin (25 µg/mouse) | 24 hr | 5-Fluorouracil | $2 \times 10^{-2}$ (at 4 hr) | AKR | Eaves and Bruce, 1974 |
| Endotoxin (25 µg/mouse) | 0–144 hr | 5-Fluorouracil | $10^{-2}$ (at 36 hr) | AKR | Eaves and Bruce, 1974 |
| Erythropoietin | 18 hr | Tritiated thymidine | 0.60 | C57BL and (C57BL × C3H)$F_1$ | Guzman and Lajtha, 1970 |

[a]Endogenous CFU-S.

extent of killing compared to normal CFU-S (Table I). A number of nonanticancer agents have been discovered which can stimulate resting CFU-S to enter cell cycle. These include stimulators of $\beta$-adrenergic receptors including isoproterenol, cholinergic activators such as acetylcholine, cyclic AMP, cyclic GMP, parathyroid hormone, prostaglandin $E_2$, and endotoxin (Byron, 1975). This latter stimulator may have therapeutic significance for bacteria-infected patients who may have concomitantly stimulated stem cells thereby making them more sensitive to chemotherapy.

We have reviewed the literature and constructed Tables III and IV from the data to provide a comprehensive review of the information available on the cytotoxic effect of anticancer agents on CFU-S. Those that are available on rapidly proliferating CFU-S and are not in Table II, are included here. In Tables III and IV we have tried to provide some estimate of cell sensitivity for the given agent. This is relatively easy with cycle-specific agents by using the conventional procedure of obtaining a measure of the slope of the dose–survival curve, expressed either as $D_0$, $D_{37}$, or $D_{1/2}$. In many cases, unfortunately, the investigator did not provide a measure of the slope of the dose–survival curve and we have therefore had to estimate it from the published figure. For phase-specific agents this cannot be done and we have resorted to defining the survival (and dose) at the plateau of the dose–survival curve at a given time, or simply the survival at the minimum of a time–survival curve at a given dose. While some investigators use doses and sensitivities in units of milligrams per kilogram, others use milligrams per mouse. If one assumes that studies are generally done on mice of about 25 g in weight, then the conversion factor is 40 mg/kg = 1 mg/mouse.

We have restricted our review essentially to results obtained with mice. Although most of the information currently available is on this species, limited data in other species, such as rat (Dunn, 1973; Dunn and Elson, 1970), are also available.

## 1.4.2. Therapeutic Implications for CFU-S

Unfortunately, most human tumors also contain nonproliferating clonogenic cells which must be destroyed and this leads to scheduling anticancer agents such that multiple courses are administered to recruit and destroy these tumor cells (Valeriote, 1978). Such scheduling also leads to the recruitment and subsequent sensitization of the stem cells as well. As expected from the preceding discussion, CFU-S become increasingly sensitive to further courses if closely spaced (Bruce et al., 1969). As indicated earlier, van Putten's group demonstrated significant proliferation-dependent cytotoxicity for alkylating agents while others have exten-

**Table III.** Cytotoxic Effect of Phase-Specific Agents on CFU-S

| Drug | Dose | Mouse strain | Fractional survival[a] | Recovery | Reference |
|---|---|---|---|---|---|
| Vinblastine | 0.1 mg/mouse[b] | AKR | 0.15 (at 24 hr) | — | Bruce *et al.*, 1969 |
| | | AKR | 0.005 (at 48 hr) | — | Bruce *et al.*, 1969 |
| | 0.5 mg/mouse[b] | AKR | 0.15 (at 24 hr) | — | Valeriote *et al.*, 1966 |
| | 0.5 mg/mouse[b] | AKR | 0.2 (at 24 hr) | — | Valeriote and Bruce, 1967 |
| | 0.5 mg/mouse[b] | AKR | 0.02 (at 24 hr)[c] | — | Valeriote and Bruce, 1967 |
| | 10 mg/kg[b] | C57BL | 0.2 | — | Millard *et al.*, 1973 |
| | 10 mg/kg[b] | C57BL | 0.05[c] | — | Millard *et al.*, 1973 |
| | 10 mg/kg | C57BL | $2 \times 10^{-4}$ (at 48 hr)[c] | 17 days | Blackett and Millard, 1976 |
| | 80 $\mu$g/mouse | C3H | 0.4 (at 24 hr) | day 2 | Chen and Schooley, 1970 |
| | 3 mg/kg | CF$_1$ | 0.24 (at 48 hr) | — | Udupa and Reissmann, 1974 |
| | 0.5 mg/mouse[b] | (C57BL $\times$ CBA)F$_1$ | $5 \times 10^{-2}$ (at 24 hr) | — | Haskill *et al.*, 1970 |
| | 4 mg/kg | (C3H $\times$ DBA/2)F$_1$ | 0.3 (at 24 hr) | By 3 days | Breivik, 1972 |
| Cytosine arabinoside | 5 mg/mouse[b] | AKR | 0.12 (at 24 hr) | — | Bruce *et al.*, 1969 |
| | | | 0.005 (at 48 hr) | — | Bruce *et al.*, 1969 |
| | 1000 mg/kg | (BALB/C $\times$ DBA)F$_1$ | 0.7 (at 24 hr) | By 3 days | Preisler and Henderson, 1971 |
| Vincristine | 0.2 mg/mouse[b] | AKR | 0.2 (at 24 hr) | — | Bruce *et al.*, 1969 |
| | | | 0.013 (at 48 hr) | — | Bruce *et al.*, 1969 |
| Methotrexate | 6 mg/mouse[b] | AKR | 0.35 (at 24 hr) | — | Blackett *et al.*, 1975 |
| | 1 mg/mouse[b] | AKR | 0.27 (at 24 hr) | — | Blackett *et al.*, 1975 |
| | | | 0.27 (at 48 hr) | — | Blackett *et al.*, 1975 |
| Hydroxyurea | 1000 mg/kg | BALB/C | 0.14 | 3–4 days | Hodgson *et al.*, 1975 |
| | | | 0.5[c] | — | Hodgson *et al.*, 1975 |
| Azaserine | 0.5 mg/mouse | AKR | 0.7 (at 24 hr) | — | Bruce *et al.*, 1966 |
| 6-Mercaptopurine | 4 mg/mouse[b] | AKR | 0.7 (at 24 hr) | — | Bruce *et al.*, 1966 |

[a]At specific assay time or else taken at minimum of time–survival curve.
[b]At plateau of dose–survival curve.
[c]CFU-S in cycle.

**Table IV.** Cytotoxic Effect of Cycle-Specific Agents on CFU-S

| Drug | Mouse strain | Sensitivity | Comment | Reference |
|---|---|---|---|---|
| Actinomycin D | AKR | 0.01 mg/mouse ($D_0$) | — | Bruce *et al.*, 1966 |
| Adriamycin | AKR | 0.27 mg/mouse ($D_{1/2}$) | — | Razek *et al.*, 1972 |
| | DBA | 6.4 mg/kg ($D_{1/2}$) | — | Alberts and van Daalen Wetters, 1976 |
| Aminochlorambucil | (C57BL × CBA)$F_1$ | 7.77 mg/kg ($D_0$) | — | van Putten *et al.*, 1972 |
| | (C57BL × CBA)$F_1$ | 3.2 mg/kg ($D_0$) | CFU-S in cycle | van Putten et al., 1972 |
| | CBA | 6.2 $\mu$mol ($D_{1/2}$) | — | Dunn, 1972 |
| BCNU | AKR | 0.28 mg/mouse ($D_{1/2}$) | — | Valeriote and Tolen, 1972 |
| | BALB/C | 31.3 $\mu$mol/liter ($D_{37}$) | — | Ogawa *et al.*, 1973a |
| | BALB/C | 26.2 $\mu$mol/liter ($D_{37}$) | CFU-S in cycle | Ogawa *et al.*, 1973a |
| | (BALB/C × CBA)$F_1$ | 0.25[a] (24 hr after 20 mg/kg) | Full recovery after 42 days | Preisler and Henderson, 1971 |
| | $CF_1$ | 0.2 (48 hr after 35 mg/kg) | — | Udupa and Reissmann, 1974 |
| | (C57BL × CBA)$F_1$ | 9 mg/kg ($D_0$) | CFU-S in cycle | van Putten *et al.*, 1972 |
| | (C57BL × CBA)$F_1$ | 13.4 mg/kg ($D_0$) | — | van Putten *et al.*, 1972 |
| | — | 15.4 mg/kg ($D_0$) | — | Blackett *et al.*, 1975 |
| Busulfan | (C57BL × CBA)$F_1$ | 20 mg/kg ($D_0$) | — | van Putten *et al.*, 1972 |
| | (C57BL × CBA)$F_1$ | 11.7 mg/kg ($D_0$) | CFU-S in cycle | van Putten *et al.*, 1972 |
| | C57BL | 0.02[a] (2 days after 40 mg/kg) | CFU-S in cycle; recovery after day 42 | Blackett and Millard, 1976 |
| | — | 27 mg/kg ($D_0$) | Shoulder region; same sensitivity for CFU-S in cycle | Blackett and Millard, 1973 |
| | $CF_1$ | <0.01 (4 days after 44 mg/kg) | Recovery later than 26 days | Udupa and Reissmann, 1974 |
| | RFM/Un | 48.2 mg/kg ($D_0$) | — | Tanaka *et al.*, 1970 |
| CCNU | (C57BL × CBA)$F_1$ | 24.5 mg/kg ($D_0$) | — | van Putten *et al.*, 1972 |
| | (C57BL × CBA)$F_1$ | 15.5 mg/kg ($D_0$) | CFU-S in cycle | van Putten *et al.*, 1972 |
| | — | 10.3 mg/kg ($D_0$) | — | Blackett *et al.*, 1975 |

| | | | | |
|---|---|---|---|---|
| Chlorambucil | AKR | 0.33 mg/kg ($D_{1/2}$) | — | Valeriote and Tolen, 1972 |
| | RFM/Un | 11.3 mg/kg ($D_0$) | — | Tanaka *et al.*, 1970 |
| | (C57BL × CBA)F$_1$ | 17.6 mg/kg ($D_0$) | — | van Putten and Lelieveld, 1971 |
| | (C57BL × CBA)F$_1$ | 9.7 mg/kg ($D_0$) | CFU-S in cycle | van Putten and Lelieveld, 1971 |
| Cyclophosphamide | AKR | 1.5 mg/mouse ($D_0$) | — | Bruce *et al.*, 1966 |
| | AKR | 0.2[a] (24 hr after 3 mg/mouse) | Recovery by 5 days | Valeriote *et al.*, 1968 |
| | AKR | 0.02[a] (24 hr after 5 mg/mouse) | Recovery by 6 days | Valeriote *et al.*, 1968 |
| | BALB/C | 2.9 mg/mouse ($D_{37}$) | — | Ogawa *et al.*, 1973a |
| | BALB/C | 1.45 mg/mouse ($D_{37}$) | CFU-S in cycle | Ogawa *et al.*, 1973a |
| | C57BL | 119 mg/kg ($D_0$) | — | Millard *et al.*, 1973 |
| | C57BL | 71 mg/kg ($D_0$) | CFU-S in cycle | Millard *et al.*, 1973 |
| | CDF$_1$ | 0.1[a] (24 hr after 275 mg/kg) | Recovery by 3 days | DeWys *et al.*, 1970 |
| | HSB | 0.1[a] (2 hr after 200 mg/kg) | Recovery by 6 days | Boyum *et al.*, 1974 |
| | CF$_1$ | 0.34 (48 hr after 200 mg/kg) | — | Udupa and Reissmann, 1974 |
| | C3H/He | 3.1 mg/mouse ($D_0$) | — | Hellman and Grate, 1971b |
| | C3H/He | 3.2 mg/mouse ($D_0$) | — | Hellman and Grate, 1971a |
| | RFM/Un | 1.6 mg/mouse ($D_0$) | — | Tanaka *et al.*, 1970 |
| | (C57BL × CBA)F$_1$ | 126 mg/kg ($D_0$) | — | van Putten and Lelieveld, 1970 |
| | (C57BL × CBA)F$_1$ | 54 mg/kg ($D_0$) | CFU-S in cycle | van Putten and Lelieveld, 1970 |
| Daunorubicin | AKR | 0.1 mg/mouse ($D_{1/2}$) | — | Razek *et al.*, 1972 |
| Dianhydromannitol | (C57BL × CBA)F$_1$ | 4.12 mg/kg ($D_0$) | — | van Putten *et al.*, 1972 |
| | (C57BL × CBA)F$_1$ | 2.65 mg/kg ($D_0$) | CFU-S in cycle | van Putten *et al.*, 1972 |
| Dimethyl Myleran | (C57BL × CBA)F$_1$ | 3.08 mg/kg ($D_0$) | — | van Putten *et al.*, 1972 |
| | (C57BL × CBA)F$_1$ | 2.07 mg/kg ($D_0$) | CFU-S in cycle | van Putten *et al.*, 1972 |
| DTIC | (C57BL × CBA)F$_1$ | 380 mg/kg ($D_0$) | — | van Putten *et al.*, 1972 |
| | (C57BL × CBA)F$_1$ | 240 mg/kg ($D_0$) | CFU-S in cycle | van Putten *et al.*, 1972 |
| 5-Fluorouracil | AKR | $1.5 \times 10^{-3}$[a] (at 24 hr after 2.5 mg/mouse) | — | Eaves and Bruce, 1974 |

**Table IV (Continued)**

| Drug | Mouse strain | Sensitivity | Comment | Reference |
|---|---|---|---|---|
|  | AKR | 1 mg/mouse ($D_0$) | Shoulder region | Bruce *et al.*, 1966 |
|  | (C57BL × CBA)$F_1$ | 49.4 mg/kg ($D_0$) | — | van Putten *et al.*, 1972 |
|  | (C57BL × CBA)$F_1$ | 12.3 mg/kg ($D_0$) | CFU-S in cycle | van Putten *et al.*, 1972 |
| Isophosphamide | (C57BL × CBA)$F_1$ | 151 mg/kg ($D_0$) | — | van Putten *et al.*, 1972 |
|  | (C57BL × CBA)$F_1$ | 96 mg/kg ($D_0$) | CFU-S in cycle | van Putten *et al.*, 1972 |
| LEO 1031 | (C57BL × CBA)$F_1$ | 125 mg/kg ($D_0$) | — | Evenaar *et al.*, 1973 |
|  | (C57BL × CBA)$F_1$ | 22.2 mg/kg ($D_0$) | CFU-S in cycle | Evenaar *et al.*, 1973 |
| Mannitol mustard | (DBA × C57BL)$F_1$ | 13.57 mg/kg ($D_0$) | — | Fuzy *et al.*, 1975 |
|  | (DBA × C57BL)$F_1$ | 8.38 mg/kg ($D_0$) | CFU-S in cycle | Fuzy *et al.*, 1975 |
| Melphalan | AKR | 0.054 mg/mouse ($D_{1/2}$) | — | Valeriote and Tolen, 1972 |
|  | BALB/C | 1.5 μg/ml ($D_{37}$) | — | Ogawa *et al.*, 1971 |
|  | CBA | $10^{-2 a}$ (48 hr after 6 mg/kg) | Recovery by day 6 | Dunn, 1974 |
|  | CBA | 2.5 μmol ($D_{1/2}$) | — | Dunn, 1972 |
|  | CBA | 1.9–3.1 mg/kg ($D_0$) | — | Dunn, 1974 |
|  | CBA | $10^{-2 a}$ (2 hr after 6 μg/kg) | CFU-S in cycle | Dunn, 1974 |
|  | CBA | 1.7 mg/kg ($D_0$) | — | Dunn, 1974 |
|  | (C57BL × CBA)$F_1$ | 4.06 mg/kg ($D_0$) | — | van Putten and Lelieveld, 1971 |
|  | (C57BL × CBA)$F_1$ | 1.65 mg/kg ($D_0$) | CFU-S in cycle | van Putten and Lelieveld, 1971 |
| Methyl CCNU | (C57BL × CBA)$F_1$ | 29 mg/kg ($D_0$) | — | van Putten *et al.*, 1972 |
|  | (C57BL × CBA)$F_1$ | 22.6 mg/kg ($D_0$) | CFU-S in cycle | van Putten *et al.*, 1972 |
|  | — | 15.4 mg/kg ($D_0$) | — | Blackett *et al.*, 1975 |
| Mitomycin C | CPB/S | 0.74 μg/ml ($D_{1/2}$) | *In vitro* (30′) | Lahiri, 1973 |
|  | CPB/S | 0.74 μg/ml ($D_{1/2}$) | CFU-S in cycle *in vitro* (30′) | Lahiri, 1973 |
| Nitrogen mustard | AKR | 0.06 mg/mouse ($D_0$) | Single doses or every 6 hr for 24 hr | Bruce *et al.*, 1966 |
|  | AKR | 0.041 mg/mouse ($D_{1/2}$) | — | Valeriote and Tolen, 1972 |

| | BALB/C | 0.15 $\mu$mol/liter ($D_{37}$) | — | Ogawa *et al.*, 1973a |
|---|---|---|---|---|
| | BALB/C | 0.15 $\mu$mol/liter ($D_{37}$) | CFU-S in cycle | Ogawa *et al.*, 1973a |
| | CBA | 2.5 $\mu$mol ($D_{1/2}$) | — | Dunn, 1972 |
| | C3H/He | 0.03 mg/mouse ($D_0$) | — | Hellman and Grate, 1971a |
| | C3H/He | 0.026 mg/mouse ($D_0$) 0.188 mg/mouse ($D_0$) | Biphasic curve | Ash *et al.*, 1972 |
| | C51/ASH | 0.1[a] (1 day after 100 $\mu$g/mouse) | Recovery by day 8 | Sharp and Thomas, 1971 |
| | (C57BL $\times$ CBA)F$_1$ | 0.79 mg/kg ($D_0$) | — | van Putten and Lelieveld, 1971 |
| | (C57BL $\times$ CBA)F$_1$ | 0.48 mg/kg ($D_0$) | CFU-S in cycle | van Putten and Lelieveld, 1971 |
| Nor-nitrogen mustard | (C57BL $\times$ CBA)F$_1$ | 21.6 mg/kg ($D_0$) | — | van Putten *et al.*, 1972 |
| | (C57BL $\times$ CBA)F$_1$ | 9.4 mg/kg ($D_0$) | CFU-S in cycle | van Putten *et al.*, 1972 |
| NSC-82196 | AKR | 2.07 mg/mouse ($D_{1/2}$) | — | Valeriote and Tolen, 1971 |
| Rubidazone | DBA | 12.4 mg/kg ($D_{1/2}$) | — | Alberts and Van Daalen Wetters, 1976 |
| Thio-TEPA | AKR | 0.048 mg/mouse ($D_{1/2}$) | — | Valeriote and Tolen, 1972 |
| Triethylenemelamine | AKR | 0.0055 mg/mouse ($D_{1/2}$) | — | Valeriote and Tolen, 1972 |
| | (C57BL $\times$ CBA)F$_1$ | 0.58 mg/kg ($D_0$) | — | van Putten *et al.*, 1972 |
| | (C57BL $\times$ CBA)F$_1$ | 0.25 mg/kg ($D_0$) | CFU-S in cycle | van Putten *et al.*, 1972 |
| | C3H | 0.58 mg/kg ($D_0$) | — | Tannock *et al.*, 1972 |
| | C3H | 0.25 mg/kg ($D_0$) | CFU-S in cycle | Tannock *et al.*, 1972 |
| Trilophosphamide | (C57BL $\times$ CBA)F$_1$ | 47.1 mg/kg ($D_0$) | — | van Putten *et al.*, 1972 |
| | (C57BL $\times$ CBA)F$_1$ | 37.7 mg/kg ($D_0$) | CFU-S in cycle | van Putten *et al.*, 1972 |

[a]Fractional survival at time indicated.

sively examined phase-specific agents and demonstrated this effect; even the antitumor antibiotics show this proliferation-dependent cytotoxicity (Twentyman and Bleehen, 1973). Proliferation-dependent cytotoxicity can be a major determinant in the toxicity of a given drug. Since the majority of stem cells are not in cell cycle, we would expect the hematopoietic system not to be seriously affected by most anticancer agents and especially by the phase-specific agents. This must be qualified for cycle-specific agents since they can destroy nonproliferating cells so that large doses could lead to hematopoietic toxicity.

It is quite surprising to us that the rate of recruitment can be as rapid as discussed previously. The kinetics of this recruitment is an important area of present-day research. One of the rationales being employed in combination therapy is to define the optimal time for a second course in such a way that the maximal recruitment of tumor cells has occurred but that few CFU-S have been so recruited or that they have subsequently moved back out of cycle. However, if therapy must be administered while these cells are still proliferating, the agents which are strongly proliferation dependent in their cytotoxic effect should not be given.

Further, there seems to be two classes of anticancer agents on the basis of hematopoietic recovery. Agents such as Myleran (or radiation) require an extended period of time before population recovery is complete and presumably stem cells are out of cycle. Agents such as cyclophosphamide require a relatively short interval following administration, as has been shown both experimentally and clinically, before recovery occurs and the initial sensitivity of the population is regained. The studies with Myleran have been most extensive and have demonstrated a defect in both CFU-S and CFU-C following its administration (Morely *et al.*, 1975). While nitrosoureas are thought to fit into the first class due to clinical responses, both CFU-S and CFU-C display rapid reproliferation following BCNU, CCNU, and MeCCNU (Blackett *et al.*, 1975).

## 1.5. CFU-GM

The first *in vitro* cell population discovered which falls into the category of progenitor cells is the one that gives rise to granulocytes and/or macrophages upon culturing; this has been termed the CFU-C (culture) or CFU-GM (granulocyte–macrophage). It is likely that this cell is the precursor of both of these functional cells as shown in Fig. 1, although the position of the CFU-Ø (discussed later) is currently unclear. The type of colony that results depends on the culture conditions employed (Bradley and Metcalf, 1966; Plusnik and Sachs, 1965).

Using tritiated thymidine suicide in a manner similar to that used by Becker for CFU-S, Iscove *et al.* (1970) demonstrated that approximately 35% of normal CFU-GM (in C3B6F$_1$ mice) were in the S phase. However, all CFU-GM were obviously not in cell cycle since their study with regenerating marrow (Iscove *et al.*, 1970) demonstrated that about 80% of CFU-GM were in the S phase. Such a potential reserve in the normal marrow might indicate a control point for a proliferative demand. Lajtha *et al.* (1969) demonstrated about 46% of CFU-GM [in (C3H × AKR)F$_1$ mice] were sensitive to tritiated thymidine; Lord *et al.* (1977) showed this fraction to be 45%.

That CFU-GM could be recruited into cycle with a tremendous change in their sensitivity was demonstrated by Eaves and Bruce (1974). Following endotoxin, cyclophosphamide, or radiation exposure, the sensitivity of CFU-GM to 5-FU increased significantly: about twofold after cyclophosphamide to over 1000-fold after endotoxin by 24 hr following the stimulus.

## 1.5.1. Cytotoxicity of Anticancer Agents to CFU-GM

To date, few investigators have carried out studies to assess the effects of anticancer agents on the survival of CFU-GM. The first large study was that of Brown and Carbone (1971). Some of these results as well as those of other investigators have been incorporated into Table V. Other studies are discussed in more detail below.

Methotrexate demonstrated a profound cytotoxic effect on CFU-GM with a CD$_{50}$ in dialyzed madia of $10^{-8}$ M and greater than 99% toxicity at about $5 \times 10^{-8}$ M (Pinedo *et al.*, 1976a,b). This *in vitro* effect was geatly decreased in media with nondialyzed serum due to reversal of toxicity by nucleosides. When studied *in vivo*, it was found that a dose of 60 mg/kg yielded an increase rather than a decrease in CFU-GM in C57BL mice (Vogler *et al.*, 1973). Repeating the injection on day 3 caused a reduction (to 44% of control) whereas on day 6 there was little if any effect. They also showed an interesting result with continued infusion of methotrexate in mice in that while CFU-S continued to fall over a 48-hr period, contrary to the results of Bruce *et al.* (1969), CFU-GM increased between 24 and 48 hr, i.e., during the methotrexate infusion, which led the authors to suggest that CFU-S differentiated to CFU-GM without division during this time period.

Haskill *et al.* (1970) compared the effect of vinblastine on both CFU-S and CFU-GM and found the latter to be significantly more sensitive to the drug. There was a suggestion of a plateau in the dose–survival curve for CFU-S at 3 to 5% of control by 0.5 mg/mouse with little change by

**Table V.**   Effect of Anticancer Agents on CFU-GM

| Drug | Dose | Mouse strain | Fractional survival | Comment | Reference |
|---|---|---|---|---|---|
| Tritiated thymidine | 0.5–3 mCi/mouse | C57BL | 0.68–1.02 | — | Blackett *et al.*, 1974 |
|  |  |  | 0.56 | Proliferating marrow | Blackett *et al.*, 1974 |
|  | 25–300 $\mu$Ci/ml |  | 0.65 | — | Blackett *et al.*, 1974 |
|  |  |  | 0.50 | Proliferating marrow | Blackett *et al.*, 1974 |
| BCNU | 10–50 $\mu$mol/liter | BALB/C | 31.3 $\mu$mol/liter | Large shoulder | Ogawa *et al.*, 1973a |
|  |  |  | 26.2 $\mu$mol/liter | Large shoulder | Ogawa *et al.*, 1973a |
|  | 35 mg/kg | CF$_1$ | 0.4 (at 48 hr) | Recovery by day 6 | Udupa and Reissmann, 1974 |
|  | 20–60 mg/kg | — | 15.4 mg/kg[a] | — | Blackett *et al.*, 1975 |
|  | 11–44 $\mu$mol/liter | C3B6F1 | 31.3 $\mu$mol/liter[b] | — | Ogawa *et al.*, 1973b |
|  | 1–100 mg/kg | C57BL/6 | 55.9 mg/kg[a] | Shoulder region | Brown and Carbone, 1971 |
| Busulfan | 40 mg/kg | C57BL | $2 \times 10^{-2}$ | Proliferating marrow | Blackett and Millard, 1976 |
| CCNU | 20–60 mg/kg | — | 10.3 mg/kg[a] | — | Blackett *et al.*, 1975 |
| Cyclophosphamide | 50–300 mg/kg | C57BL | 176 mg/kg[a] | — | Millard *et al.*, 1973 |
|  |  |  | 119 mg/kg[a] | Regenerating marrow | Millard *et al.*, 1973 |
|  | 3–300 mg/kg |  | 67.2 mg/kg[a] | Shoulder region | Brown and Carbone, 1971 |
|  | 200 mg/kg |  | 0.07 mg/kg (1 hr) | Partial recovery at 4 days | Brown and Carbone, 1971 |
|  | 0–200 mg/kg |  | 51 mg/kg[a] | — | Gordon and Blackett, 1976 |
|  | 2–6 mg/mouse | BALB/C | 2.9 mg/mouse[b] | — | Ogawa *et al.*, 1973a |
|  |  |  | 1.45 mg/mouse[a] | CFU-GM in cycle | Ogawa *et al.*, 1973a |
| Cytosine arabinoside | 1–44 $\mu$g/ml | C57BL | 0.77 | — | Millard and Okell, 1975 |
|  | 15, 20, 40 $\mu$g/ml |  | 0.46 | Proliferating marrow | Millard and Okell, 1975 |
|  | 100–300 mg/kg |  | 0.8[c] | — | Gordon and Douglas, 1976 |
|  |  |  | 0.2–0.3[c] | Proliferating | Gordon and Douglas, 1976 |
| 5-FU | 50–300 $\mu$mol/ liter | BALB/C | 25.4 mg/kg[a] | Proliferating marrow | Blackett *et al.*, 1975 |
|  |  |  | 104 $\mu$mol/liter[b] | — | Ogawa *et al.*, 1973a |
|  |  |  | 25.4 $\mu$mol/liter[b] | CFU-GM in cycle | Ogawa *et al.*, 1973a |

| | | | | | |
|---|---|---|---|---|---|
| | 0–50 mg/kg | C57BL | 12.8 mg/kg[a] | — | Gordon and Blackett, 1976 |
| | 0.1–0.3 mmol/liter | C3B6F1 | 0.104 mmol/liter[b] | — | Ogawa et al., 1973b |
| | 2.5 mg/mouse | AKR | $5 \times 10^{-2}$ (at 24 hr) | — | Eaves and Bruce, 1974 |
| | | | $<10^{-4}$ (at 24 hr) | Endotoxin stimulated | Eaves and Bruce, 1974 |
| Hydroxyurea | 900 mg/kg | CF$_{1s}$ | 0.5 (2 hr) | — | Rickard et al., 1970 |
| | | | 0.70 (2 hr) | Proliferating marrow | Rickard et al., 1971 |
| Methotrexate | 250 mg/kg | C57BL/6 | 0.5 (24 hr)[c] | — | Brown and Carbone, 1970 |
| | 0–300 mg/kg | C57BL | ~0.6[c] | — | Gordon and Blackett, 1976 |
| MeCCNU | 20–40 mg/kg | — | 15.4 mg/kg[a] | — | Blackett et al., 1975 |
| Melphalan | 1.6–64 $\mu$mol/liter | C3B6F1 | 4.2 $\mu$mol/liter[b] | — | Ogawa et al., 1973b |
| | 0.02–0.1 mg/mouse | BALB/C | 0.14 mg/mouse[b] | — | Ogawa et al., 1971 |
| | 0.02–1 $\mu$g/ml | | 1.5 $\mu$g/ml[b] | — | Ogawa et al., 1971 |
| | 0.5–1 $\mu$g/ml | | 1.5 $\mu$g/ml[b] | CFU-GM in cycle | Ogawa et al., 1971 |
| 6-Mercaptopurine | 40 mg/kg × 4 every 12 hr | CD2F1 | 0.3 (at 2 days) | Nearly recovered by day 8 | Ragab et al., 1974 |
| Nitrogen mustard | 0.13–0.52 $\mu$mol/liter | C3B6F1 | 0.21 $\mu$mol/liter[b] | — | Ogawa et al., 1973b |
| | 5–20 mg/kg | C57BL/6 | 2.7 mg/kg[a] | Shoulder region | Brown and Carbone, 1971 |
| | 0.1–0.6 $\mu$mol/liter | BALB/C | 0.15 $\mu$mol/liter[b] | Same for proliferating CFU-GM | Ogawa et al., 1973a |
| VLB | 10 mg/kg | C57BL | $<3 \times 10^{-5}$ | Proliferating marrow | Blackett and Millard, 1976 |
| | 0.2–30 mg/kg | C57BL | 0.18 (10 mg/kg)[c] | — | Millard et al., 1973 |
| | | | $<0.005$ (10 mg/kg)[c] | Regenerating marrow | Millard et al., 1973 |
| | 50 mg/kg | C57BL/6 | 0.04 (24 hr)[c] | — | Brown and Carbone, 1971 |
| | 80 $\mu$g/mouse | C3H | 0.22 (24 hr) | Recovery ~day 3 | Chen and Schooley, 1970 |
| | 0.05–1 mg/mouse | (C57BL × CBA)F$_1$ | 0.09 mg/mouse | Biphasic dose–survival curve | Haskill et al., 1970 |
| | 0–30 mg/kg | C57BL | about 0.5[c] | — | Gordon and Blackett, 1976 |

[a] $D_0$ value.
[b] $D_{37}$ dose.
[c] Plateau value.

1 mg/mouse. For CFU-GM, survival was about 0.6% of control at the former dose and decreased to 0.07% at the latter dose.

The ansamycin antibiotics were found to be effective against CFU-GM, appearing to yield an exponential killing over the dose range studied with $LD_{50}$ values for rifamycin SV, streptovaricin complex, and streptovaricin C present continuously in culture at doses of about 0.25, 0.5–1.0, and 5 mg/ml, respectively (Horoczewicz and Carter, 1974). In the same study, on human CFU-GM, the same agents were 10- to 40-fold less effective.

A recent surprising result is the wide variability observed in the response of human CFU-GM to ara-C cytotoxicity (Niho *et al.*, 1976). Most investigators likely think *a priori* that while significant differences in response may exist between tumors, within any species, the response to normal cells should be similar. If this difference were similar for other arms of the hematopoietic system, then this should correlate strongly with toxicity for those agents whose dose is limited by hematopoietic toxicity. Further, pretherapy dose–survival curves for CFU-GM might then allow a better "tailoring" of the drug dose to the individual patient.

Ogawa *et al.* (1973b) compared the response of a number of anticancer agents to both human and mouse CFU-GM *in vitro* and found the cell populations to differ in sensitivity when compared to each other. The authors caution against extrapolating mouse results to humans since differences even between strains of mice have been noted (Millard *et al.*, 1973).

### 1.5.2. Therapeutic Implications for CFU-GM

The therapeutic implications for CFU-GM are similar to those discussed previously for CFU-S; however, because a larger fraction of this population is proliferating, one would expect to find it more sensitive than CFU-S to anticancer agents. Such an effect is certainly true for the phase-specific agents as seen by comparing Tables I, III, and V, although for agents such as Myleran the opposite has been noted (Blackett and Millard, 1973).

A possible important effect observable in some dose–survival curves (Brown and Carbone, 1971) is the existence of a shoulder region for CFU-GM indicating that little if any cell killing occurs at low doses. If recruitment also does not occur, and if the tumor cells do *not* have a similar shoulder region, fractionation of the drug would be an effective regimen.

As has been noted for the CFU-S, when CFU-GM are examined in proliferating marrow, they are significantly more sensitive to the cytotoxic effects of anticancer agents. This is a consequence of recruitment of the nonproliferating fraction into cell cycle and is well demonstrated by the phase-specific agent VLB (Millard *et al.*, 1973).

Unlike the CFU-S, it is possible to culture human CFU-GM and study its response to agents. In an elegant study by Gordon and Douglas (1976), they show not only the expected plateau-type dose–response curve of human CFU-GM to ara-C, but also their increase in sensitivity shortly following the initiation of chemotherapy and a subsequent return to normal sensitivity. The similarity between the human and mouse system and expectations from our animal models are most encouraging. While absolute values for sensitivies to drug may not be identical between human and mouse progenitor cells (Gordon and Blackett, 1976), it is dangerous to draw conclusions about such differences based on a comparison with one mouse strain; Table III demonstrates for cyclophosphamide a difference of more than two-fold in sensitivity between AKR and C3H mice.

## 1.6. CFU-E

The first systematic study which demonstrated the ability to produce colonies from progenitors of the erythroid series was by Stephenson *et al.* (1971). Murine fetal liver as well as adult bone marrow in the presence of erythropoietin in a plasma clot culture yielded Lepehne-positive colonies of 10 to 20 cells in number by day 2, reaching 60 to 70 cells by day 4. These were termed CFU-E (CFU-E3 by our terminology, Fig. 1).

Further studies with a modified plasma clot system showed 2 days to be the optimum time to score CFU-E3 (McLeod *et al.*, 1974). That the progenitor cell is separate from the CFU-GM is demonstrated by CSF not affecting CFU-E3 number nor erythropoietin affecting CFU-GM number. It has been well demonstrated that CFU-E3 differ from CFU-GM and CFU-S. CFU-E3 were shown to decrease upon erythrocyte-induced transfusion plethora but this does not affect CFU-S and CFU-GM (Gregory *et al.*, 1974). The morphology of the *in vivo* spleen colonies and the relation to the number of CFU-E3 and their lack of correlation with the CFU-S content support the notion that the CFU-E3 appear to be in a much later stage of hematopoietic differentiation than the CFU-GM. The majority of these cells are in cycle since 77% of these cells are killed upon exposure to [$^3$H]-TdR (Singer and Adamson, 1977). Their growth kinetics, ability to respond to erythropoietin, and dose response to ionizing radiation also characterize these progenitors (Gregory *et al.*, 1974). In general, CFU-E3 are considered to be a more differentiated cell population than CFU-GM. Furthermore, the number of CFU-E3 did not correlate with the number of either CFU-GM or CFU-S assayed in individual spleen colonies whereas the latter two cell populations showed a more positive correlation.

Axelrad and co-workers (1974) substantiated that CFU-E3 were relatively differentiated progenitors in the erythroid series by showing that much larger (>500 cells) erythroid colonies appeared later in culture (day 7) after repeated additions of erythropoietin to plasma culture over a 3- to 4-day period. These colonies were coined burst-forming units, erythroid (or BFU-E; CFU-E1 in our terminology), to distinguish them from CFU-E3. CFU-E1 were shown to be progenitors having a more extensive proliferative capacity than CFU-E3 and that in all probability were composed of clusters of CFU-E3.

A third category of erythropoietin-sensitive colony-forming cells has recently been demonstrated (termed day 3 BFU-E; CFU-E2 by our terminology) (Gregory, 1976) which seems to be intermediate in state of differentiation to the CFU-E1 and CFU-E3. It is a burst-type colony and reaches maximum size by day 3 then disappears from culture. This population has been noted in humans as well as in mice (Gregory and Eaves, 1977).

Studies of erythrocytic progenitors were recently done in humans. Using the plasma clot system or the methyl cellulose system and waiting 7 to 9 days before analysis, erythropoietin-dependent erythrocytic colonies were observed (Tepperman *et al.*, 1974; Iscove *et al.*, 1974). Two different populations of colony-forming cells were obtained by sedimentation separation and their proliferative capacity correlated well with murine CFU-E1 and CFU-E3.

Unfortunately, at present there is no major study on the effects of anticancer agents on any of these cell populations.

## 1.7. CFU-M

Recently, techniques have become available whereby megakaryocyte progenitors from murine femora can be grown as colonies *in vitro*. This type of progenitor may be cultured in modified plasma cultures (Nakeff and Daniels-McQueen, 1976; McLeod *et al.*, 1976) as well as in agar (Nakeff *et al.*, 1975; Metcalf *et al.*, 1975a). CFU-M yield colonies averaging from 4 to 12 cells which can be stained for acetylcholinesterase activity as a specific cytochemical marker for rodent megakaryocytes. To date, no drug studies on this population have appeared in the literature; however, the effect for cyclophosphamide is described subsequently herein.

## 1.8. CFU-BL

A class of colony-forming cells has been identified which is derived from lymphoid tissue (Metcalf *et al.*, 1975b, 1976). It requires $\beta$-mercap-

toethanol for its expression; the progeny are greatly stimulated by endotoxin (Metcalf, 1976) and have the characteristics of B-lymphocytes. The
only drug they have been tested against has been cortisone acetate to
which they are sensitive, showing a surviving fraction of about $1.8 \times 10^{-1}$
at 2 mg/mouse (Metcalf *et al.*, 1976).


## 1.9. CFU-O

A class of colony-forming cells which gives rise to macrophages was
described recently by Lin and Stewart (1973) and termed PCFC (peritoneal colony-forming cells). These authors have subsequently shown that
there are subclasses of this population with different physical and culturing characteristics. As indicated in Fig. 1, it is not known whether this is a
separate progenitor cell or whether it arises from the CFU-GM. Extensive
experimentation is currently in progress to understand the biology of this
population and its response to physical and chemical agents.


## 1.10. Nonclonogenic Assays

In the past, a great deal of study on drug effects has employed
nonclonogenic assays such as the erythrocytic repopulation ability assay
(Hodgson, 1962), the erythroid responsive cell assay (Hellman and Grate,
(1967), or the platelet repopulating ability assay (Goodman *et al.*, 1977) of
a host. It is not the purpose of this chapter to discuss these studies both
because Marsh (1976) has recently completed such a comprehensive
review and because we think the clonogenic assays are much more precise;
they are better quantitatively and much more amenable to modeling and
testing.


## 1.11. Cytotoxic Effect of Cyclophosphamide on Progenitor Cells

Most investigators who examine the effects of anticancer agents on
progenitor cells generally do so only on one of the cells. We believe it is
important to examine the effects of one drug in a single strain of mouse,
but upon as many of the progenitor populations in bone marrow as
possible. In this manner, more valid comparisons could be obtained of
differential drug cytotoxicities and degrees of competition and inhibition
between the committed progenitors and their common stem cell. Since it
is important to control as many variables as possible in *in vitro* assay
systems if a valid comparison is to be made among the various clonogenic

populations in a drug-treated host marrow, the use of a common culture system has obvious advantages. In addition, the ability to use cytochemical or cytological markers as an aid in rapidly and unequivocally identifying different colonies *in situ* is a distinct asset in quantitating different committed progenitors. The plasma culture system satisfies these requirements. In addition, the small size of the cultures (0.1 ml) necessitates small amounts of all culture ingredients, in particular stimulating factor(s), and makes it possible to fix and store cultures for subsequent analysis and comparison with later cultures.

We have initiated a series of studies to define in detail the dose– and time–response relationship of both pluripotent stem cells (CFU-S) assayed *in vivo* and committed clonogenic progenitors (CFU-GM, -M, and -E3) assayed in plasma culture to a series of different chemotherapeutic agents in normal mice. Figure 2 presents preliminary dose–response curves obtained for marrow CFU-S, -E3, -GM, and -M following a single dose of cyclophosphamide (Nakeff and Valeriote, 1977) showing approximately equivalent exponential cell killing for CFU-S, -E3, and -M. CFU-GM,

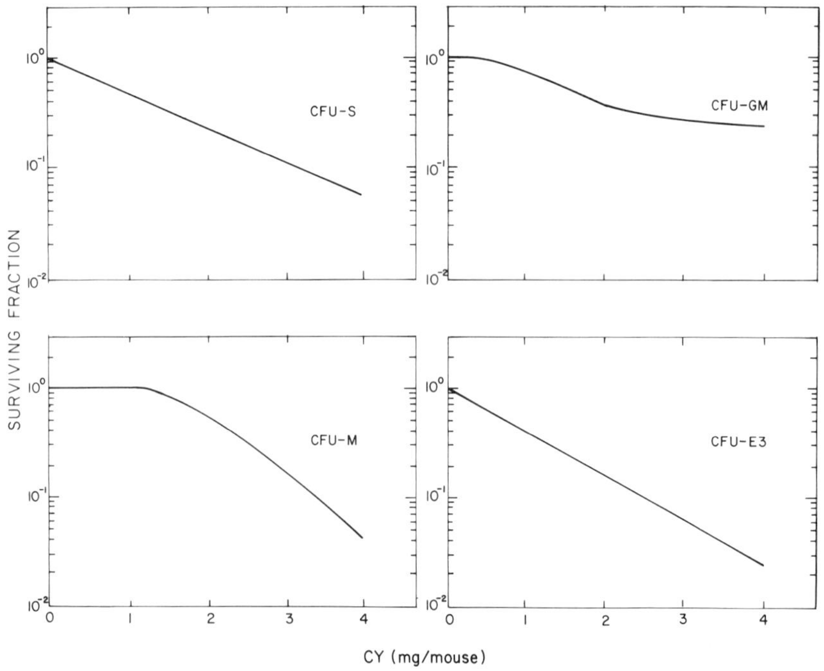


**Fig. 2.** Dose–response relationship for femoral marrow CFU-S, -M, -GM, and -E3 to cyclophosphamide administered as a single intraperitoneal injection to male donor B6D2F1 mice and assayed 24 hr later.

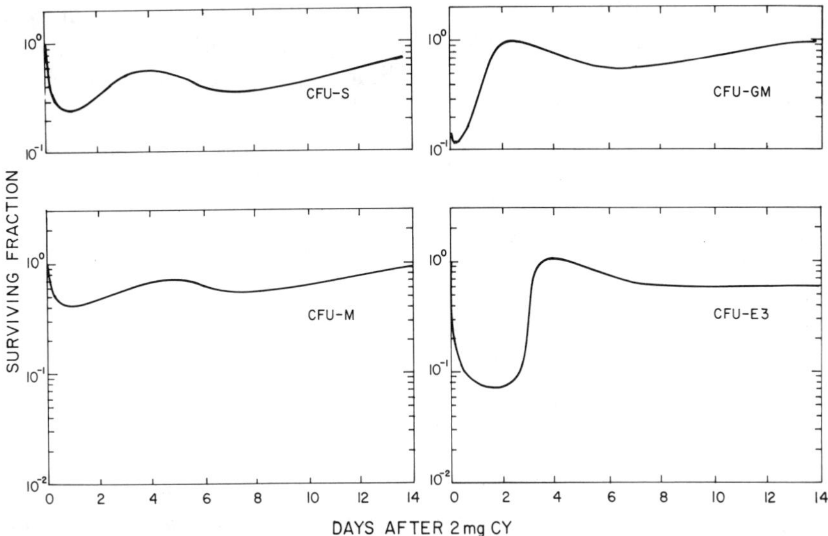



**Fig. 3.** Fractional survival of CFU-S, -M, -GM, and -E3 in the marrow of B6D2F1 mice as a function of time following a single intraperitoneal injection of 2 mg cyclophosphamide.

however, not only is much less sensitive than the other progenitor populations but demonstrates a plateau effect with increasing dose as well as a shoulder region at low dose. Although this form of curve was not found by others, the overall sensitivity was quite similar (see Table V). These data yield a $D_0$ for CFU-S of 1.4 mg cyclophosphamide/mouse, a value similar to that found by other investigators (Table IV).

A comparison of the cell recovery patterns for these progenitors following a single dose of 2 mg/mouse of cyclophosphamide revealed interesting similarities and differences (Fig. 3). For example, the responses for CFU-S and -M were remarkably similar with respect to the initial level of depletion and rate of recovery. This may reveal a close developmental relationship between these two classes of progenitors and imply that CFU-M are probably very immature progenitors not far removed in terms of differentiation from CFU-S. CFU-GM, on the other hand, were initially slightly more sensitive to cyclophosphamide at this dose than the previous two progenitors but recovered more rapidly and completely. CFU-E3 were the most sensitive but reached their nadir somewhat later than CFU-GM; their recovery after this point was most rapid and complete by day 4. One difficulty in the interpretation of these studies is knowing the extent of depletion due to cyclophosphamide cytotoxicity compared to that due to differentiation. Since it is known from clonogenic studies with tumor cells that cyclophosphamide cytotoxicity is complete within a few hours following 2 mg/mouse, then an early time point (4 hr) would indicate the extent of drug-induced cytotoxicity. The early time points for CFU-S indicate significantly greater survival than that found at 24 hr, indicating CFU-S loss due to differentiation. This was also found for CFU-E3, indicating that part of the apparently high drug sensitivity was due to loss through differentiation. We will be better able to understand the kinetics of the erythroid system after examining the effects of cyclophosphamide upon CFU-E1 and -E2. For CFU-GM and CFU-M, minimum survival is noted early following drug administration with recovery immediately thereafter. These results indicate that any loss due to differentiation is more than balanced by input from earlier cell compartments.

## 1.12. Conclusion

The study of drug effects on progenitor cells and their analysis both as a function of dose and time is important for several reasons. First, therapeutically, results of the kind reported herein may demonstrate the possibility of subclassifying chemotherapeutic agents on the basis of differential cytotoxicities toward various normal progenitors. This would permit a more rational approach to the choice of appropriate agents in drug combinations such that they would not have extensive cytotoxicities to the same progenitor cell population yet be synergistic in their killing of tumor cells. This approach may permit more of one drug, or more drugs, to be used without the limitation of critically depleting the normal marrow progenitors. Although the cytotoxicity of various agents has been quantitated clinically for end cells from changes in the number of circulating blood cells, little information is available on damage expression at the level of the progenitor cells.

Second, the prospect of culturing human marrow under uniform culture conditions to assay for committed progenitors will represent a substantial advance since it would then become possible to screen for cytotoxicities of specific agents on a sample of a patient's marrow prior to treatment. In addition, samples of marrow could be cultured for the level of the various progenitors as a function of time after treatment had commenced. This would be a more effective predictor of normal cell toxicity than the blood cell count alone since it would monitor important cellular changes before they would be manifest in the blood at which time therapy must be discontinued and blood transfusions commenced.

Finally, from the point of view of the basic cell biology of the hematopoietic system, the use of drugs with well-defined mechanisms of action can be used effectively as probes to elucidate complex interrelationships among progenitor cells and provide concepts as well as specific kinetic information in the modeling of the hematopoietic system. Further, the sensitivities of perturbed populations following therapy are important to define. This type of data is necessary for better scheduling of anticancer agents, particularly those that display a proliferation-dependent cytotoxicity.

As a result of the development of clonogenic assays for the progenitor populations of the hematopoietic system, the cell biology of this complex cell system is going through a major advancement. The cellular components and their control mechanisms are being sharply defined and this should have a major impact on many facets of hematology. We expect this to be true for medical oncology where this knowledge and that of drug effects at the progenitor level will lay a more scientific foundation to therapy and provide for a further advance toward the goal of cure.

ACKNOWLEDGMENT

This investigation was supported by Grant Number 5P01CA13053-05 from the National Cancer Institute, DHEW.

# References

Alberts, D. S., and van Daalen Wetters, T., 1976, Rubidazone vs. adriamycin: An evaluation of their differential toxicity in the spleen colony assay system, *Br. J. Cancer* **34**:64.

Ash, R., Chaffey, J. T., and Hellman, S., 1972, The effects of nitrogen mustard on the survival of murine hematopoietic stem cells, *Cancer Res.* **32**:1695.

Axelrad, A. A., McLeod, D. L., Shreeve, M. M., and Heath, D. S., 1974, Properties of cells that produce erythrocytic colonies *in vitro*, in *Proceedings of the Second International Workshop on Hemopoiesis in Culture* (W. A. Robinson, ed.), pp. 226–234, U.S. Govt. Printing Office, Washington, D.C.

Becker, A. J., McCulloch, E. A., Siminovitch, L., and Till, J. E., 1965, The effect of differing demands for blood cell production on DNA synthesis by hemopoietic colony-forming cells of mice, *Blood* **26**:296.

Bhuyan, B. K., Fraser, T. J., and Day, K. J., 1977, Cell proliferation kinetics and drug sensitivity of exponential and stationary populations of cultured L1210 cells, *Cancer Res.* **37**:1057.

Blackett, N. M., and Millard, R. E., 1973, Differential effect of Myleran on two normal haematopoietic progenitor cell populations, *Nature* **244**:300.

Blackett, N. M., and Millard, R. E., 1976, Different recovery patterns of mouse haematopoietic stem cells in response to cytotoxic agents, *J. Cell. Physiol.* **89**:473.

Blackett, N. M., Millard, R. E., and Belcher, H. M., 1974, Thymidine suicide *in vivo* and *in vitro* of spleen colony-forming and agar colony-forming cells of mouse bone marrow, *Cell Tissue Kinet.* **7**:309.

Blackett, N. M., Courtenay, V. D., and Mayer, S. M., 1975, Differential sensitivity of colony-forming cells of hemopoietic tissue, Lewis lung carcinoma, and B16 melanoma to three nitrosoureas, *Cancer Chemother. Rep.* **59**:929.

Boyum, A., Carsten, A. L., and Laerum, O. D., 1974, Hematopoiesis measured by spleen colony and diffusion chamber techniques in mice treated with one or two injections of cyclophosphamide. *Br. J. Haematol.* **26**:605.

Bradley, T. R., and Metcalf, D., 1966, The growth of mouse bone marrow cells *in vitro*, *Aust. J. Exp. Biol. Med. Sci.* **44**:287.

Breivik, H., 1972, Response of multipotent (CFU) and granulocyte (diffusion chamber assay) progenitor cells and differentiating cells of murine haematopoietic tissues to a perturbation of the steady state, *J. Cell. Physiol.* **79**:171.

Brown, C. H., and Carbone, P. P., 1971, Effects of chemotherapeutic agents on normal mouse bone marrow grown *in vitro*, *Cancer Res.* **31**:185.

Bruce, W. R., and Meeker, B. E., 1967, Comparison of the sensitivity of hematopoietic colony-forming cells in different proliferative states to 5-fluorouracil, *J. Natl. Cancer Inst.* **38**:401.

Bruce, W. R., Meeker, B. E., and Valeriote, F. A. , 1966, Comparison of the sensitivity of normal hematopoietic and transplanted lymphoma colony-forming cells to chemotherapeutic agents administered *in vivo*, *J. Natl. Cancer Inst.* **37**:233.

Bruce, W. R., Meeker, B. E., Powers, W. E., and Valeriote, F. A., 1969, Comparison of the dose- and time-survival curves for normal hematopoietic and lymphoma colony-forming cells exposed to vinblastine, vincristine, arabinosylcytosine, and amethoptecin, *J. Natl. Cancer Inst.* **42**:1015.

Byron, J. W., 1972, Comparison of the action of $^3$H-thymidine and hydroxyurea on testosterone-treated hemopoietic stem cells, *Blood* **40**:198.

Byron, J. W., 1975, Manipulation of the cell cycle of the hemopoietic stem cell, *Exp. Hematol.* **3**:44.

Chen, M. G., and Schooley, J. C., 1970, Recovery of proliferative capacity of agar colony-forming cells and spleen colony-forming cells following ionizing radiation or vinblastine, *J. Cell. Physiol.* **75**:89.

Croizat, H., Frindel, E., and Tubiana, M., 1970, Proliferative activity of the stem cells in the bone marrow of mice after single and multiple irradiations (total- or partial-body exposure), *Int. J. Radiat. Biol.* **18**:347.

DeWys, W. D., Goldin, A., and Mantel, N., 1970, Hematopoietic recovery after large doses of cyclophosphamide: Correlation of proliferative state with sensitivity, *Cancer Res.* **30**:1692.

Dunn, C. D. R., 1972, The effect of certain nitrogen mustard derivatives on bone marrow colony-forming units and erythroid repopulating ability. II. Mice, *Euro. J. Cancer* **8**:517.

Dunn, C. D. R., 1973, The proliferative capacity of haemopoietic colony-forming units in the rat, *Cell Tissue Kinet.* **6**:55.

Dunn, C. D. R., 1974, Effect, with time, of melphalan on hematopoietic stem cells proliferating at different rates, *J. Natl. Cancer Inst.* **52**:173.

Dunn, C. D. R., and Elson, L. A., 1970, The comparative effect of busulphan (myleran) and aminochlorambucil on haemopoietic colony forming units in the rat, *Cell Tissue Kinet.* **3**:131.

Eaves, A. C., and Bruce, W. R., 1974, Altered sensitivity of hematopoietic stem cells to 5-fluorouracil (NSC-19893) following endotoxin (NSC-189681) and cyclophosphamide (NSC-26271), or irradiation, *Cancer Chemother. Rep.* **58**:813.

Evenaar, A. H., Wins, E. H. R., and van Putten, L. M., 1973, Cell killing effectiveness of an alkylating steroid (Leo 1031), *Eur. J. Cancer* **9**:773.

Fuzy, M., Lelieveld, P., and van Putten, L. M., 1975, The effect of cytostatic hexitol derivatives on hematopoietic stem cells, the L1210 leukaemia and C22LR osteosarcoma, *Eur. J. Cancer* **11**:169.

Giadali, J., Fehr, I., and Antal, S., 1974, Some properties of the circulating hemopoietic stem cells, *Blood* **43**:573.

Goodman, R., Grate, H., Hannon, E., and Hellman, S., 1977, Hematopoietic stem cells: Effect of preirradiation, bleeding and erythropoietin on thrombopoietic differentiation, *Blood* **49**:253.

Gordon, M. Y., and Blackett, N. M., 1976, The sensitivities of human and murine hemopoietic cells exposed to cytotoxic drugs in an *in vivo* culture system, *Cancer Res.* **36**:2822.

Gordon, M. Y., and Douglas, I. D. C., 1976, Changes in proliferative rate of human bone marrow colony-forming cells measured by a cytosine arabino-side-diffusion chamber method, *Eur. J. Cancer* **12**:551.

Gregory, C. J., 1976, Erythropoietin sensitivity as a differentiation marker in the hemopoietic system: Studies of three erythropoietic colony responses in cultures, *J. Cell. Physoil.* **89**:289.

Gregory, C. J., McCulloch, E. A., and Till, J. E., 1974, Erythropoietic progenitors capable of colony formation in culture: State of differentiation, *J. Cell. Physiol.* **81**:411.

Gregory, C. J., and Eaves, A. C., 1977, Human marrow cells capable of erythropoietic differentiation *in vitro:* Definition of three erythroid colony responses, *Blood* **49**:855.

Guzman, E., and Lajtha, L. G., 1970, Some comparisons of the kinetic properties of femoral and splenic haemopoietic stem cells, *Cell Tissue Kinet.* **3**:91.

Hanks, G. E., 1972, Recruitment and altered recovery in noncycling bone marrow stem cells, *Radiology* **103**:691.

Haskill, J. S., McNeil, T. A., and Moore, M. A. S., 1970, Density distribution analysis of *in vivo* and *in vitro* colony forming cells in bone marrow, *J. Cell. Physiol.* **75**:167.

Hellman, S., and Grate, H. E., 1967, Production of granulocytic progeny by transplanted bone marrow in irradiated mice. *Blood* **30**:103.

Hellman, S., and Grate, H. E., 1971a, X-ray and alkaylating agents alter differentiation of surviving hematopoietic stem cells, *Blood* **38**:174.

Hellman, S., and Grate, H. E., 1971b, Effect of cyclophosphamide on the murine hematopoietic stem cells compartment as measured by different assay techniques, *Blood* **38**:706.

Hodgson, G., 1962, Erythrocyte $^{59}$Fe uptake as a function of bone marrow dose injected in lethally irradiated mice, *Blood* **19**:460.

Hodgson, G., Bradley, T. R., Martin, R. F., Summer, M., and Fry, P., 1975, Recovery of proliferating haemopoietic progenitor cells after killing by hydroxyurea, *Cell Tissue Kinet.* **8**:51.

Horoczewicz, J. S., and Carter, W. A., 1974, Responses of the murine myeloid colony-forming cell to ansamycin antibiotics, *Antimicrob. Agents Chemother.* **5**:196.

Iscove, N. N., Till, J. E., and McCulloch, E. A. , 1970, The proliferative state of mouse granulopoietic progenitor cells, *Proc. Soc. Exp. Biol. Med.* **134**:33.

Iscove, N. N., Sieber, F., and Winterhalter, K. H., 1974, Erythroid colony formation in cultures of mouse and human bone marrow: Analysis of the requirement for erythropoiesis by gel filtration and affinity chromatography on agarose-concanavalin A, *J. Cell. Physiol.* **83**:309.

Lahiri, S. K., 1973, Response of mouse bone marrow colony forming units in different stages of the cell cycle to *in vitro* incubation with mitomycin-C. *Cell Tissue Kinet.* **6**:509.

Lajtha, L. G., Oliver, R., and Gurney, C. W., 1962, Kinetic model of a bone marrow stem-cell population, *Br. J. Haematol.* **8**:442.

Lajtha, L. G., Pozzi, L. V., Schofield, R., and Fox, M., 1969, Kinetic properties of haemopoietic stem cells, *Cell Tissue Kinet.* **2**:39.

Levin, J., 1972, Chemotherapy and thrombopoiesis, in *Cancer Chemotherapy II. 22nd Hahnenmann Symposium* (I. Brobsky, S. B. Kahn, and J. H. Moyer, eds.), pp. 263–273, Grune & Stratton, New York.

Lin, H., and Stewart, C. C., 1973, Colony formation by mouse peritoneal exudate cells *in vitro*, *Nature New Biol.* **127**:176–177.

Lord, B. I., Lajtha, L. G., and Gidali, J., 1974, Measurement of the kinetic status of bone marrow precursor cells: Theee cautionary tales, *Cell Tissue Kinet.* **7**:507.

Lord, B. I., Testa, N. G., Wright, E. G., and Banerjee, R. K., 1977, Lack of effect of a granulocyte proliferation inhibitor on their committed precursor cells, *Biomedicine* **26**:163.

Marsh, J. C., 1976, The effects of cancer chemotherapeutic agents on normal hematopoietic precursor cells: A review, *Cancer Res.* **36**:1853.

McLeod, D. L., Shreeve, M. M., and Axelrad, A. A., 1974, Improved plasma culture system for production of erythrocytic colonies *in vitro:* Quantitative assay method for CFU-E, *Blood* **44**:517.

McLeod, D. L., Shreeve, M. M., and Axelrad, A. A., 1976, Induction of megakaryocyte colonies with platelet formation *in vitro*, *Nature* **261**:492.

Metcalf, D., 1976, Role of mercaptoethanol and endotoxin in stimulating B lymphocyte colony formation *in vitro*, *J. Immunol.* **116**:635.

Metcalf, D., MacDonald, H. R., Odartchenko, N., and Sordat, B., 1975a, Growth of mouse megakaryocyte colonies *in vitro*, *Proc. Natl. Acad. Sci. U.S.A.* **72**:1744.

Metcalf, D., Warner, N. L., Nossal, G. J. V., Miller, J. F. A. P., Shortman, K., and Rabellino, E., 1975b, Growth of B lymphocyte colonies *in vitro* from mouse lymphoid organs, *Nature* **255**:630.

Metcalf, D., Wilson, J. W., Shortman, K., Miller, J. F. A. P., and Stocker, J., 1976, The nature of the cells generating B-lymphocytes colonies *in vitro*, *J. Cell. Physiol.* **88**:107.

Millard, R. E., and Okell, S. F., 1975, The effect of cytosine arabinoside *in vitro* on agar colony-forming cells and spleen colony forming cells of C57BL mouse bone marrow, *Cell Tissue Kinet.* **8**:33.

Millard, R. E., Blackett, N. M., and Okell, S. F., 1973, A comparison of the effect of cytotoxic agents on agar colony forming cells, spleen colony forming cells, and the erythrocytic repopulating ability of mouse bone marrow, *J. Cell. Physiol.* **82**:309.

Monette, F. C., Gilio, M. J., and Chalifoun, P., 1974, Separation of proliferating CFU from $G_0$ cells of mouse of murine bone marrow, *Cell Tissue Kinet.* **7**:443.

Morley, A., Trainor, K., and Blake, J., 1975, A primary stem cell lesion in experimental chronic hypoplastic marrow failure, *Blood* **45**:681.

Nakeff, A., and Daniels-McQueen, S., 1976, *In vitro* colony assay for a new class of megakaryocyte precursor: Colony-forming unit megakaryocyte (CFU-M), *Proc. Soc. Exp. Biol. Med.* **151**:587.

Nakeff, A., and Valeriote, F. A. 1977, Use of *in vitro* cell colony assays for measuring the cytotoxicity of chemotherapeutic agents to hematopoietic progenitor cells committed to myeloid, erythroid and megakaryocytoid differentiation, in *Cell Culture and Its Applications* (R. Acton, ed.), pp. 433–448, Academic Press, New York.

Nakeff, A., Dicke, K. A. , and van Noord, M. J., 1975, Megakaryocytes in agar cultures of mouse bone marrow, *Ser. Haematol.* **8**:4.

Necas, E., and Neuwirt, J., 1976, Control of hematopoietic stem cell proliferation by cells in DNA synthesis, *Br. J. Haematol.* **33**:395.

Necas, E., Ponka, P., and Neuwit, J., 1976, Study on the proliferative state of haemopoietic stem cells (CFU), *Cell Tissue Kinet.* **9**:223.

Niho, Y., Till, J. E., and NcCulloch, E. A., 1976, Effect of arabinosyl cytosine on granulopoietic colony formation by marrow cells from leukemic and nonleukemic patients, *Exp. Hematol.* **4**:63.

Nowell, P. C. , and Wilson, D. B., 1971, Lymphocytes and hemic stem cells, *Am. J. Pathol.* **65**:641.

Ogawa, M., Bergsagel, D. E., and McCulloch, E. A., 1971, Differential effects of melphalan on mouse myeloma (adj. PC-5) and hemopoietic stem cells, *Cancer Res.* **31**:2116.

Ogawa, M., Bergsagel, D. E., and McCulloch, E. A., 1973a, Chemotherapy of mouse myeloma: Quantitative cell cultures predictive of response *in vivo*, *Blood* **41**:7.

Ogawa, M., Bergsagel, D. E., and McCulloch, E. A., 1973b, Sensitivity of human and murine hemopoietic precursor cells to chemotherapeutic agents assessed in cell culture, *Blood* **42**:851.

Pinedo, H. M., Chabner, B. A., Zaharko, D. S., and Bull, J. M., 1976a, Evidence for early recruitment of granulocyte precursors during high-dose methotrexate infusions in mice, *Blood* **48**:301.

Pinedo, H. M., Zaharko, D. S., Bull, J. M., and Chabner, B. A., 1976b, The reversal of methotrexate cytotoxicity to mouse bone marrow cells by leucovorin and nucleosides, *Cancer Res.* **36**:4418.

Plusnik, D. H., and Sachs, L., 1965, The cloning of normal "mast" cells in tissue culture, *J. Cell. Comp. Physiol.* **66**:319.

Preisler, H. D., and Henderson, E. E. , 1971, Effect of cytosine arabinoside and 1,3-bis(2-chlorethyl)-1-nitrosourea on hematopoietic precursors in the mouse, *J. Natl. Cancer Inst.* **47**:971.

Ragab, A. H., Gilkerson, E., and Myers, M., 1974, The effect of 6-mercaptopurine and allopurinol on granulopoiesis, *Cancer Res.* **34**:2246.

Razek, A., Valeriote, F., and Vietti, T., 1972, Survival of hematopoietic and leukemic colony-forming cells *in vivo* following the administration of daunorubicin or adriamycin, *Cancer Res.* **32**:1496.

Rickard, K. A., Shadduck, R. K., Howard, D. F., and Stohlman, F., Jr., 1970, A differential effect of hydroxyurea on hemopoietic stem cell colonies *in vitro* and *in vivo*, *Proc. Soc. Exp. Biol. Med.* **134**:152.

Rickard, K. A., Morley, A., Howard, D., and Stohlman, F., Jr., 1971, The *in vitro* colony-forming cell and the response to neutropenia, *Blood* **37**:6.

Sensenbrenner, L. L., Owens, A. H., Jr., Jeiby, J. R., and Jeejeebhoy, H. F., 1973, Comparative effects of cytotoxic agents on transplanted hematopoietic and antibody-producing cells, *J. Natl. Cancer Inst.* **50**:1027.

Sharp, J. G. and Thomas, D. B., 1971, The effects of mustine hydrochloride on the colony forming units of murine bone marrow, *Acta Haematol.* **46**:271.

Singer, J. W., and Adamson, J. W., 1977, Steroids and hematopoiesis. II. The effect of steroids on *in vivo* erythroid colony growth evidence for different target cells for different classes of steroids, *J. Cell. Physiol.* **88**:135.

Stephenson, J. T., Axelrad, A. A., McLeod, D. L., and Shreeve, M. M., 1971, Induction of colonies of hemoglobin-synthesizing cells by erythropoietin *in vitro*, *Proc. Natl. Acad. Sci. U.S.A.* **68**:1542.

Tanaka, T., Craig, A. W., and Lajtha, L. G., 1970, A kinetic study on murine myeloid leukaemia, *Br. J. Cancer* **24**:138.

Tannock, I. F., Marshall, N., and van Putten, L. M., 1972, An attempt at selective chemotherapy of hypoxic cells: Triethylenemelamine and irradiation of a C3H mouse mammary tumour, *Eur. J. Cancer* **8**:501.

Tepperman, A. D., Curtis, J. E., and McCulloch, E. A., 1974, Erythropoietic colonies in cultures of human marrow, *Blood* **44**:659.

Till, J. E., and McCulloch, E. A., 1961, A direct measurement of the radiation sensitivity of normal mouse bone marrow cells, *Radiat. Res.* **14**:213.

Twentyman, P. R., and Bleehen, N. M., 1973, The sensitivity to bleomycin of spleen colony-forming units in the mouse, *Br. J. Cancer* **28**:66.

Udupa, K. B., and Reissman, K. R., 1974, Acceleration of granulopoietic recovery by androgenic steroids in mice made neutropenic by cytotoxic drugs, *Cancer Res.* **34**:2517.

Valeriote, F., 1978, The use of cell kinetics in the development of drug combinations, *J. Pharmacol. Exp. Ther.*, Part A (in press).

Valeriote, F. A., and Bruce, W. R., 1967, Comparison of the sensitivity of hematopoietic colony-forming cells in different proliferative states to vinblastine, *J. Natl. Cancer Inst.* **38**:393.

Valeriote, F. A., and Edelstein, M. B., 1977, The role of cell kinetics in cancer chemotherapy, *Semin Oncol.* **4**:217.

Valeriote, F. A., and Tolen, S., 1971, Comparison of the cytotoxicity of 5-[3,3-bis(2-chloroethyl)-1-triazeno] imidazole-4-carboxamide] (NSC-82196) on normal and leukemic colony-forming cells, *Cancer Chemother. Rep.* **55**:43.

Valeriote, F. A., and Tolen, S. J., 1972, Survival of hematopoietic and lymphoma colony-forming cells *in vivo* following the administration of a variety of alkylating agents, *Cancer Res.* **32**:470.

Valeriote, F. A., and van Putten, L., 1975, Proliferation-dependent cytotoxicity of anticancer agents: A review, *Cancer Res.* **35**:2619.

Valeriote, F. A., Bruce, W. R., and Meeker, B. E., 1966, Comparison of the sensitivity of normal hematopoietic and transplanted lymphoma colony-forming cells of mice to vinblastine administered *in vivo*, *J. Natl. Cancer Inst.* **36**:21.

Valeriote, F. A., Collins, D. C., and Bruce, W. R., 1968, Hematological recovery in the mouse following single dose of gamma radiation and cyclophosphamide, *Radiat. Res.* **33**:501.

van Putten, L. M., and Lelieveld, P., 1970, Factors determining cell killing by chemotherapeutic agents *in vivo*—1-cyclophosphamide, *Eur. J. Cancer* **6**:313.

van Putten, L. M., and Lelieveld, P., 1971, Factors determining cell killing by chemotherapeutic agents *in vivo* II. Melphalan, chlorambucil and nitrogen mustard, *Eur. J. Cancer* **7**:11.

van Putten, L. M., Lelieveld, P., and Kram-Idsenga, L. K. J., 1972, Cell-cycle specificity and therapeutic effectiveness of cytostatic agents, *Cancer Chemother. Rep.* **56**:691.

Vassort, F., Frindel, E., and Tubiana, M., 1971, Effects of hydroxyurea on the kinetics of colony-forming units of bone marrow in the mouse, *Cell Tissue Kinet.* **44**:423.

Vassort, F., Winterholer, M., Frindel, E., and Tubiana, M., 1973, Kinetic parameters of bone marrow stem cells using *in vivo* suicide by tritiated thymidine or by hydroxyurea, *Blood* **41**:789.

Vogler, W. R., Mingioli, E. S., and Garwood, F. A., 1973, The effect of methotrexate on granulocyte stem cells and granulopoiesis, *Cancer Res.* **33**:1628.

2

# Culture of Granulocytic Stem Cells and Its Application to Clinical Problems

## Malcolm A. S. Moore

## 2.1. Characteristics of Granulocyte–Macrophage Stem Cells

The development of a semisolid agar culture system for cloning murine granulocyte–macrophage committed stem cells (CFU-C) (Bradley and Metcalf, 1966), and its subsequent adaptation for human studies (Pike and Robinson, 1970) has resulted in the accumulation of much information on this committed stem cell population in health and disease. The bipotentiality of the majority of CFU-C has been demonstrated in single-cell micromanipulation studies which confirmed that the mixed population of neutrophil granulocytes, monocytes, and macrophages developing within a colony was indeed derived from a common precursor cell which, in turn, is derived from the pluripotential stem cell (Moore *et al.*, 1972).

MALCOLM A. S. MOORE  •  Sloan-Kettering Institute for Cancer Research, New York, New York.

Several types of bone marrow colony-forming assays are being used currently. In many laboratories double-layer cultures are used, where peripheral blood leukocytes are in an underlayer to stimulate bone marrow cells in a semisolid agar overlayer. Other laboratories use a single semisolid layer containing both the bone marrow cells and an exogenous source of conditioned medium containing colony-stimulating factor. Two supporting media, agar or methylcellulose, are used routinely, the latter being preferable when the studies require the harvesting of colony cells for morphological or cytogenetic study, but the agar culture system is essential when assessment of cluster as well as colony numbers is required. Colony or cluster formation may be scored between 7 and 14 days and, although there is no agreement as to the number of cells which constitute colonies or clusters, it is usually accepted that colonies contain at least 20 cells, although many laboratories only count colonies with more than 40 cells. The results of the CFU-C assay are dependent on the definition of colony size and the day on which the colonies are scored. The number of human colonies may be maximal at day 10 and colonies scored on day 7 and 14 are not necessarily generated from the same population of precursor cells. When colonies are scored for morphology of the component cells, neutrophil–monocyte colonies account for 97% of all colonies at day 7 but only 75% at day 14, with the remaining colonies being composed of eosinophils (Moore $et$ $al.$, 1977). While recognizing the differences in culture techniques and scoring criteria, there is general agreement that the incidence of CFU-C in normal human marrow is in the range of 30 to $50/10^5$ nucleated cells. Although the frequency may range from 20 to 120 CFU-C/$10^5$ on any particular patient, the mean frequencies all fall within the narrow range just given. Despite the low incidence of CFU-C in normal marrow, considerable enrichment of the population has proved possible using density and sedimentation separation. The relative homogeneity and light density of CFU-C in monkey bone marrow allowed extensive enrichment using a two-step density separation procedure, and in this study morphological identification of CFU-C as transitional mononuclear cells was possible (Moore $et$ $al.$, 1972). In the majority of species, however, CFU-C are heterogeneous by biophysical and functional criteria. Sedimentation velocity sedimentation of human marrow has shown that CFU-C predominantly responsible for colony formation at day 7 had a peak sedimentation rate of 7.1 mm/hr with a high proportion of cells in DNA synthesis and could be separated from a population of smaller, more slowly cycling CFU-C predominantly forming colonies by day 14. Comparison of these two populations with cells forming granulocytic colonies in diffusion chambers implanted in irradiated mice (CFU-D) has revealed significant differences (Jacobsen $et$ $al.$, 1977). CFU-D had a peak sedimentation rate of 5.2 to 5.4 mm/hr and could be largely separated from CFU-C. Additional differences were found in the cycle status of the CFU, since only 8% of CFU-D were in DNA synthesis in contrast to 35–45% of CFU-C. Culturing marrow cell fractions enriched for CFU-D, either in suspension culture or diffusion chambers, resulted in generation of greatly increased numbers of CFU-C, suggesting that the CFU-D is a pre-CFU-C but not a pluripotent stem cell.

Granulopoiesis *in vitro* is dependent on diffusible activities termed colony-stimulating factors (CSF). Addition of CFUs to cultures at concentrations as low as $10^{-12}$ to $10^{-14}$ M will promote colony formation. The factor is not a simple inducing agent, since its presence is continually required throughout the growth of the colony in addition to promoting CFU-C survival, proliferation, and differentiation (Metcalf and Moore, 1971). Recently, purified CSF preparations have also been shown to act as macrophage growth-stimulating or mitogenic factors, stimulating extensive peritoneal macrophage or blood monocyte proliferation in agar culture (Stanley *et al.*, 1976; Lin and Freeman, 1977). Extensive functional and biochemical studies on CSFs obtained from a number of sources have revealed considerable heterogeneity of material with colony-stimulating activity. The CSFs most extensively characterized are glycoproteins of varying molecular weights and, although the apparent sedimentation coefficients of the various molecules indicate that they are not exact multiples of the discrete basic unit, a polymeric subunit structure is tenable if the molecules are also polydispersed due to the presence of variable amounts of carbohydrate. The most highly purified CSFs have been obtained from human urine, mouse L cell conditioned medium, and endotoxin-treated mouse lung conditioned medium, and are glycoproteins of molecular weights 45,000, 65,000, and 20,000, respectively (Stanley *et al.*, 1975; Burgess *et al.*, 1977a; Moore *et al.*, 1977). The specific activity of pure mouse L cell CSF was $3 \times 10^8$ colonies/mg protein. The purity of the protein was analyzed by discontinuous polyacrylamide gel electrophoresis in both the presence and absence of sodium dodecyl sulfate. A single protein band was observed associated with all the CSF activity. Isoelectric focusing (pH 3–8) indicated some charge heterogeneity but CSF was associated with all protein species. None of the preceding sources of CSF stimulate human colony formation; however, human urine and L cell CSF stimulate predominantly macrophage differentiation of murine CFU-C, whereas lung conditioned medium stimulates granulocytic or mixed colonies.

Preparations of CSF-containing conditioned medium which will stimulate growth from human bone marrow have been obtained from human peripheral blood leukocytes, PHA-stimulated lymphocytes, human embryro kidneys, human monocyte–macrophages, human placenta and lung tissue (Price *et al.*, 1975; Shah *et al.*, 1977; Burgess *et al.*, 1977b;

Moore *et al.*, 1977). In general, these concentrated conditioned media stimulate a similar number of colonies to peripheral blood underlayers, but the size of the colonies is invariably smaller with conditioned media. Partial purification of CSF from these sources, while again demonstrating heterogeneity of the activity, has revealed a common protein of ~30,000 molecular weight which does not appear to bind to concanavalin A-Sepharose.

## 2.2. Positive and Negative Feedback Control of CFU-C Proliferation and Differentiation

Recognition that CSF is produced by monocytes and macrophages (Moore and Williams, 1972; Moore *et al.*, 1974a; Golde and Cline, 1972) and that it acts to promote increased monocyte production and macrophage proliferation introduces the problem of mechanisms designed to counterbalance this positive feedback drive. A number of mechanisms have been revealed in *in vitro* studies and many, if not all, may be of physiological significance *in vivo*. The functional heterogeneity of the phagocytic mononuclear cell population must first be considered, since marked variation in CSF-producing capacity exists. "Virgin" macrophages developing in agar culture from CFU-C and macrophages generated in continuous marrow culture are not constitutive producers of CSF; however, exposure of these cells to macrophage-activating agents such as lipopolysaccharide or BCG rapidly induces CSF synthesis and secretion (M. A. S. Moore, unpublished observation). In this sense, CSF recruitment of additional monocytes and macrophages would not, *ipso facto*, lead to increased CSF production in the absence of an exogenous source of stimulation such as endotoxemia due to gram-negative bacterial infection. Neoplastic monocyte or macrophage cell lines also retain the capacity to produce CSF; however, in some cases the leukemic cell lines are constitutive producers and in other cases CSF production is observed only after LPS stimulation, suggesting retention of a degree of normal responsiveness by the transformed cells (Ralph *et al.*, 1977).

A second feature of monocyte–macrophage CSF production resides in the functional heterogeneity of the activities. Medium conditioned by human monocytes contains two species of CSF, one of apparent molecular weight 30,000, is a true human CSF, stimulating human granulocyte–macrophage colony formation. A high-molecular-weight (150,000) factor is also produced which stimulates mouse marrow colony formation but not human (Shah *et al.*, 1977). This latter CSF may be identical to the CSF species purified from human urine (Stanley *et al.*, 1975). The physiological significance of these two species of CSF resides in the temporal course of their production. Human active CSF is produced early in monocyte cultures but production ceases in 1 to 2 weeks, whereas mouse active CSF is produced continuously for many weeks. The paradox of human cells producing a CSF active only in a different species is resolved if the heterogeneity of the responding cell populations in mouse and human marrow culture is considered. The spectrum of CFU-C in the mouse can be defined by biophysical heterogeneity with respect to cell size and buoyant density. This heterogeneity is also reflected in the dose responsiveness of CFU-C to different species of CSF and in the morphology of the colonies (Van Den Engh *et al.*, 1977; Williams and Jackson, 1977). Human urinary and human macrophage CSF stimulate predominantly macrophage colony formation in mouse marrow culture and appear to act on a more differentiated CFU-C subset than do other species of CSF which stimulate predominantly granulocytic colony formation. Indeed, these macrophage-stimulating CSFs are capable of promoting macrophage colony formation in agar cultures of thioglycollate-activated mouse peritoneal macrophages (Stanley *et al.*, 1976). Assay systems equivalent to the mouse peritoneal macrophage colony assay have not been developed for human use, but it is of relevance that the high-molecular-weight species of CSF produced by human monocytes and macrophages stimulates macrophage cluster formation in human bone marrow culture (Shah *et al.*, 1977). The apparent species specificity may therefore be related to the arbitrary criteria established for a colony (>40 cells) and to differences in the rate of proliferation of human versus mouse cells *in vitro*. The temporal change in production of the two species of CSF by human monocytes and macrophages may thus represent a regulatory mechanism whereby the acute response involves systemic recruitment of additional monocytes and granulocytes by elaboration of a CSF active at the marrow stem cell level and a chronic local response involving continual elaboration of a CSF which exclusively promotes macrophage proliferation.

There is increasing evidence that mature granulocytes and their products participate as one of the regulators of myelopoiesis. Negative feedback control of granulopoiesis has been reported in various systems and the concept of a granulocyte chalone specifically inhibitory to CFU-C or to more differentiated myeloid cells has received some experimental support (Rytomaa, 1973; Lord *et al.*, 1974). The studies of Broxmeyer have indicated a more indirect mechanism of granulocyte negative feedback which recognizes the implications of the bipotentiality of the granulocyte–monocyte committed stem cell (Broxmeyer *et al.*, 1977a,b). "Spontaneous" colony formation in the absence of an exogenous source of CSF is observed in marrow cultures of all species so far investigated when the cells are cultured at a sufficiently high concentration (Moore and Williams, 1972). This spontaneous colony formation is due to endogenous elaboration of CSF by marrow monocytes and macrophages and is considerably enhanced by removal of mature granulocytes from the cultured cell population. Addition of mature granulocytes, granulocyte extracts, or medium conditioned by incubation with granulocytes markedly inhibits spontaneous colony formation (Broxmeyer *et al.*, 1977a). This granulocyte-derived colony inhibitory activity (CIA) acts in a non-species-specific manner to suppress CSF production by monocytes and macrophages. CIA is not inhibitory to monocyte–macrophage proliferation and is clearly distinct from granulocyte chalone, since no inhibition of granulocytic colony formation is observed in the presence of an exogenous source of CSF.

The existence of a negative feedback from the mature granulocyte acting to modulate CSF production may explain steady state balance of granulocytes and monocytes, but does not adequately account for the neutrophil leukocytosis, monocytosis, and extensive macrophage proliferation associated with infection, inflammation, or immune responses. In this context, granulocyte-derived CIA does not inhibit CSF production by endotoxin-stimulated monocytes and macrophages nor by mitogen-stimulated lymphocytes (Broxmeyer *et al.*, 1977a). The existence of override mechanisms permitting increased CSF production in the face of neutrophil leukocytosis introduces the complexity of additional self-limiting mechanisms for which experimental evidence is available.

Activation of normal or neoplastic B- and T-lymphocytes by an appropriate mitogenic or antigenic stimulus leads to induction of CSF production (Ruscetti and Chervenick, 1975). Similar activation protocols also lead to increased production of interferon, which has been shown to be profoundly inhibitory to human and murine granulocyte–macrophage colony formation *in vitro* (Fleming *et al.*, 1972). Thus, interferon may play a physiological role in counteracting the stimulatory activity of lymphocyte-derived CSF.

The regulatory interactions involving diffusible stimulatory and inhibitory activities elaborated by granulocytes, lymphocytes, and phagocytic mononuclear cells can clearly involve specific macromolecules or, alternatively, nonspecific modulating activities. Pharmacological studies have shown that prostaglandins of the E series (PGE) and other agents capable of elevating intracellular levels of cAMP profoundly inhibit granulopoiesis and macrophage proliferation *in vitro* (Kurland and Moore, 1977a). Just as CSF promotes continued replication of the CFU-C and its progeny, PGE limits this effect by an opposing action on the responsiveness of the myeloid stem cell and its proliferative progeny to stimulation by CSF. Kurland and Moore (1977a,b) have shown that prostaglandin synthesized by phagocytic mononuclear cells may be of central importance in the modulation of hematopoiesis. Measurement of prostaglandin

E production by murine macrophages and human monocytes has been performed using a sensitive radioimmunoassay and has shown a linear relationship between the number of phagocytic mononuclear cells and the concentration of PGE in the conditioned medium (Kurland, *et al.*, 1978). This observation explains the lack of correlation between the numbers of monocytes and macrophages used to stimulate granulocyte–macrophage colony formation and the incidence of colonies. Titration of varying numbers of adherent macrophages or blood monocytes as a source of stimulus for human or murine marrow CFU-C has clearly shown that colony formation is stimulated by low numbers of phagocytic mononuclear cells ($0.05–2 \times 10^5$) and inhibited if higher concentrations are used. Parallel studies using monocytes or macrophages treated with indomethacin, a potent inhibitor of prostaglandin synthesis, have revealed a linear relationship between the number of colonies stimulated and the number of phagocytic mononuclear cells used as the source of CSF (Kurland *et al.*, 1977). These observations point to the unique ability of the macrophage to control the proliferation of its own progenitor cell by elaboration of opposing regulatory influences. Macrophages activated by *in vitro* exposure to LPS show marked enhancement of prostaglandin synthesis and a concomitant increased capacity to inhibit granulocytic colony formation (J. Kurland and M. A. S. Moore, unpublished observation). It may appear paradoxical that LPS stimulation which elicits a marked increase in macrophage CSF production should also induce increased production of an opposing activity which can effectively neutralize CSF action. This paradox can be resolved if the temporal sequence of events is considered. LPS *in vivo* and *in vitro* induces increased macrophage/CSF production very rapidly with significant changes observed within minutes, whereas increased prostaglandin synthesis is delayed for 18 to 24 hr (J. Kurland and M. A. S. Moore, unpublished observation). Indeed, the stimulus for increased PGE production is not directly due to LPS but rather to the increased levels of CSF induced which, in turn, activate macrophage prostaglandin synthetase. Incubation of nonactivated macrophages with increasing concentrations of CSF in the absence of LPS leads to a proportional increase in prostaglandin synthesis, indicating a very direct relationship between CSF levels and induction of an opposing activity (Kurland and Moore, 1977b; Kurland *et al.*, 1977). These observations point to the macrophage as a surveillance cell which, under steady state conditions, is elaborating basal levels of CSF and prostaglandin E. The extreme lability of the PGE molecule provides a further physiological control, since the CSF elaborated by fixed tissue macrophages can act systemically to stimulate CFU-C proliferation. The local influence of PGE under basal conditions may thus be limited to inhibition of CSF-dependent proliferation of fixed tissue macrophages. The constitutive contribution of CSF to granulopoiesis and monocyte production is rapidly increased under physiologically perturbed circumstances such as infection. Progressive increases in CSF levels would promote recruitment of additional granulocytes and monocytes by an action on the marrow CFU-C population and would also promote local macrophage proliferation. This process would be self-limiting, since a progressive increase in CSF beyond a critical concentration within the local milieu of the macrophage is ultimately sensed and serves to stimulate the coincident production and release of PGE which opposes the stimulatory action of CSF.

## 2.3. *In Vitro* Culture Studies in the Acute Leukemias

*In vitro* proliferation of leukemic marrow cells in agar culture may be observed in 95% of untreated or relapse cases of AML (and its morphological variants). Cytogenetic analysis of *in vitro* cultures has confirmed the relationship of the *in vitro* colonies or clusters to the *in vivo* leukemic clone (Moore and Metcalf, 1973). The most characteristic defect seen in AML culture was the impaired proliferation of leukemic CFU-C in the presence of optimal or supraoptimal concentrations of CSF (Greenberg *et al.*, 1971; Bull *et al.*, 1973; Moore *et al.*, 1973a,b, 1974b; Spitzer *et al.*, 1976). In cultures of normal or remission bone marrow, a spectrum of clones of different sizes is observed, ranging from colonies containing many hundreds of cells to small clusters of 3 to 40 cells. The ratio between clusters and colonies is very constant despite variation in plating efficiency. In contrast, this growth pattern is abnormal in 91% of AML cases with a spectrum ranging from nongrowing, cluster formation only, to small colonies with an excess of clusters. In addition, plating efficiency of the leukemic blast cells varied widely with, in some cases, 50 to 100% of the blast cells proliferating; however, the average plating efficiency was generally in the range of 1 to 10% (Moore *et al.*, 1974b). This spectrum thus provides a direct measure of the proliferative defects of clonogenic leukemic cells. The qualitative defects observed *in vitro* did not correlate with conventional morphological subdivisions of the acute nonlymphoid leukemias; however, reclassification of leukemia on the basis of *in vitro* growth pattern has proved to be of predictive value in determining patient response to therapy and subsequent remission rate (Moore *et al.*, 1974b).

Standardized culture and scoring criteria were used in a study of 250 cases of untreated AML and its morphological variants (acute monocytic, myelomonocytic, promyelocytic, stem cell, and erythroleukemia). All cultures were stimulated by feeder layers of $1 \times 10^6$ normal white blood cells

(WBC) and were scored at 7 days for the presence of colonies larger than 40 cells and clusters of 3 to 40 cells (Moore, 1976). In this survey, classification of leukemia was performed on the basis of the *in vitro* growth pattern, and the following categories of growth pattern were observed:

1. Nongrowing: 2% of cases. Absence of persisting cells in CSF-stimulated cultures with no colony or cluster formation detected.
2. Microcluster formation: 52% of cases. Absence of colonies and presence of varying numbers of clusters of 3 to 20 cells. The great majority of these cases exhibit a pattern of small clusters in marrow culture, generally only 3 to 10 cells with dispersion and degeneration. Included in this category are examples of extensive persistence of leukemic cells in CSF-stimulated cultures without evidence of cluster formation at 7 days. Marrow cultures from these latter patients, when scored prior to 7 days, show cluster formation with premature dispersion and degeneration of clusters. The majority of microcluster-forming leukemias would be considered nongrowing if scored later than 7 days.
3. Macrocluster formation: 22% of cases. Absence of colonies and presence of varying numbers of clusters approaching the lower limit of colony size, i.e., up to 40 cells. If the cultures are scored later than 7 days, the majority of cases would show evidence of colony formation and merge with the fourth type of classification.
4. Small colonies (microcolonies) with an abnormal cluster-to-colony ratio: 13% of cases. Maximum colony size in this group is less than in control cultures, and an abnormal excess of aggregates of less than 40 cells is seen (the normal ratio of colonies to clusters is 2:10).
5. Colony forming with a normal cluster-to-colony ratio at 7 days of culture: 9% of cases. This category can be further subdivided into cases showing a lower than normal colony incidence and cases with a marked elevation in marrow colony formation invariably associated with a pronounced increase in circulating CFU-C. Both groups share a similar prognosis; however, the former category is mainly comprised of cases in which colony growth is nonleukemic and thus is similar to the pattern seen in acute lymphoblastic leukemia, whereas the latter category merges with the growth pattern seen in chronic myeloid leukemia.

A simple relationship between degree of impairment of *in vitro* proliferation and differentiation and refractoriness to therapy was not observed; however, it was evident that two growth patterns were associated with good prognosis. This group comprised 63% of all cases and included the examples of cluster formation in the absence of colonies with maximum cluster size not exceeding 20 cells by 7 days incubation. In the majority of these cases, clusters were in the range of 3 to 10 cells and did not continue to grow after 7 days. Good prognosis was also associated with examples of colony-forming leukemia with normal colony size and cluster-to-colony ratio. Bad prognosis was associated with complete absence of *in vitro* proliferation, examples of absence of colony formation, but with large clusters developing (bordering on the 40-cell lower limit accepted for colony classification), and examples of small colony formation with an excess of clusters (i.e., an abnormal cluster-to-colony ratio). The complete remission rate in the good prognosis group was 73%, rising to 94% in patients under the age of 40 years, and in the bad prognosis group was only 13% overall and only 14% in the under-40 age group. These differences in response to therapy were highly significant ($p > 0.0001$) in both a retrospective study of 108 cases and a prospective study of a further 142 cases. The association of bad prognosis with certain growth patterns was noted with a variety of remission induction regimens.

Although growth pattern is not an absolute predicator of potential responsiveness of patients to therapy, it provides one of the most significant predictive parameters; however, other factors (such as the labeling index of the blast cell population, age of patient, or previous history of a preleukemic phase) provide additional and interacting prognostic factors. Ten patients included in this survey had acute undifferentiated or stem cell leukemia, and classification into myeloblastic or lymphoblastic type was not possible on the basis of morphology, cytochemistry, or surface markers. Three of these cases showed a myeloid cluster-forming growth pattern in marrow culture, whereas the remainder showed a colony-forming pattern with low plating efficiency and normal granulocytic maturation. The indication that colony formation seen in these cases was due to persisting normal CFU-C coexisting with a nonmyeloid acute leukemia was supported by cell separation studies (Moore, 1975, 1976).

Buoyant density distribution of colony- or cluster-forming cells has been studied by a continuous bovine serum albumin (BSA) density gradient (Moore *et al.*, 1973a,b) or by a simplified density cut technique in which marrow or blood cells were centrifuged in BSA of a density of 1.062 g/cm$^3$ (Moore *et al.*, 1974b). The distribution of CFU-C in the supernatant and pellet fractions was determined by subsequent agar culture. Of cluster-forming cells in untreated AML patients, 56 ± 4% were of a density less than 1.062 g/cm$^3$ (in contrast to the normal distribution of CFU-C, 1–10% less than 1.062 g/cm$^3$). This light density distribution of CFU-C was also observed in the microcolony and high-cloning-efficiency colony-forming acute leukemias (96 ± 5% less than 1.062 g/cm$^3$). In contrast, the CFU-C in patients with low-cloning-efficiency colony-forming acute leukemia had a normal density distribution (1.5 ± 1% less than 1.062 g/cm$^3$), as did the CFU-C in untreated acute lymphoblastic leukemia (Moore, 1975, 1976). The light density abnormality characterizing acute myeloid leukemic cells could not be attributed to the cycle status of the cells or to the influence of therapy. It would appear to be a highly reproducible marker which offers the possibility of biophysical separation of coexisting normal and leukemic stem cells.

In complete remission, density cut determinations consistently reveal a normal CFU-C density distribution until relapse occurs or is imminent. Analysis of CFU-C density distribution in remission using the more analytical continuous density gradient equilibrium centrifugation process suggests that changes in density profiles may be of value in predicting early onset of relapse. Three of nine continuous gradient analyses performed during complete remission showed an increased proportion of abnormal light density CFU-C, followed within 3 months by relapse (Heller and Greenberg, 1978).

The correlation between return of normal colony formation in marrow culture and onset of remission has been investigated in a study of 57 patients serially analyzed throughout the induction and consolidation phase of therapy (Moore, 1976). Patients were selected on the basis of marrow growth characteristics prior to therapy, and only examples of non-colony-forming AML were studied, since appearance of normal colony formation during remission induction would provide a simple parameter for detection of nonleukemic progenitor cells. Of the 30 patients who showed return of colony formation at some point during induction, 29 achieved complete remission on the average of 21 days after first detection of colony formation. No examples were observed of a leukemic growth pattern persisting in complete clinical remission. There was no correlation between actual number of colonies observed and the time to remission; however, preliminary analysis indicates some correlation between initial colony incidence and duration of remission. The value of marrow culture analysis in predicting the onset of relapse has been investigated in a large group of patients in whom complete remission had been achieved (Moore, 1976). In this analysis four patterns of relapse emerged:

1.  Most frequently observed was a concordance of a clinical diagnosis of relapse with a complete return to a cluster-forming leukemic growth pattern.
2.  Loss of colony formation and return to a cluster-forming growth pattern 1 to 4 weeks prior to clinical and hematological evidence of relapse.
3.  Coexistence of normal and leukemic colony- or cluster-forming cells for varying periods preceding overt relapse. Discrimination between normal and leukemic cells was possible in these cases on the basis of colony size, cell morphology, and the dispersion or degeneration of the leukemic clusters. Density separation and cytogenetic analysis of individual colonies and clusters have further confirmed the coexistence of normal and leukemic CFU-C in marrow cultures prior to clinical evidence of relapse.

4.  This category comprised patients who showed evidence of early relapse based on hematological criteria, including elevated marrow blast cell incidence (without detectable Auer rods); presence of immature cells in the circulation; and, in the case of patients presenting with acute monocytic or myelomonocytic leukemia, abnormal monocytoid cells in marrow and blood with qualitatively normal colony and cluster formation. In this category there is a clear discrepancy between the interpretation of marrow morphology and the *in vitro* culture parameters which showed no evidence of leukemic cell proliferation. This paradox was largely resolved by sequential analysis of CFU-C in the marrow of patients in prolonged remission. A striking variation in the incidence of marrow CFU-C was observed in a number of patients which could not be attributed to technical variation or, in any direct sense, to the maintenance protocol. Correlated with the periodicity of marrow CFU-C in many patients was a fluctuation in marrow blast cell incidence (Moore, 1976). A marked increase in the CFU-C was frequently associated with or closely followed by an increase in marrow blast count to levels compatible with early relapse. The majority of such cases were treated with intensive reinduction therapy; however, a number were continued on maintenance therapy. In the latter type of cases, both blast cell and CFU-C incidence returned to normal levels in subsequent marrow aspirates, and the patients remained in complete remission. In the former cases, a number of patients went on to full leukemic relapse; however, it appears possible that agressive therapy coinciding with episodes of reactive or regenerating marrow as determined by CFU-C analysis can severely compromise the status of the normal stem cell compartment, possibly to the extent of allowing the acute leukemic clone to have a proliferative advantage.

## 2.4. Regulatory Interactions in Acute Leukemia

One of the most consistent observations with the *in vitro* cloning of AML cells is their total dependence on the presence of a source of CSF (Metcalf *et al.*, 1974; Moore *et al.*, 1974b). Differences in the dose responsiveness of leukemic versus normal or remission CFU-C may be observed but no examples of truly autonomous cloning of leukemic cells have been reported. In this context, AML may be considered as a dependent rather than an autonomous neoplasm and humoral regulators may play a role in the development and progression of the disease. In untreated patients with AML, the leukemic CFU-C population in marrow and blood is largely noncycling and resistant *in vitro* to the killing effects of high doses of high-specific-activity tritiated thymidine. If, however, the leukemic cells are subjected to a brief 1- to 3-hr exposure to a source of CSF, 50 to 90%

of the cells enter DNA synthesis, indicating the cycle-activating role of the factor and suggesting that a considerable degree of cell cycle synchronization may be obtained (Moore *et al.*, 1976). The apparent low cycling status of the leukemic population is thus not an intrinsic property of the leukemic state but possibly reflects retention, to some degree, of a population size control mechanism. This conclusion is reinforced by the observations that the fraction of leukemic CFU-C in DNA synthesis increases as the tumor burden is decreased by chemotherapy. Such cycling populations of CFU-C may be rendered noncycling following *in vitro* incubation for 18 hr at high cell concentrations in the absence of an exogenous source of CSF.

If AML and CML are considered to be diseases involving regulatory disorders, then possible therapeutic intervention with appropriate regulatory macromolecules may be considered. It has been suggested that the *in vivo* maturation of AML cells may be facilitated by infusion of CSF. Depletion of the growing stem cell fraction of the leukemic population by increased differentiation pressure may play a role in therapy. In this context, the capacity of CSF to promote leukemic cell differentiation as well as proliferation must be investigated in detail, particularly since there are conflicting reports in the literature of the differentiation-promoting action of CSF. When large numbers of patients with AML in relapse have been investigated, it has become evident that a spectrum of potentials for *in vivo* differentiation has been observed. In morphological analysis of leukemic colonies or clusters developing in agar culture, less than 10% of the cases showed evidence of normal neutrophil maturation; the majority showed various degrees of maturation arrest at the blast–promyelocyte level, together with variable production of cells with macrophage or monocytoid features (Moore *et al.*, 1974b). In a study of AML cells cultured in suspension in the presence of CSF, differentiation obtained in 15% of cases could not be clearly distinguished from that observed with normal bone marrow, since blast cells disappeared and numerous peroxidase-positive granulocytes developed (Morley and Higgs, 1974). However, in the remaining 85% of the cases, differentiation appeared to be impaired both qualitatively and quantitatively. The most common pattern observed was persistence of blast cells, with delayed development of more differentiated cells exhibiting abnormalities such as asynchrony of nuclear-cytoplasmic maturation or gross disorganization. Cells resembling myelocytes or metamyelocytes were a frequent feature of cultures; however, their nuclear chromatin tended to remain primitive and their cytoplasm was often peroxidase negative. Polymorphic cells resembling abnormal polymorphs also developed in culture, but their morphological characterization is frequently difficult, and many of these cells may have been abnormal monocytes. Increasing the CSF concentration in cultures did not appear to influence the degree of differentiation observed. Since the operational definition of CSF is based on colony formation (a property which ultimately depends on stimulation of cell proliferation and not necessarily differentiation), and in view of the *in vivo* evidence suggesting that AML cells can indeed show a degree of differentiation, it appears most likely that CSF is not capable of overcoming to any major degree the maturation arrest or maturation imbalance characteristic of the leukemic clone both *in vivo* and *in vitro*.

The existence of activities which uniquely stimulate leukemic rather than normal hematopoiesis is suggested by the studies of Gallo *et al.* (1976). Continuous maintenance of human myeloid leukemic cell proliferation and differentiation in suspension culture was sustained by a conditioned medium obtained from a first trimester human embryro cell culture. This stimulatory activity did not sustain normal marrow cell proliferation and did not act as a colony-stimulating factor in agar culture. A uniquely leukemic proliferative response has also been reported involving 13 to 24 hr incubation of leukemic cells in liquid culture in the presence of phytohemagglutinin (Dicke *et al.*, 1976). Subsequent culture of such cells in agar resulted in the formation of colonies which developed in the absence of CSF. The leukemic nature of these colonies was confirmed by cytogenetic and ultrastructural criteria. The activation of AML cells by PHA is dependent on the density of cells in the preincubation, suggesting that cell–cell interactions are involved in the activation of leukemic CFU-C. Once the cells are placed in agar, there is a linear relationship between the number of cells plated and the number of colonies which appear at 14 days. A similar assay has been devised based on studies of the proliferation of leukemic blast cells in suspension culture. Stimulation of proliferation is observed in cultures containing media conditioned by normal or leukemic leukocytes in the presence of PHA (Moore *et al.*, 1977). Based on this information, PHA-stimulated leukocyte conditioned medium (PHA-LCM) was tested for its capacity to promote colony formation by cells from the peripheral blood of patients with AML or CML. Colony formation was obtained in leukemic peripheral blood cultures where colony formation was not observed in the presence of a conventional source of CSF. The colonies contained peroxidase-negative cells unlike the colonies stimulated by CSF, but were, in some cases, clearly identified as of leukemic origin by cytogenetic analysis. Interestingly, it was not possible to obtain colonies from leukemic marrow similar to those observed in cultures of leukemic peripheral blood. The active molecule in PHA-LCM appeared to be different from the CSF activity in the conditioned medium. Preliminary separation on Sephadex G-150 indicated a molecular weight of 44,000. This molecular species could be dissociated by 2-mercaptoethanol into 27,000 and 15,000 molecular weight moieties.

In some PHA-LCM preparations, the 27,000 molecular weight activity can be present without the larger molecular species.

The myeloid leukemic cell population is heterogeneous with respect to capacity to respond to CSF and to produce CSF. The production of CSF by leukemic leukocytes is variable and is a particularly prominent feature of acute monocytic and myelomonocytic leukemia (Moore *et al.*, 1973b; Golde *et al.*, 1974b). When peripheral leukocytes from newly diagnosed leukemic patients are used to prepare conditioned medium only one of the three species of high-molecular-weight CSF produced by normal leukocytes is detected in the medium (Price *et al.*, 1975; Senn *et al.*, 1976). The cellular origin of the three high-molecular-weight CSFs has been identified as the cell surface membrane. Whereas leukemic leukocyte conditioned medium yields only a single high-molecular-weight species (generally 36,500 mol.wt.), the leukemic cell membrane contains all three species.

Early studies on CSF levels in the serum of patients with leukemia were conducted before it was understood that CSF inhibitors must be removed before assay (Foster *et al.*, 1968). Nevertheless, elevated CSF levels were reported in 20 to 25% of patients with AML. In more recent surveys, 30% of AML sera showed elevated CSF levels and 53% of patients had an elevated 24-hr urine CSF output (Metcalf *et al.*, 1971). Indeed, all patients exhibited serum or urine CSF levels at some stage of the disease. Very low or absent urine CSF levels have been reported in 60% of patients with untreated AML and elevated levels in 15% (Robinson and Pike, 1970). During the course of treatment, patients presenting with low urine CSF output frequently showed a marked rise in urine CSF.

Some correlation between CSF levels and disease status has been observed but it is likely that serum or urine levels of CSF will not accurately reflect the regulatory factors impinging on the leukemic cell population within the hematopoietic organs. Furthermore, the majority of the earlier studies on CSF levels in patients were performed using assays involving mouse bone marrow rather than normal human marrow. In a recent study of the CSF-producing capacity of adherent marrow cells from leukemic patients, decreased CSF production was associated with failure of remission induction or short remission, whereas complete remissions occurred in patients exhibiting normal CSF production (Greenberg and Mara, 1977). Furthermore, sequential studies indicated that patients with prolonged remission had repeated normal or increased CSF production, whereas intermittent low marrow CSF production was found in patients with short remissions. These findings suggest that adequate marrow CSF production may be essential to sustaining normal hematopoiesis in AML and that this may reflect clonal persistence of normal monocyte–macrophage progeny.

Defects in candidate negative feedback control mechanisms have been reported in AML. One such defect involves impaired production of a granulocyte chalone which is a granulocyte-derived cell-line-specific, non-species-specific inhibitor of granulopoiesis. It has, however, been shown that malignant cells retain responsiveness to the chalone of their tissue of origin; in particular, when extracts containing granulocyte chalone were injected into rats with transplantable granulocytic leukemia, the leukemia regressed, sometimes permanently (Rytomaa, 1973). In clinical studies utilizing partially purified granulocytic chalone, intravenous injection inhibited proliferation of leukemic cells in patients with myeloid leukemia. In five of seven cases, inhibition was followed by actual regression of the leukemia, lasting up to several months in the absence of any maintenance therapy and, in one case, the treatment was associated with a complete remission (Rytomaa *et al.*, 1976).

Granulocyte-derived colony inhibitory activity (CIA) is markedly reduced or absent in patients with AML in relapse. Of interest is the observation that this deficiency persists in the majority of patients with AML in remission (Broxmeyer *et al.*, 1976). It is unlikely that this persisting defect resulted from chemotherapy, since it was also present in patients who had been without therapy for prolonged periods. In addition, granulocytes from patients with acute lymphoblastic leukemia, multiple myeloma, or lymphoma exhibited a normal content of CIA despite extensive chemotherapy. In contrast to the defect in CIA production, the leukemic cells elaborating CSF retain responsiveness to the inhibitory action of CIA derived from normal granulocytes. Indeed, in one study, normal responsiveness to CIA was shown to be retained by a murine myelomonocytic leukemic cell which had been adapted to continuous culture and was a high constitutive producer of CSF (Broxmeyer and Ralph, 1977).

Leukemia is clinically and experimentally associated with replacement of normal hematopoiesis by cells with abnormal growth and maturation properties, suggesting the operation of some as yet unknown interactions leading to suppression of normal stem cell differentiation. In this regard, there have been numerous attempts to test the hypothesis that leukemic cells can suppress normal CFU-C. Negative results have been reported by some (Greenberg *et al.*, 1971; Robinson *et al.*, 1971), while others have demonstrated via mixing experiments with intact cells that leukemic cells inhibit normal CFU-C (Chiyoda *et al.*, 1975, 1976; Knudtzon and Mortensen, 1976). Broxmeyer *et al.* (1978a,b) have reported an inhibitory activity released following lysis of leukemic cells or present in media conditioned by leukemic cells. This leukemic inhibitory activity (LIA) was present in a subpopulation of nonadherent, light density, slowly sedimenting cells in leukemic marrow or blood. LIA acts in a non-species-specific manner to inhibit CFU-C proliferation, either spontaneous or stimulated by an exogenous source of CSF. Inhibition was observed with as short a period as 10 min exposure of marrow cells to LIA at 37°C. Comparison of the degree of inhibition of colony formation obtained following preincubation of marrow cells with LIA, high-specific-activity tritiated thymidine, or both revealed that LIA inhibits CFU-C exclusively when they are in DNA synthesis. This observation together with the extreme lability of the inhibition at 37°C accounts for the fact that inhibition is in the range of 30 to 60% rather than 100% following a single addition of LIA. Repeated daily administration of LIA to agar cultures does, however, lead to 90 to 100% inhibition of colony formation. Inhibitory activity obtained from acute leukemic marrow could be titrated over $10^5$- to $10^6$-fold and still exhibit inhibitory activity; however, LIA preparations obtained from patients with chronic leukemia were significantly less potent. The assay for LIA has proved to be extremely reproducible and extracts of marrow cells from 76 of 85 untreated or relapse patients with AML, blastic CML, acute lymphoblastic leukemia, and certain lymphomas demonstrated LIA. Control extracts obtained from a variety of normal hematopoietic cell types, or of light density slowly sedimenting cells from normal or regenerating bone marrow all failed to inhibit colony formation even when prepared at up to 10 times the concentration of leukemic test extracts. Specificity of the action of LIA is suggested by the observation that extracts from leukemic cells containing $10^4$ to $10^6$ times as much LIA as that necessary to inhibit CFU-C from normal donors were inactive when assayed against CFU-C obtained from patients with acute or chronic leukemia. In addition, even though cells from most leukemic remission patients lacked detectable LIA, the remission CFU-C population, unlike normal CFU-C, were generally resistant to LIA from other leukemic donors. This lack of inhibition was not related to the cycle status of leukemic CFU-C.

Various reports have failed to demonstrate leukemic cell inhibition of normal CFU-C (Greenberg *et al.*, 1971; Robinson *et al.*, 1971). A possible explanation is provided by the cell-cycle-specific action of LIA and the heterogeneity of the CFU-C population. Colony formation at day 7 is due to the proliferation of a subpopulation of CFU-C biophysically distinct from CFU-C which form the majority of colonies scored at days 10 to 14. The latter are derived from more slowly sedimenting cells which proliferate later. Hence, addition of LIA at day 0 will lead to inhibition of colony formation at day 7 but not at days 10 to 14. Only by adding LIA at later stages during the proliferative phase of the smaller cells could inhibition be seen at days 10 to 14.

## 2.5. *In Vitro* Studies in Chronic Myeloid Leukemia (CML)

In untreated CML the colony-forming capacity of marrow is normal to increased and greatly increased numbers of CFU-C are present in the circulation (Paran *et al.*, 1970; Moore *et al.*, 1973a; Moberg *et al.*, 1974). In a study of 103 patients, the incidence of colony- and cluster-forming cells in the marrow was increased on average 15-fold and circulating CFU-C were increased 500 times (Moore, 1977a,b). Unlike the situation in AML, colony size is normal and the ratio of clusters to colonies is consistently within the lowest range of normal (3:1–10:1). A correlation exists between the leukocyte count and total circulating CFU-C; however, the magnitude of the absolute increase in the granulocyte committed stem cell compartment is quite out of proportion to the 5- to 20-fold increase in granulocyte production, suggesting that inappropriate overproduction of committed stem cells rather than their excessive differentiation is the underlying defect in CML.

Cytogenetic studies of CML-derived colonies have generally shown the exclusive presence of Philadelphia chromosome (Ph[1]) positive metaphases (Shadduck and Nankin, 1971; Moore and Metcalf, 1973). However, Chervenick *et al.* (1971) reported Ph[1]-negative colonies in cultures from two patients in relapse and in one patient rendered aplastic following myleran therapy. This observation suggests the presence of normal stem cells in CML and is supported by evidence of normal CFU-C in marrow cultures of CML patients who have partially reverted to a Ph[1]-negative state following intensive chemotherapy (Moore, 1977a,b).

In contrast to cultures of acute myeloid leukemic bone marrow, normal maturation of CFU-C is observed in CML with colonies composed of mature neutrophils, eosinophils, monocytes, and macrophages (Moberg *et al.*, 1974; Moore, 1977a,b). The proliferation of CML bone marrow in liquid culture is two- to threefold greater than normal, presumably reflecting the increased incidence of committed stem cells (Golde *et al.*, 1974a). Cellular maturation in such cultures is normal with granulocytes and actively replicating macrophages which are functionally indistinguishable from normal. The presence of the Ph[1] chromosome in all metaphases in cultures containing large numbers of proliferating macrophages confirmed the *in vitro* colony data that monocytes and macrophages are derived from Ph[1]-positive stem cells. This observation suggests that large segments of the tissue macrophage population may be replaced by cells derived from the leukemic clone and since tissue macrophages also have proliferative capacity they may participate in further clonal evolution (Golde *et al.*, 1977).

In addition to the quantitative abnormality of marked increase in CFU-C numbering, other qualitative abnormaltities serve to characterize leukemic CFU-C. Separation of marrow and peripheral blood leukocytes in density gradients has revealed a markedly reproducible light density shift of leukemic CFU-C. This difference in buoyant density of colony- and cluster-forming cells is observed in both marrow and blood and persists in patients undergoing therapy (Moore *et al.*, 1973a; Moore, 1977a,b). In untreated CML, density separation produces sufficient enrichment of CFU-C to permit their morphological characterization (Moore *et al.*, 1973a) and, in one study, cultures of density fractions of CML peripheral blood containing 93% myeloblasts revealed that 60% of these cells were capable of forming colonies and clusters in culture. The difference in morphology of CFU-C in normal and leukemic hemato- poiesis is intriguing, since in the former case the cells are predominantly transitional lymphocyte-like rather than myeloblastic. Possibly one of the contributing defects in CML is retention of stem cell properties by cells that normally would have lost this function as a consequence of maturation.

The abnormal light density of CFU-C persists in patients whose peripheral blood values have returned to normal and also in the majority of patients whose marrow and blood CFU-C numbers were in the normal range. This suggests that total granulocyte mass or CFU-C population size does not influence the CFU-C density distribution. Only very rarely has CFU-C density returned to normal in CML, in one case in a patient in prolonged, unmaintained remission, and in a second case in a patient who had received intensive therapy and had a predominantly Ph[1]-negative marrow.

The light density abnormality of CML CFU-C places these cells in a density region occupied by CFU-C present in human fetal liver between 9 and 14 weeks gestation (Moore and Williams, 1973). This observation and comparison of other characteristics of fetal versus CML CFU-C suggest that leukemogenesis involves an oncofetal transformation (Moore, 1974). The fetal transition in CML would require the development of a multipo- tential stem cell clone displaying fetal growth characteristics which, in the adult environment, would respond abnormally to regulatory influences and generate mature cells with features adapted to the fetal environment. In juvenile CML, it is probable that erythropoiesis and granulopoiesis are of fetal type. In typical Ph[1]-positive CML there is little evidence that erythropoiesis is grossly abnormal and consequently the multipotential stem cell clone marked by the Ph[1] chromosome may be biased in favor of generation of fetal-type granulocytic progenitor cells and the adult-type erythroid progenitors. The competitive advantage of the Ph[1] clone could be explained by fetal transformation of stem cells since, during competitive marrow regeneration, fetal stem cells always outgrow adult stem cells (Micklem and Loutit, 1966).

## 2.6. *In Vitro* Culture Studies in Accelerated Phase and Blastic Transformation of CML

Clonal evolution in CML is reflected in changing *in vitro* growth characteristics most frequently associated with loss of colony formation (Paran *et al.*, 1970; Chervenick *et al.*, 1971; Moore *et al.*, 1973a). However, cases of persisting colony-forming capacity in blastic transformation have been reported (Paran *et al.*, 1970). Analysis of the *in vitro* growth characteristics of marrow or blood from 42 patients at the time of clinical diagnosis of blastic transformation revealed, in every case, defects in proliferation and maturation which served to distinguish this phase from the chronic phase of the disease (Moore, 1977a,b). Blastic CML exhibited the same spectrum of proliferative abnormalities as has been reported in untreated acute myeloid leukemic marrow cultures (Moore *et al.*, 1974b; Moore, 1977a,b). In only one case was complete absence of growth in bone marrow and blood culture found, corresponding to the very low incidence of this variant in acute myeloid leukemia (AML; 2%). The most common pattern was that of absence of normal colony formation with persistence of clusters of up to 40 cells (macrocluster type) or presence of small colonies with an excess of clusters (microcolony type). In both categories *in vitro* maturation was markedly defective, with blasts, promyelocytes, and macrophages predominating and mature neutrophils generally absent. These variants accounted for 50% of the cases studied. Patients with the macrocluster variant tended to present after a shorter duration of chronic phase disease than did the microcolony variant. They had higher leukocyte counts, higher blast incidence, and lower platelet counts. Minimal response to therapy was shown in both categories, remissions were not observed, and survival in blastic crisis was brief. The next most common variants were cases with absence of colony formation in marrow culture with persistence of clusters of 3 to 10 cells (microcluster variant, 14% of cases) and examples of persisting colony formation with high plating efficiency in marrow and blood culture (19%). This latter category cannot be distinguished from chronic phase disease on the basis of growth pattern alone, but morphological analysis of the colonies revealed maturation arrest at the blast–promyelocyte level. The colony-forming category had a high platelet count and a considerably lower blast count in marrow and blood than did any other category and generally the patients had a more subacute course reflected in their longer survival in blast crisis. Patients in the microcluster category were, on the average, younger than those in the other groups and had the longest average survival after diagnosis of blast crisis due to the fact that 50% achieved complete remission which, in two cases, was prolonged. The relatively short mean duration of chronic phase disease in the microcluster group can be attributed to the fact that two of six cases presented at first diagnosis in blastic crisis with no antecedent history of chronic phase disease. A final category comprising 14% of cases generally presented with a low leukocyte count and high blast count in marrow and had a very low incidence of colonies and clusters in marrow and blood with normal colony maturation and normal colony-to-cluster ratio. The blast cells in these patients possessed no discernible myeloblastic features as determined by marrow culture; they neither responded to nor produced CSF and had the buoyant density characteristics of leukemic lymphoblasts rather than myeloblasts (Moore, 1975). A similar growth pattern is seen in acute undifferentiated leukemias (Moore, 1975). In these latter leukemic states granulocytic colony formation reflects the persistence of low numbers of normal CFU-C coexisting with a nonmyeloid leukemic blast population which cannot totally suppress normal granulopoiesis. It appears probable that a similar situation exists in this variant of blastic transformation and that the low incidence of colonies reflects residual chronic phase CFU-C coexisting with an acute leukemic blast population which is either lymphoblastic or so undifferentiated that it lacks the capacity to proliferate in response to CSF.

The characteristics of the terminal acute phase clone are clearly not always expressed morphologically or functionally in myeloblastosis; promyelocytes may predominate as may monocytes and, occasionally, proerythroblasts. In a minority of cases the blast cells have a lymphoid appearance (Boggs, 1974), and it is of significance that such patients responded to prednisone and vincristine, agents with little effect in AML. In this context the patients with a nonmyeloid blastic CML by *in vitro* culture criteria achieved 50% remission using protocols including vincristine and prednisone. Recent studies in the blastic crisis of CML have reinforced the possibility of a lymphoblastic transformation by demonstrating that in some cases the blast cells contained terminal deoxynucleotidyl transferase, which is also found predominantly in normal thymus and acute lymphoblastic leukemic cells but not in AML cells (McCaffrey *et al.*, 1975; Sarin *et al.*, 1976). In a study of 14 cases of blastic transformation in CML, all were negative for surface markers for thymocytes and T- or B-lymphocytes; however, five cases reacted with an antiserum specific for acute lymphoblastic leukemia (ALL) of non-T or non-B type and were weakly reactive with a lymphocyte-reactive serum (Janossy *et al.*, 1976). A sixth patient whose blast cells were anti-ALL negative at presentation subsequently developed central nervous system leukemia with anti-ALL positive blast cells in the cerebrospinal fluid. It may be argued that acquisition by the blastic CML clone of one of the phenotypic characteristics of a lymphoblastic leukemia may represent an inappropriate genotypic expression resulting from neoplastic transformation and thus would not be a reliable index of cell lineage. However, the inability to distinguish the blast cells in a variant of transformed CML from those of the common form of ALL by morphological criteria, membrane markers, enzymatic studies, and functional analysis *in vitro* suggests that the Ph[1] stem cell has lymphoid as well as myeloid potentiality.

While the majority of studies of CML have shown that terminal transferase is not present at detectable levels in the chronic phase of the disease, Saffhill *et al.* (1977) reported high levels of terminal transferase in the peripheral blood leukocytes of a 1-year-old child with Ph[1]-positive CML. Hematological, clinical, and *in vitro* culture parameters were all compatible with chronic phase disease, and following chemotherapy spleen size, WBC, and incidence of circulating CFU-C all fell appreciably; in contrast, there was no change in the level of terminal transferase, indicating that in this case chemotherapy is not selectively removing the terminal transferase positive cells from the peripheral blood. Childhood Ph[1]-positive CML is rare; however, failure to detect terminal transferase in another case of pediatric CML (R. Mertelsmann and M. A. S. Moore, unpublished observation) suggests that terminal transferase is not invariably associated with this variant of CML.

A discrepancy exists between the incidence of blastic transformations which are terminal transferase positive (~30%) and the incidence of cases displaying lymphoblastic *in vitro* culture characteristics (10–15%). While this discrepancy may be accounted for by inappropriate expression of terminal transferase in acute myeloblastic leukemia, an alternative explanation may be the coexistence of two blastic phase clones—a lymphoblastic variant lacking *in vitro* proliferative capacity but being terminal transferase positive, and the other responsive to CSF *in vitro* and being terminal transferase negative. The latter possibility would suggest that in approximately 15% of blastic CML, therapy designed specifically for AML and ALL would have to be combined to achieve a remission.

Some generalizations can be made concerning the early detection of acute leukemic clones in CML. A progressive increase in the cluster-to-colony ratio in marrow or blood cultures may precede by weeks or months clinical or hematological evidence of blastic transformation. During this period chronic phase colony- and cluster-forming cells coexist with emerging acute clones characterized by a microcluster, macrocluster, or microcolony growth pattern. The rate of progression of the disease may be determined by the relative proportions of the coexisting clones as determined by an increasing cluster-to-colony ratio. Physical separation by density gradient centrifugation of coexisting acute and chronic CFU-C in CML marrow has not proved possible because the acute phase CFU-C have a similar abnormal light density distribution to chronic phase cells. Velocity sedimentation separation has proved of value in distinguishing between acute and chronic phase CFU-C; in one study, separation of marrow and blood revealed two populations of CFU-C some 10 months before blastic transformation, one characteristic of the chronic phase and a second minor population of greater sedimentation rate which formed clusters of 3 to 10 cells with maturation abnormalities (Moore, 1975). This latter population comprised less than 2% of the clonogenic cells in the marrow when first detected and rose to approximately 75% in the month preceding clinical evidence of transformation.

Prediction of blast transformation in patients who will terminate with a colony-forming acute leukemia with high cloning efficiency cannot be made on the basis of progressive abnormality in cluster-to-colony ratio. It can, however, be predicted on the basis of a progressive increase in circulating colony- and cluster-forming cells not associated with subsequent rise in the leukocyte count. Further confirmation can be obtained by morphological analysis of colonies in order to detect maturation arrest at the blast–promyelocyte stage.

A declining incidence of both colony- and cluster-forming cells in marrow and blood with a normo- to hypercellular marrow and normal to elevated leukocyte count and an increase in blast cell incidence precedes clinical evidence of a terminal blast crisis associated with the development of a nonmyeloid acute leukemia. A subnormal incidence of marrow CFU-C with normal cluster-to-colony ratio and normal maturation may also be seen in CML patients with myelofibrosis; however, in such cases circulating CFU-C are increased in number.

The presence of hyperdiploid metaphases at low frequency in the marrow in some patients in clincially stable CML some months prior to blastic transformation (Pedersen, 1973) suggests the possible predictive value of cytogenetic analysis in detecting early onset of blastic transformation. However, cytogenetic change is not invariably associated with blastic transformation or, if it is, may not be manifest prior to clinical changes associated with an accelerated disease course. In contrast, qualitative *in vitro* culture changes, compatible with early blastic transformation, are almost invariably detected prior to blastic transformation, and in a recent survey of 50 patients in stable chronic phase disease abnormal culture characteristics were detected a median of 8 months prior to transformation (M. A. S. Moore, unpublished observation).

A discordant pattern of chromosome change and colony-forming capacity has been reported in a patient presenting with extramedullary manifestations of blastic transformation apparently localized in the lymphatic system (Gall *et al.*, 1976). New chromosome abnormalities, in addition to the existing Ph[1], were revealed in lymph node, blood, and bone marrow at a time when 70% of the cells from the lymph node were blasts and promyelocytes, yet marrow and blood showed a morphology compatible with typical chronic phase disease. Colony formation in semi-solid cultures of blood and marrow at the time of initial blast crisis yielded growth patterns characteristic of CML. On recurrence of the blast crisis after therapy growth patterns were characteristic of CML in blast crisis of a microcolony-forming type even though the blood and marrow still showed relatively low levels of myeloblasts and promyelocytes.

## 2.7. Regulatory Defects in CML

Spontaneous colony formation in cultures of CML marrow and peripheral blood is frequently reported; however, cell separation techniques have shown that endogenous elaboration of CSF from colony-stimulating cells is responsible for this spontaneous growth and that leukemic CFU-C retain an absolute requirement for CSF for their proliferation and differentiation (Moore *et al.*, 1973a). Comparison of the sensitivity of leukemic versus normal or remission CFU-C to CSF stimulation has revealed that CFU-C from CML patients in blastic transformation have a lower threshold for CSF stimulation than do normal CFU-C, while CFU-C from patients with CML in the chronic phase have a higher threshold (Metcalf *et al.*, 1974). Retention of CSF responsiveness by leukemic stem cells supports the view that the myeloid leukemias are dependent rather than autonomous neoplasms in that they remain under the influence of a candidate humoral regulatory macromolecule. Differences in the threshold for stimulation of leukemic versus normal CFU-C, while slight, may be of major importance in providing selective proliferative advantages for leukemic clones and may play a role in the progression from the chronic to the acute phase in CML.

The concept of defective negative feedback control has particular attractiveness as an explanation for the granulocytic hyperplasia associated with CML. CML cells have been reported to respond to the inhibitory effects of granulocyte chalones (Rytomaa, 1973). However, CML polymorphs (PMN) appear to be defective in the production and/or release of this chalone (Boyum *et al.*, 1976). The inhibitory action of granulocyte chalones is directed at the proliferation of the granulocyte committed stem cell.

The alternative negative feedback involving a granulocyte-derived inhibitory activity (CIA) which suppresses CSF production by monocytes and macrophages is also defective in CML. In a study of 58 patients with CML at all stages of the disease, Broxmeyer *et al.* (1977b) reported that extracts of PMN from the patients were quantitatively deficient in CIA. An additional regulatory defect in CML was the reduced responsiveness of CSF-producing cells to inhibitory activity derived from normal PMN. The combination of these two defects may, in part, play a role in the profound granulocytic hyperplasia associated with CML.

## 2.8. Marrow Culture Studies in Myeloproliferative Disorders

The neutropenic disorders provide a clinical setting for evaluating abnormalities of granulopoietic regulation and numerous studies have been carried out to determine CFU-C incidence in such disease states. Greenberg and Schrier (1973) utilized the thymidine suicide technique to determine the proportion of granulocytic progenitor cells in S phase in order to correlate *in vitro* proliferative activity of neutrophil precursors with peripheral demand in various neutropenic states. The clearest example of such a correlation was observed in cyclic neutropenia. When peripheral blood neutrophil counts were at their peak level both CFU-C and the percentage of these cells in S phase were comparable to controls, whereas at the neutrophil nadir both of these values were strikingly increased. Measurement of CSF production and serum CSF levels in cyclic neutropenia has also revealed a cyclic fluctuation with peak CSF levels coinciding with the neutrophil nadir (Moore *et al.*, 1974a).

In patients with splenomegaly and neutropenia due to accelerated neutrophil removal the incidence of CFU-C and the percentage in S phase is increased, suggesting the existence of a compensated state characterized by enhanced granulocytic turnover (Greenberg and Schrier, 1973). Decreased production appears to contribute significantly to the neutropenia present in patients with myeloid hypoplasia, Felty's syndrome, and some patients with idiopathic neutropenia, and marked decreases in CFU-C incidence are found even when corrected for the number of granulocytic precursors plated.

Patients presenting with refractory cytopenia of one or more cell lines with cellular marrows for which no hematinic deficiency or extramyeloid cause can be detected may progress to overt acute leukemia, to a "smoldering" leukemic state, or lead a benign course. Marrow culture offers a potential method for distinguishing patients with hematopoietic dysplasias who will ultimately progress to overt leukemia from clinically similar cases who will not progress.

In a study of 37 patients with idiopathic acquired sideroblastic anemia (Moore, 1977c), eight cases had refractory anemia only, whereas the remaining cases also had neutropenia, thrombocytopenia, or both. In all cases the marrow was normo- to hypercellular as determined by marrow biopsy and the blast incidence in no case exceeded 5% at the time of initial study. Marrow colony and cluster incidence was within the normal range in the eight cases with refractory anemia only. Of the remaining cases, 17 showed a markedly reduced incidence of colony- and cluster-forming cells with normal *in vitro* granulocytic maturation and a ratio of clusters to colonies within the normal range. Over a period of 6 months to 3 years only one of these cases has progressed to overt acute leukemia and then only after showing qualitative defects in marrow culture consistent with those seen in the remaining 12 patients. These latter exhibited one or more qualitative defects similar to those observed in AML. Six of 12 cases showed no colony formation with a persisting micro- or macrocluster growth pattern and three cases showed a pattern of small colonies with an excess of clusters (microcolony type). Of the remaining three cases, low numbers of colonies were present of normal size and maturation, but the cluster-to-colony ratio exceeded the normal range. Sequential studies of these latter patients revealed a progressive loss in colony-forming capacity and increase in cluster incidence, suggesting that at the time of initial observation normal colony-forming cells and leukemic cluster-forming cells were coexisting. Eight of the 12 patients showing an abnormal cluster-to-colony ratio progressed to acute leukemia between 3 and 14 months after first detection of this *in vitro* defect. Two patients died without evidence of leukemia and two have remained clinically unchanged over periods of 4 and 11 months. Progression to overt leukemia was generally associated with an increasing incidence of cluster-forming cells in the marrow.

Greenberg *et al.* (1976) have also reported abnormal *in vitro* marrow growth patterns and abnormally light CFU-C buoyant density of CFU-C in preleukemic patients a median of 10 months prior to acute transformation. Acute transformation was not observed in patients with idiopathic ineffective erythropoiesis characterized by a normal incidence and density distribution pattern of marrow CFU-C and normal urinary CSF output (Greenberg *et al.*, 1976).

The biochemical characteristics of CSF produced by leukemic leukocytes have been shown to differ from CSF elaborated from normal leukocytes and this difference has been used to identify patients with preleukemic disorders at high risk of progression to acute leukemia. Senn *et al.* (1976) reported that the normal three species of nondialyzable CSF were regularly purified from media prepared from the leukocytes of patients with secondary or hereditary sideroblastic anemia and three out of six patients with idiopathic acquired sideroblastic anemia. Of this latter group, three more patients released only one species of CSF; of these, two subsequently developed AML and one died shortly after study, whereas the three other cases remained clinically unchanged for 13 to 19 months.

A further variant of the preleukemic state is the chronic myelomonocytic syndrome. Patients with this disorder are predominantly elderly males presenting with chronic monocytosis, generally associated with refractory anemia, neutrophil leukocytosis, splenomegaly, and markedly elevated serum and urine lysozyme. Cytogenetic analysis shows all cases to be Ph[1] negative, but in some patients a 45XO karyotype may predominate on direct marrow examination.

In a study of 14 such cases, Moore (1977c) showed an increased incidence of colonies and clusters in marrow and/or blood culture with, in most instances, a normal colony-to-cluster ratio. Biophysical characterization of the CFU-C in these patients was performed using continuous gradient centrifugation in bovine serum albumin or a modified density "cut" procedure in albumin of density 1.062 $g/cm^3$. The CFU-C were of abnormal light density with $58 \pm 3\%$ less dense than 1.062 $g/cm^3$ in contrast to the 0 to 10% of normal CFU-C in this density region. A similar light density characterizes CFU-C in patients with chronic myeloid leukemia. Maturation defects were observed in colonies derived from 3 of 14 patients and an abnormal colony-to-cluster ratio in four cases. These additional qualitative defects identified the cases of chronic myelomonocytic syndrome which subsequently progressed to acute monocytic or myelomonocytic leukemia associated with loss of colony formation and appearance of a cluster-forming acute leukemic growth pattern in marrow and blood culture.

It is apparent that the manifestations of preleukemic states involve detectable intrinsic stem cell defects and alterations in the availability of bioactive molecules involved in regulatory interactions. The heterogeneity of preleukemic manifestations may be resolved in part by considering that, in some patients, clonal evolution occurs with development of progressively more abnormal clones as a function of time. Other cases may simply be early stages of expansion of a true leukemic clone coexisting with normal stem cells as in a partial remission state. The therapeutic strategies to be employed in these two manifestations of the preleukemic phase could conceivably be very different.

Extensive marrow culture studies have been carried out in aplastic anemia, a syndrome characterized by marrow hypoplasia and severe pancytopenia. In almost all cases studied, the severe defect in myelopoiesis is associated with absent or very reduced numbers of CFU-C in marrow culture although occasionally patients may present with severe aplastic anemia and normal CFU-C incidence indicating the possible heterogeneous nature of the disease (Kagan *et al.*, 1977). On theoretical grounds three fundamentally different mechanisms may lead to aplastic anemia: (1) an absent or defective hematopoietic stem cell population, (2) a defect intrinsic to the hematopoietic microenvironment (including defects in humoral regulation), or (3) suppression of hematopoiesis by other host systems. Until recently, most instances of aplastic anemia have been attributed to either congenital or acquired stem cell defects and bone marrow transplantation has been a logical therapeutic approach which corrects the disease in about 50% of cases (Van Bekuum *et al.*, 1976). A small proportion of patients, however, who have received either HL-A identical or haploidentical marrow transplants reject their allograft and then spontaneously recover their autologous marrow function (Thomas *et al.*, 1976; Jeannet *et al.*, 1974). Such patients were treated prior to transplantation by cytotoxic drugs and/or antilymphocyte globulin. Reversal of the aplastic anemia following this pretreatment with immunosuppressive therapy is consistent with the elimination of an immunologic suppressor of marrow stem cells. Experimental support for this concept was provided by correction of the severe defect in granulocytic colony formation by removal of small lymphocytes from aplastic anemic bone marrow by velocity sedimentation prior to agar culture (Kagan *et al.*, 1976). Treatment of the patient's marrow *in vitro* with antithymocyte globulin and complement also resulted in normal numbers of colonies in the CFU-C assay, suggesting that the suppressor cell in this patient was a T-lymphocyte (Ascensao *et al.*, 1976). These suppressor cells were also identified by their ability to inhibit normal CFU-C when marrow from the patient was cocultured with marrow from a normal donor in the CFU-C assay. In a more extensive analysis of 15 patients with aplastic anemia, Kagan *et al.* (1977) demonstrated a suppressor cell involvement in six cases using coculture of patient marrow with normal marrow. Treatment with antithymocyte globulin was effective in eliminating the suppressor cell in only one case and in other cases with documented suppressor cells in coculture were ineffective in restoring normal colony formation *in vitro*. The role of a suppressor lymphocyte in some cases of aplastic anemia has been recently confirmed by Haak and Goselink (1977) and by Speck *et al.* (1978). In the latter study restoration of normal colony formation *in vitro* was observed in over half the cases of aplastic anemia following *in vitro* pretreatment of the marrow with an anti-human thoracic duct lymphocyte serum. Therapy of these patients with the antiserum led to marked clinical and hematologic improvement.

Suppressor cells directed at granulocytic or erythroid committed stem cells may be involved in other hematologic diseases. Peripheral blood mononuclear cells capable of suppressing myelopoiesis have been reported in patients with agranulocytosis (Lutton *et al.*, 1976) and lymphocyte-mediated suppression of erythropoiesis has been reported in aplastic anemia (Hoffman *et al.*, 1977), the Blackfan–Diamond syndrome (Hoffman *et al.*, 1976), and pure red cell aplasia with thymoma (Zanjani *et al.*, 1975).

## 2.9. Conclusions

The development of *in vitro* methodologies for detection of human granulocytic and erythroid stem cells has resulted in improved insight into neoplastic, idiopathic, or acquired hematologic disease. Increased understanding of the biology of the disease process, particularly the nature of the stem cell defect or associated humoral or microenvironmental imbalance, may ultimately lead to the development of new therapeutic strategies. At the present time, however, the culture systems can serve to improve diagnosis and functional classification of a wide variety of hematological disease and, as illustrated in acute and chronic myeloid leukemia and preleukemia, can provide a prognostic index of value in patient management. Ultimately, however, *in vitro* assays are required for detection and characterization of human pluripotential stem cells if a complete understanding of hematologic diseases is to be obtained. The recently developed technique of Dexter *et al.* (1977) allows prolonged *in vitro* pluripotential stem cell renewal and differentiation in a continuous mouse bone marrow culture system, suggesting the feasibility of a similar system for *in vitro* characterization of human pluripotential stem cells.

ACKNOWLEDGMENTS

This work was supported in part by National Cancer Institute Grants CA-17353, CA-17085, and CA-20194, and the Gar Reichman Foundation.

## References


Ascensao, J., Pahwa, R., Kagan, W., Hansen, J., Moore, M. A. S., and Good, R. A., 1976, Aplastic anemia: Evidence for an immunological mechanism, *Lancet* i:669.

Boggs, D. R., 1974, Hematopoietic stem cell theory on relation to possible lymphoblastic conversion of CML, *Blood* **44**:449.

Boyum, A., Lovhaug, D., and Boecker, W. R., 1976, Regulation of bone marrow cell growth in diffusion chambers: The effect of adding normal and leukemic CML PMN granulocytes, *Blood* **48**:373.

Bradley, T. R., and Metcalf, D., 1966, The growth of mouse bone marrow cells *in vitro*, *Aust. J. Exp. Biol. Med. Sci.* **44**:287.

Brown III, C. H., and Carbone, P. P., 1971, *In vitro* growth of normal and leukemic human bone marrow, *J. Natl. Cancer Inst.* **46**:989.

Broxmeyer, H. E., and Ralph, P., 1977, *In vitro* regulation of a mouse myelomonocytic leukemia line adapted to culture, *Cancer Res.* **37**:3578.

Broxmeyer, H. E., Baker, F. L., and Galbraith, P. R., 1976, *In vitro* regulation of granulopoiesis in human leukemia: Application of an assay for colony inhibiting cells, *Blood* **47**:389.

Broxmeyer, H. E., Moore, M. A. S., and Ralph, P., 1977a, Cell-free granulocyte colony inhibiting activity derived from human PMN, *Exp. Hematol.* **5**:87.

Broxmeyer, H. E., Mendelsohn, N., and Moore, M. A. S., 1977b, Abnormal granulocyte feedback regulation of colony stimulating activity-producing cells from patients with chronic myelogenous leukemia, *Leukemia Res.* **1**:3.

Broxmeyer, H. E., Grossbard, E., Jacobsen, N., and Moore, M. A. S., 1978a, Evidence for a proliferative advantage of human leukemic CFU-c *in vitro*, *J. Natl. Cancer Inst.* **60**:513.

Broxmeyer, H. E., Jacobsen, N., Kurland, J., Mendelsohn, N., and Moore, M. A. S., 1978b, *In vitro* suppression of normal granulocytic stem cells by inhibitory activity derived from human leukemic cells, *J. Natl. Cancer Inst.* **60**:497.

Bull, J. M., Duttera, M. J., Stashick, E. D., Northup, J., Henderson, E., and Carbone, P. P., 1973, Serial *in vitro* marrow culture in acute myelocytic leukemia, *Blood* **42**:679.

Burgess, A. W., Camakaus, J., and Metcalf, D., 1977a, Purification and properties of colony stimulating factor from mouse lung-conditioned medium, *J. Biol. Chem.* **252**:1998.

Burgess, A. W., Wilson, E. M. A., and Metcalf, D., 1977b, Stimulation by human placental conditioned medium of hemopoietic colony formation by human marrow cells, *Blood* **49**:573.

Chervenick, P. A., Ellis, L. D., Pan, S. F., and Lawson, A. L., 1971, Human leukemic cells: *In vitro* growth of colonies containing the Philadelphia chromosome, *Science* **174**:1134.

Chiyoda, S., Mizoguchi, H., Kosaka, K., Takaku, F., and Miura, Y., 1975, Influence of leukemic cells on the colony formation of human bone marrow cells *in vitro*, *Br. J. Cancer* **31**:355.

Chiyoda, S., Mizoguchi, H., Asano, S., Takaku, F., and Miura, Y., 1976, Influence of leukemic cells on the colony formation of human bone marrow cells *in vitro* II. Suppressive effects of leukemic cell extracts, *Br. J. Cancer* **33**:379.

Dexter, T. M., Allen, T. D., and Lajtha, L. G., 1977, Conditions controlling the proliferation of hemopoietic stem cells *in vitro*, *J. Cell. Physiol.* **91**:335.

Dicke, K. A., Spitzer, G., Scheffer, H. M., Cork, A., Ahearn, M. J., Lowenberg, B., and McCredie, K. B., 1976, *In vitro* colony growth of acute myelogenous leukemia, *in Modern Trends in Human Leukemia II* (R. Neth, R. C. Gallo, K. Mannweiler, and W. C. Moloney, eds.), p. 63, Lehmans Verlag, Munich.

Fleming, W. A., McNeill, T. A., and Killen, M., 1972, Effects of inhibitory factor (interferon) on the *in vitro* growth of granulocyte-macrophage colonies, *Immunology* **23**:429.

Foster, R., Metcalf, D., Robinson, W. A., and Bradley, T. R., 1968, Bone marrow colony stimulating activity in human sera: Results of two independent surveys in Buffalo and Melbourne, *Br. J. Haematol.* **15**:147.

Gall, J. A., Boggs, D. R., Chervenick, P. A., Pan, S., and Fleming, R. B., 1976, Discordant patterns of chromosome changes in myeloblast proliferation during the terminal phase of CML, *Blood* **47**:347.

Gallo, R. C., 1976, RNA tumor virus and leukemia: Evaluation of present results supporting their presence in human leukemias, *in Modern Trends in Human Leukemia II* (R. Neth, R. C. Gallo, K. Mannweiler, and W. C. Moloney, eds.), p. 431, Lehmans Verlag, Munich.

Golde, D. W., and Cline, M. J., 1972, Identification of CSC in human peripheral blood, *J. Clin. Invest.* **51**:2981.

Golde, D. W., Byers, L. A., and Cline, M. J., 1974a, CML cell growth and maturation in liquid culture, *Cancer Res.* **34**:419.

Golde, D. W., Rothman, B., and Cline, M. J., 1974b, Production of CSF by malignant leukocytes, *Blood* **43**:749.

Golde, D. W., Burgaleta, C., Sparkes, R. S., and Cline, M. J., 1977, The Philadelphia chromosome in human macrophages, *Blood* **49**:367.

Greenberg, P. L., and Mara, B., 1977, Alteration of marrow colony stimulating activity (CSA) in acute myeloid leukemia, Proceedings American Society of Hematology Meeting, Boston, p. 146.

Greenberg, P. L., and Schrier, S. L., 1973, Granulopoiesis in neutropenic disorders, *Blood* **41**:753.

Greenberg, P. L., Nichols, W. C., Nichols, B. A., and Schrier, S. L., 1971, Granulopoiesis in acute myeloid leukemia and preleukemia, *N. Engl. J. Med.* **284**:1225.

Greenberg, P., Mara, B., Box, I., Brassel, R., and Schrier, S., 1976, The myeloproliferative disorders: Correlation between clinical evolution and alterations of granulopoiesis, *Am. J. Med.* **61**:878.

Haak, H. L., and Goselink, H. M., 1977, Mechanisms in aplastic anemia, *Lancet* **1**:194.

Heller, P., and Greenberg, P., 1978, Density distribution patterns of marrow colony forming cells during remission of acute myelogenous leukemia, *J. Natl. Cancer Inst.*, in press.

Hoffman, R., Zanjani, E. D., and Vila, J., 1976, Diamond–Blackfan syndrome: Lymphocyte-mediated suppression of erythropoiesis, *Science* **193**:899.

Hoffman, R., Zanjani, E. D., and Lutton, J. D., 1977, Suppression of erythroid colony formation by lymphocytes from patients with aplastic anemia, *N. Engl. J. Med.* **296**:10.

Jacobsen, N., Broxmeyer, H. E., and Moore, M. A. S., 1977, Demonstration of human granulopoietic stem cell diversity, *in Experimental Hematology Today*, Vol. II (S. Baum and G. Ledney, eds.), Springer-Verlag, Berlin.

Janossy, G., Greaves, M. F., Revesz, T., Lister, T. A., Roberts, M., Durrant, J., Kirk, B., Catovsky, D., and Beard, M. E. J., 1976, Blast crisis of chronic myeloid leukemia II. Cell surface marker analysis of "lymphoid" and myeloid cases, *Br. J. Haematol.* **34**:179.

Jeannet, M., Rubinstein, A., and Pelet, B., 1974, Prolonged remission of severe aplastic anemia after ALG pretreatment and HLA semi-incompatible bone marrow cell transfusion, *Transplant. Proc.* **6**:359.

Kagan, W., Ascensao, J., Pahwa, R., Hansen, J., Goldstein, G., Moore, M. A. S., and Good, R. A., 1976, Aplastic anemia: Presence in human bone marrow of cells capable of suppressing myelopoiesis, *Proc. Natl. Acad. Sci. U.S.A.* **73**:2890.

Kagan, W. A., Ascensao, J. L., Fialk, M. A., Coleman, M., Valera, E. B., and Good, R. A., 1977, Aplastic anemia: At least three different diseases, submitted for publication.

Knudtzon, S., and Mortensen, B. T., 1976, Interaction between normal and leukemic human cells in agar culture, *Scand. J. Haematol.* **17**:369.

Kurland, J., and Moore, M. A. S., 1977a, Modulation of hemopoiesis by prostaglandins, *Exp. Hematol.* **5**:357.

Kurland, J., and Moore, M. A. S., 1977b, The regulatory role of the macrophage in normal and neoplastic hemopoiesis, *in Experimental Hematology Today*, Vol. II (S. Baum and G. Ledney, eds.), p. 51, Springer-Verlag, Berlin.

Kurland, J., Bockman, R., Broxmeyer, H., and Moore, M., 1978, Limitation of excessive myelopoiesis by the intrinsic modulation of macrophage-derived prostaglandin E, *Science* **199**:552.

Lin, H. S., and Freeman, P. G., 1977, Peritoneal exudate cells IV: Characterization of CFC, *J. Cell. Physiol.* **90**:407.

Lord, B. I., Cercek, L., Cercek, B., Shah, G. P., Dexter, T. M., and Lajtha, L. G., 1974, Inhibitors of hemopoietic cell proliferation? Specificity of action on the hemopoietic system, *Br. J. Cancer* **29**:168.

Lutton, J. D., Hoffman, R., and Greenberg, M. L., 1976, Lymphocyte-mediated neutropenia in man, 19th Annual American Society of Hematology Meetings, Boston, p. 65.

McCaffrey, R., Harrison, T. A., Parkman, D., and Baltimore, D., 1975, Terminal deoxynucleotidyl transferase activity in human leukemic cells and in normal human thymocytes, *N. Engl. J. Med.* **292**:775.

Metcalf, D., and Moore, M. A. S., 1971, *Haemopoietic Cells*, ASP—Biological and Medical Press (North-Holland Division), Amsterdam.

Metcalf, D., Chan, S. H., Gunz, F. W., Vincent, P., and Ravich, R. B. M., 1971, Colony-stimulating factor and inhibitor levels in acute granulocytic leukemia, *Blood* **38**:143.

Metcalf, D., Moore, M. A. S., Sheridan, J. W., and Spitzer, G., 1974, Responsiveness of human granulocyte leukemic cells to CSF, *Blood* **43**:847.

Micklem, H. S., and Loutit, J. F., 1966, *Tissue Grafting and Radiation*, Academic Press, New York.

Moberg, C., Oloffson, T., and Olson, I., 1974, Granulopoiesis in CML I: *In vitro* cloning of blood and bone marrow cells in agar culture, *Scand. J. Haematol.* **12**:381.

Moore, M. A. S., 1974, *In vitro* studies in the myeloid leukaemias, *in Advances in Acute Leukaemia* (F. J. Cleton, D. Crowther, and J. S. Malpas, eds.), p. 161, ASP—Biological and Medical Press, Amsterdam.

Moore, M. A. S., 1975, Marrow culture—A new approach to classification of leukemias, *Blood Cells* **1**:149.

Moore, M. A. S., 1976, Prediction of relapse and remission in AML by marrow culture criteria, *Blood Cells* **2**:109.

Moore, M. A. S., 1977a, *In vitro* culture studies in chronic granulocytic leukemia, *Clin. Haematol.* **6**:97.

Moore, M. A. S., 1977b, Agar culture studies in CML and blastic transformation, *Semin. Hematol.* **8**:11.

Moore, M. A. S., 1977c, Marrow culture studies in preleukemia, Proceedings, XVI Congress International Society of Hematology, Kyoto, p. 99, Excerpta Medica, Amsterdam.

Moore, M. A. S., and Metcalf, D., 1973, Cytogenetic analysis of human acute and CML cells cloned in agar culture, *Int. J. Cancer* **11**:143.

Moore, M. A. S., and Williams, N., 1972, Physical separation of CSC from *in vitro* CFC in hemopoietic tissues, *J. Cell. Physiol.* **80**:195.

Moore, M. A. S., and Williams, N., 1973, Analysis of proliferation and differentiation of foetal granulocyte-macrophage progenitor cells in monkey haemopoietic tissue, *J. Cell. Physiol.* **82**:81.

Moore, M. A. S., Williams, N., and Metcalf, D., 1972, Purification and characterization of the *in vitro* colony-forming cell in monkey haemopoietic tissue, *J. Cell. Physiol.* **79**:283.

Moore, M. A. S., Williams, N., and Metcalf, D., 1973a, *In vitro* colony formation by normal and leukemic hematopoietic cells: Characterization of the colony-forming cell, *J. Natl. Cancer Inst.* **50**:603.

Moore, M. A. S., Williams, N., and Metcalf, D., 1973b, *In vitro* colony formation by normal and leukemic human hematopoietic cells: Interaction between colony forming and colony stimulating cells, *J. Natl. Cancer Inst.* **50**:591.

Moore, M. A. S., Spitzer, G., Metcalf, D., and Penington, D. G., 1974a, Monocyte production of colony-stimulating factor in familial cyclic neutropenia, *Br. J. Haematol.* **27**:47.

Moore, M. A. S., Spitzer, G., Williams, N., Metcalf, D., and Buckley, J., 1974b, Agar culture studies in 127 cases of untreated acute leukemia: Prognostic value of reclassification of leukemia according to *in vitro* growth characteristics, *Blood* **44**:1.

Moore, M. A. S., Kurland, J., and Broxmeyer, H., 1976, The granulocyte-monocyte stem cell, *in Stem Cells of Renewing Cell Populations* (A. B. Cairnie and D. Osmond, eds.), p. 181, Academic Press, New York.

Moore, M. A. S., Burgess, A. W., Metcalf, D., McCulloch, E. A., Robinson, W. A., Dicke, K. A., Chervenich, P. A., Bull, J. M., Wu, A. M., Stanley, E. R., Goldman, J., and Testa, N., 1977, Report of a workshop on standardization of selective cultures for normal and leukemic cells, *Br. J. Cancer* **35**:500.

Morley, A., and Higgs, D., 1974, *In vitro* differentiation of leukemic cells, *in Hemopoiesis in Culture: Second International Workshop* (W. A. Robinson, ed.), DHEW Publication No. (NIH) 74:205. p. 359.

Paran, M., Sachs, L., Barak, Y., and Resnitzky, P., 1970, *In vitro* induction of granulocyte differentiation in hematopoietic cells from leukemic and nonleukemic patients, *Proc. Natl. Acad. Sci. U.S.A.* **57**:1542.

Pedersen, B., 1973, Annotation: The blastic crisis of chronic myeloid leukemia: Acute transformation of a preleukemic condition, *Br. J. Haematol.* **25**:141.

Pike, B. L., and Robinson, W. A., 1970, Human bone marrow colony growth *in vitro, J. Cell. Physiol.* **76**:77.

Price, G. B., Senn, J. S., McCulloch, E. A., and Till, J. E., 1975, The isolation and properties of granulocytic colony-stimulating activities from medium conditioned by human peripheral leukocytes, *Biochem. J.* **148**:209.

Ralph, P., Broxmeyer, H. E., and Nakoinz, I., 1977, Immunostimulators induce granulocyte-macrophage colony-stimulating activity and block proliferation in a monocytic tumor cell line, *J. Exp. Med.* **146**:611.

Robinson, W. A., and Pike, B. L., 1970, Leukopoietic activity in human urine: The granulocytic leukemias, *N. Engl. J. Med.* **282**:1291.

Robinson, W. A., Kurnick, J. E., and Pike, B. L., 1971, Colony growth of human leukemic peripheral blood cells *in vitro, Blood* **38**:500.

Ruscetti, F. W., and Chervenick, P. A., 1975, Regulation of the release of colony-stimulating activity from mitogen-stimulated lymphocytes, *J. Immunol.* **114**:1513.

Rytomaa, T., 1973, Annotation: Role of chalone in granulopoiesis, *Br. J. Haematol.* **24**:141.

Rytomaa, T., Vilpo, J. A., Levanto, A., and Jones, W. A., 1976, Effect of granulocytic chalone on acute and chronic granulocytic leukemia in man. Report of 7 cases, *Scand. J. Haematol. Suppl.* **27**:5.

Saffhill, R., Dexter, T. M., Muldal, S., and Testa, N. G., 1977, Terminal deoxynucleotidyl transferase in a case of Ph[1] positive infant chronic myelogenous leukemia, submitted for publication.

Sarin, P. S., Anderson, P. N., and Gallo, R. C., 1976, Terminal deoxynucleotidyl transferase in human leukemias and lymphoblastoid cell lines, *Blood* **47**:11.

Senn, J. S., Pinkerton, P. H., Price, G. B., Mak, T. W., and McCulloch, E. A., 1976, Human preleukemia cell culture studies in sideroblastic anemia, *Br. J. Cancer* **33**:299.

Shadduck, R. K., and Nankin, H. R., 1971, Cellular origin of granulocyte colonies in chronic myeloid leukemia, *Lancet* **ii**:1097.

Shah, R. G., Caporale, L. H., and Moore, M. A. S., 1977, Characterization of colony stimulating activity produced by human monocytes and PHA stimulated lymphocytes, *Blood* **50**:811.

Speck, B., Cornu, P., Sartorius, J., Nissen, C., Groff, P., Burri, H. P., and Jeannet, M., 1978, Immunologic aspects of aplasia, *Transplant. Proc.* **10**:131.

Spitzer, G., Dicke, K. A., Gehan, E. A., Smith, T., McCredie, K. B., Boulogie, B., and Freireich, E. J., 1976, A simplified *in vitro* classification for prognosis in adult acute leukemia, *Blood* **48**:795.

Stanley, E. R., Hansen, G., Woodcock, J., and Metcalf, D., 1975, Colony stimulating factor and the regulation of granulopoiesis and macrophage production, *Fed. Proc.* **34**:2272.

Stanley, E. R., Cifone, M., Heard, P. M., and Defendi, V., 1976, Factors regulating macrophage production and growth: Identity of CSF and macrophage growth factor, *J. Exp. Med.* **143**:631.

Thomas, E. D., Storb, R., and Giblett, E. R., 1976, Recovery from aplastic anemia following attempted marrow transplantation, *Exp. Hematol.* **4**:97.

Van Bekkum, D. W., Bach, F. H., and Bergan, J. J., 1976, Bone marrow transplantation from histocompatible allogeneic donors for aplastic anemia. A report from the ACS/NIH bone marrow transplant registry, *JAMA* **236**:1131.

Van Den Engh, G., Mulder, D., Williams, N., and Bol, S., 1977, Physical characterization of a sub-population of granulocyte-monocyte progenitor cells (CFU-c), *in Experimental Hematology Today,* Vol. II (S. Baum and G. Ledney, eds.), p. 157, Springer-Verlag, Berlin.

Williams, N., and Jackson, H., 1977, Analysis of population of macrophage-granulocytic progenitor cells stimulated by activities in mouse lung conditioned medium, *Exp. Hematol.* **5**:523.

Zanjani, E. D., Litwin, S. D., and Zalusky, R., 1975, Impairment of erythroid colony formation by lymphocytes from patients with variable immunodeficiency, *Blood* **46**:1038.

# Abnormalities of Red Cell Membrane Lipids: Clinical–Biophysical Correlates

## Richard A. Cooper

## 3.1. Introduction

Among mammalian cells, mature red cells are unique in that they possess only one membrane, their surface membrane. Other membranes are lost during the process of cellular maturation (Shattil and Cooper, 1972). All of the lipid present in mature red cells is in this surface membrane.

The organization of lipids in red cell membranes has been the subject of intensive investigation. This stems from two basic areas of inquiry. One relates to the structure and function of cell surface membranes, the red cell being a convenient and suitable model for certain aspects of all cell surface membranes. The second relates to the pathogenesis of hemolytic diseases, abnormalities of the red cell membrane being a cause of premature red cell destruction *in vivo*. This chapter discusses the structure, organization, and turnover of red cell membrane lipids, the role played by

RICHARD A. COOPER • Hematology–Oncology Section, Department of Medicine, University of Pennsylvania School of Medicine, Philadelphia, Pennsylvania.

membrane lipids in the functional characteristics of red cell membranes, and the abnormalities that exist in red cell membranes in human disease.

## 3.2. Membrane Lipid Composition

Lipids account for approximately 50% of the weight of red cell membranes. Cholesterol and phospholipid are the major lipids (Table I). Small amounts of glycolipids are also present in human red cells, and larger amounts are found in the red cells of other mammalian species. Both glycolipids and phospholipids are polar, whereas cholesterol is a neutral lipid. Small amounts of free fatty acids are also present. Neither triglycerides nor cholesterol esters are constituents of red cell membranes (Cooper, 1970).

A constant feature of mammalian red cell membranes is that the mole ratio of neutral lipid (cholesterol) to polar lipid (phospholipid + glycolipid) is always approximately 0.9 to 1.0 (Rouser *et al.*, 1968). However, the relative amounts of glycolipid and phospholipid vary considerably as do the relative amounts of the various major phospholipid classes. Four phospholipids predominate in human red cell membranes: lecithin (phosphatidylcholine), sphingomyelin, phosphatidylserine, and phosphatidylethanolamine. Small amounts of lysolecithin, phosphatidylinositol, and phosphatidic acid are also present. Lecithin is absent from red cells obtained from ruminants, such as the sheep, cow, and goat. In these

**Table I.**  Lipids of the Normal Human Red Cell Membrane

|  | $\mu$mol/$10^{11}$ cells |
| --- | --- |
| Cholesterol | 36.1 |
| Phospholipid | 38.0 |
| Glycolipid | 1.0 |
| Free fatty acid | 2.6 |
|  | % of total phospholipids |
| Sphingomyelin | 26.0 |
| Lecithin | 30.5 |
| Phosphatidylserine (+ phosphatidylinositol) | 13.2 |
| Phosphatidylethanolamine | 27.3 |
| Lysolecithin | 1.3 |
| Other (polyglycerol phosphatide, phosphatidic acid) | 1.7 |
|  | Mol/mol |
| Cholesterol/phospholipid | 0.95 |
| Sphingomyelin/lecithin | 0.85 |

instances, there is an increase in the amount of sphingomyelin. In general, lecithin and sphingomyelin together account for 50 to 60% of the total phospholipids in various mammalian red cells.

## 3.3. Cholesterol–Phospholipid Interactions

The importance of the association between polar lipids and sterols is emphasized by the fact that the membranes of all higher organisms, including plants and animals, contain both. In those few instances in which sterols are known not to occur in prokaryotes and lower eukaryotes, molecules are present which appear to mimic the sterol structure (Nes, 1974). For example, caratenols are found in certain Mycoplasma and tetrahymanol occurs in *Tetrahymena piriformis*. Cholesterol is the predominant sterol in all cells within the animal kingdom, whereas sterols with an alkylated side chain predominate in plants. Van Deenen and others have shown that the structural requirements for sterols in cell membranes are quite specific. They must possess a $\beta$-OH on the third carbon, a $\Delta$5 double bond, alternating trans-antistereochemistry creating a planar ring structure, and an uncyclized side chain at C-17 (Nes, 1974; Demel *et al.*, 1972). The molecular interactions which occur between sterols and polar lipids in membranes are not completely understood. Huang (1977) has recently proposed that hydrogen bonding occurs between the carbonyl oxygen of the phospholipid acyl side chains and the $3\beta$-OH of the sterol. This particular model permits an efficient alignment between the acyl chains of phospholipids and the planar sterol nucleus. In most biologic membranes, one phospholipid acyl chain is saturated and the other has at least one unsaturated double bond, a *cis* double bond at C-9–C-10. This asymmetry of acyl chain structure accommodates the asymmetry of the sterol molecule, caused by the protrusion of two angular methyl groups (C-18 and C-19) from one face of the sterol nucleus. Models of the sterol–phospholipid interaction suggest that a 1:1 molar ratio of cholesterol to phospholipid is readily achieved, that phospholipids are capable of accommodating up to 2 moles of cholesterol per mole of phospholipid, and that for amounts of sterol in excess of a cholesterol/phospholipid (C/PL) ratio of 2.0, some other molecular configuration is required. This concept is supported by an increasing body of experimental data (Cooper *et al.*, 1978). It should be noted that, although cholesterol is the usual sterol present in red cell membranes, other sterols which have the structural requirements just described may also gain access to the membrane. This has been observed in patients who accumulate cholesterol due to an inherited metabolic derangement (Salen and Grundy, 1973) and in patients who absorb inappropriate quantities of dietary plant sterols, such as $\beta$-sitosterol (Salen *et al.*, 1970).

The interactions between sterols and phospholipids have a number of important consequences for membrane structure. For example, sterols increase the efficiency of packing of phospholipids in artificial membranes (Demel and De Kruyff, 1976). The close interpositioning of sterols with phospholipids causes a degree of immobility to be imposed upon the 10 acyl carbon atoms nearest the membrane's surface, while increasing the freedom of motion deep within the hydrophobic core of the membrane (Rothman and Engelman, 1972), thus creating what Chapman (1968) has called an "intermediate fluid state." One manifestation of this, which is seen when sterols are added to pure phospholipids, is a diminution and finally eradication of the endothermic gel to liquid crystal phase transition which is normally seen upon cooling. Another manifestation of this, which is discussed later, is the effect that sterols have on the fluidity of lipid bilayers.

## 3.4. Organization of Lipids in Red Cell Membranes

There is an increasing amount of evidence which establishes that the lipids of red cell membranes are not randomly distributed but rather that their disposition within the membrane follows an organizational pattern. Evidence for three types of lipid segregation has been obtained. The first, and largest, body of data concerns the asymmetrical distribution of lipids on the two sides of the membrane bilayer. The second concerns the presence of boundary lipids (or annular lipids) which surround membrane proteins and create an interface between proteins and the broad areas which are presumed to be the bulk lipid bilayer. The third, and least well established, type of lipid segregation within naturally occurring membranes is clustering and phase separation with the creation of distinct lipid domains.

The concept that lipids within the membrane are asymmetrically distributed was introduced by Bretscher (1972), who observed that reagents which are most reactive with amino groups reacted better with phosphatidylethanolamine and phosphatidylserine in red cell ghosts as compared with intact red cells. This suggested that these two phospholipids were primarily situated on the inner surface of the membrane. Subsequent work both with phospholipases and with the phospholipid exchange protein confirms this concept (Verkleij *et al.*, 1973; Bloj and Zilversmit, 1976; Rothman and Lenard, 1977). From these studies, it appears that all the phosphatidylserine and 80% of the phosphatidyle-thanolamine of human red cell membranes are present on the inner surface, whereas 70% of the lecithin and 80% of the sphingomyelin are present on the outer surface.

The extent to which phospholipids are capable of moving from one side of the membrane to the other ("flip-flop") is still controversial. For example, some workers have determined that the rate of flip-flop is very slow and consistent with the anisotropic distribution of phospholipids in the red cell membrane during the life of the cell (Kahlenberg *et al.*, 1974; Rousselet *et al.*, 1976). In contrast, others have found that the transposition rate for lecithin across rat red cell ghosts has a half-time for equilibration of several hours (Bloj and Zilversmit, 1976). In contrast, it appears that the transmembrane movement of cholesterol in human red cells is quite rapid, with a half-time of less than 1 hr (Lange *et al.*, 1977).

Although phase separations have been readily documented in mixtures of cholesterol with synthetic phospholipids with markedly different fatty acid compositions (Shimshick and McConnell, 1973), it has been more difficult to identify phase separations when phospholipids contain fatty acids that are less dissimilar. Evidence for phase separations in naturally occurring biologic membranes is only scanty. Nonetheless, many workers in this field attribute the paucity of evidence to limitations in current technology rather than to the absence of phase separations in some regions of naturally occurring membranes. The requirement for specific lipids which are necessary for the optimal activity of a variety of membrane enzymes supports the concept that some segregation of the lipids in membranes results from their necessary association with such proteins (Gennis and Jonas, 1977). In certain instances, it appears that a lipid annulus exists which is composed of a single layer of phospholipids surrounding the protein complex (Jost *et al.*, 1973; Warren *et al.*, 1975). In artificial systems *in vitro*, it has been demonstrated that cholesterol preferentially associates with sphingomyelin in mixed lecithin–sphingomyelin membranes and with lecithin in mixed lecithin–phosphatidylethanolamine bilayers (Van Dijck *et al.*, 1976; Demel *et al.*, 1977). A careful examination of nearest neighbor lipids suggests that phosphatidylserine and phosphatidylethanolamine occur as small clusters in a nonrandom array in red cell membranes and that phosphatidylserine preferentially associates with spectrin (Marinetti, 1977; Van Zoelen *et al.*, 1977). It is evident that we are just beginning to learn the intricacies of lipid structure in membranes.


## 3.5. Membrane Lipid Fluidity

Under physiologic conditions the lipids of biologic membranes are in a liquid crystalline state. Although the hydrophobic interactions and the hydrogen bonding which occur between lipids maintain the integrity of the lipid bilayer, they also permit appreciable amounts of molecular motion within that bilayer. This motion appears to be greatest within the hydrophobic core of the membrane and least near the hydrocarbon–water interface. It is the process of molecular motion within the membrane that is referred to as "fluidity." This property of membrane lipids is most readily assessed in terms of the motion of small, hydrophobic probes that insert into the membrane and are detectable by means of nuclear magnetic resonance, magnetic resonance, or fluorescence. The random motion of these probes within the membrane is referred to as rotational diffusion, and this motion is influenced by the viscosity of the microenvironment in which the probe resides. Therefore, measurement of the movement of hydrophobic probes is a means of assessing molecular interactions among membrane lipids.

Concepts of membrane fluidity must not be confused with recent studies which have begun to define membrane viscoelastic properties. Whereas both lipids and proteins have viscous properties, only proteins have elastic properties. The surface viscoelasticity of red cells results from the character of certain membrane proteins, spectrin being the most important, and not from the fluidity of membrane lipids (Evans and Hochmuth, 1977).

Membrane fluidity is strongly influenced by the composition of membrane lipids. For example, the number of saturated double bonds within the phospholipid acyl chains in membranes is an important determinant of the membrane's fluid qualities. Indeed, variation in acyl chain saturation is the most common determinant of membrane fluidity in nature. Saturated acyl chains form highly ordered membranes in which fluidity is of low magnitude. Conversely, phospholipids with unsaturated acyl chains form fluid disordered membranes. Red cell membrane fluidity is also influenced by the amount of cholesterol relative to phospholipid (Kroes *et al.*, 1972; Vanderkooi *et al.*, 1974; Cooper *et al.*, 1978) and by the relative amounts of the various phospholipids (Cooper *et al.*, 1977a). Amphiphilic molecules, such as soaps, alcohols, and detergents, partition between aqueous and lipid phases, and have a fluidizing effect on membrane lipids. Lysophosphatides are a naturally occurring amphipathic substance. Local anesthetics, such as procaine, and psychotropic drugs, such as chlorpromazine, also exert a fluidizing effect under physiologic conditions (Feinstein *et al.*, 1975). Recent studies have suggested that the process of complement lysis is associated with the generation of amphipathic molecules which increase the fluidity of the hydrophobic core of membranes (Shattil *et al.*, 1977).

The asymmetry of the red cell membrane lipids suggests that fluidity may also be asymmetrical. Indeed, evidence supporting this concept has been presented using electron spin resonance probes (Tanaka and Ohnishi, 1976). It has been suggested that the differential effects which anionic and cationic amphiphilic molecules have on membrane structure may relate to the differential concentrations of anionic molecules on the inner lamella of the membrane and cationic molecules on the other lamella (Sheetz *et al.*, 1976).

Because lipid fluidity is very sensitive to temperature, a demand is imposed upon nature to control fluidity under conditions in which temperature changes, for example, in cold-blooded animals exposed to varying ambient temperatures or warm-blooded animals during torpor or hibernation. Similar needs exist in plants which are cold insensitive. In eukaryotes, sterols buffer the effects of temperature on fluidity by decreasing the activation energy for viscosity, thus permitting less change in fluidity per degree change in temperature than would occur in the absence of sterols. The concept of homeoviscous adaptation is derived from the observation that simple organisms, as diverse as bacteria and tetrahymena, are able to maintain membranes having a constant fluidity at a variety of growth temperatures (Sinensky, 1974; Cronan and Gelmann, 1975; McElhaney and Souza, 1976; Kitajima and Thompson, 1977). This is achieved by varying the degree of saturation and branching of acyl fatty acids. A similar process of adaptation has been demonstrated in eukaryotic organisms, such as crustacean plankton, which grows in water of widely varying temperatures while maintaining a degree of fatty acid saturation such that the gel-to-liquid crystal phase transition of its membrane lipids is always approximately 2° lower than the ambient temperature (Farkas and Herodek, 1964). Fish and frogs also vary the saturation/ unsaturation ratio of their acyl fatty acids during cold adaptation (Knipprath and Mead, 1966; Baranska and Wlodawer, 1969), and this has also been observed in the red cell and mitochondrial membranes of echidna, a primitive mammal, during periods of torpor (McMurchie and Raison, 1975). Additional mechanisms have been observed in high mammals during hibernation. For example, ground squirrels increase the lysophosphatide content of their cardiac mitochondria (Keith *et al.*, 1975), and hamsters decrease the C/PL of their brain lipids (Goldman, 1975). All these changes in membrane lipid composition serve to permit a normal fluidity under conditions of decreased temperature.

## 3.6. Synthesis and Exchange

Mature red cells lack specific adaptative processes with which to control membrane fluidity. Instead, they depend on the lipid composition of plasma lipoproteins. Similarities exist between membranes and lipoproteins in the sense that both contain cholesterol and phospholipid in close association with proteins. In addition, plasma lipoproteins contain cholesterol esters and triglycerides. More than two-thirds of the sterol in plasma lipoproteins is in the form of cholesterol esters. From the specific structural requirements for sterols in membranes described earlier, it is clear that cholesterol esters are incapable of associating with phospholipids in the membrane bilayer. When studied in aqueous systems *in vitro,* phospholipids are able to solubilize only 4 moles/100 ml of cholesterol ester, and similar data exist for triglycerides (Small and Shipley, 1974). Recent studies support the concept that cholesterol esters and triglycerides are enclosed within lipoproteins as microdroplets, presumably surrounded by quasi-membranous cholesterol–phospholipid–protein structures (Deckelbaum *et al.,* 1975). Whereas cholesterol esters and triglycerides are incapable of interacting with cell membranes, the cholesterol and phospholipid of plasma lipoproteins interact strongly. These interactions are particularly important for red cells since they lack the enzymatic apparatus necessary for cholesterol synthesis or esterification or for phospholipid synthesis *de novo,* although they are able to bring about fatty acid chain lengthening (Pittman and Martin, 1966).

### 3.6.1. Phospholipid Turnover

Plasma free fatty acids rapidly exchange into red cell membranes and are actively incorporated into lysophosphatides utilizing ATP and coenzyme A (CoA) (Oliveria and Vaughan, 1964; Shohet *et al.,* 1968). Since lysophospholipids also rapidly exchange between plasma and red cell membranes, the acylation of lysophospholipids within the membrane provides one mechanism for the renewal of membrane phospholipids which have been degraded.

A second mechanism of phospholipid renewal utilizing lysophospholipids, but not requiring energy, occurs by a dismutation of lysolecithin resulting in the generation of lecithin and glycerophosphorylcholine (Mulder *et al.,* 1965; Tarlov and Mulder, 1967). Both the energy-requiring acylation and the dismutation of lysophospholipid involve predominantly lecithin.

Phospholipid renewal within red cell membranes may also occur by a direct exchange of the intact molecule with its counterpart in plasma. Studies *in vitro* utilizing red cell and plasma phospholipids labeled with $^{32}$P *in vivo* have demonstrated that both lecithin and sphingomyelin participate in this exchange, resulting in a 9% turnover of lecithin and a 4% turnover of sphingomyelin in 12 hr (Reed, 1968). Exchange data suggest that these two phospholipids are not homogeneous in the red cell membrane, but rather that only a portion of each is exchangeable, amounting to 60% of lecithin and 30% of sphingomyelin in human red cells, a finding consistent with the asymmetric distribution of phospholipids on the two sides of the bilayer. The presence of this direct exchange process would predict that, since lecithin is plentiful in sheep plasma, sheep red cell membranes would have substantial amounts of lecithin. However, as noted earlier, sheep red cells lack lecithin. This appears to be due to the presence of a lecithinase in sheep red cell membranes (Kramer *et al.*, 1974).

The turnover of red cell lecithin by the three mechanisms just discussed was studied in rat red cells (Tarlov and Mulder, 1967). The total turnover was 5.8% in 3 hr: 1.2% resulted from the acylation of lysolecithin utilizing fatty acids, ATP, and CoA; 1.6% resulted from the dismutation (or condensation) of two molecules of lysolecithin; and 3% resulted from a direct exchange with plasma lecithin.

### 3.6.2. Glycolipid Turnover

Glycolipids are complex molecules containing sphingosine, a long-chain fatty acid, and one or more molecules of hexose or hexosamine. The presence of sphingosine and a fatty acid makes this class of compounds similar to sphingomyelin. Indeed, like sphingomyelin, the fatty acids are predominantly 24:0 and 24:1. Sphingosine and fatty acid together are referred to as ceramide.

The glycolipids of mammals can be divided into two major classes. Those that contain glucose, galactose, and *N*-acetylgalactosamine (GalNAc) or *N*-acetylglycosamine (GluNAc) are termed globosides, and those that contain glucose, galactose, and *N*-acetylneuraminic acid (NANA) or *N*-glycolylneuraminic acid (NGNA) are termed hematosides. Human red cell membranes contain glycolipids of the globoside (GL) type with one to four (GL-1 to GL-4) hexose residues (Sweeley and Dawson, 1969).

The stability of red cell membrane glycolipids *in vivo* has been studied in the pig (Sweeley and Dawson, 1969) and the rabbit (Krivit and Kern, 1969). Following the injection of $^{14}$C-labeled glucose, membrane GL-1 rapidly exchanges with plasma, primarily with low density lipoproteins. GL-4 in the pig and GL-5 in the rabbit do not undergo exchange, labeled GL-4 and GL-5 of red cell origin appearing in plasma only at the time of red cell destruction. GL-2 and GL-3 appear to behave in an intermediate way with 40 to 60% of the labeled molecules being lost from the membrane over the first few days, indicating exchange with plasma, and the remainder being released at the time of red cell destruction. The Lewis blood group glycolipids, complex lipids containing glucose, galactose, fucose, and GluNAc, are transported by plasma high- and low-density lipoproteins and are in exchange equilibrium with the red cell membrane (Marcus and Cass, 1969).

### 3.6.3. Cholesterol Turnover

Two types of exchange diffusion are necessary to describe the movement of cholesterol between plasma lipoproteins and red cell membranes.

The first is simple equilibrium exchange in which one molecule of membrane cholesterol exits into plasma in exchange for one molecule of cholesterol in plasma which enters the membrane. This process of equilibrium exchange has a half-time of 2 hr, and was first described with isotopically labeled cholesterol by Gould more than 25 years ago (Hagerman and Gould, 1951). Studies with whole plasma and with isolated plasma lipoproteins *in vitro* and *in vivo* have demonstrated that the equilibrium involves the entire free cholesterol pools of both plasma lipoproteins and red cell membranes (London and Schwartz, 1953; Gould *et al.*, 1955; Murphy, 1962; Ashworth and Green, 1964; Basford *et al.*, 1964).

The second type of exchange diffusion between cholesterol in membranes and plasma lipoproteins concerns the partition of cholesterol within this exchangeable pool; i.e., how much cholesterol is in lipoproteins and how much is in membranes? The nature of this partition is best appreciated when it is recognized that cholesterol does not exist as a solute in water, nor does it by itself form micelles or liposomal membranes, as is the case for fatty acids and phospholipids. Sterols are virtually insoluble in water. They are solubilized in lipoproteins and in membranes by amphipathic lipids, such as phospholipids. Therefore, the partition of cholesterol between membranes and lipoproteins is determined by the amount of phospholipid relative to the amount of cholesterol within each compartment i.e., the cholesterol/phospholipid ratio (C/PL). This has been confirmed by studies in a variety of systems *in vivo* and *in vitro* (Cooper *et al.*, 1972, 1975, 1978). It is of particular interest because it underlies the pathogenesis of spur cell anemia in man (Cooper *et al.*, 1975) and it may play a role in the development of atherosclerosis in animals fed cholesterol-rich atherogenic diets (Arbogast *et al.*, 1976).

## 3.7. Cholesterol Effects in Red Cells

### 3.7.1. Spur Cells

The syndrome of spur cell anemia represents an abnormality of red cell membrane cholesterol content which results from a primary disorder of plasma lipoprotein metabolism (Cooper, 1969). It occurs in patients with severe liver disease, usually cirrhosis of the alcoholic. Red cells have bizarrely spiculated shapes, and they undergo premature destruction *in vivo*, primarily in the spleen. Of the two major lipids of the red cell membrane, phospholipids are present in normal amounts but cholesterol is increased by 25 to 65% (Cooper *et al.*, 1972). This results in an increase in membrane C/PL from normal values of 0.95 to values as high as 1.60. It is of interest to compare this to values that can be achieved *in vitro* when cholesterol is mixed with purified phospholipids in water. Under conditions of high lipid concentration and gentle agitation, multilamellar liposomes form in which the maximum C/PL is 1.0 (Bourgès *et al.*, 1967). This value has been considered to be the upper limit of C/PL, and normal membranes have C/PL values which are below 1.0. Values greater than 1.0 can be achieved *in vitro* when lipids are suspended at a low concentration in water and energy is added, usually in the form of sonication (Horwitz *et al.*, 1971; Cooper *et al.*, 1975, 1978; Freeman and Finean, 1975). Thus, although values of less than 1.0 are preferred, values of C/PL greater than 1.0 can be achieved *in vitro* and are found in disease states *in vivo*.

Clinical observation has demonstrated that the spur cell membrane phenomenon is acquired, since normal transfused blood develops the abnormality (Silber *et al.*, 1966). Similar observations have been made *in vitro* (Cooper, 1969). Since cholesterol is transferred from plasma lipoproteins to cell membranes, it was of interest to examine the role of plasma cholesterol concentration in this process. It was observed that the transfer of cholesterol from plasma lipoproteins to cell membranes is independent of serum cholesterol concentration but is strongly dependent on the C/PL of low density lipoproteins (Cooper *et al.*, 1975). Thus, by means of equilibrium partition, red cells acquire cholesterol from lipoproteins which have an increased C/PL.

The syndrome of spur cell anemia is not unique to man, but has been described in rodents (guinea pigs and rabbits) (Westerman *et al.*, 1970; Sardet *et al.*, 1972) and recently in dogs (Cooper *et al.*, 1977b) fed cholesterol-rich atherogenic diets. The accumulation of cholesterol is not confined to red cell membranes. In man and in dogs, platelet membranes are affected as well (Cooper, 1969; Cooper *et al.*, 1977b), and in rodents an increase in C/PL has been observed in the surface membranes of macrophages (Dianzani *et al.*, 1976), liver cells (Grandison and Green, 1976), and both lymphocytes and lymphoblasts (Ip *et al.*, 1978). Nor are changes isolated to surface membranes. Cholesterol equilibrates between cell surface membranes and internal membranes (Bell, 1975), causing an increase in the C/PL of microsomal membranes in cholesterol-fed animals (Lang, 1976). Thus, an increase in the C/PL of plasma lipoproteins leads to an increase in the C/PL of many cell membranes.

### 3.7.2. Cholesterol Enrichment *In Vitro*

In order to avoid the complexities inherent in dealing with human disease states or animal models of disease, studies of the equilibrium partition of cholesterol have been extended to sonicated lipid dispersions containing various quantitites of cholesterol (Cooper *et al.*, 1975, 1978). The C/PL of red cell membranes is directly influenced by the C/PL of lipid dispersions containing cholesterol cosonicated with various lecithins and with sphingomyelin. In each case, red cell cholesterol is unaffected by dispersions with a C/PL of 1.0 and is directly proportional to the C/PL of the dispersions over a range of membrane C/PL from 0.4 to 2.7. Moreover, the addition of cholesterol esters to these dispersions had no influence on the partition of cholesterol. Thus, studies with pure lipid dispersions confirm the conclusions reached with human and experimental spur cell anemia.

If the equilibrium partition of cholesterol in terms of phospholipid was the sole determinant of the C/PL of membranes and lipoproteins, then all structures involved in this exchange should have identical C/PL values. Yet red cells, which have a C/PL of 0.95, are in equilibrium with various phospholipid dispersions with a C/PL of 1.0, and also with low density lipoprotein which has a C/PL of 0.8 and high density lipoprotein with a C/PL of 0.2. Platelet membranes have a C/PL of 0.6, and the surface membranes of nucleated cells have C/PL values of 0.4 to 0.8. Both are in equilibrium with plasma lipoproteins. When high density lipoprotein is incubated with various phospholipid dispersions, its C/PL remains unchanged in the presence of dispersions with a C/PL of 1.0, and it increases in the presence of dispersions with C/PL values of greater than 1.0 (Cooper *et al.*, 1975). A part of this seeming disparity results from variable quantities of glycolipids in membranes and lipoproteins. Like phospholipids, these are polar lipids capable of solubilizing cholesterol. In red cells of various mammalian species, glycolipids represent up to 15% of the total membrane lipids. Large amounts are present in the central nervous system. However, glycolipids alone do not account for the wide range of C/PL values observed. It is likely that the association between phospholipids and proteins, which are essential for certain functional and structural properties of both membranes and lipoproteins, occupies some phospholipids in a way which precludes their availability to solubilize cholesterol.

The ubiquitous nature of sterols in membranes of all but the most primitive life forms implies that they serve an essential role. The influence of sterols on membrane structure has been studied in a number of ways. The recent use of hydrophobic probes has permitted an analysis of lipid–lipid interactions at physiologic temperatures. These studies show that cholesterol decreases fluidity. Moreover, by interposing itself between adjacent phospholipid acyl fatty acid chains, it increases the degree of order within the membrane bilayer. Indeed, a direct correlation has been observed between the amount of cholesterol present in red cell membranes and the fluidity of membrane lipids (Vanderkooi *et al.*, 1974; Shinitzky and Inbar, 1976). This effect of cholesterol on membrane

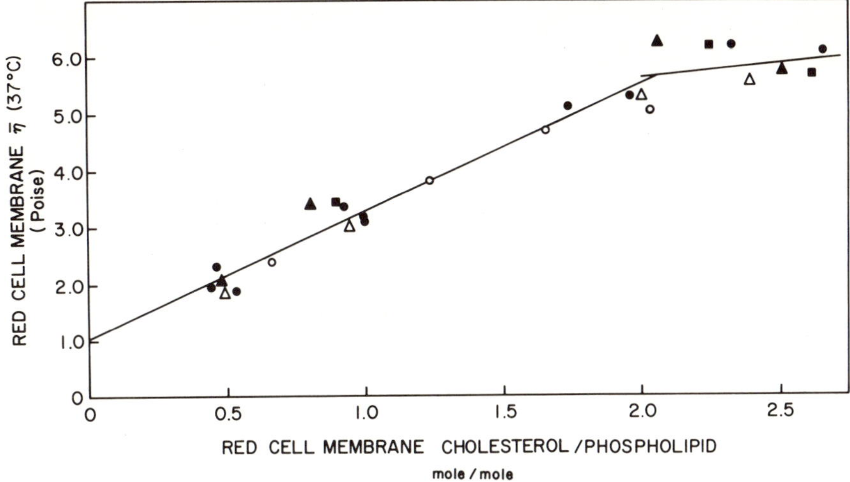

**Fig. 1.** The effective membrane viscosity ($\bar{\eta}$) in red cells in which the cholesterol/ phospholipid mole ratio (C/PL) has been altered by incubation with lipid dispersions containing cholesterol together with one of a series of synthetic and naturally occurring phospholipids. The symbols represent different phospholipids. A linear relationship exists between $\bar{\eta}$ and C/PL to a maximum $\bar{\eta}$ at a C/PL of 2.0. (From Cooper *et al.*, 1978.)

fluidity appears to be maximum when cholesterol is present at a membrane C/PL of 2.0 (approximately twice normal) (Cooper *et al.*, 1978); see Fig. 1. Thus, the equilibrium partition of cholesterol has a direct effect on the fluidity of red cell membranes.

### 3.7.3. Cholesterol Effects on Cell Contour

Striking changes in cell contour occur in association with increases in membrane cholesterol. These are characterized by a folding and scalloping of the cell margins (Fig. 2). Similar changes occur when normal red cells are enriched with cholesterol by incubation with cholesterol-rich lecithin dispersions or with serum from patients with spur cells (Cooper, 1969; Cooper *et al.*, 1975). Moreover, a similar morphology was observed in a patient with spur cells who had undergone splenectomy (Cooper *et al.*, 1974). The addition of cholesterol to red cells under these circumstances also increases membrane surface area in proportion to the contribution that cholesterol makes to the surface area of normal red cells. The magnitude of this increase in surface area is 0.20 to 0.25% for each 1.0% increase in membrane cholesterol (Cooper *et al.*, 1972). Thus, the effect of added cholesterol is to increase surface area and alter cell contour.

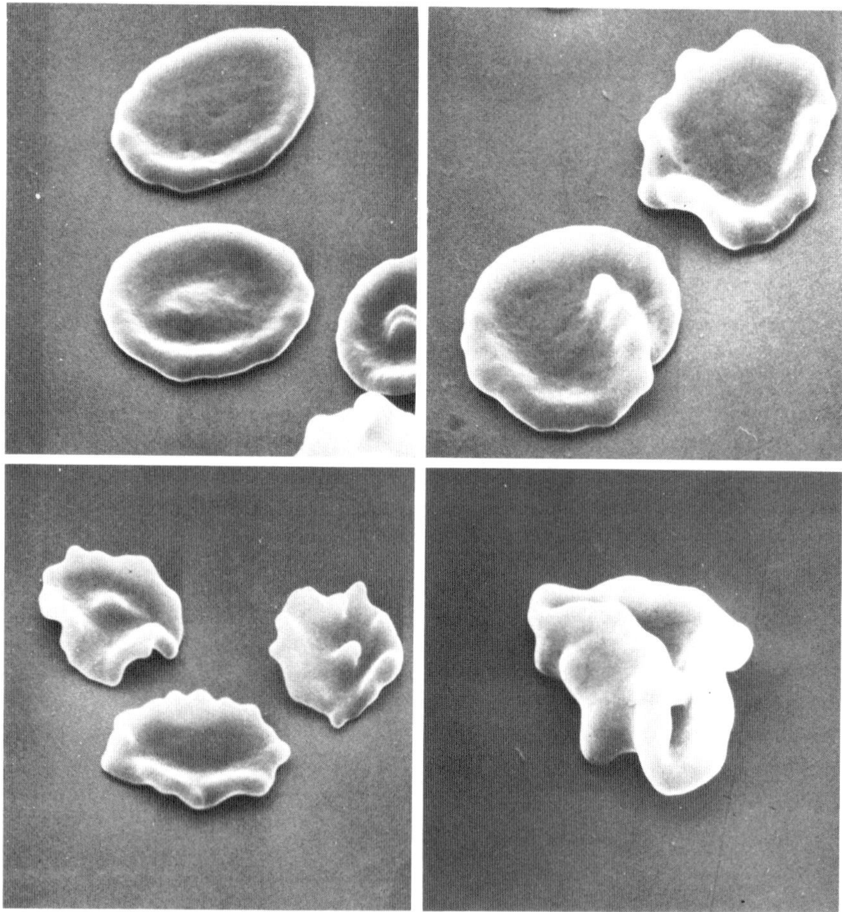

**Fig. 2.**  Morphology of red cells enriched with cholesterol *in vitro* (membrane C/PL = 2.0). All cells are from the same preparation. (From Cooper *et al.*, 1975.)

Whether due to these gross physical changes in the membrane or whether due to the more subtle changes in fluidity which are also caused by added cholesterol, the flow properties of cholesterol-rich red cells are impaired. This is seen *in vitro* by a decrease in the red cell's ability to traverse filters of small pore size (Cooper, 1969; Cooper *et al.*, 1975). *In vivo*, spur cells are retarded in their circulation through the spleen, where they lose a portion of their surface membrane and undergo changes in cell contour (Cooper, 1969; Cooper *et al.*, 1974). This results in a thorny appearing red cell (the "spur cell"), for which this disorder is named. Membrane remodeling in spur cell anemia is analogous to the loss of membrane which hereditary spherocytes undergo under similar conditions, and has been called splenic conditioning (Emerson *et al.*, 1956).

### 3.7.4. Cholesterol Effects on Membrane Function

The enrichment of membranes with cholesterol has a number of effects on the permeability, transport, and enzymatic activities of the membrane and on the availability of membrane surface receptors. An effect of cholesterol on permeability was first demonstrated using lecithin liposomes containing various sterols, and these studies helped to establish the structural requirements for sterols in membranes (De Gier *et al.*, 1968). Although not all studies utilizing red cells are in agreement, it appears that increases in membrane cholesterol reduce the passive permeability and facilitate diffusion of a number of electrolytes and nonelectrolytes, whereas cholesterol depletion increases permeability. In contrast, changes in membrane cholesterol do not appear to influence directly the active transport of Na or K. Thus, for example, cholesterol depletion increases the passive permeability of red cells to glycerol, acetate, and Na (Grunze and Deuticke, 1974; Cooper *et al.*, 1975). An apparent increase in active Na flux also accompanies cholesterol depletion. However, this is best explained in terms of a response to the increase in passive Na permeability rather than the primary effect on the transport mechanism (Cooper *et al.*, 1975), although an effect of cholesterol on the affinity of the pump for Na has also been demonstrated (Giraud *et al.*, 1976). In contrast, cholesterol enrichment inhibits the furosemide-sensitive diffusion of Na + K (Wiley and Cooper, 1975) as well as the diffusion of glycerol, erythritol, acetate, and propionate (Deuticke and Ruska, 1976). Similar decreases in nonelectrolyte permeability have been observed in cholesterol-rich guinea pig red cells (Kroes and Ostwald, 1971). We have not observed any effect of cholesterol enrichment on active Na or K transport (Cooper *et al.*, 1975), although a decrease in active Na flux of very small magnitude was reported in cholesterol-rich guinea pig cells (Kroes and Ostwald, 1971). Thus, modulation of membrane cholesterol has a substantial effect on the cell's permeability to small molecules.

The effect of cholesterol on membrane enzymes has been analyzed in rats fed a corn oil diet supplemented with cholesterol (Bloj *et al.*, 1973). Cholesterol enrichment was found to increase the sensitivity of acetylcholine esterase to fluoride inhibition, decrease the fluoride sensitivity of the Na, K-ATPase, and cause no change in the fluoride sensitivity of Mg-ATPase. An effect of cholesterol on membrane enzymes is supported by studies of adenylate cyclase activity in human platelets with varying membrane cholesterol content. For example, human platelets which were enriched with cholesterol by incubation with cholesterol-rich lipid dispersion showed a complex effect of cholesterol on the membrane enzyme, adenylate cyclase (Sinha *et al.*, 1977). The basal level of this enzyme was increased two- to three-fold in cholesterol-rich platelets, and the opposite was seen in platelets with a decreased membrane cholesterol content. Moreover, the stimulation of adenylate cyclase which normally occurs with fluoride or with prostaglandin $E_1$ was not observed in cholesterol-rich platelets, and prostaglandin $E_1$ was relatively ineffective in inhibiting platelet aggregation. Effects of membrane cholesterol on membrane enzymes have also been observed in mycoplasma membranes (Rottem *et al.*, 1973a; De Kruyff *et al.*, 1973).

Three general concepts relate to the mechanism of these cholesterol-induced changes in membrane properties. First is the role of cholesterol influence on bulk membrane fluidity. Changes in fluidity may be translated across short distances and influence the range of motion or the potential volume available to a membrane enzyme and its substrate during the enzymatic process. Second is the lipid composition of the immediate environment of the enzyme. Studies with both cytochrome oxidase from mitochondria (Jost *et al.*, 1973) and Ca-ATPase from sarcoplasmic reticulum (Warren *et al.*, 1975) have demonstrated a specific boundary layer, or annulus, of phospholipid. Moreover, it appears that cholesterol is specifically excluded from the annulus in sarcoplasmic reticulum. Therefore, in a manner quite distinct from its bulk influence on membrane fluidity, cholesterol may influence membrane enzymes by directly interacting with these boundary lipids.

A third general mechanism by which the cholesterol content of membranes may influence membrane enzyme and transport properties relates to the potential effect of membrane lipid composition on the position of proteins, such as enzymes, transport proteins, and receptors, in the plane of the membrane. Shinitzky has recently presented evidence which suggests that enrichment of red cell membranes with cholesterol causes an increase in the exposure of membrane proteins to their aqueous environment (Borochov and Shinitzky, 1976; Shinitzky and Rivnay, 1977). If these conclusions can be supported by other techniques, this concept provides a subtle mechanism for the modulation of many membrane events by a primary modulation of membrane lipid composition.

These effects of cholesterol on the permeability and enzymatic properties of membranes emphasize the importance for normal physiology of maintaining membrane cholesterol within narrow limits. Razin has shown that mycoplasma which had been adapted to low levels of membrane cholesterol compensate for this by increasing the amount of unsaturated fatty acids associated with their membrane phospholipids (Rottem *et al.*, 1973b). In contrast, it appears that most mammalian cell membranes adapt poorly when exposed to lipoproteins with an increased C/PL. This is evidenced by the accumulation of cholesterol in the membranes of red cells, platelets, liver cells, and macrophages in animals fed a cholesterol-rich diet, as discussed earlier. These animals also accumulate cholesterol esters in their vessel walls in the form of fatty streaks and atheromatous plaques. The genesis of these lesions is undoubtedly multifactorial, and vessel injury may play an important role. Indeed, it is possible that cholesterol enrichment of endothelial cell membranes may contribute to the process of injury (Ross and Harker, 1976). It is likely that a need exists within cells lining vessel walls to adapt to cholesterol-induced changes in membrane fluidity. Cholesterol esters represent an end product with no functional role. They do serve to divert cholesterol from a form which is available to enter membranes to a form which is excluded from the membrane structure. Cholesterol esterification may represent a form of adaptation to an excess C/PL just as cholesterol synthesis represents an adaptation to a low level of membrane C/PL (Fogelman *et al.*, 1977). Evidence for this mechanism of cholesterol ester accumulation has been derived from studies of mammalian cells in tissue culture in which it has been shown that the rate of cholesterol esterification bears no relation to the cholesterol concentration of the medium, but rather is directly related to the C/PL presented to the cells (Arbogast *et al.*, 1976). Thus, it appears that the elevated C/PL of lipoproteins in various animals fed cholesterol-rich atherogenic diets may call forth an adaptative process by some cells whose membranes have become less fluid due to an increase in membrane cholesterol, and that this adaptative process results in the accumulation of cholesterol esters within such cells.

## 3.8. Sphingomyelin–Lecithin Effects in Red Cells

### 3.8.1. Physical Properties

Lecithin and sphingomyelin represent two of the major lipids in mammalian red cells. Together, they represent the bulk of phospholipid on the exterior surface of the cell. Although the relative amounts of lecithin and sphingomyelin vary, these two phospholipids always represent 50 to 60% of the total membrane phospholipids (Rouser *et al.*, 1968). Moreover, together they account for more than 90% of the phospholipids in plasma. Both contain choline. Using space-filling models, both appear to relate to cholesterol in a similar fashion (Vandenheuvel, 1966). However, in recent years it has become apparent that the physical properties of lecithin and sphingomyelin are quite different (Shinitzky and Barenholz, 1974; Shipley *et al.*, 1974; Cooper *et al.*, 1977a). The fact that these two lipids may not be functionally interchangeable is emphasized by the presence of a lecithinase in sheep red cells which serves to maintain high levels of sphingomyelin and to prevent the entry of lecithin into the membrane (Kramer *et al.*, 1974).

Compared with lecithin from natural sources, sphingomyelin is highly ordered and possesses a low fluidity (Shinitzky and Barenholz, 1974; Cooper *et al.*, 1977a), and in the absence of added cholesterol it undergoes a phase transition upon cooling (Shinitzky and Barenholz, 1974; Shipley *et al.*, 1974). Its high degree of order and low magnitude of fluidity are preserved in the presence of equimolar cholesterol (Cooper *et al.*, 1977a).

Variations in sphingomyelin and lecithin content have been observed in a number of tissues. For example, the sphingomyelin/lecithin ratio rises in association with aging and with atherosclerosis (Small and Shipley, 1974). In contrast, an abrupt fall in the sphingomyelin/lecithin ratio of human pulmonary surfactant lipids occurs during the final days of gestation, coincident with an increase in surfactant fluidity (Shinitzky *et al.*, 1976), and the failure to complete this process prior to birth is associated with a high incidence of the respiratory distress syndrome.

### 3.8.2. Acanthocytes

Red cells in human abetalipoproteinemia (acanthocytes) have a reciprocal increase in sphingomyelin and decrease in lecithin. In a group of patients studied in our laboratory, the sphingomyelin/lecithin ratio was increased from a normal value of 0.85 to an average value of 1.50 (Cooper *et al.*, 1977a). In addition, the cholesterol content of acanthocytes is normal or slightly increased and the total phospholipid content is normal or slightly decreased, leading to an average increase in membrane C/PL of approximately 10% (Cooper and Jandl, 1977). Changes in red cell sphingomyelin and lecithin appear to reflect the changes which exist in the phospholipid composition of HDL, the only plasma lipoprotein in this disorder (Jones and Ways, 1967). Attempts to induce or reverse this red cell abnormality *in vitro* have not been successful, presumably because of the slow exchange processes involving sphingomyelin and lecithin. However, normal red cells transfused into a patient with abetalipoproteinemia acquired the morphologic defect (Frezal *et al.*, 1961).

Recent studies have demonstrated that the fluidity of acanthocyte membranes is decreased and that this results from the presence of excessive amounts of sphingomyelin at the expense of lecithin (Cooper *et al.*, 1977a) (Fig. 3). Conversely, sheep red cells which lack lecithin become more fluid when lecithin is acquired *in vitro* at the expense of sphingomyelin (Borochov *et al.*, 1977). It is of interest to relate these changes in fluidity to the abnormal contour and impaired filterability of acanthocytes

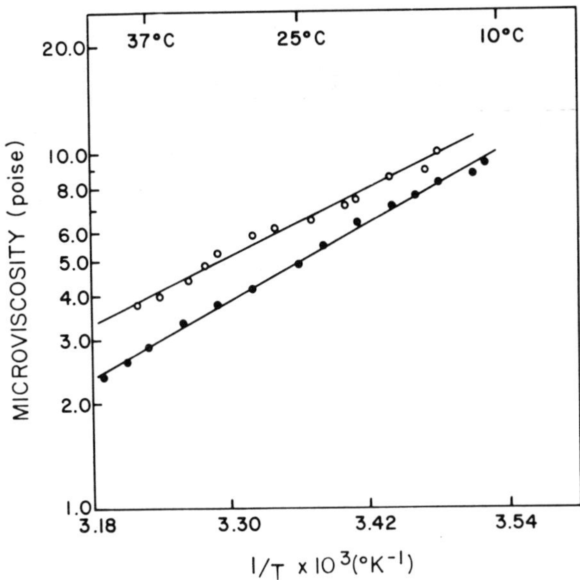

**Fig. 3.** Fluidity of red cell membranes from a patient with abetalipoproteinemia (○) and a normal subject (●). The microviscosity of acanthocytes in abetalipoproteinemia is greater than normal due to their increased sphingomyelin/lecithin ratio. (From Cooper *et al.*, 1977a.)

(McBride and Jacob, 1970; Cooper *et al.*, 1977a) since both findings are characteristic of spur cells as well and since red cell membrane fluidity in both clinical disorders is similar. In contrast to specific physical measurements such as fluidity of lipids or viscoelasticity of proteins, filterability simply measures the deformability of whole red cells as they flow through small orifices which are meant to mimic the spleen filter. Filterability is known to be influenced by cell surface viscosity as well as by hemoglobin viscosity, and it is sensitive to changes in the surface area-to-volume ratio of cells (La Celle, 1970). Since cell surface viscosity is primarily a function of membrane proteins and is influenced only minimally by membrane lipid fluidity, it seems unlikely that decreased deformability of these red cells results from the change in the fluidity of lipids, *per se.* Nor is there reason to believe that the hemoglobin of acanthocytes or spur cells has abnormal physical properties. Finally, when evaluated in terms of osmotic fragility, the surface area-to-volume ratio of both acanthocytes and spur cells is normal. In the case of red cells enriched with cholesterol *in vitro*, the surface area-to-volume ratio is actually increased, a factor which theoretically should aid rather than impair deformability. It is possible that the poor filterability of acanthocytes, spur cells, and cholesterol-enriched red cells is related to the distorted membrane contour which is present under each condition. However, the mechanism by which filterability is decreased in red cells in which membrane fluidity is also decreased remains to be defined.

The sphingomyelin/lecithin ratio of older acanthocytes is greater than that of younger cells (Ways and Dong, 1965), a fact consistent with the genesis of the red cell abnormality through equilibration with plasma lipoproteins. Therefore, the fluidity of older cells is probably less than that of younger cells, and the premature destruction of these older cells may account for the somewhat shortened red cell survival observed in abetalipoproteinemia (Ways *et al.*, 1963; Simon and Ways, 1964). Nonetheless, red cell survival in abetalipoproteinemia is not shortened as profoundly as in spur cell anemia (Silber *et al.*, 1966; Cooper, 1969). As indicated earlier, the spleen conditions spur cells, transforming them from a scalloped contour to a thorny shape and then destroying them. It is likely that the same process affects acanthocytes. However, patients with spur cells have spleens which are congested and hyperplastic, in association with cirrhosis and portal hypertension. In contrast, neither splenomegaly nor portal hypertension is a feature of abetalipoproteinemia, probably explaining the longer survival of these physically similar red cells.

### 3.8.3. Stomatocytes

Effects of sphingomyelin and lecithin on membrane-associated events have not been extensively studied. In a correlative study of K influx in the red cells of various mammalian species, a progressive decrease in K influx was observed in red cells with higher sphingomyelin content and lower lecithin content (Kirk, 1977). Whether these lipids actually play a role in regulating K influx or whether phospholipid composition merely correlates for reasons which are not casually related is as yet unknown. In this regard, we have observed that the K influx of hereditary acanthocytes is within the normal range. However, studies in still another hereditary abnormality of human red cells implicate lecithin and sphingomyelin in the control of monovalent cation transport. This is the syndrome of hereditary stomatocytosis.

Hereditary stomatocytosis, in its broadest definition (Wiley *et al.*, 1975), includes a number of related red cell abnormalities which include, in most patients, an increased cell Na content and decreased K content, increased active transport of Na and K, and an increase in membrane lecithin content (Zarkowsky *et al.*, 1968; Jaffe and Gottfried, 1968; Oski *et al.*, 1969; Honig *et al.*, 1971; Miller *et al.*, 1971, Shohet *et al.*, 1973; Glader *et al.*, 1974; Wiley *et al.*, 1975). Red cells are bowl shaped in wet preparations. On dried smears, those red cells in which the abnormality of K and

Na permeability has led to a net increase in Na + K content take on the appearance of true stomatocytes. In contrast, red cells in which the decrease in K exceeds the increase in Na (therefore causing cellular dehydration) take on the appearance of target cells. In five patients studied in our laboratory, the sphingomyelin/lecithin ratio was decreased from the normal value of 0.85 to 0.72. Although in itself this decrease in sphingomyelin/lecithin did not cause a significant change in the bulk fluidity of the entire membrane, it may have caused critical changes within specific domains of the membrane and these domains may be involved in the regulation of monovalent cation permeability.

## 3.9. Transfer of Cholesterol Plus Lecithin to Red Cells

### 3.9.1. Target Cells

In most patients with liver disease, cholesterol-rich spur cells are not observed. Rather, red cells become targeted in appearance and acquire an excess of both cholesterol and phospholipid in proportional amounts (Cooper *et al.* 1972; Verkleij *et al.*, 1976) (Fig. 4). Patients with various forms of liver disease, including hepatitis, cirrhosis, and obstructive jaundice, have red cells with an increased content of both cholesterol and phospholipid (Cooper and Jandl, 1968; Neerhout, 1968; Westerman *et*

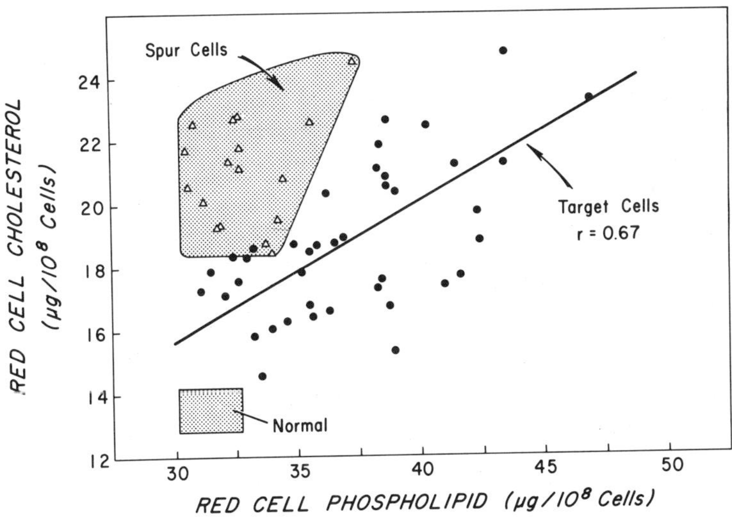



**Fig. 4.** The cholesterol and phospholipid content of red cell membranes from patients with liver disease and either spur cells or target cells. (From Cooper *et al.*, 1972.)

*al.*, 1968). These changes are most striking in patients with obstructive jaundice or with other forms of liver disease with an obstructive component. The cholesterol increase may be as great as 75% but more commonly ranges between 25 and 50% above normal. Although there is variability from patient to patient, the percent increase in phospholipid is approximately 60% of the percent increase in cholesterol, resulting in an increase in the C/PL of approximately 15%. The phospholipid increase is not distributed among the various phospholipids but rather is confined to lecithin. Thus, cholesterol and lecithin are not only the most exchangeable of the major red cell lipids, but their membrane compartments also undergo the greatest quantitative change in liver disease. In several patients with target cells studied by us thus far, membrane fluidity is normal or actually increased slightly as a result of the acquisition of both cholesterol, which tends to decrease fluidity, and lecithin, which is a very fluid lipid.

It is of interest that a similar abnormality in red cells has been observed in patients with a congenital absence of the serum enzyme lecithin–cholesterol acyltransferase (LCAT) (Gjone *et al.*, 1968). LCAT deficiency of a variable degree is also quite common in patients with liver disease. However, we have not been able to find any correlation between the serum LCAT activity of patients with liver disease and the abnormalities of lipids within their red cells (Cooper *et al.*, 1972).

Two processes appear to participate in determining the amounts of cholesterol and lecithin in target cells. First is a process analogous to, if not identical with, the isolated transfer of cholesterol from lipoproteins to red cells as dictated by the C/PL of the lipoprotein. Since the C/PL of LDL in most patients with liver disease is increased only mildly (Cooper *et al.*, 1972), this accounts for only a small amount of the additional membrane cholesterol. However, this process is readily demonstrable *in vitro* (Cooper and Jandl, 1968), and it accounts for the increased C/PL of target cells in liver disease (Cooper *et al.*, 1972).

The larger amount of cholesterol and lecithin which is acquired by red cells may involve an independent transfer of lecithin followed by a process of equilibrium during which the C/PL of the red cell (now transiently decreased because of this added lecithin) comes into equilibrium with the increased C/PL of LDL by means of a transfer of cholesterol from LDL to cells. In this regard, it is of interest that the normal phospholipid/protein weight ratio of LDL is approximately 1.0, but it is increased 25% in patients with liver disease (Cooper *et al.*, 1972). Although an *in vitro* system has not yet been established to test the importance of phospholipid/protein interactions on the transfer of phospholipid from LDL to cell membranes, it appears likely that the elevated phospholipid/protein of LDL in liver disease underlies the increased lecithin content of target cells. The LDL in patients with spur cells also has a high phospholipid/protein ratio and lecithin also accumulates in spur cells. The fact that the total phospholipid content is not increased in spur cells *in vivo* appears to result from a loss of membrane phospholipid together with other membrane components as these red cells are conditioned during circulation *in vivo* (Cooper, 1969; Cooper *et al.*, 1974). Only the relative increase in lecithin compared with other phospholipids remains in spur cells (Cooper *et al.*, 1972). Thus, the total content of cholesterol in red cell membranes appears to be a function of, *first,* the membrane phospholipid content (possibly as influenced by the phospholipid/protein of LDL); *second,* the fraction of phospholipid which is available within each membrane for solubilizing cholesterol (as determined by the amount of membrane phospholipid which is in the form of boundary lipids and other structures strongly related to proteins within the membrane but excluding cholesterol); and *third,* by the C/PL of LDL which is in equilibrium with these membranes.

### 3.9.2. Vesicle Fusion

An alternative mechanism for cholesterol and lecithin accumulation in target cells has been suggested by DeGier and his co-workers (Verkleij *et al.*, 1976). This mechanism takes cognizance of the fact that many patients with liver disease, particularly of the obstructive variety, have a discrete lipoprotein (LP-X) which is discoidal in appearance and which is composed primarily of cholesterol and lecithin in equimolar amounts (Switzer, 1967; Hamilton *et al.*, 1971). Similar structures have been observed in LCAT deficiency (Glomset *et al.*, 1973). De Gier and associates have proposed that these lipoprotein vesicles fuse with the red cell membrane and in this way transfer equivalent quantities of cholesterol and lecithin to the red cell membrane. Moreover, these workers have presented electron micrographs which are interpreted as showing fusion occurring within 2 hr *in vitro*. Although fusion of artificial vesicles with red cells has also been reported, it appears that the presence in the vesicle of a negatively charged phospholipid, such as phosphatidylserine, is an essential requirement for fusion to occur (Papahadjopoulos *et al.*, 1973). Lecithin–cholesterol vesicles in liver disease and in LCAT deficiency are neutral. Furthermore, the time course of lipid acquisition by target cells *in vivo* is slow, with a $T_{1/2}$ of 24 hr, whereas fusion leading to a 15% increase in surface area was observed with LP-X *in vitro* in only 2 hr (Verkleij *et al.*, 1976). Finally, the process of target cells is totally reversible *in vivo* (Cooper and Jandl, 1968), whereas a fusion process would be irreversible. Thus, it appears unlikely that vesicle fusion with red cells represents a major mechanism whereby large excess of lecithin is acquired by target cells, and direct transfer of lecithin, followed by equilibration with cholesterol, appears more likely. Further work is needed to resolve this problem.

## 3.10. Other Red Cell Membrane Abnormalities

### 3.10.1. Hereditary Spherocytosis

Abnormalities in red cell membrane lipid composition or fluidity have been described in several other human diseases. One disorder studied extensively is hereditary spherocytosis. Membrane lipid content is decreased in this disorder (Cooper and Jandl, 1969). This is most readily evaluated in patients who have previously undergone splenectomy, since reticulocytes are rich in lipid and their presence in large numbers makes quantitation of membrane lipids difficult to interpret. Following splenectomy, hereditary spherocytosis red cells have approximately 15% less cholesterol and phospholipid than otherwise normal red cells in individuals who have undergone splenectomy. Although a report to the contrary exists (Aloni *et al.*, 1975), we have found that the fluidity of hereditary spherocytosis red cells is normal both before and after splenectomy (Leslie *et al.*, 1978). This is to be anticipated, since fluidity is a function of lipid composition, and although total lipids are decreased in hereditary spherocytosis red cells, the relative amounts of the various lipids are normal.

### 3.10.2. Membrane Lipid Oxidation

Membrane lipids are subject to damage by oxidative processes within the red cell. Most sensitive are the polyunsaturated fatty acids which are usually present in all phospholipids but particularly in phosphatidylethanolamine. When Vitamin E is deficient, lipid peroxidation is readily demonstrated *in vitro* (Dodge *et al.*, 1967). This is striking in patients with abetalipoproteinemia, since they are both deficient in vitamin E and possess an increased quantity of polyunsaturated fatty acids in their red cell membranes. Similar patterns of lipid peroxidation involving phosphatidylethanolamine and, to a lesser extent, phosphatidylserine have been demonstrated in vitamin E-deficient animals (Dodge *et al.*, 1967). We have observed that peroxidation of membrane lipids under these conditions leads to a decrease in membrane fluidity.

The classical oxidative disease is glucose-6-phosphate dehydrogenase (G6PD) deficiency. Although a great deal is known about the oxidation of cellular protein in this disorder, the role of lipid oxidation in the hemolytic process is uncertain. However, a disorder in which the oxidation of membrane lipids is known to occur is erythropoietic protoporphyria

(Lamola *et al.*, 1973). It appears that the photoactivation of porphyrins within the membrane gives rise to a long-lived species of singlet oxygen which is capable of oxidizing cholesterol to cholesterol hydroperoxide (Lamola *et al.*, 1973; Suwa *et al.*, 1977).

### 3.10.3. Muscle Disorders

Abnormalities of red cell membrane fluidity have also been described in patients and experimental animals with muscular disorders. For example, membrane fluidity is increased in red cells from patients with both myotonic muscular dystrophy and congenital myotonia, but not in Duchenne muscular dystrophy (Butterfield *et al.*, 1976). Fluidity is also increased in muscle membranes from mice with congenital muscular dystrophy (Rubsamen *et al.*, 1976), whereas it is decreased in muscular dystrophic chicks (Sha'afi *et al.*, 1975). In chicks, this decrease in fluidity correlates with an elevated membrane C/PL. It is of interest in this regard that the accumulation of desmosterol in man and in animals fed 20,25-diazacholesterol is associated with the development of myotonia (Peter and Fiehn, 1973) and red cells in such animals manifest an increase in membrane fluidity (Butterfield and Watson, 1977).

## 3.11. Conclusion

The organization of lipids in cell membranes requires specific molecular interactions. Many cell processes occur within the fluid environment created by these membrane lipids. As evolution has proceeded from prokaryotes to eukaryotes and from poikilotherms to homeotherms, cells have developed a decreased tolerance for fluctuations in membrane fluidity. Adaptative mechanisms have developed in order to maintain a normal cell membrane fluidity under conditions which might cause it to change, such as variations in the lipid composition or temperature of the cell's environment. Disease states result when human cells fail to adapt. Red cells are particularly vulnerable to abnormalities in membrane fluidity since they lack specific adaptive mechanisms of their own and must depend for adaptation on the lipid composition of plasma lipoproteins.

ACKNOWLEDGMENT

The author's studies were supported by research grant AM-15541 from the National Institutes of Health.

## References


Aloni, B., Shinitzky, M., Moses, S., and Livne, A., 1975, Elevated microviscosity in membranes of erythrocytes affected by hereditary spherocytosis, *Br. J. Haematol.* **31**:117.

Arbogast, L. Y., Rothblat, G. H., Leslie, M. H., and Cooper, R. A., 1976, Cellular cholesterol ester accumulation induced by free cholesterol-rich lipid dispersions, *Proc. Natl. Acad. Sci. U.S.A.* **73**:3680.

Ashworth, L. A. E., and Green, C., 1964, The transfer of lipids between human α-lipoprotein and erythrocytes, *Biochim. Biophys. Acta* **84**:182.

Baranska, J., and Wlodawer, P., 1969, Influence of temperature on the composition of fatty acids and on lipogenesis in frog tissues, *Comp. Biochem. Physiol.* **28**:553.

Basford, J. M., Glover, J., and Green, C., 1964, Exchange of cholesterol between human β-lipoproteins and erythrocytes, *Biochim. Biophys. Acta* **84**:764.

Bell, F. P., 1975, Cholesterol exchange between microsomal, mitochondrial and erythrocyte membranes and its enhancement by cytosol, *Biochim. Biophys. Acta* **398**:18.

Bloj, B., and Zilversmit, D. B., 1976, Asymmetry and transposition rates of phosphatidylcholine in rat erythrocyte ghosts, *Biochemistry* **15**:1277.

Bloj, B., Morero, R. D., and Farias, R. N., 1973, Membrane fluidity cholesterol and allosteric transitions of membrane-bound $Mg^{2+}$-ATPase, $(Na^+ + K^+)$-ATPase and acetylcholinesterase from rat erythrocytes, *FEBS Lett.* **38**:101.

Borochov, H., and Shinitzky, M., 1976, Vertical displacement of membrane proteins mediated by changes in microviscosity, *Proc. Natl. Acad. Sci. U.S.A.* **73**:4526.

Borochov, H., Zahler, P., Wilbrandt, W., and Shinitzky, M., 1977, The effect of lecithin-to-spingomyelin male ratio on the dynamic properties of sheep erythrocyte membranes, *Biochim. Biophys. Acta* **470**:382.

Bourgès, M., Small, D. M., and Dervichian, D. G., 1967, Biophysics of lipidic associations II. The ternary systems cholesterol-lecithin-water, *Biochim. Biophys. Acta* **137**:157.

Bretscher, M. S., 1972, Asymmetrical lipid bilayer structure for biological membranes, *Nature New Biol.* **236**:11.

Butterfield, D. A., and Watson, W. E., 1977, Electron spin resonance studies of an animal model of human congenital myotonia: Increased erythrocyte membrane fluidity in rats with 20,25-diazacholesterol-induced myotonia, *J. Membrane Biol.* **32**:165.

Butterfield, D. A., Chesnut, D. B., Appel, S. H., and Roses, A. D., 1976, Spin label study of erythrocyte membrane fluidity in myotonic and Duchenne muscular dystrophy and congenital myotonia, *Nature* **263**:159.

Chapman, D., 1968, Recent physical studies of phospholipids and natural membranes, *in Biological Membranes: Physical Fact and Function* (D. Chapman, ed.), pp. 125–202, Academic Press, New York.

Cooper, R. A., 1969, Anemia with spur cells: A red cell defect acquired in serum and modified in the circulation, *J. Clin. Invest.* **48**:1820.

Cooper, R. A., 1970, Lipids of human red cell membrane: Normal composition and variability in disease, *Semin. Hematol.* **7**:296.

Cooper, R. A., and Jandl, J. H., 1968, Bile salts and cholesterol in the pathogenesis of target cells in obstructive jaundice, *J. Clin. Invest.* **47**:809.

Cooper, R. A., and Jandl, J. H., 1969, The role of membrane lipids in the survival of red cells in hereditary spherocytosis, *J. Clin. Invest.* **48**:736.

Cooper, R. A., and Jandl, J. H., 1977, Acanthocytosis, *in Hematology* (W. Williams, E. Beutler, A. J. Erslev, and R. W. Rundles, eds.), pp. 461–465, McGraw-Hill, New York.

Cooper, R. A., Diloy-Puray, M., Lando, P., and Greenberg, M. S., 1972, An analysis of lipoproteins, bile acids, and red cell membranes associated with target cells and spur cells in patients with liver disease, *J. Clin. Invest.* **51**:3182.

Cooper, R. A., Kimball, D. B., and Durocher, J. R., 1974, Role of the spleen in membrane conditioning and hemolysis of spur cells in liver disease, *N. Engl. J. Med.* **290**:1279.

Cooper, R. A., Arner, E. C., Wiley, J. S., and Shattil, S. J., 1975, Modification of red cell membrane structure by cholesterol-rich lipid dispersions, *J. Clin. Invest.* **55**:115.

Cooper, R. A., Durocher, J. R., and Leslie, M. H., 1977a, Decreased fluidity of red cell membrane lipids in abetalipoproteinemia, *J. Clin. Invest.* **60**:115.

Cooper, R. A., Leslie, M. H., Knight, D., Shattil, S. J., and Detweiler, D. K., 1977b, Decreased fluidity of red cell membrane lipids in dogs fed an atherogenic diet, *Clin. Res.* **25**:454A.

Cooper, R. A., Leslie, M. H., Fischkoff, S., Shinitzky, M., and Shattil, S. J., 1978, Factors influencing the lipid composition and fluidity of red cell membranes *in vitro:* Production of red cells possessing more than two cholesterols per phospholipid, *Biochemistry* **17**:327.

Cronan, J. E., Jr., and Gelmann, E. P., 1975, Physical properties of membrane lipids: Biological relevance and regulation, *Bacteriol. Rev.* **39**:232.

Deckelbaum, R. J., Shipley, G. G., Small, D. M., Lees, R. S., and George, P. K., 1975, Thermal transitions in human plasma low density lipoproteins, *Science* **190**:392.

De Gier, J., Mandersloot, J. G., and Van Deenen, L. L. M., 1968, Lipid composition and permeability of liposomes, *Biochim. Biophys. Acta* **150**:666.

De Kruyff, B., Van Dijck, P. W. M., Goldbach, R. W., Demel, R. A., and Van Deenen, L. L. M., 1973, Influence of fatty acid and sterol composition on the lipid phase transition and activity of membrane-bound enzymes in *Acholeplasma laidlawii, Biochim. Biophys. Acta* **330**:269.

Demel, R. A., and De Kruyff, B., 1976, The function of sterols in membranes, *Biochim. Biophys. Acta* **457**:109.

Demel, R. A., Bruckdorfer, K. R., and Van Deenen, L. L. M., 1972, Structural requirements of sterols for the interaction with lecithin at the air-water interface, *Biochim. Biophys. Acta* **255**:311.

Demel, R. A., Jansen, J. W. C. M., Van Dijck, P. W. M., and Van Deenen, L. L. M., 1977, The preferential interaction of cholesterol with different classes of phospholipids, *Biochim. Biophys. Acta* **465**:1.

Deuticke, B., and Ruska, C., 1976, Changes of nonelectrolyte permeability in cholesterol-loaded erythrocytes, *Biochim. Biophys. Acta* **433**:638.

Dianzani, M. U., Torrielli, M. V., Canuto, R. A., Garcea, R., and Feo, F., 1976, The influence of enrichment with cholesterol on the phagocytic activity of rat macrophages, *J. Pathol.* **118**:193.

Dodge, J. T., Cohen, G., Kayden, H. J., and Phillips, G. B., 1967, Peroxidative hemolysis of red blood cells from patients with abetalipoproteinemia (acanthocytosis), *J. Clin. Invest.* **46**:357.

Emerson, C. P., Jr., Shen, S. C., Ham, T. H., Fleming, E. M., and Castle, W. B., 1956, Studies on the destruction of red blood cells. IX. Quantitative methods for determining the osmotic and mechanical fragility of red cells in the peripheral blood and splenic pulp; the mechanism of increased hemolysis in hereditary spherocytosis (congenital hemolytic jaundice) as related to the functions of the spleen, *Arch. Intern. Med.* **97**:1.

Evans, E. A., and Hochmuth, R. M., 1977, A solid-liquid composite model of the red cell membrane, *J. Membrane Biol.* **30**:351.

Farkas, T., and Herodek, S., 1964, The effect of environmental temperature on the fatty acid composition of crustacean plankton, *J. Lipid Res.* **5**:369.

Feinstein, M. B., Fernandez, S. M., and Sha'afi, R. I., 1975, Fluidity of natural membranes and phosphatidylserine and ganglioside dispersions. Effects of local anesthetics, cholesterol and protein, *Biochim. Biophys. Acta* **413**:354.

Fogelman, A. B., Seager, J., Edwards, P. A., and Popjak, G., 1977, Mechanism of induction of 3-hydroxy-3-methylglutaryl coenzyme A reductase in human leukocytes, *J. Biol. Chem.* **265**:644.

Freeman, R., and Finean, J. B., 1975, Cholesterol:lecithin association at molecular ratios of up to 2:1, *Chem. Phys. Lipids* **14**:313.

Frezal, J., Rey, J., Polonovski, J., Levy, G., and Lamy, M., 1961, L'absence congénitale de β-lipoprotéins: Etude de l'absorption des graisses après exsanguino-transfusion mesuré de la demi-vie des β-lipoprotéins injectées, *Rev. Fr. Clin. Biol.* **6**:677.

Gennis, R. B., and Jonas, A., 1977, Protein-lipid interactions, *Annu. Rev. Biophys. Bioeng.* **6**:195.

Giraud, F., Claret, M., and Garay, R., 1976, Interactions of cholesterol with the Na pump in red blood cells, *Nature* **264**:646.

Gjone, E., Torsvik, H., and Norum, K. R., 1968, Familial plasma cholesterol ester deficiency, *Scand. J. Clin. Lab. Invest.* **21**:327.

Glader, B. E., Fortier, N., Albala, M. M., and Nathan, D. G., 1974, Congenital hemolytic anemia associated with dehydrated erythrocytes and increased potassium loss, *N. Engl. J. Med.* **291**:491.

Glomset, J. A., Nichols, A. V., Norum, K. R., King, W., and Forte, T., 1973, Plasma lipoproteins in familial lecithin: Cholesterol acyltranferase deficiency, *J. Clin. Invest.* **52**:1078.

Goldman, S. S., 1975, Cold resistance of the brain during hibernation. III. Evidence of a lipid adaptation, *Am. J. Phys.* **228**:834.

Gould, R. G., Le Roy, G. V., Okita, G. T., Kabara, J. J., Keegan, P., and Bergenstal, D. B., 1955, The use of $C^{14}$-labeled acetate to study cholesterol metabolism in man, *J. Lab. Clin. Med.* **46**:372.

Grandison, A. S., and Green, C., 1976, Cholesterol in plasma-membrane subfractions from livers of control and cholesterol-fed guinea pigs, *Biochem. Soc. Trans.* **4**:645.

Grunze, M., and Deuticke, B., 1974, Changes of membrane permeability due to extensive cholesterol depletion in mammalian erythrocytes, *Biochim. Biophys. Acta* **356**:125.

Hagerman, J. S., and Gould, R. G., 1951, The *in vitro* interchange of cholesterol between plasma and red cells, *Proc. Soc. Exp. Biol. Med.* **78**:329.

Hamilton, R. L., Havel, R. J., Kane, J. P., Blaurock, A. E., and Sata, T., 1971, Cholestasis: Lamellar structure of the abnormal human serum lipoprotein, *Science* **172**:475.

Honig, G. R., Lacsow, P. S., and Maurer, H. S., 1971, A new familial disorder with abnormal erythrocyte morphology and increased permeability of the erythrocytes to sodium and potassium, *Pediatr. Res.* **5**:159.

Horwitz, C., Krut, L., and Kaminsky, L., 1971, Cholesterol uptake by egg-yolk phosphatidylcholine, *Biochim. Biophys. Acta* **239**:329.

Huang, C.-H., 1977, A structural model for the cholesterol-phosphatidylcholine complexes in bilayer membranes, *Lipids* **12**:348.

Ip, S. H., Pomazon, J. B., and Cooper, R. A., 1978, Decreased fluidity of lymphocyte membranes induced by cholesterol, *Clin. Res.* **26**:505A.

Jaffe, E. R., and Gottfried, E. L., 1968, Hereditary non-spherocytic hemolytic disease associated with an altered phospholipid composition of the erythrocytes, *J. Clin. Invest.* **47**:1375.

Jones, J. W., and Ways, P., 1967, Abnormalities of high density lipoproteins in abetalipoproteinemia, *J. Clin. Invest.* **46**:1151.

Jost, P. C., Griffith, O. H., Capaldi, R. A., and Vanderkooi, G., 1973, Evidence for boundary lipid in membranes, *Proc. Natl. Acad. Sci. U.S.A.* **70**:480.

Kahlenberg, A., Walker, C., and Rohrlick, R., 1974, Evidence for an asymmetric distribution of phospholipids in the human erythrocyte membrane, *Can. J. Biochem.* **52**:803.

Keith, A. D., Aloia, R. C., Lyons, J., Snipes, W., and Pengelley, E. T., 1975, Spin label evidence for the role of lysoglycerophosphatides in cellular membranes of hibernating mammals, *Biochim. Biophys. Acta* **394**:204.

Kirk, R. G., 1977, Potassium transport and lipid composition in mammalian red blood cell membranes, *Biochim. Biophys. Acta* **464**:157.

Kitajima, Y., and Thompson, G. A., Jr., 1977, Tetrahymèna strives to maintain the fluidity interrelationships of all its membranes constant, *J. Cell Biol.* **72**:744.

Knipprath, W. G., and Mead, J. F., 1966, Influence of temperature on the fatty acid pattern of mosquito fish *(Gumbusia affinis)* and guppies *(Legistes reticulatus)*, *Lipids* **1**:113.

Kramer, R., Jungi, B., and Zahler, P., 1974, Some characteristics of a phospholipase $A_2$ from sheep red cell membranes, *Biochim. Biophys. Acta* **373**:404.

Krivit, W., and Kern, L., 1969, Intravascular membrane dehiscence of red cell: Model survival curve using glycolipid labeled with $C^{14}$ glucose in rabbits, *Blood* **34**:858.

Kroes, J., and Ostwald, R., 1971, Erythrocyte membranes—Effect of increased cholesterol content on permeability, *Biochim. Biophys. Acta* **249**:647.

Kroes, J., Ostwald, R., and Keith, A., 1972, Erythrocyte membranes—Compression of lipid phases by increased cholesterol content, *Biochim. Biophys. Acta* **274**:71.

La Celle, P. L., 1970, Alterations of membrane deformability in hemolytic anemias, *Semin. Hematol.* **7**:355.

Lamola, A. A., Yamane, T., and Trozzolo, A. M., 1973, Cholesterol hydroperoxide formation in red cell membranes and photohemolysis in erythropoietic protoporphyria, *Science* **179**:1131.

Lang, M., 1976, Dietary cholesterol caused modification in the structure and function of rat hepatic microsomes, studied by fluorescent probes, *Biochim. Biophys. Acta* **455**:947.

Lange, Y., Cohen, C. M., and Poznansky, M. J., 1977, Transmembrane movement of cholesterol in human erythrocytes, *Proc. Natl. Acad. Sci. U.S.A.* **74**:1538.

Leslie, M. H., Gill, F., and Cooper, R. A., 1978, Fluidity of hereditary spherocytosis red cell membranes is normal, *Clin. Res.* **26**:351A.

London, I. M., and Schwartz, H., 1953, Erythrocyte metabolism. The metabolic behavior of the cholesterol of human erythrocytes, *J. Clin. Invest.* **32**:1248.

Marcus, D. M., and Cass, L. E., 1969, Glycosphingolipids with Lewis blood group activity: Uptake by human erythrocytes, *Science* **164**:553.

Marinetti, G. V., 1977, Arrangement of phosphatidylserine and phosphatidylethanolamine in the erythrocyte membrane, *Biochim. Biophys. Acta* **465**:198.

McBride, J. A., and Jacob, H. S., 1970, Abnormal kinetics of red cell membrane cholesterol in acanthocytosis: Studies in genetic and experimental abetalipoproteinemia and in spur cell anemia. *Br. J. Haematol.* **18**:383.

McElhaney, R. N., and Souza, K. A., 1976, The relationship between environmental temperature, cell growth and the fluidity and physical state of the membrane lipids in *Bacillus stearothermophilus, Biochim. Biophys. Acta* **443**:348.

McMurchie, E. J., and Raison, J. K., 1975, Hibernation and homeothermic status of the echidna *(Tachyglossus aculeatus), J. Thermal Biol.* **1**:113.

Miller, D. R., Rickles, F. R., Lichtman, M. A., LaCelle, P. L., Bates, J., and Weed, R. I., 1971, A new variant of hereditary hemolytic anemia with stomatocytosis and erythrocyte cation abnormality, *Blood* **38**:184.

Mulder, E., Van den Berg, J. W. O., and Van Deenen, L. L. M., 1965, Metabolism of red cell lipids. II. Conversions of lysophosphoglycerides, *Biochim. Biophys. Acta* **106**:118.

Murphy, J. R., 1962, Erythrocyte metabolism. IV. Equilibration of cholesterol-4-$C^{14}$ between erythrocytes and variously treated sera, *J. Lab. Clin. Med.* **60**:571.

Neerhout, R. C., 1968, Abnormalities of erythrocyte stromal lipids in hepatic disease: Erythrocyte stromal lipids in hyperlipemic states, *J. Lab. Clin. Med.* **71**:438.

Nes, W. R., 1974, Role of sterols in membranes, *Lipids* **9**:596.

Oliveria, M. M., and Vaughan, M., 1964, Incorporation of fatty acids into phospholipids of erythrocyte membranes, *J. Lipid Res.* **5**:156.

Oski, F. A., Naiman, J. L., Blum, S. F., Zarkowsky, H. S., Whaun, J., Shohet, S. B., Green, A., and Nathan, D. G., 1969, Congenital hemolytic anemia with high-sodium, low-potassium red cells, *N. Engl. J. Med.* **280**:909.

Papahadjopoulos, D., Poste, G., and Schaeffer, B. E., 1973, Fusion of mammalian cells by unilamellar lipid vesicles: Influence of lipid surface charge, fluidity and cholesterol, *Biochim. Biophys. Acta* **323**:23.

Peter, J. B., and Fiehn, W., 1973, Diazacholesterol myotonia: Accumulation of demosterol and increased adenosine triphosphatase activity of sarcolemma, *Science* **179**:910.

Pittman, J. G., and Martin, D. B., 1966, Fatty acid biosynthesis in human erythrocytes: Evidence in mature erythrocytes for an incomplete long chain fatty acid synthesizing system, *J. Clin. Invest.* **45**:165.

Reed, C. F., 1968, Phospholipid exchange between plasma and erythrocytes in man and the dog. *J. Clin. Invest.* **47**:749.

Ross, R., and Harker, L., 1976, Hyperlipidemia and atherosclerosis, *Science* **193**:1094.

Rothman, J. E., and Engelman, D. M., 1972, Molecular mechanism for the interaction of phospholipid with cholesterol, *Nature New Biol.* **237**:42.

Rothman, J. E., and Lenard, J., 1977, Membrane asymmetry, *Science* **195**:743.

Rottem, S., Cirillo, V. P., De Kruyff, B., Shinitzky, M., and Razin, S., 1973a, Cholesterol in mycoplasma membranes: Correlation of enzymic and transport activities with physical state of lipids in membranes of *Mycoplasma mycoides* var. *capri* adapted to grow with low cholesterol concentrations, *Biochim. Biophys. Acta* **323**:509.

Rottem, S., Yashouv, J., Ne'eman, Z., and Razin, S., 1973b, Cholesterol in mycoplasma membranes: Composition. Ultrastructure and biological properties of membranes from *Mycoplasma mycoides* var. *capri* cells adapted to grow with low cholesterol concentrations, *Biochim. Biophys. Acta* **323**:495.

Rouser, G., Nelson, G. J., Fleischer, S., and Simon G., 1968. Lipid composition of animal cell membranes, organelles and organs, *in Biological Membranes* (D. Chapman, ed.), pp. 6–69, Academic Press, New York.

Rousselet, A., Guthmann, C., Matricon, J., Bienvenue, A., and Devaux, P. F., 1976, Study of the transverse diffusion of spin labeled phospholipids in biological membranes. I. Human red blood cells, *Biochim. Biophys. Acta* **426**:357.

Rubsamen, H., Barald, P., and Podleski, T., 1976, A specific decrease of the fluorescence depolarization of perylene in muscle membranes from mice with muscular dystrophy, *Biochim. Biophys. Acta* **455**:767.

Salen, G., and Grundy, S. M., 1973, The metabolism of cholestanol, cholesterol, and bile acids in cerebrotendinous xanthomatosis, *J. Clin. Invest.* **52**:2822.

Salen, G., Ahrens, E. H., Jr., and Grundy, S. M., 1970, Metabolism of $\beta$-sitosterol in man, *J. Clin. Invest.* **49**:952.

Sardet, C., Hansma, H., and Ostwald, R., 1972, Effects of plasma lipoproteins from control and cholesterol-fed guinea pigs on red cell morphology and cholesterol content: An *in vitro* study, *J. Lipid Res.* **13**:705.

Sha'afi, R. I., Rodan, S. B., Hintz, R. I., Fernandez, S. M., and Rodan, G. A., 1975, Abnormalities in membrane microviscosity and ion transport in genetic muscular dystrophy, *Nature* **254**:525.

Shattil, S. J., and Cooper, R. A., 1972, Maturation of macroreticulocyte membranes *in vito, J. Lab. Clin. Med.* **79**:215.

Shattil, S. J., Cines, D. B., and Schreiber, A. D., 1977, Membrane events during human antibody and complement-mediated platelet injury, *Clin. Res.* **25**:347A.

Sheetz, M. P., Painter, R. G., and Singer, S. J., 1976, Biological membranes as bilayer couples. III. Compensatory shape changes induced in membranes, *J. Cell Biol.* **70**:193.

Shimshick, E. J., and McConnell, H. M., 1973, Lateral phase separation in phospholipid membranes, *Biochemistry* **12**:2351.

Shinitzky, M., and Barenholz, Y., 1974, Dynamics of the hydrocarbon layer in layer in liposomes of lecithin and sphingomyelin containing diacetylphosphate, *J. Biol. Chem.* **249**:2652.

Shinitzky, M., and Inbar, M., 1976, Microviscosity parameters and protein mobility in biological membranes, *Biochim. Biophys. Acta* **433**:133.

Shinitzky, M., and Rivnay, B., 1977, Degree of exposure of membrane proteins determined by fluorescence quenching, *Biochemistry* **16**:982.

Shinitzky, M., Goldfisher, A., Bruck, A., Goldman, B., Stern, E., Barkai, G., Mashiach, S., and Serr, D. M., 1976, A new method for assessment of fetal lung maturity, *Br. J. Obstet. Gynaecol.* **83**:838.

Shipley, G. G., Avecilla, L. S., and Small, D. M., 1974, Phase behavior and structure of aqueous dispersions of sphingomyelin, *J. Lipid Res.* **15**:124.

Shohet, S. B., Nathan, D. G., and Karnovsky, M. L., 1968, Stages in the incorporation of fatty acids into red blood cells, *J. Clin. Invest.* **47**:1096.

Shohet, S. B., Nathan, D. G., Livermore, B. M., Feig, S. A., and Jaffe, E. R., 1973, Hereditary hemolytic anemia associated with abnormal membrane lipid. II. Ion permeability and transport abnormalities, *Blood* **42**:1.

Silber, R., Amorosi, E., Lhowe, J., and Kayden, H. J., 1966, Spur-shaped erythrocytes in Laennec's cirrhosis, *J. Engl. J. Med.* **275**:639.

Simon, E. R., and Ways, P., 1964, Incubation hemolysis and red cell metabolism in acanthocytosis, *J. Clin. Invest.* **43**:1311.

Sinensky, M., 1974, Homeoviscous adaptation: A homeostatic process that regulates the viscosity of membrane lipids in *Escherichia coli, Proc. Natl. Acad. Sci. U.S.A.* **71**:522.

Sinha, A. K., Shattil, S. J., and Colman, R. W., 1977, Cyclic AMP metabolism in cholesterol-rich platelets, *J. Biol. Chem.* **252**:3310.

Small, D. M., and Shipley, G. G., 1974, Physical-chemical basis of lipid deposition in atherosclerosis, *Science* **185**:222.

Suwa, K., Kimura, T., and Schaap, A. P., 1977, Reactivity of singlet molecular oxygen with cholesterol in a phospholipid membrane matrix. A model for oxidative damage of membranes, *Biochem. Biophys. Res.* **75**:785.

Sweeley, C. C., and Dawson, G., 1969, Lipids of the erythrocyte, *in Red Cell Membrane Structure and Function* (G. A. Jamieson and T. J. Greenwalt, eds.), pp. 172–197, Lippincott, Philadelphia.

Switzer, S., 1967, Plasma lipoproteins in liver disease. I. Immunologically distinct low-density lipoproteins in patients with biliary obstruction, *J. Clin. Invest.* **46**:1855.

Tanaka, K.-I., and Ohnishi, S.-I., 1976, Heterogeneity in the fluidity of intact erythrocyte membrane and its homogenization upon hemolysis, *Biochim. Biophys. Acta* **426**:218.

Tarlov, A. R., and Mulder, E., 1967, Phospholipid metabolism in rat erythrocytes: Quantitative studies of lecithin biosynthesis, *Blood* **30**:853.

Vandenheuvel, F. A., 1966, Lipid-protein interactions and cohesional forces in the lipoprotein systems of membranes, *J. Am. Oil Chem.* **43**:258.

Vanderkooi, J., Fischkoff, S., Chance, B., and Cooper, R. A., 1974, Fluorescent probe analysis of the lipid architecture of natural and experimental cholesterol-rich membranes, *Biochemistry* **13**:1589.

Van Dijck, P. W. M., De Kruijff, B., Van Deenen, L. L. M., De Gier, J., and Demel, R. A., 1976, The preference of cholesterol for phosphatidylcholine in mixed phosphatidylcholine-phosphatidylethanolamine bilayers, *Biochim. Biophys. Acta* **455**:576.

Van Zoelen, E. J. J., Zwaal, R. F. A., Reuvers, F. A. M., Demel, R. A., and Van Deenen, L. L. M., 1977, Evidence for the preferential interaction of glycophorin with negatively charged phospholipids, *Biochim. Biophys. Acta* **464**:482.

Verkleij, A. J., Zwaal, R. F. A., Roelofsen, B., Comfurius P., Kastelijn, D., and Van Deenen, L. L. M., 1973, The asymmetric distribution of phospholipids in the human red cell membrane: A combined study using phospholipases and freeze-etch electron microscopy, *Biochim. Biophys. Acta* **323**:178.

Verkleij, A. J., Nauta, I. L. D., Werre, J. M., Mandersloot, J. G., Reinders, B., Ververgaert, P. H. J. Th., and De Gier, J., 1976, The fusion of abnormal plasma lipoprotein (LP-X) and the erythrocyte membrane in patients with cholestasis studied by electronmicroscopy, *Biochim. Biophys. Acta* **436**:366.

Warren, G. B., Houslay, M. D., Metcalfe, J. C., and Birdsall, N. J. M., 1975, Cholesterol is excluded from the phospholipid annulus surrounding an active calcium transport protein, *Nature* **255**:684.

Ways, P., and Dong, D., 1965, Etiology of the RBC phospholipid abnormalities in abetalipoproteinemia, *Clin. Res.* **13**:283.

Ways, P., Reed, C. F., and Hanahan, D. J., 1963, Red cell and plasma lipids in acanthocytosis, *J. Clin. Invest.* **42**:1248.

Westerman, M. P., Balcerzak, S. P., and Heinle, E. W., Jr., 1968, Red cell lipids in Zieve's syndrome: Their relation to hemolysis and to red cell osmotic fragility, *J. Lab. Clin. Med.* **72**:663.

Westerman, M. P., Wiggans, R. G., III, and Mao, R., 1970, Anemia and hypercholesterolemia in cholesterol-fed rabbits, *J. Lab. Clin. Med.* **75**:893.

Wiley, J. S., and Cooper, R. A., 1975, Inhibition of cation cotransport by cholesterol enrichment of human red cell membranes, *Biochim. Biophys. Acta* **413**:425.

Wiley, J. S., Ellory, J. C., Shuman, M. A., Shaller, C. C., and Cooper, R. A., 1975, Characteristics of the membrane defect in the hereditary stomatocytosis syndrome, *Blood* **46**:337.

Zarkowsky, H. S., Oski, F. A., Sha'afi, R., Shohet, S. B., and Nathan, D. G., 1968, Congenital hemolytic anemia with high sodium, low potassium red cells. I. Studies of membrane permeability, *N. Engl. J. Med.* **278**:573.

# Hemoglobin Switching in Sheep and Man

## Neal S. Young and Arthur W. Nienhuis

## 4.1. Introduction

Hemoglobin switching is the regulated replacement of one hemoglobin type by another in the peripheral blood of an animal. During the normal development of most animals, selective expression of individual globin genes results in the sequential appearance of different hemoglobin types—embryonic, fetal, and adult. Globin gene expression may be viewed as a mammalian regulatory system with possible analogy to the better understood regulatory mechanisms of lower animals, such as bacteria and phage viruses. The approach to globin gene regulation at the molecular level has extended understanding of important events of protein synthesis in higher animals, although many features responsible for the pattern of hemoglobin switching have remained elusive. Regulation of the individual globin genes is far more complex than the selective expression of genes in prokaryotic cells since the globin genes are expressed in a cellular system, the erythron, which is characterized by continual proliferation, differentiation, and maturation of cells. Current evidence indicates that commitment to expression of particular globin genes may occur in

NEAL S. YOUNG and ARTHUR W. NIENHUIS • Clinical Hematology Branch, National Heart, Lung, and Blood Institute, National Institutes of Health, Bethesda, Maryland 20014.

early progenitor cells, while synthesis of specific globin mRNAs occurs in maturing erythroblasts. The recent development of adequate cell culture techniques for erythroid tissues has promoted the study of regulation at the cellular level, allowing an analytical approach to this problem.

This chapter emphasizes both studies at the molecular level, which are directed toward understanding why particular genes are expressed in maturing erythroblasts, and studies at the cellular level, which have led to the concept that commitment to expression of particular globin genes occurs during earlier erythroid cell differentiation. Two well-studied hemoglobin switching models, the Hb A to Hb C switch induced by anemia in sheep and goats, and the Hb F to Hb A switch in higher animals, particularly man, form the basis for our discussion. The switching model in sheep and goats is particularly useful since induction of Hb C synthesis can be accomplished routinely both *in vitro* and *in vivo* by elevating the concentration of erythropoietin. Hb F synthesis in man is clearly of clinical relevance. It also has provided a major body of useful information through detailed hematological and genetic analysis of the hereditary syndromes characterized by persistent synthesis of fetal hemoglobin in adult life.

## 4.2. Multiple Globin Genes in Man and Sheep

The genomes of higher organisms contain sequences encoding for several closely related globins. The globin genes in men and sheep and the relevant hemoglobin switches, which occur because of differential expression of these genes, are outlined in Fig. 1. In general, there are two types of globins: $\alpha$-globin, which is synthesized continuously from early intrauterine life, and non-$\alpha$-globins, the differential synthesis of which forms the basis for the various hemoglobin switching phenomena. In addition there are genes for various embryonic globins expressed early in gestation in primitive yolk sac erythroblasts. The relationship of these embryonic genes to the $\alpha$ genes and the non-$\alpha$ complex remains unknown.

In human cells, the $\alpha$- and non-$\alpha$-globin genes are known to be on separate chromosomes (Deisseroth *et al.*, 1976); the $\alpha$ genes are on chromosome 16 (Deisseroth *et al.*, 1977) and non-$\alpha$-globin genes are on chromosome 11 (Deisseroth *et al.*, 1978). The linkage relationship of the $\gamma$–$\delta$–$\beta$ genes has been established by genetic analysis and the occurrence of certain fusion globins resulting from meiotic crossover events (Benz and Forget, 1975; Nienhuis and Benz, 1977). For example, hemoglobin Lepore contains a non-$\alpha$-globin, the amino-terminal portion of which has the sequence of $\delta$-globin while the carboxyl-terminal portion of the molecule has the sequence of $\beta$-globin.

All humans have at least two types of $\gamma$-globin, one having glycine in

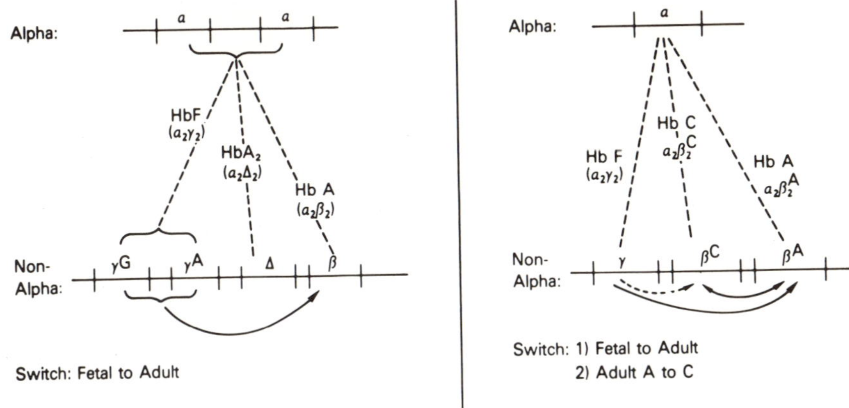


**Fig. 1.** Multiple globin genes in man and sheep. The combination of the individual gene products to form various hemoglobins is emphasized. In man (left), duplication of the $\alpha$ and $\gamma$ genes, the arrangement of the genes of the non-$\alpha$ complex, and the presence of the $\alpha$ and non-$\alpha$ genes on separate chromosomes have been experimentally established. The number, linkage, and chromosomal assignment of the globin genes in sheep (right) are not known.

position 136 ($^{G}\gamma$) and the other having alanine at that position ($^{A}\gamma$). Thus there are two loci for $\gamma$-globin (Huisman *et al.*, 1974). In addition, a $\gamma$-globin having threonine rather than isoleucine at position 75 has recently been found in many patients homozygous for $\beta$-thalassemia, certain newborns with sickle cell anemia, and in some normal individuals (Ricco *et al.*, 1976; Huisman *et al.*, 1977). These observations may imply a third locus for $\gamma$-globin, although further genetic analysis is necessary. The ratio of $^{G}\gamma$- to $^{A}\gamma$-globin in fetal red cells is 7:3, in adult red cells it is 2:3, and in cord blood it is 3:2. Thus in addition to the switch from mainly $\gamma$-globin synthesis in fetal life to mainly $\beta$-globin synthesis in adult life, there is an alteration in the relative amounts of the two types of $\gamma$-globin produced during this transition.

The chromosomal assignment and linkage relationship of the sheep globin genes are not known in the same detail as in humans. Similar to humans, there appear to be two separately inherited gene complexes encoding for the $\alpha$- or non-$\alpha$-globins.

## 4.3. Structure of Hemoglobins in Sheep and Goats

Prior to discussing the basic molecular and cellular mechanisms of the Hb A to Hb C switch in sheep and goats, it is necessary to review the structural features and the classification of the several hemoglobins in these animals. In sheep, the adult $\beta$-globin locus has two alleles, the $\beta^A$- and $\beta^B$-globin genes. The $\beta^A$- and $\beta^B$-globins differ in sequence at 8 of the 146 positions in the polypeptide chain (Huisman *et al.*, 1965). Animals homozygous for the $\beta^A$-globin gene have predominantly Hb A ($\alpha_2\beta_2^A$) in the circulating blood and animals homozygous for the $\beta^B$ gene have predominantly Hb B ($\alpha_2\beta_2^B$). Animals that are heterozygous for the $\beta^A$ and $\beta^B$ genes produce equal amounts of Hb A and Hb B. In addition, rare animals have Hb D; this hemoglobin has a structural formula $\alpha_2^D\beta_2^A$. The $\alpha^D$ is a rare allele at the $\alpha$ gene locus which differs from the usual $\alpha$- globin by a single substitution at position 15 (Huisman *et al.*, 1968). This amino acid substitution in the $\alpha$ chain does not change the electrophoretic mobility of the hemoglobin (Vaskov and Efremov, 1967).

Hemoglobin C of sheep has the structural formula $\alpha_2\beta_2^C$. The $\beta^C$-globin has a shorter length than $\beta^A$- and $\beta^B$-globins, 141 amino acids compared to 146. The "missing" amino acids are those found at the *N*-terminal end of the molecule. Also, there are at least 16 additional amino acid sequence differences between the $\beta^A$- and $\beta^C$-globins and at least 21 differences between the $\beta^B$- and $\beta^C$-globins. From analysis of these amino acid sequence differences, it has been inferred that the origin of the $\beta^C$-globin gene antedated the divergence of the $\beta^A$ and $\beta^B$ genes (Boyer *et al.*, 1966). Only sheep having a $\beta^A$-globin gene, either homozygotes (AA) or heterozygotes (AB), produce Hb C during the neonatal period and with erythropoietic stress, as outlined later. Direct analysis of DNA from animals homozygous for the $\beta^B$ gene has shown that the $\beta^C$ genes is absent from the genomes of these animals (Benz *et al.*, 1977a).

The primary structural differences among the various globins appear to produce differences in oxygen affinity (VanVliet and Huisman, 1964; Huisman and Kitchens, 1968). Hb A has a higher oxygen affinity than Hb B whereas purified Hb C has an oxygen disassociation curve which is identical to that of Hb A. However, the oxygen affinity of Hb C is far more sensitive to $P_{CO_2}$ than that of Hb A. At high $P_{CO_2}$, the oxygen affinity of red cells containing Hb C is less than that of red cells containing Hb A, while lowering of the $P_{CO_2}$ increases the oxygen affinity of the Hb C-containing cells more than the Hb A-containing cells (M. Swenberg and R. Winslow, unpublished observations). Presumably this ability to respond to differing $CO_2$ tensions *in vivo* is advantageous to an anemia or hypoxic animal. The subsequent evolution of the North American sheep population toward members which lack the $\beta^C$ gene suggests that the selective advantage of this hemoglobin is no longer important.

The basic scheme of hemoglobin phenotypes is similar but slightly more complicated in goats than in sheep, due in part to the addition of a nonallelic $\alpha$ gene (Huisman *et al.*, 1967b,1968). There are three separate alleles which may be present at the adult $\beta$ locus, $\beta^A$, $\beta^D$, and $\beta^E$, resulting in Hb A ($\alpha_2\beta_2^A$), Hb D ($\alpha_2\beta_2^D$), and Hb E ($\alpha_2\beta_2^E$) (Huisman *et al.* 1967a; Wrightstone *et al.*, 1970; Adams *et al.*, 1969). The $\beta^A$- and $\beta^D$-globins differ from one another by only a single amino acid, whereas the $\beta^E$ differs from $\beta^A$ by a minimum of three amino acid residues. The $\beta^A$-globins of sheep and goat differ by only four amino acid residues, whereas the $\beta^A$ of goat differs from the $\beta^B$ of sheep by seven. All goats produce Hb C ($\alpha_2\beta_2^C$) during neonatal life and during periods of erythropoietic stress. The $\beta^C$-globins of sheep and goat are almost identical, differing only at a single amino acid residue (Huisman, 1974).

In goats there are two gene loci for $\alpha$-globin. The first locus has two alleles, designated number I$\alpha$ and I$_\alpha^B$; they differ in a single amino acid residue (Huisman *et al.*, 1967b,1968). Hb B in goats is therefore determined by the nature of the $\alpha$ globin. The other $\alpha$ locus has only a single allele, the globin for which is designated as II$\alpha$. This globin differs at four positions from I$\alpha$. The hemoglobin tetramers formed from the II$\alpha$-globins and the $\beta$-globins comigrate with the I$\alpha$-containing hemoglobins on standard electrophoretic analysis (Huisman *et al.*, 1967b, 1968; Adams *et al.*, 1969).

## 4.4. General Patterns of Hemoglobin Switching in Sheep and Goats

Sheep and goats demonstrate a sequential switching of hemoglobins during embryonic, fetal, and neonatal life (Fig. 2) which has many features in common with the pattern in humans. Only embryonic hemoglobins are present in sheep embryos under 25 days' gestational age; during this period, embryonic hemoglobin synthesis is associated with yolk sac erythropoiesis and large, nucleated erythrocytes in the primitive circulation (Hammerburg *et al.*, 1974). In sheep fetuses under 3 cm in of length, Hb Gower ($\epsilon_4$) and subsequently Hb Gower II ($\alpha_2\epsilon_2$) are detectable on starch gel electrophoresis (Kleihauer and Stöffler, 1968). In older embryos, the major site of erythropoiesis changes from the yolk sac to the fetal liver. The absence of embryonic hemoglobins in the erythropoietic fetal liver has not been established (Hammerburg *et al.*, 1974). Nevertheless, Hb F is found first on day 25 of gestation and becomes the major hemoglobin species by day 27 (Hammerburg *et al.*, 1974), and embryonic hemoglobins are not detectable in embryos larger than 4 cm in crown rump length (Kleihauer and Stöffler, 1968).

At the time of birth, Hb F levels are 95 to 99% of total hemoglobin (Huisman *et al.*, 1969). The transition from fetal to adult hemoglobin synthesis is more rapid in sheep than in man, with a sharp decrease in the proportion of Hb F in the first two postnatal weeks (Huisman, 1974). In sheep, the switch from Hb F to Hb A requires a 2-month period, from 1

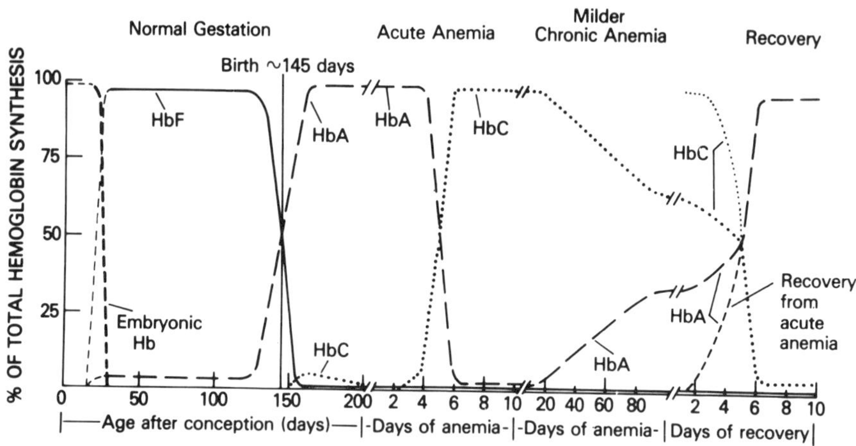


**Fig. 2.** Physiology of hemoglobin switching in sheep. The switching events include sequential replacement of embryonic by fetal hemoglobin early in gestation and replacement of Hb F by Hb A at about the time of birth. A small amount of Hb C appears in the circulation early in neonatal life. Hb A is promptly replaced with Hb C during acute severe anemia while mild chronic anemia results in partial replacement of Hb A with Hb C. During recovery from anemia, Hb C disappears from the circulation.

month prior to birth until 1 month after, compared to a human transition from 9 weeks prenatal to 4 to 5 months postnatal (Bard *et al.*, 1972). Similar patterns of embryonic and fetal hemoglobin synthesis and switching are found in goats (Kitchen and Brett, 1974).

During the neonatal period, all goats and those sheep which are either homozygous or heterozygous for Hb A have transient Hb C production (Huisman *et al.*, 1969; Huisman, 1974). In neonatal caprines, as in many other mammals, hemoglobin levels fall during the first 20 to 30 days following birth. In sheep, however, during the same period Hb C levels, near zero at birth, rise to 5 to 15% of the total hemoglobin in circulating red cells. As total hemoglobin rises to normal adult levels by day 50, Hb C levels fall. In newborn goats, Hb C rises more dramatically with the fall in total hemoglobin during the first 40 days of life, and it may account for 80 to 99% of the total hemoglobin in circulating red cells by day 50. Levels of Hb C in both sheep and goats then fall over the subsequent 2 months to reach levels found in adult nonanemic animals: 0 to 5% in the sheep and 3 to 10% in the goat.

## 4.5. The Hb A to Hb C Switch in Anemic Sheep

### 4.5.1. General Features

A change in hemoglobin phenotype was first noted in anemic sheep by Huisman *et al.* (1958). Several years later, three groups identified the hemoglobin species which increased with anemia as Hb C by starch gel electrophoresis (Blunt and Evans, 1963; VanVliet and Huisman, 1964; Braend *et al.*, 1964). This change in hemoglobin phenotype occurred not only in response to phlebotomy-induced anemia, but also in the presence of naturally occurring parasites which cause anemia (Braend *et al.*, 1964), drug-induced hemolysis (Gabuzda *et al.*, 1968), and exposure to real or simulated high altitude (Blunt *et al.*, 1970; Boyer *et al.*, 1968b). The percentage of Hb A replaced by Hb C depends on the severity and acuteness of the anemic stress, with complete replacement following severe stress. Only Hb A is replaced by Hb C; sheep homozygous for Hb B do not produce Hb C because they lack the $\beta^C$-globin gene (Benz *et al.*, 1977a). All animals heterozygous for Hb A and Hb B replace only the Hb A component in their red cells. Hb C first appears 3 to 6 days following initiation of stress, and 7 to 10 days after onset of anemia all circulating reticulocytes synthesize only Hb C. Animals that are maintained in a chronic state of moderate anemia for long periods may exhibit only partial replacement of Hb A with Hb C and the proportion of Hb A may increase with time (Fig. 2). However, reexposure to more severe stress during a period of chronic anemia may increase the proportion of Hb C again to 100% (Moore *et al.*, 1966).

## 4.5.2. Molecular Mechanism of the Hb A to Hb C Switch

The general rationale in investigating the molecular mechanism of this switch has been to examine the nature of chromatin structure, RNA molecules, and patterns of hemoglobin synthesis in extracts from bone marrow cells or reticulocytes from peripheral blood. To date it has not been possible experimentally to approach the actual molecular mechanism by which one or more of the individual genes is activated during early erythroid differentiation. The schematic representation of an early erythroblast in Fig. 3 depicts the various sites at which differential regulation of the individual globin genes might occur. These include the levels of chromatin structure, transcription of the globin genes, processing of molecules containing mRNA sequences in the nucleus, and translation of mRNA in the cytoplasm. As protein synthesis was initially studied in the reticulocyte, the earliest experimental data pertinent to the Hb A to Hb C switch concern the mechanisms of translation of the individual globin mRNAs.

### 4.5.2.1. Translational Regulation

The hypothesis that regulation of synthesis of $\beta^A$- and $\beta^C$-globin might occur at the translational level seemed especially attractive because of the marked differences in amino acid sequence at the $N$-terminal

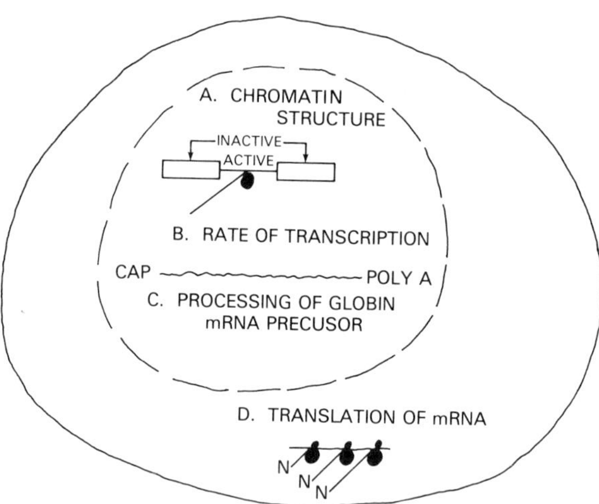


**Fig. 3.** Potential mechanism for regulation of the individual globin genes. Synthesis of a specific globin in a particular erythroblast might be due to regulation at any of the following levels: A, differences in chromatin structure among the globin genes; B, variable rates of transcription of the individual globin genes; C, selective processing of RNA molecules containing the sequences of one of the globin mRNAs; or D, preferential translation of one globin mRNA species compared to another in the cytoplasm. As discussed in the text, commitment to synthesis of a particular hemoglobin is accompanied by accumulation of a specific globin mRNA, probably due to differences in the rate of transcription of the individual genes or processing of RNA molecules in the nucleus.

portion of $\beta^C$-globin (Pro–Asn–Lys) compared to the $N$-terminal portion of the $\beta^A$- and $\beta^B$-globins (Met–Leu–Thr), which suggested the possibility of control at the site of initiation of polypeptide synthesis on the ribosome. However, Elson *et al.* (1974) found that synthesis of $\alpha$-, $\beta^B$-, and $\beta^C$-globin was initiated with methionine, derived from the initiator tRNA, Met–tRNA$_f$, by a mechanism common to initiation of most proteins in eukaryotic cells. The methionine residue is cleaved from $\beta^C$-globin leaving proline as the $N$-terminal amino acid, while the methionine remains as the $N$-terminal amino acid of the completed $\beta^B$-globin polypeptide. The initial dipeptide bond formed during the synthesis of $\beta^C$-globin is methionine–proline; thus, there is no evidence for posttranslational cleavage of amino acids other than methionine from the $\beta^C$-globin to account for its shorter length compared to the $\beta^A$- and $\beta^B$-globins.

Sheep $\beta^A$-globin has two methionine residues compared to none in $\beta^C$-globin, and $\beta^C$-globin contains an isoleucine not present in $\beta^A$-globin. Regulation of synthesis of these globins might occur at the translational level by modulation of the quantities of specific tRNA molecules in erythroid cells. Litt and Kabat (1972) found low levels of isoleucine tRNA in reticulocytes making only $\beta^A$-globin although there was a sharp increase in isoleucine tRNA shortly after onset of $\beta^C$-globin synthesis. It seemed possible that a transient period might exist during which a relative deficiency of isoleucine tRNA retarded translation of the $\beta^C$-globin mRNA early in hemoglobin switching. However, erythroid cells active in the synthesis of $\beta^C$-globin contained adequate quantities of isoleucine tRNA.

Messenger RNA may be assayed functionally by measurement of the protein product formed by cell-free extracts capable of protein synthesis using exogenous mRNA. In mRNA-dependent cell-free extracts there was an excellent correlation between the synthesis of specific $\beta$ chains *in vitro* and the globins synthesized by the cells from which the mRNAs were isolated (Baldy *et al.*, 1972; Nienhuis and Anderson, 1972). Thus, hemoglobin switching would appear to require changes in the amounts of functional mRNA in the cytoplasm. It does not depend on "specific" initiation factors or tRNA molecular species.

### 4.5.2.2. Direct Measurement of mRNA and DNA Sequences Relevant to the Switch

Quantitation of the absolute amounts of the various mRNA species in extracts from erythroid cells has relied on the development of specific complementary DNAs (cDNA) for the individual sheep globins. This has been accomplished by utilizing viral reverse transcriptase to synthesize cDNA (Verma *et al.*, 1972; Kacian *et al.*, 1972; Ross *et al.*, 1972) followed by purification of the individual $\beta$ and $\gamma$ cDNAs by techniques which have recently been described in detail (Benz *et al.*, 1977b). Measurement of the $\beta^A$ and $\beta^C$ mRNA sequence concentration in reticulocytes during induction of anemia in neonatal sheep has yielded the observation that there is quantitative replacement of the $\beta^A$ mRNA with $\beta^C$ mRNA. There was very close correspondence between the quantity of the two mRNA species as measured by hybridization analysis and their functional activity as determined by translation in frog oocytes (Benz *et al.*, 1978). These data provide formal proof that the Hb A to Hb C switch is accompanied by quantitative change in the mRNA species in erythroid cells. Thus a translational mode of regulation has been excluded.

Kabat (1972) proposed that selective gene excision might be the mechanism of regulation of the individual globin genes and immunoglobin genes. According to his model, genes might be selectively excised by specific enzymes so that a single controller or promoter sequence assumed a position physically adjacent to a particular gene, allowing expression of only one globin gene. One possible prediction of this model is that maturing erythroblasts from an anemic sheep homozygous for the $\beta^A$-globin gene would lack the gene sequences for the $\gamma$- and $\beta^A$-globins if these cells were making only Hb C. We have directly tested this hypothesis by extracting DNA from the erythroid bone marrow of such a sheep. The concentration of $\beta^C$-, $\beta^A$-, and $\gamma$-globin genes in DNA from these cells was exactly that found in spleen, indicating that destruction of gene sequences does not play a role in regulation of these genes (Benz *et al.*, 1977a). A similar conclusion was reached by a different analytical technique with regard to the human $\gamma$- and $\beta$-globin genes and their selective expression during erythroid maturation (Papayannopoulou *et al.*, 1977a). These observations do not, however, bear on the possibility that genes may be excised from one chromosomal location and reinserted into another region of the same chromosome or into a different chromosome or episome.

### 4.5.2.3. Transcriptional Regulation

Chromatin is a nuclear protein complex resulting from the noncovalent binding of DNA strands to both histone and nonhistone proteins in the nucleus. Functionally, it consists of a transcriptionally active or open fraction (euchromatin) and an inactive or condensed fraction (heterochromatin). Current evidence indicates that the primary structural unit of chromatin is the "Nu" body, which is a complex formed by eight histones (two each of H2A, H2B, H3, and H4) and approximately 200 base pairs of DNA (Kornberg, 1974; Olins and Olins, 1974; Weintraub *et al.*, 1976; reviewed by Nieuhuis and Benz, 1977). Nu bodies appear to be present on transcriptionally active genes although their structure may be somewhat modified to permit RNA polymerase binding and transcription of mRNA. Higher orders of chromatin structure appear to occur by supercoiling of the primary filament of DNA associated with these histone octamers.

Weintraub and Groudine (1976) developed an assay which utilized an enzyme, pancreatic deoxyribonuclease I (DNAse I), to selectively digest the DNA sequences representing transcriptionally active genes in isolated nuclei. In these initial important experiments, exposure of nuclei isolated from chick reticulocytes to DNAse I for a brief period resulted in solubilization of 5 to 10% of the total DNA but led to virtually complete digestion of the transcriptionally active globin genes. Similar results have been obtained with DNAse I in the analysis of the structure of the ovalbumin gene in nuclei from oviduct (Garel and Axel, 1976) and the integrated but expressed murine leukemia genome in chick fibroblasts (Panet and Cedar, 1977).

We have utilized the DNAse I assay for transcriptionally active genes to compare the structure of the $\gamma$-, $\beta^A$-, and $\beta^C$-globin genes in nuclei isolated from the erythroblasts of anemia sheep producing predominantly

Hb C and no Hb F (N. Young, E. Benz, R. Croissant, P. Turner, and A. Nienhuis, unpublished observations). Solubilization of 10% of the total nuclear DNA resulted in an eightfold reduction in the concentration of the $\beta^C$-globin sequences. However, the $\beta^A$ and $\gamma$ gene sequences were also destroyed by this limited nuclease digestion. These observations suggest that the $\gamma$ and $\beta^A$ in addition to the $\beta^C$-globin genes in this animal may have been in a potentially active configuration in chromatin.

### 4.5.2.4. Transcriptional Regulation or Selective Processing

With regard to the potential levels of regulation depicted in Fig. 3, current evidence tends to exclude both chromatin structure and translational regulation as the bases for the differential expression of the individual globin genes. Differential rates of transcription of the individual genes and selective processing of RNA molecules containing the individual globin mRNA sequences remain the most likely mechanisms by which individual cells might accumulate one of the mRNA species.

Recent studies have yielded many insights into the metabolism of nuclear RNA species containing globin mRNA sequences (Aviv *et al.*, 1976; Bastos *et al.*, 1977; Bastos and Aviv, 1977; Ross, 1976; Kwan *et al.*, 1977; Strair *et al.*, 1977; Curtis and Weismann, 1976). A precursor containing $\beta$-globin mRNA sequences which is three times larger than the cytoplasmic mRNA has been reported; the precursor containing $\alpha$ mRNA sequences is only 30% larger than cytoplasmic $\alpha$ mRNA (Curtis *et al.*, 1977). The initial product of transcription of the globin genes may be even larger than these nuclear RNA species (Spohr *et al.*, 1976; Strair *et al.*, 1977). Modification at the 5' end, referred to as "capping" (Perry and Kelley, 1976), and addition of a 150- to 200-nucleotide tail of adenosines (poly A) at the 3' end (Perry, 1976) are other steps in the processing of nuclear RNA molecules containing globin mRNA sequences. These complex metabolic events are obviously amenable to regulation which might control the nature and amount of the individual mRNA species which accumulate in the cytoplasm.

We have analyzed nuclear RNA prepared from nonanemic sheep synthesizing only Hb A; $\beta^A$-globin mRNA sequences were present but to the limits of the sensitivity of these measurements, $\beta^C$ globin mRNA was absent (Nienhuis *et al.*, 1978). However, a short-lived high-molecular-weight precursor present in very low concentration would not be detected by these methods of analyses. Short pulse labeling periods are required and techniques suitable for detecting a labeled mRNA species must be utilized to adequately test the hypothesis that there is equivalent transcription of all of the individual globin genes regardless of the final hemoglobin which is made in erythroblasts.

### 4.5.3. Kinetics of Induction of Hb C Synthesis

Following imposition of an anemic stress, synthesis of Hb C in the bone marrow is initially detected after 3 days and reaches a maximum at 5 days (Gabuzda *et al.*, 1968). A similar time course of switching may be demonstrated in nonanemic sheep following injection of plasma from anemic animals (Boyer *et al.*, 1968a), and partially purified human urinary erythropoietin (Thurmon *et al.*, 1970). From these early experiments, it appeared likely that erythropoietin induced Hb C synthesis by action on an erythroid precursor cell rather than on a cell already active in hemoglobin synthesis.

Results consistent with this hypothesis have been obtained in tissue culture experiments. Establishment of cultures of sheep bone marrow containing high concentrations of erythropoietin resulted in the formation of erythroid colonies which make Hb C (Barker *et al.*, 1976). However, during the initial 3 days in semisolid culture only Hb A was detected; a small amount of Hb C was made between 72 and 96 hr and only between 96 and 120 hr did Hb C become the predominant hemoglobin species synthesized. These results suggest that the initial colonies formed *in vitro* might be derived from precursor cells already committed to $\beta^A$-globin synthesis and that subsequent synthesis of Hb C represents the generation of colonies from an earlier precursor cell.

Injection of erythropoietin into a nonanemic neonatal animal and subsequent serial sampling of the bone marrow allowed more accurate definition of the temporal relationship of the commitment of the progenitor cell, the accumulation of $\beta^C$-globin mRNA, and the onset of Hb C synthesis (Nienhuis *et al.*, 1978a). Bone marrow obtained 12, 24, 48, and 72 hr after the injection of erythropoietin was cultured in plasma clot at a low concentration of erythropoietin (0.01 unit/ml). This concentration is sufficient to support the development of erythroid colonies but will not independently induce colonies which make Hb C. Nonetheless, at 12 hr this assay detected progenitor erythroid cells which made Hb C *in vitro*. Thus within 12 hr commitment had occurred to the subsequent expression of the $\beta^C$-globin gene. A second aliquot of each bone marrow sample was fractionated by isopycnic centrifugation to obtain cell populations containing predominantly early or late erythroblasts. RNA was extracted from the nuclei and cytoplasm of these cell populations and analyzed by annealing to $\beta^A$- and $\beta^C$-globin cDNA; $\beta^C$-globin mRNA was initially detected in the nuclei of early erythroblasts 48 hr after the injection of erythropoietin *in vivo*. Although commitment of the early progenitor cells, as detected by the *in vitro* colony-forming assay, occurred within 12 hr of erythropoietin stimulation, the appearance of the $\beta^C$-globin mRNA required 48 hr. Synthesis of Hb C *in vivo* paralleled the appearance of the $\beta^C$-globin mRNA species.

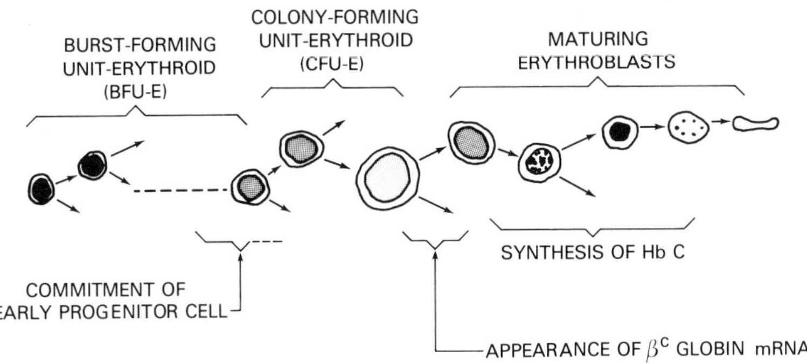


**Fig. 4.** Kinetics of induction of Hb C synthesis. Exposure of an early erythroid progenitor cell (possibly a BFU-E) to a high concentration of erythropoietin results in the commitment of the cell to generate erythroblasts which make $\beta^C$-globin. There appears to be an approximately 24- to 36-hr interval between this commitment event and the appearance in the bone marrow of erythroblasts which contain $\beta^C$-globin mRNA. Hb C accumulates in the cytoplasm during subsequent phases of erythroid maturation.

These experimental data and the earlier results cited previously lead to the concept of induction of Hb C synthesis depicted in Fig. 4. Erythropoietin acts on an early progenitor cell, activating it to form erythroblasts which express the $\beta^C$-globin gene. Subsequently these erythroblasts appear in the bone marrow and Hb C synthesis begins. There is an approximately 24- to 36-hr lag between the commitment event and the onset of Hb C synthesis in maturing erythroblasts.

### 4.5.3.1. Cellular Analysis of the Hb A to Hb C Switch

It is possible to at least tentatively integrate the cellular aspects of Hb A to Hb C switching into a general scheme of erythroid cellular differentiation derived from tissue culture experimentation. Stephenson, Axelrad, and co-workers (Stephenson *et al.*, 1971) first described an assay for erythroid stem cells in which benzidine-positive erythroid colonies containing 8 to 64 cells were generated from murine erythropoietic tissue in plasma clot cultures. Similar colonies have been generated from the erythroid tissue of other animals including man (Iscove *et al.*, 1975; Papayannapoulou *et al.*, 1976; Ogawa *et al.*, 1976; Tepperman *et al.*, 1974) and sheep and goats (Barker *et al.*, 1975, 1976). These colonies descend from an erythroid stem cell termed the CFU-E, or erythroid colony-forming unit, and require a relatively low concentration of erythropoietin (0.1–0.5 unit/ml). *In vitro* evidence of an earlier erythroid stem cell than the CFU-E depended on the generation of large macroscopic colonies derived from the erythroid burst-forming unit (BFU-E) (Axelrad *et al.*, 1974; Iscove and Sieber, 1975). These appeared after 7 days in mouse culture and 14 days in human culture and required a high concentration of erythropoietin (0.5–3.0 units/ml) for growth. That burst colonies are derived from single cells has been established for humans (Papayannopoulou *et al.*, 1977b) and seems likely in the case of other species. Erythroid stem cells intermediate between the BFU-E and CFU-E in colony size, time required for *in vitro* development, and erythropoietin requirement have been described in mouse (Gregory, 1976) and humans (Gregory and Ezaves, 1977). There is probably a continuum of erythroid progenitor cells which may be cultured *in vitro* beginning with the BFU-E, which is closely related to the pluripotential stem cell, and ending with the CFU-E, which is presumably the immediate precursor to cells within the maturing erythron (Fig. 4).

Several lines of evidence support the thesis that erythropoietin induces the Hb A to Hb C switch by acting on the immediate precursor to the CFU-E. Injection of ESF into a neonatal sheep resulted in a five-fold increase in the number of CFU-E over a period of 24 hr following the injection (Barker *et al.*, 1976). These CFU-E were committed to generate colonies which made Hb C, even when these colonies were grown at low erythropoietin concentration (0.1 unit/ml). More direct evidence that the cell which responds to ESF is not identical to the majority of CFU-E was derived from fractionation of goat bone marrow (Barker *et al.*, 1976). The highest level of Hb C synthesis (50% of the total) between 72 and 96 hr *in vitro* was found in cultures derived from the most slowly sedimenting subset of the CFU-E population. Finally, culture of sheep bone marrow at high erythropoietin concentration resulted in initial formation of small erythroid colonies which synthesize Hb A. The appearance of Hb C synthesis coincided with the maturation of larger erythroid colonies between 96 and 120 hr *in vitro* (Barker *et al.*, 1976).

Although it seems likely that erythropoietin acts on a stem cell earlier than the CFU-E in mediating the Hb A to Hb C switch, there remain several possible mechanisms by which this might occur. Three general schemes are outlined in Fig. 5. The first depicts the possibility that there might be several distinct subclasses of stem cells. Under conditions of low

**Fig. 5.** Possible mechanisms for hemoglobin switching. Erythropoietin might promote the development of erythroblasts which make Hb C by one of three mechanisms: A, selection among distinct erythroid stem cells which are precommitted with regard to the potential for expression of the $\beta^C$-globin gene (phenotypic selection); B, selection among erythroid progenitor cells all derived from a common stem cell pool but which are at various stages in the process of erythroid stem cell differentiation (developmental selection); or C, direct modulation of the commitment to expression of the $\beta^C$-globin gene in individual erythroid stem cells (intracellular modulation).

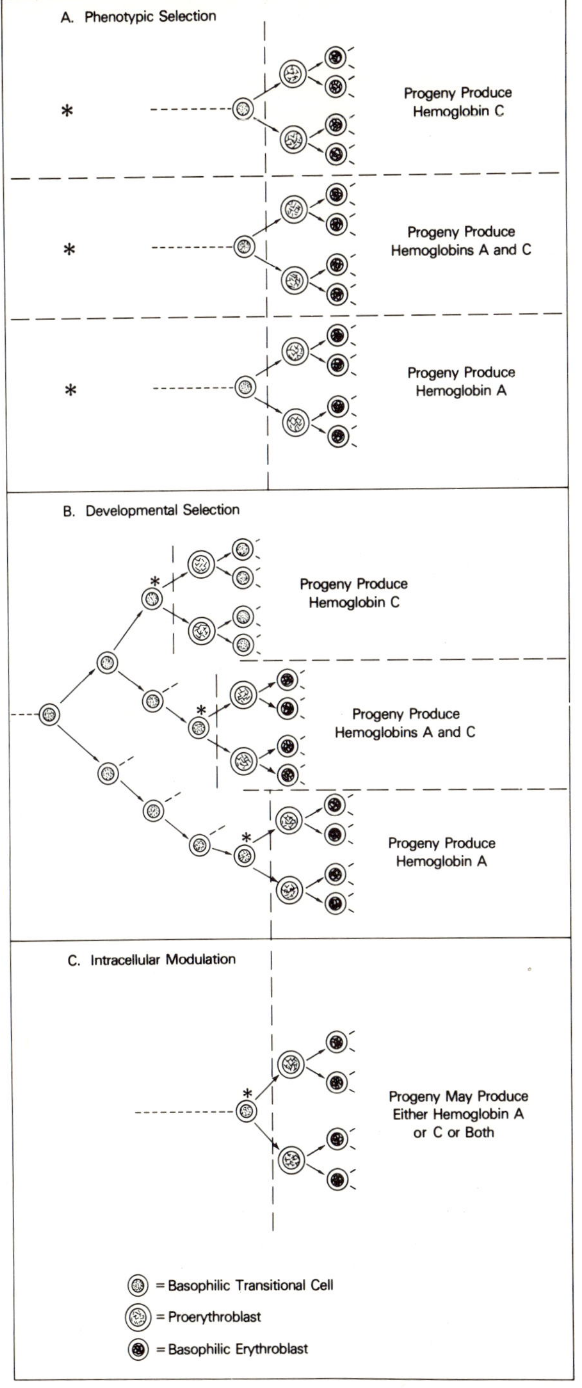


A. Phenotypic Selection
Progeny Produce Hemoglobin C
Progeny Produce Hemoglobins A and C
Progeny Produce Hemoglobin A
B. Developmental Selection
Progeny Produce Hemoglobin C
Progeny Produce Hemoglobins A and C
Progeny Produce Hemoglobin A
C. Intracellular Modulation
Progeny May Produce Either Hemoglobin A or C or Both
= Basophilic Transitional Cell
= Proerythroblast
= Basophilic Erythroblast

ESF concentration (nonanemic animals), only those already committed to generate erythroblasts which synthesize Hb A might be activated and enter the maturing erythron. In the anemic or hypoxic animal with a higher ESF concentration, other stem cells with a potential for producing erythroblasts which make Hb C might be activated.

A very simple clonal selection model is unlikely since both Hb A and Hb C have been shown to be present in the same peripheral blood cells. Using specific immunofluorescent antisera to Hb A and Hb C, smears of peripheral blood from a goat recently induced to switch from Hb A to C production were examined for the presence of the two Hb species (Garrick *et al.*, 1973). The sum of the fraction of cells staining with anti-Hb A and the fraction staining with anti-Hb C exceeded 100%. During switching from Hb C to Hb A production, almost all of the cells stained with anti-Hb C and over half with anti-Hb A. The presence of both hemoglobins in a single cell was confirmed by detecting the asymmetrical hybrid hemoglobin with the structure $\alpha_2\beta^A\beta^C$ in a erythrocytes of switching animals (Nienhuis and Bunn, 1974). If a clonal selection mechanism is responsible for Hb switching, then committed early cells must give rise to descendant erythroblasts which synthesize varying proportions of Hb A and Hb C.

An alternative clonal model, developmental selection (Fig. 5), is based on the fact that there is a horizontal array of stem cells at various stages of development with differing sensitivities to erythropoietin (Lajtha and Schofield, 1974; Nienhuis *et al.*, 1977). The most sensitive of these might be the CFU-E, which at low physiological ESF concentration generates maturing erythroblasts which make Hb A. In the presence of anemia, earlier progenitor cells might bypass later cell divisions in the maturational sequence of erythroid stem cells and directly enter the maturing erythron. The erythroblasts derived from these earlier stem cells might then make varying proportions of Hb A and Hb C. Finally, under the most severe anemic stress and highest ESF concentration, an even earlier erythroid stem cell might be triggered directly into the maturing erythron. These erythroblasts would synthesize only Hb C.

The simplest mechanism of Hb A to Hb C switching is intracellular modulation (Fig. 5). All erythroid progenitor cells at the level of the immediate precursor to the CFU-E might have an equal potential to develop erythroblasts which make varying proportions of Hb A and Hb C. The ESF concentration to which these stem cells are exposed before entering the maturing erythron would then determine the amounts of Hb A and Hb C made in their progeny. While this simple and direct mechanism is consistent with all the experimental data, no direct proof exists to support this hypothesis and some clonal selection mechanism is equally likely.

## 4.6. Mechanism of Action of Erythropoietin in Inducing Hb C Synthesis

The primary mechanism of action of erythropoietin during normal erythropoiesis is to support the development of an adequate number of red cells to meet the oxygen requirement of the organism (Nienhuis *et al.*, 1977). Erythropoietin regulates the number of erythroid stem cells in the bone marrow and triggers these cells to enter the maturing erythron (Paul, 1976). Many intracellular effects have been ascribed to erythropoietin, including enhanced heme and globin synthesis (Glass *et al.*, 1975), increased synthesis of globin mRNA (Ramirez *et al.*, 1975; Conkie *et al.*, 1975), stimulation of RNA polymerase activity (Piantadosi *et al.*, 1976), and enhanced synthesis of nonhistone chromosomal proteins (Spivak, 1976). These biochemical actions, however, may be the indirect consequences of the fact that ESF stimulates cells to enter the maturing erythron (Nienhuis *et al.*, 1977). As the hormone increases the number of cells engaged in hemoglobin synthesis it is problematic whether it directly affects the intracellular mechanisms of protein synthesis.

Similar considerations apply to the role of erythropoietin in stimulating Hb C synthesis in sheep. Its role in the Hb A to Hb C switch may be indirect by virtue of the variable sensitivity of stem cells to erythropoietin action. Even if intracellular modulation of gene activity is the hormone's mechanism of action, the commitment event, as defined both *in vivo* and *in vitro*, does not require a continued high concentration of erythropoietin to sustain $\beta^C$-globin synthesis. It seems unlikely that erythropoietin has a direct role in modulating the intracellular events which result in the accumulation of $\beta^C$-globin mRNA and the synthesis of Hb C.

## 4.7. The Hb F to Adult Hemoglobin Switch in Sheep

The general pattern of the transition from Hb F to adult hemoglobin synthesis in sheep has been described in an earlier section. Little is known about the stimuli which result in the abrupt transition from Hb F synthesis to adult hemoglobin synthesis during the perinatal period. Fetal erythropoiesis appears to be dependent on erythropoietin, at least during the last trimester of pregnancy (Zanjani *et al.*, 1974). Phlebotomy has been reported to accelerate the switch from Hb F to adult hemoglobin synthesis in late gestation sheep (Kazazian *et al.*, 1976) although others have been unable to confirm this result (Barker *et al.*, 1977). Hypophysectomy of a fetal sheep resulted in delayed and incomplete switching from Hb F to adult hemoglobin production, suggesting that hormones other than erythropoietin might be involved in this hemoglobin switch (Wood *et al.*, 1976a). Many hormones have been demonstrated to affect erythropoiesis *in vitro,* including androgens (Moriyama and Fisher, 1975), corticosteroids (Singer and Adamson, 1976; Golde *et al.*, 1976), cyclic nucleotides (Brown and Adamson, 1977a), thyroxine (Popovic *et al.*, 1977), and $\beta$-adrenergic agents (Brown and Adamson, 1977b). The specific role of these agents in modulating Hb F or Hb A synthesis either *in vivo* or *in vitro* has yet to be investigated.

Attempts to simulate the production of Hb C synthesis in fetal sheep known to be homozygous for the $\beta^A$-globin gene has yielded the observation that while a switch from Hb F to Hb C synthesis may be obtained *in vitro,* such a switch does not appear to occur *in vivo* (Barker *et al.*, 1977). Culture of fetal erythroid liver in plasma clot resulted in the generation of erythroid colonies which at high ESF concentration make substantial amounts of Hb C after 4 to 5 days *in vitro.* Both the erythropoietin dependence and kinetics of the Hb F to Hb C switch by colonies derived from fetal tissues appear similar to these features of the Hb A to Hb C switch which occurs in cultures of neonatal and adult bone marrow. However, erythropoietic stresses, including phlebotomy and injection of erythropoietin into the fetus *in utero,* did not stimulate Hb C production until shortly before birth (in two of the six late gestation animals tested). Although the presence of a responsive erythroid progenitor cell could be demonstrated *in vitro,* these cells could not be induced to generate erythroblasts which made Hb C *in vivo.* Perhaps some component of the culture media was necessary for the development of colonies which made Hb C. Alternatively, certain microenvironmental, cellular, or hormonal factors in the fetus might have been unfavorable and prevented the development of erythroblasts making Hb C. In any case, these results point out that multiple factors may interact to modulate hemoglobin switching phenomena.

## 4.8. The Hb F to Hb A Switch in Man

Gamma globin has been detected in the youngest human embryos examined (1.6 cm crown rump length), and by 8 weeks of gestational age (4.6 cm), Hb F represents 90% of the hemoglobin present in the embryo (Weatherall and Clegg, 1975). Gamma globin is also part of Hb Portland, an embryonic hemoglobin composed of two $\zeta$ chains and two $\gamma$ chains. The appearance of Hb F in the embryo is associated with the transition of the major site of erythropoiesis from the yolk sac to the liver.

Adult Hb A is present in fetuses as young as 11 weeks of gestational age (8 cm) and remains at levels between 5 and 10% of total hemoglobin until weeks 32 to 34 (Pataryas and Stamatoyannopoulos, 1972), although there is a gradual increase in the $\beta$:$\gamma$ synthetic ratio during the first and second trimester (Cividalli *et al.*, 1974). Hb A synthesis has been observed *in vitro* in reticulocytes obtained from fetuses of 55 days of age (Kazazian and Woodhead, 1973). Cells which contain Hb A as well as Hb F, measured by the acid elution technique, first appear at gestational week 34 and rise steadily to peak levels at 8 weeks postnatal (Weatherall *et al.*, 1974). Hb A has been detected in 25% of peripheral blood erythrocytes of fetuses of 13 to 18 weeks gestational age by a single-cell microscopic immunodiffusion technique; a further 25% of cells showed a faint "dust" precipitate. Occasional fetal red blood cells showed large quantities of Hb A as well as Hb F (Boyer *et al.*, 1974). Using the more sensitive immunofluorescent method, Hb A has been observed in the majority of hepatic erythroblasts in fetuses as small as 8.5 cm in crown rump length (T. Papayannopoulou and G. Stamatoyannopoulos, unpublished observations). Although there is a shift in the major site of erythropoiesis from the liver to bone marrow late in fetal life, there is no evidence that fetal hemoglobin synthesis is related to the site of erythropoiesis. There is no difference in the relative proportions of Hb F and Hb A synthesized by liver, spleen, and bone marrow from fetuses 13 to 34 weeks of age (Wood and Weatherall, 1973).

While Hb F remains the predominant hemoglobin of fetuses until 40 weeks of gestational age, at about 30 weeks $\gamma$-globin synthesis decreases and $\beta$-globin synthesis increases. By term, 50 to 60% of the non-$\alpha$-globin synthesized is $\gamma$. The proportion of $\gamma$ chain synthesis falls rapidly to 25% at 4 to 5 weeks of postnatal age and more gradually to 5% at 4 months postnatal age (Bard, 1975). During this period of declining $\gamma$ synthetic rate, the levels of fetal hemoglobin remain constant in neonates at about 60% of total hemoglobin during the 2 to 3 weeks following birth. Hb F levels then decrease linearly until approximately age 100 days (to a level of 5%) and at a slower rate to normal adult levels by 200 days (Colombo *et al.*, 1976). The temporary discrepancy between the plateau levels of the amount of Hb F present in the first few weeks of life and the progessive decline in synthesis of $\gamma$-globin is due to the sharp decline in total erythropoiesis which accompanies birth.

The most important determinant of switching from fetal to adult hemoglobin synthesis is postconceptional age, with the sharpest period of transition between weeks 30 and 52 (Bard, 1975). The fetal to adult switch appears unrelated to the birth event itself and unaffected by intrauterine transfusion of adult blood (Bard *et al.*, 1970). Perinatal hemolytic anemias accelerate the disappearance of Hb F from the blood, but the relative amounts of $\beta$- and $\gamma$-globin synthesis are unaffected (Jonxis, 1965). However, a real effect on the fetal to adult switching phenomena is observed in children with gross chromosomal abnormalities: In $D_1$ trisomy, embryonic hemoglobins are present at birth and Hb F disappearance is delayed by 7 to 8 weeks (Bard *et al.*, 1972; Jensen and Murken, 1976). Infants with trisomy G (Down's syndrome) (Wilson *et al.*, 1968) and C/D translocation (Weller *et al.*, 1966) have a pattern of accelerated switching, with lower than normal levels of Hb F and higher than normal levels of Hb A at term.

## 4.9. Persistence of Fetal Hemoglobin beyond the Neonatal Period

### 4.9.1. F Cells

Low concentrations of fetal hemoglobin, determined by chemical methods, are present in all normal individuals, although the concentration of Hb F is usually less than 1% of the total hemoglobin (Schroeder *et al.*, 1970). This small amount of Hb F is restricted to only a small fraction of the total red cells as revealed by the acid elution technique (Kleihauer *et al.*, 1957, quoted in Weatherall *et al.*, 1974). Highly specific immunofluorescent antibodies to Hb F provide a much more sensitive method for detecting and localizing Hb F. Cells that contain Hb F, termed F cells, as defined by this technique are present in all individuals: The F cell frequency has been reported as 0.02 to 5% (Boyer *et al.*, 1975a) or 0.5 to 7% (Wood *et al.*, 1975) of all erythrocytes. There is a linear correlation between the F cell frequency and the quantity of Hb F in the blood. The amount of Hb F in each F cell is 14 to 28% of the mean cell hemoglobin. The number of F cells in an individual is fairly constant but increases during the midtrimester of pregnancy (Pembrey *et al.*, 1973; Boyer *et al.*, 1975b), and during sickle cell crises (Bhattacharya *et al.*, 1976).

F cells must be differentiated from the erythrocytes present in the fetal circulation (Dover *et al.*, 1977). F cells are characterized only by an increased quantity of fetal hemoglobin as determined by immunofluorescent staining. True fetal erythrocytes, in contrast, differ from normal adult erythrocytes in the quantity of many intracellular enzymes and the antigenic properties of the cell membrane, as well as the type of hemoglobin. For example, carbonic anhydrase levels are lower in fetal than in adult red cells. Fetal erythrocytes demonstrate an antigen on their cell surface, termed the i antigen, which is absent on adult cells, while adult erythrocytes are characterized by an antigen absent on fetal cells, termed I. While F cells are normally present in adult blood, fetal erythrocytes in adults are observed only in pathologic conditions.

What is the origin of F cells? F cells might be the progeny of a unique stem cell population; alternatively, they might arise from random, incomplete suppression of γ-globin synthesis during erythroid cell maturation (Weatherall *et al.*, 1976). Recent observations of F cell frequency in two hematologic disorders characterized by clonal proliferation of hematopoietic cells are informative with regard to the possible origin of F cells. In a patient with an elevated number of F cells who developed chronic myelocytic leukemia, the number of F cells did not change with the onset of the disease or chemotherapy directed at proliferating cells (Papayannopoulou *et al.*, 1978a). Chronic myelocytic leukemia is a disease in which a clone of abnormal hematopoietic cells (erythroid, myeloid, and megakaryocytic) is marked by the presence of the Philadelphia chromosome (Fialkow *et al.*, 1967). In this patient, the replacement of the normal hematopoietic cells with the progeny of the stem cell containing the Philadelphia chromosome did not change the F cell frequency, suggesting that F cells as well as red cells which contain only Hb A share an early common ancestor. In another clonal disorder, paroxysmal nocturnal hemoglobinuria, abnormal clones of erythroid cells are characterized by a cell membrane defect resulting in a heightened susceptibility to complement-mediated lysis. In patients with born normal and abnormal erythrocytes in the circulation, the proportion of F cells present in both populations was the same (Papayannopoulou *et al.*, 1978b). This observation also suggests that F cells arise by regulatory events during the development of the two erythroid populations, rather than from a distinctive stem cell line.

## 4.9.2. Hereditary Persistence of Fetal Hemoglobin

A group of genetic abnormalities characterized by elevated levels of Hb F in persons without gross hematologic disease has been characterized as the hereditary persistence of fetal hemoglobin (HPFH) syndromes. By their very complexity and diversity, these syndromes have provided important clues concerning the mechanism of globin gene regulation. A convenient division of HPFH into pancellular and heterocellular varieties has been proposed (Boyer *et al.*, 1977). In the heterozygous form of pancellular HPFH, Hb F is uniformly distributed among the peripheral blood erythrocytes as determined by the acid elution technique. In the heterocellular form, there is a variable distribution of fetal hemoglobin among the erythrocytes.

### 4.9.2.1. Pancellular HPFH

The Negro form of pancellular HPFH has been found to be due to a deletion of the genes coding for β- and δ-globin (Forget *et al.*, 1976; Kan *et al.*, 1975). Homozygotes for this defect do not produce either δ- or βglobin and thus have 100% Hb F. While this syndrome does not produce symptoms, the red cells of affected persons are not normal. The peripheral smear may be characterized by target cells, microcytosis, anisocytosis, and poikilocytosis. Anemia is absent, but the mean corpuscular volume and mean corpuscular hemoglobin may be decreased. The $^{G}\gamma{:}^{A}\gamma$-globin ratio in Negro pancellular HPFH is usually near the 2:3 ratio found in normal adults. In addition, patients with homozygous HPFH of the Negro type may demonstrate a slight imbalance in globin synthesis similar to a mild form of $\beta$-thalassemia (Friedman *et al.*, 1976; Charache *et al.*, 1976). Heterozygotes for the Negro form of HPFH have 10 to 30% Hb F. Heterozygotes for both HPFH and Hb S or Hb C disease have higher Hb F levels, 20 to 35% (Weatherall *et al.*, 1975).

A variety of other syndromes characterized by elevated fetal hemoglobin levels in the pancellular distribution have been described and are summarized in Table I (Huisman *et al.*, 1970; Stamatoyannopoulos *et al.*, 1975). Beta chain production may be present *cis* to the HPFH locus in association with pancellular HPFH (Huisman *et al.*, 1975; Friedman and Schwartz, 1976). In some forms of pancellular HPFH either $^{G}\gamma$ or $^{A}\gamma$ chains are exclusively synthesized. For example, in the Greek variety of HPFH, observed only in the heterozygous state or in combination with $\beta$-thalassemia, only $^{A}\gamma$-globin is produced and Hb F levels are lower than in the Negro form of HPFH. Based on globin synthesis studies, some $\beta$-globin synthesis *cis* to the HPFH deletion must occur, although it is inadequate to "compensate" for the deficiency due to the $\beta$-thalassemia gene (Sfofroniadou *et al.*, 1975).

**Table I.**  Hereditary Persistence of Fetal Hemoglobin

| | Characteristics of $\gamma$ globin | Status of linked $\delta$ and $\beta$ genes | % Hb F | |
| --- | --- | --- | --- | --- |
| | | | Heterozygotes | Homozygotes |
| Normal | $^{G}\gamma{:}^{A}\gamma = 2{:}3$ | Active | Less than 1 | — |
| Pancellular | | | | |
|   Negro | $^{G}\gamma{:}^{A}\gamma$ usually 2:3, rarely $^{G}\gamma$ only | Deleted Rarely active | 25–30 | 100 |
|   Greek | $^{A}\gamma$ | Active | 10–20 | None described |
|   Hb Kenya | $^{G}\gamma$ | $\gamma^{A}$-B fusion, $\delta$ deleted | 6–7 | None described |
| Heterocellular | | | | |
|   British | Mainly $^{A}\gamma$ | Active | 6–12 | 20 |
|   Seattle | $^{G}\gamma{:}^{A}\gamma = 2{:}3$ | Active | 3–8 | None described |
|   Georgia | $^{A}\gamma$ | Active | 4–7 | None described |
|   Swiss | — | Active | 1–3 | None described |

Further evidence that deletion within the $\gamma$–$\delta$–$\beta$ complex results in $\gamma$-globin production beyond neonatal life is also derived from studies of Hb Kenya (Huisman *et al.*, 1972; Smith *et al.*, 1973; Nute *et al.*, 1976). This hemoglobin variant results from fusion of the $\gamma$ and $\beta$ genes, presumably by a crossover event occurring during meiosis leading to production of a globin with the amino-terminal sequence of $\gamma$-globin and the carboxyl-terminal sequence of $\beta$-globin. The fusion has occurred at a point between amino acid residues 81 and 86. Heterozygotes for Hb Kenya have increased levels of Hb F of the $^G\gamma$ type and pancellular distribution of fetal hemoglobin. The crossover event which gives rise to the Hb Kenya gene may result in the deletion of a nucleotide sequence which affects $\gamma$ gene expression. Persistence of fetal hemoglobin may thus result from deletion of a specific set of nucleotides, as in Hb Kenya, or deletion of the entire $\delta$–$\beta$ complex, as in Negro pancellular HPFH. Although it seems likely that the other forms of pancellular HPFH (Table I) are also due to deletions of genetic material, other types of mutations might also be responsible.

### 4.9.2.2. Heterocellular HPFH

A pronounced increase in Hb F levels in which the fetal hemoglobin has a variable distribution among the erythrocytes has been described in a British family (Weatherall *et al.*, 1975). Affected members of this family could be distinguished by the Hb F levels as homozygotes (20%) and heterozygotes (9%). Hb $A_2$ levels were reduced in the homozygotes. Although the amount of $^G\gamma$ chain was reduced, $\alpha/\beta + \gamma$ chain synthesis was balanced. A milder elevation of fetal hemoglobin levels, also associated with a heterocellular distribution, has been termed Swiss-type HPFH and is present in about 2% of adult Europeans (Knox-Macaulay *et al.*, 1973; Weatherall *et al.*, 1974). The characteristics of these and other varieties of HPFH are summarized in Table I.

The high Hb F levels in heterocellular HPFH result from an increase in the number of F cells rather than the proportion of Hb F in individual cells (Wood *et al.*, 1976b; Stamatoyannopoulos *et al.*, 1975; Boyer *et al.*, 1977). In addition, the genetic site that regulates the number of F cells appears to be closely linked to the $\beta$ and $\delta$ structural genes and to the mutation which results in $\beta$-thalassemia. In studies of families in which both heterocellular HPFH and either sickle cell trait or $\beta$-thalassemia trait were present, the segregation of these characters was analyzed for gene linkage (Wood *et al.*, 1976b; Bethlenfalvey *et al.*, 1975). The incidence of phenotypes resulting from recombination between the gene for heterocellular HPFH and either the $\beta$-globin structural locus or the $\beta$-thalassemia locus was very low, implying a close physical proximity of these genes on a chromosome.

Persons heterozygous for $\delta$–$\beta$-thalassemia have increased quantities of Hb F in a heterocellular distribution (Weatherall and Clegg, 1972). A heterogeneous distribution of the capacity for Hb F synthesis is also implied by the ineffective erythropoiesis which characterizes the homozygote for $\delta$–$\beta$-thalassemia; those cells with a low capacity for Hb F synthesis have a marked excess of $\alpha$-globin and are destroyed in the bone marrow, while the "F cell precursors" produce the circulating erythrocytes. $\delta$–$\beta$-thalassemia is due to a depletion of the $\delta$- and $\beta$-globin genes (Ottolenghi et al., 1976). In Negro pancellular HPFH, the deletion of the $\delta$- and $\beta$-globin structural genes appears to include that region of the chromosome which is involved in suppressing $\gamma$-globin synthesis in adult red cells. In $\delta$–$\beta$-thalassemia the deletion results in an enhanced capacity for F cell formation but not in a uniform capacity for Hb F synthesis in all erythroblasts. Thus in $\delta$–$\beta$-thalassemia the deletion appears to affect a putative controller locus for F cell frequency.

### 4.9.3. Elevated Hb F Levels in Other Hematologic Diseases

#### 4.9.3.1. Hemoglobinopathies

Increased Hb F levels are common in persons with congenital anemias, including $\beta$-thalassemia and sickle cell anemia. As in the genetically determined heterocellular HPFH syndromes, elevated Hb F in these disorders is due to an increased number of F cells (Wood et al., 1975). Increased fetal hemoglobin synthesis in hereditary anemias has been assumed to represent "compensation" for abnormal or decreased $\beta$-globin production, analogous to the reciprocal relationship between $\beta$ and $\gamma$ chain synthesis in fetal and neonatal life. However, in some persons with hemoglobinopathies, high Hb F levels are probably genetic rather than physiologic in origin. For example, family studies indicate that certain Arabs with sickle cell disease have inherited the ability to make large amounts of Hb F (Perrine et al., 1972). Unusually high levels of fetal hemoglobin have also been associated with sickle cell trait in some American Negro families (Stamatoyannopoulos et al., 1975).

The combination of sickle cell anemia and elevated fetal hemoglobin levels may have been selectively favored: the altered hemoglobin increasing resistance to hemolysis by malarial parasites, and the high F cell number ameliorating the thrombotic effects of sickle hemoglobin, offering the doubly heterozygous individual significant survival advantage under the appropriate conditions. There is a characteristic tail at the upper end of the distribution of Hb F levels in normal populations (Weatherall *et al.*, 1974) further implying a genetic polymorphism with regard to F cell number. Higher than normal Hb F levels are more common in particular races, as for example among certain Oriental populations, and within certain genetically closed groups, such as some Saudi Arabian Arabs. As described in the preceding section, the tight linkage between the $\beta$ structural gene, the thalassemia mutations, and the HPFH heterocellular locus would favor inheritance of these genes in combination.

### 4.9.3.2. Acquired Elevations of Hb F

Increased Hb F levels have been associated with a wide variety of hematologic disorders, as, for example, frequently with juvenile chronic myelogenous leukemia and Fanconi's anemia, and less often with aplastic anemia, erythroleukemia, paroxysmal nocturnal hemoglobinuria, refractory normoblastic anemia, the leukemias, and many malignancies (reviewed by Weatherall *et al.*, 1974). In contrast to HPFH syndromes, fetal hemoglobin production in these disorders is not congenital or under apparent genetic control, and, in addition, in certain instances it has been associated with striking features of fetal or primitive erythropoiesis.

Increased Hb F levels are frequent in juvenile chronic myelogenous leukemia (JCML) and are associated with a poor prognosis (Sheridan *et al.*, 1976). Many patients with elevated Hb F levels also demonstrate decreased erythrocyte carbonic anhydrase levels and increased i antigen on the cell surface. Thus, the erythrocytes of some patients may have some or all of the characteristics of fetal erythrocytes. In the same patient with JCML, cell lines may appear which differ in the completeness and degree of abnormality of their fetal erythropoietic characteristics (Dover *et al.*, 1977). Another anomaly of reversion to the fetal pattern of hemoglobin erythropoiesis is imbalanced synthesis of globin (Pagnier and Labie, 1975). The clonal nature of cells with fetal erythropoietic characteristics and high Hb F levels has been demonstrated by separation of two fractions of red cells from a single patient on the basis of erythrocyte surface antigens (Pagnier *et al.*, 1977).

Erythropoiesis which is characterized by high Hb F production, a fetal rather than adult $^A\gamma:^G\gamma$ ratio, and i antigenicity of the erythrocyte surface may also be present during recovery from bone marrow transplantation in either homologous or autologous marrow cells (Alter *et al.*, 1976) and also following intensive chemotherapy for leukemia. In these instances, it may be postulated that F-producing cells have a selective advantage over adult hemoglobin-producing cells in the peculiar environment of the regenerating bone marrow.

### 4.9.4. *In Vitro* Hb F Synthesis

Stamatoyannopoulos and his collaborators have undertaken an extensive investigation of Hb F synthesis in cultures of adult marrow *in vitro* (Hermodson *et al.*, 1976; Papayannopoulou *et al.*, 1976, 1977a–c). In these studies, the $\gamma$-globin synthesized was well characterized chemically and the conditions for enhanced $\gamma$-globin production were partially defined. Fetal hemoglobin was identified in colonies using specific fluorescent antibodies, and the synthesis of $\gamma$-globin was measured by the incorporation of a radioactive precursor amino acid. Production of fetal hemoglobin was 5- to 14-fold higher in cultures containing erythroid colonies compared to the synthesis of Hb F measured at the initiation of culture or in reticulocytes from peripheral blood. Fetal hemoglobin synthesis also correlated with the erythropoietin concentration in bone marrow cultures maintained for 8 to 9 days.

An attempt was made to characterize the erythroid progenitor cell pivotal to the enhanced synthesis of Hb F observed in culture. Conditions were chosen to optimize growth of CFU-Es and BFU-Es. BFU-E colony production was noted with longer periods of cultivation (14–16 days) and at higher erythropoietin concentrations (2 units/ml). CFU-E production was optimal at 8 to 9 days at lower erythropoietin concentrations (0.2–0.5 unit/ml). Under these culture conditions, fetal hemoglobin production was more common among cells resulting from BFU-Es (34%) compared to cells resulting from CFU-E culture (13%) (Papayannopoulou *et al.*, 1977b). This difference was due to an increased frequency of Hb F-producing colonies among the late developing colonies. The increased number of fetal hemoglobin-producing cells in BFU-E-derived colonies was also observed when they were developed at low erythropoietin concentrations (0.25–0.5 unit/ml). While both BFU-Es and CFU-Es were shown to be clonal in origin, the pattern of fluorescent anti-Hb F staining of the cells in the colonies was different. Fetal hemoglobin-producing colonies derived from CFU-Es showed uniform staining with the anti-Hb F antibody. While some BFU-E colonies stained uniformly, others showed significant variation in the intensity levels among and within subcolonies. As in the studies of sheep and goat erythropoiesis *in vitro* (Barker *et al.*, 1976, 1977), a stem cell at the level between the BFU-E and CFU-E was implicated as the probable site at which regulation of expression of the individual globin genes occurred. A role for erythropoietin in modulating the Hb F to Hb A switch *in vitro* was also suggested in the experiments with human marrow cells.

In studies employing fetal tissues, the role of erythropoietin appeared uncertain. Human fetal liver maintained in cell suspension synthesized 84% $\gamma$ chain and 11% $\beta$ chains. Non-$\alpha$-globin synthesis remained balanced with respect to $\alpha$ production, but $\beta$ chain synthesis increased sharply after about 1 week in culture (Shchory and Weatherall, 1975). Cultured fetal liver and fetal spleen cells show a peak in responsiveness of total globin synthesis to erythropoietin at 16 and 19 weeks of fetal age, respectively (Basch, 1972); no effect of erythropoietin on the relative proportions of Hb F and Hb A was noted. As with studies of fetal to adult switching in fetal sheep, cited in Section 4.7, these studies are consistent with a complex mechanism of regulation of Hb F to Hb A switching which may include erythropoietin among other factors.

## 4.10. A Model for Fetal to Adult Hemoglobin Switching and Hb F Production in Adults

Several important observations concerning hemoglobin switching and the synthesis of Hb F in adult humans may be summarized by the following statements:

1. Hb F in the fetus is contained in fetal erythrocytes which differ from adult erythrocytes with regard to enzyme content and cell surface antigens. In adults, Hb F is contained in a subpopulation of adult erythrocytes, the F cells.
2. Hb F elevation in certain HPFH syndromes and in congenital anemias is mediated by an increase in the number of F cells. Increased Hb F levels due to reactivation of fetal erythropoiesis, a much rarer occurrence, is found in some leukemic conditions and following bone marrow transplantation or chemotherapy.
3. The number of F cells in normal individuals is genetically determined.
4. A regulatory locus for F cell number is closely linked to the $\beta$ structural gene and mutations which cause $\beta$-thalassemia.
5. F cells arise from a committed stem cell, probably at the level of BFU-E.
6. F cells and adult erythrocytes which lack Hb F appear to arise from a common stem cell pool.

In the model outlined in Fig. 6, events of regulatory importance are assumed to occur at both the intracellular and cellular levels. This scheme has certain features in common with those proposed by others (Weatherall et al., 1976; Papayannopoulou et al., 1977b). Erythroid stem cell maturation, symbolized by $BFU\text{-}E_1 \rightarrow BFU\text{-}E_2 \rightarrow BFU\text{-}E_3$, occurs prior to commitment of the progenitor cells to terminal erythroid maturation. Terminal maturation is characterized morphologically by development of mature normoblasts from early erythroblasts and functionally by multiple cell divisions, accumulation of globin mRNA, and synthesis of hemoglo-

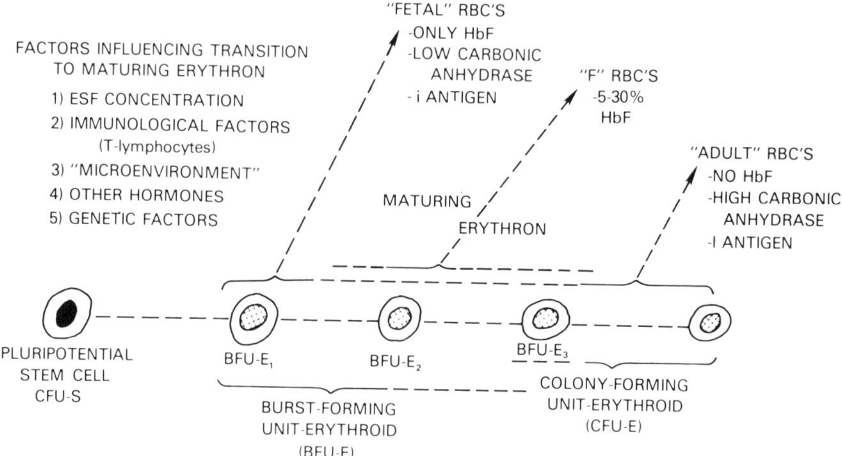



**Fig. 6.** Hb F synthesis: Potential relationship to erythroid stem cell development. This model incorporates the knowledge that erythroid stem cells mature with an increase in erythropoietin sensitivity and a decrease in proliferative potential and the idea that stem cells might be triggered to enter terminal erythroid maturation at various points in their differentiation, thereby giving rise to fetal erythrocytes, F cells, or normal adult red blood cells. The factors which potentially regulate entry of stem cells into the maturing erythron are listed.

bin. In contrast, stem cell differentiation lacks readily recognized morphological and functional features, although there is probably an increase in the number of erythropoietin receptors and changes in cell surface antigens. Stem cells at an early stage of maturation (BFU-E₁) in this model are less likely to give rise to progeny with adult red cell characteristics than more mature stem cells (BFU-E₃).

Intracellular regulation at the stem cell level may involve a coordinated series of regulatory loci analogous to the promoter and controller genes of bacteria. Mutations and deletions within such loci have been proposed to account for varying patterns of hemoglobin synthesis (Huisman *et al.,* 1974; Nigon and Godet, 1976). The mechanism by which cell surface characteristics resulting in altered reactivity with erythropoietin, cellular mediators, various hormones, etc., could influence the expression of particular globin genes remains unknown. By analogy to the sheep Hb A to Hb C switch, the difference in commitment to globin synthesis of one cell compared to another might reflect the presence of an RNA processing apparatus which promotes the accumulation of $\beta$ mRNA in favor of $\gamma$. Alternatively, the molecular process might involve adjustment in the rate of transcription of the individual globin genes.

The stage of stem cell differentiation at which commitment to terminal erythroid maturation occurs could determine the character of the resulting erythrocytes with respect both to their surface and enzymatic properties and their Hb F content. In the normal adult, development of increasing numbers of erthropoietin receptors on the cell surface of stem cells might ultimately modulate entry into the maturing erythron. Most cells would contain only Hb A. In conditions of bone marrow stress associated with elevated erythropoietin levels, such as congenital anemias, some BFU-Es might prematurely enter the maturing erythron. Propensity for this to occur might also reflect a polymorphism at the putative controller locus for F cell number.

Cells unrelated morphologically and functionally to erythroid cells may play a role in the regulation of erythroid stem cell development. For example, T-lymphocytes have defined and complex regulatory functions in the immunological system, but also produce a diffusible factor which stimulates hematopoiesis (Cerny, 1974). Cells capable of giving rise to erythroid colonies *in vitro* may be obtained from the "null fraction" of human peripheral blood lymphocytes. These cells lack the surface markers of B- and T-lymphocytes. In the presence of erythropoietin, but in the absence of T cells, these erythroid stem cells (BFU-E) give rise to small undifferentiated colonies. Upon addition of T cells or of T-cell-conditioned media, typical hemoglobinized colonies develop (Nathan *et al.*, 1978).

Erythroid stem cells might be characterized by membrane antigens that are recognized by T cells. There is evidence for such an age-dependent surface marker in early erythroid cells of mice as determined by their susceptibility to rabbit anti-mouse brain serum (Rosendaal, 1977). In humans, the I–i antigen system might also be an example of such marker differentiation. Specific antigens on the cell surface could allow recognition followed by either inhibition or stimulation of proliferation by specific T cells. The HPFH gene product might be a membrane antigen or an enzyme that alters such an antigen, which is recognized by a specific T cell. The gross abnormality of T cell function that occurs in leukemia or following intensive chemotherapy could result in fetal erythropoiesis. Conceivably a change either in the T cell lymphocyte population or an erythroid stem cell surface marker might be responsible for the physiological switch from Hb F to Hb A synthesis in neonatal humans.

## 4.11. Summary

In both the Hb A to Hb C switch in sheep and goats and the Hb F to Hb A switch, there is evidence for regulation at both the cellular and intracellular levels. In many ways, studies of these two sytems complement one another. In sheep and goats the Hb A to Hb C switch is linked to the hormone erythropoietin. The mechanism of accumulation of specific mRNA is either through selective transcription of certain genes or at an immediate post-transcriptional site, the processing of molecules containing globin mRNA sequences. Intracellular alterations reflected in the commitment to synthesize specific globins must occur prior to onset of terminal maturation of erythroid cells. However, these intracellular changes may represent aspects of normal development in all erythroid cells. Switching would then involve selection of cells at various stages of intracellular development.

In both switch systems, a simple clonal selection of a unique stem cell line appears unlikely. A model is proposed in which development alterations in the character of the human stem cell membrane may result in a difference in the sensitivity to hormones, such as erythropoietin, or regulator cells, possibly T cells. In either case, erythroid stem cells at varying stages of development would be stimulated to enter the maturing erythron yielding either fetal erythrocytes, F cells, or normal adult red blood cells.

It is likely that research over the next several years will concentrate on the mechanisms of cell–cell interaction which may bear similarity to such interactions in the immune system and have broad implications for cell differentiation. A second major line of investigation will certainly be the mechanism of action of erythropoietin, including its membrane binding properties and the mode of stimulation of protein synthesis and cell proliferation. The goal of activation of fetal hemoglobin production as a therapy for hematologic disease may now be approached equally well from the cellular as from the intracellular orientation.

## References

Adams, E., Wrightstone, R., Miller, A., and Huisman, T., 1969, Quantitation of hemoglobin alpha chains in adult and fetal goats: Gene duplication in the production of polypeptide chains, *Arch. Biochem. Biophys.* **132**:223.

Alter, B., Rappeport, J., Huisman, T., Schroeder, W., and Nathan, D., 1976, Fetal erthropoiesis following bone marrow transplantation, *Blood* **48**:843.

Aviv, H., Voloch, Z., Bastos, R., and Levy, S., 1976, Biosynthesis and stability of globin mRNA in cultured erythroleukemic Friend cells, *Cell* **8**:495.

Axelrad, A., McLeod, D., Shreeve, M., and Heath, D., 1974, Properties of cells that produce erythrocytic colonies *in vitro, in Proceedings Second International Workshop in Hemopoiesis in Culture* (W. Robinson, ed.), pp. 226–234, U.S. Govt. Printing Office, Washington, D.C.

Baldy, M., Gaskill, P., and Kabat, D., 1972, Expression of the silent hemoglobin gene in sheep. Studies of the globin messenger ribonucleic acids, *J. Biol. Chem.* **247**:6665.

Bard, H., 1972, Postnatal fetal and adult hemoglobin synthesis in $D_1$ trisomy syndrome, *Blood* **40**:523.

Bard, H., 1975, The postnatal decline of Hb F synthesis in normal full-term infants, *J. Clin. Invest.* **55**:395.

Bard, H., Makowski, E., Meschia, G., and Battaglia, F., 1970, The relative rates of synthesis of Hb A and F in immature red cells of newborn infants, *Pediatrics* **45**:766.

Bard, H., Battaglia, F., Makowski, E., and Meschia, G., 1972, The synthesis of adult and fetal hemoglobin in sheep during the perinatal period, *Proc. Soc. Exp. Biol. Med.* **139**:1148.

Barker, J., Anderson, W., and Nienhuis, A., 1975, Hemoglobin switching in sheep and goats. V. Effect of erythropoietin concentration on *in vitro* erythroid colony growth in globin synthesis, *J. Cell Biol.* **64**:515.

Barker, J., Pierce, J., and Nienhuis, A., 1976, Hemoglobin switching in sheep and goats. VI. Commitment of erythroid colony-forming cells to the synthesis of $\beta^C$ globin, *J. Cell Biol.* **71**:715.

Barker, J., Pierce, J., Kefauver, B., and Nienhuis, A., 1977, Hemoglobin switching in sheep and goats: Induction of Hb C synthesis in cultures of sheep fetal erythroid cells, *Proc. Natl. Acad. Sci. U.S.A.* **74**:5078.

Basch, R., 1972, Hemoglobin synthesis in short-term cultures of human fetal hematopoietic tissues, *Blood* **39**:530.

Bastos, R., and Aviv, H., 1977, Globin RNA precursor molecules: Biosynthesis and processing in erythroid cells, *Cell* **11**:641.

Bastos, R., Volloch, Z., and Aviv, H., 1977, Messenger RNA population analysis during erythroid differentiation: A kinetical approach, *J. Mol. Biol.* **110**:191.

Benz, E., and Forget, B., 1975, The molecular genetics of the thalassemia syndromes, *Prog. Hematol.* **9**:107.

Benz, E., Turner, P., Barker, J., and Nienhuis, A., 1977a, Stability of the individual globin genes during erythroid differentiation, *Science* **196**:1213.

Benz, E., Geist, C., Steggles, A., Barker, J., and Nienhuis, A., 1977b, Hemoglobin switching in sheep and goats. Preparation and characterization of complementary DNAs specific for the alpha-, beta-, and gamma-globin messenger RNAs of sheep, *J. Biol. Chem.* **252**:1908.

Benz, E., Steggles, A., Geist, C., and Nienhuis, A., 1978, Hemoglobin switching in sheep: Quantitation of $\beta^A$ and $\beta^C$ mRNA sequences in nuclear and cytoplasmic RNA during the Hb A to Hb C switch, *J. Biol. Chem.*, in press.

Bethlenfalvey, N., Motulsky, A., Ringelhann, B., Lehmann, H., Humbert, J., and Konotey-Ahulu, F., 1975, Hereditary persistence of fetal hemoglobin, $\beta$-thalassemia, and the hemoglobin $\delta\beta$ locus: Further family data and genetic interpretations, *Am. J. Hum. Genet.* **27**:140.

Bhattacharya, S., Anyaibe, S., and Headings, V., 1976, Biological variation in the heterogeneous distribution of Hb F among erythrocytes, *Br. J. Haematol.* **33**:401.

Blunt, M., and Evans, J., 1963, Changes in the concentration of potassium in the erythrocytes and in the hemoglobin type in Merino sheep under a severe anemic stress, *Nature* **200**:1215.

Blunt, M., Perry, M., and Lane, R., 1970, The production of Hb C by sheep at simulated high altitude, *Res. Vet. Sci.* **11**:191.

Boyer, S., Hathaway, P., Pascasio, F., Orton, C., Bordley, J., and Naughton, M., 1966, Hemoglobins in sheep: Multiple differences in amino acid sequences of three beta-chains and possible origins, *Science* **153**:1539.

Boyer, S., Crosby, E., and Noyes, A., 1968a, Hemoglobin switching in non-anemic sheep. I. Mediation by plasma from anemic animals, *Johns Hopkins Med. J.* **123**:85.

Boyer, S., Crosby, E., Noyes, A., Kaneko, J., Keeton, K., and Zinkl, J., 1968b, Hemoglobin switching in non-anemic sheep. II. Response to high altitude, *Johns Hopkins Med. J.* **123**:92.

Boyer, S., Boyer, M., Noyes, A., and Belding, T., 1974, Immunological basis for detection of sickle cell hemoglobin phenotypes in amniotic fluid erythrocytes, *Ann. N.Y. Acad. Sci.* **241**:699.

Boyer, S., Belding, T., Margolet, L., and Noyes, A., 1975a, Fetal hemoglobin restriction to a few erythrocytes (F cells) in normal human adults, *Science* **188**:361.

Boyer, S., Belding, T., Margolet, L., Noyes, A., Burke, P., and Bell, W., 1975b, Variations in the frequency of fetal hemoglobin-bearing erythrocytes (F-cells) in well adults, pregnant women, and adult leukemics, *Johns Hopkins Med. J.* **137**:105.

Boyer, S., Margolet, L., Boyer, M., Huisman, T., Schroeder, W., Wood, W., Weatherall, D., Clegg, J., and Cartner, R., 1977, Inheritance of F cell frequency in heterocellular hereditary persistence of fetal hemoglobin: An example of allelic exclusion, *Am. J. Hum. Genet.* **29**:256.

Braend, M., Efremov, G., and Helle, O., 1964, Abnormal hemoglobin in sheep, *Nature* **204**:700.

Brown, J., and Adamson, J., 1977a, Studies of the influence of cyclic nucleotides on *in vitro* hemoglobin synthesis, *Br. J. Haematol.* **35**:193.

Brown, J., and Adamson, J., 1977b, Modulation of *in vitro* erythropoiesis. The influence of beta-adrenergic agonists on erythroid colony formation, *J. Clin. Invest.* **60**:70.

Cerny, J., 1974, Stimulation of bone marrow hemopoietic stem cells by a factor from activated T cells, *Nature* **249**:63.

Charache, S., Clegg, J., and Weatherall, D., 1976, The Negro variety of hereditary persistence of fetal hemoglobin is a mild form of thalassemia, *Br. J. Haematol.* **34**:527.

Cividalli, G., Nathan, D., Kan, Y., Santamarina, B., and Frigoletto, F., 1974, Relationship of beta to gamma synthesis during the first trimester: An approach to prenatal diagnosis of thalassemia, *Pediatr. Res.* **8**:553.

Colombo, K., Colombo, B., Kim, B., Perez Atencio, R., Molina, C., and Terrenato, L., 1976, The pattern of fetal hemoglobin disappearance after birth, *Br. J. Haematol.* **32**:79.

Conkie, D., Kleiman, L., Harrison, P., and Paul, J., 1975, Increase in the accumulation of globin mRNA in immature erythroblasts in response to erythropoietin *in vivo* or *in vitro*, *Exp. Cell Res.* **93**:315.

Curtis, P., and Weissmann, C., 1976, Purification of globin messenger RNA from dimethylsulfoxide-induced Friend cells on detection of a putative globin messenger RNA precursor, *J. Mol. Biol.* **106**:1061.

Curtis, P., Mantei, N., VanDenBerg, J., and Weissmann, C., 1977, Presence of a putative 15S precursor to beta-globin mRNA but not to alpha-globin mRNA in Friend cells, *Proc. Natl. Acad. Sci. U.S.A.* **74**:3184.

Deisseroth, A., Velez, R., and Nienhuis, A., 1976, Hemoglobin synthesis in somatic cell hybrids: Independent segregation of the human alpha- and beta-globin genes, *Science* **191**:1262.

Deisseroth, A., Nienhuis, A., Turner, P., Velez, R., Anderson, W., Ruddle, R., Lawrence, J. Creagan, R., and Kucherlapati, R., 1977, Localization of the human alpha-globin structural gene on chromosome 16 in somatic cell hybrids by molecular hybridization assay, *Cell* **12**:205.

Deisseroth, A., Nienhuis, A., Lawrence, J., Giles, R., Turner, P., and Ruddle, F., 1978, Chromosomal localization of the human beta globin gene to human chromosome 11 in somatic cell hybrids, *Proc. Natl. Acad. Sci. U.S.A.* **75**:1456.

Dover, G., Boyer, S., Zinkham, W., Kazazian, H., Pinney, D., and Sigler, A., 1977, Changing erythrocyte populations in juvenile chronic myelocytic leukemia: Evidence for disordered regulation, *Blood* **49**:355.

Elson, N., Brewer, H., and Anderson, W., 1974, Hemoglobin switching in sheep and goats. II. Cell-free initiation of sheep globin synthesis, *J. Biol. Chem.* **249**:5227.

Fialkow, P., Gartler, S., and Yoshida, A., 1967, Clonal origin of chronic myelocytic leukemia cells in man, *Proc. Natl. Acad. Sci. U.S.A.* **58**:1468.

Forget, B., Hillman, D., Lazarus, H., Barrell, E., Benz, E., Caskey, C., Huisman, T., Schroeder, W., and Housman, D., 1976, Absence of messenger RNA in gene DNA for beta-globin chains in hereditary persistence of fetal hemoglobin, *Cell* **7**:323.

Friedman, S., and Schwartz, E., 1976, Hereditary persistence of fetal hemoglobin with beta-chain synthesis in *cis* position ($^{G}$gamma-beta$^{+}$-HPFH) in a Negro family, *Nature* **259**:138.

Friedman, S., Schwartz, E., Ahern, E., and Ahern, V., 1976, Variations in globin chain synthesis in hereditary persistence of fetal hemoglobin, *Br. J. Haematol.* **32**:357.

Gabuzda, T., Schuman, M., Silver, R., and Lewis, H., 1968, Erythropoietic kinetics in sheep studied by means of induced changes in hemoglobin phenotype, *J. Clin. Invest.* **47**:1895.

Garel, A., and Axel, R., 1976, Elective digestion of transcriptionally active ovalbumin genes from oviduct nuclei, *Proc. Natl. Acad. Sci. U.S.A.* **73**:3966.

Garrick, M., Reichlin, M., Mattioli, N., and Manning, R., 1973, The anemia-induced reversible switch from Hb A to Hb C in caprine ruminants: Immunochemical evidence that both hemoglobins are found in the same cell, *Dev. Biol.* **30**:1.

Glass, J., Labidor, L., and Robinson, S., 1975, Use of cell preparation and short-term culture techniques to study erythroid cell development, *Blood* **46**:705.

Golde, D., Bersch, N., and Cline, M., 1976, Potentiation of erythropoiesis *in vitro* by dexamethasone, *J. Clin. Invest.* **57**:57.

Gregory, C., 1976, Erythropoietin sensitivity as a differentiation marker in the hemopoietic system: Studies of three erythropoietic responses in culture, *J. Cell. Physiol.* **89**:289.

Gregory, C., and Ezaves, A., 1977, Human marrow cells capable of erythropoietic differentiation *in vitro:* Definition of three erythroid responses, *Blood* **49**:855.

Hammerburg, B., Brett, I., and Kitchen, H., 1974, Ontogeny of hemoglobins in sheep, *Ann. N.Y. Acad. Sci.* **241**:672.

Hermodson, M., Papayannopoulou, T., Kurachi, S., and Stamatoyannopoulos, G., 1976, Structural evidence for gamma globin chain synthesis in adult bone marrow cultures, *Biochem. Biophys. Res. Commun.* **72**:991.

Huisman, T., 1974, The *in vivo* production of Hb C in ruminants, *Ann. N.Y. Acad. Sci.* **241**:549.

Huisman, T., and Kitchens, T., 1968, Oxygen equilibria studies of the hemoglobins from normal and anemic sheep and goats, *Am J. Physiol.* **215**:140.

Huisman, T., van Vliet, G., and Sebens, T., 1958, Hemoglobin types in different species of sheep, *Nature* **182**:172.

Huisman, T., Reynolds, C., Dozy, A., and Wilson, J., 1965, The structure of sheep hemoglobins. The amino acid composition of the alpha and beta chains of Hbs A, B, and C, *J. Biol. Chem.* **240**:2455.

Huisman, T., Adams, H., Dimmock, M., Edwards, W., and Wilson, J., 1967a, The structure of goat hemoglobins. I. Structural studies of the beta chains of the hemoglobins of normal and anemic goats, *J. Biol. Chem.* **242**:2534.

Huisman, T., Wilson, J., and Adams, H., 1967b, The heterogeneity of goat hemoglobin: Evidence for the existence of two non-allelic and one allelic alpha chain structural genes, *Arch. Biochem. Biophys.* **121**:528.

Huisman, T., Brandt, G., and Wilson, J., 1968, The structure of goat hemoglobins. II. Studies of the alpha chains of Hbs A and B, *J. Biol. Chem.* **243**:3675.

Huisman, T., Lewis, J., Blunt, M., Adams, H., Miller, A., Dozy, A., and Boyd, E., 1969, Hb C in newborn sheep and goats: A possible explanation for its function and biosynthesis, *Pediatr. Res.* **3**:189.

Huisman, T., Schroeder, W., Adams, H., Shelton, J., Shelton, J., and Appell, G., 1970, A possible subclass of the hereditary persistence of fetal hemoglobin, *Blood* **36**:1.

Huisman, T., Schroeder, W., and Kendall, A., 1972, Hb Kenya, the product of nonhomologous cross-over of $\gamma$ and $\beta$ genes, *Blood* **40**:947.

Huisman, T., Schroeder, W., Efremov, G., Duma, H., Mladnovski, B., Hyman, C., Rachmilewitz, E., Bouver, N., Miller, A., Brodie, A., Shelton, J., Shelton, J., and Appell, G., 1974, The present status of the heterogeneity of fetal hemoglobin in beta thalassemia: An attempt to unify some observations of thalassemia and related conditions, *Ann. N.Y. Acad. Sci.* **232**:107.

Huisman, T., Miller, A., and Schroeder, W., 1975, A G[gamma] type of hereditary persistence of fetal hemoglobin with beta chain production in *cis, Am. J. Hum. Genet.* **27**:765.

Huisman, T. H. J., Schroeder, W. A., Reese, J. B., Wilson, J., Lam, H., Shelton, J., Shelton, J., and Baker, S., 1977, The [T]gamma chain of human fetal hemoglobin at birth and in several abnormal hematological conditions, *Pediatr. Res.* **11**:1102.

Iscove, N., and Sieber, F., 1975, Erythroid progenitors in mouse bone marrow detected by macroscopic colony formation in culture, *Exp. Hematol.* **3**:32.

Iscove, N., Sieber, F., and Winterhalter, K., 1975, Erythroid colony formation in cultures of mouse and human bone marrow: Analysis of the requirement for erythropoietin by gel filtration and affinity chromatography on agarose-conconavalin A, *J. Cell. Physiol.* **83**:309.

Jensen, M., and Murken, J.-D., 1976, Hemoglobin chain synthesis in two children with trisomy 13. Evidence for temporary imbalance during switch from gamma to beta chain synthesis, *Eur. J. Pediatr.* **122**:151.

Jonxis, J., 1965, The development of hemoglobin, *Pediatr. Clin. North Am.* **12**:535.

Kabat, D., 1972, Gene selection in hemoglobin and in antibody-synthesizing cells, *Science* **175**:134.

Kacian, D., Spiegelman, S., Bank, A., Terada, M., Metafora, S., Dol, L., and Marks, P., 1972, *In vitro* synthesis of DNA components of human genes, *Nature New Biol.* **235**:167.

Kan, Y., Holland, J., Dozy, A., Charache, S., and Kazazian, H., 1975, Deletion of the beta-globin structure gene in hereditary persistence of fetal hemoglobin, *Nature* **258**:162.

Kazazian, H., and Woodhead, A., 1973, Hb A synthesis in the developing fetus, *N. Engl. J. Med.* **289**:58.

Kazazian, H., Silverstein, A., Snyder, P., and VanBeneden, R., 1976, Increasing beta-chain synthesis in fetal development as associated with the declining gamma to alpha mRNA ratio, *Nature* **260**:67.

Kitchen, H., and Brett, I., 1974, Embryonic and fetal hemoglobins in animals, *Ann. N.Y. Acad. Sci.* **241**:653.

Kleihauer, E., and Stöffler, G., 1968, Embryonic hemoglobins of different animal species. Quantitative and qualitative data about production in properties of hemoglobins during early developmental stages of pig, cattle, and sheep, *Mol. Gen. Genet.* **101**:59.

Knox-Macaulay, H., Weatherall, D., Clegg, J., and Pembrey, M., 1973, Thalassemia in the British, *Br. Med. J.* **III**:150.

Kornberg, R. B., 1974, Chromatin structure: A repeating unit of histones in DNA, *Science* **184**:868.

Kwan, S., Wood, T., and Lingrel, J., 1977, Purification of a putative precursor of globin messenger RNA from mouse nucleated eythroid cells, *Proc. Natl. Acad. Sci. U.S.A.* **74**:178.

Lajtha, L., and Schofield, R., 1974, On the problem of differentiation in hemopoiesis, *Differentiation* **2**:313.

Litt, M., and Kabat, D., 1972, Studies of transfer ribonucleic acids and of hemoglobin synthesis in sheep reticulocytes, *J. Biol. Chem.* **237**:6659.

Moore, S., Godley, W., VanVliet, G., Lewis, J., Boyd, E., and Huisman, T., 1966, The production of hemoglobin C in sheep carrying the gene for hemoglobin A: Hematological aspects, *Blood* **28**:314.

Moriyama, Y., and Fisher, J., 1975, Effects of testosterone and erythropoietin on erythroid colony formation and their human bone marrow cultures, *Blood* **45**:665.

Nathan, D., Chess, L., Hillman, D., Clarke, B., Braerd, J., Merler, E., and Housman, D., 1978, Human erythroid burst forming units (BFU-E): T cell requirement for erythroid proliferation *in vitro*, *J. Exp. Med.* **147**:324.

Nienhuis, A., and Anderson, W., 1972, Hemoglobin switching in sheep and goats: Changes in functional globin messenger RNA in reticulocytes and bone marrow cells, *Proc. Natl. Acad. Sci. U.S.A.* **69**:2184.

Nienhuis, A., and Benz, E., 1977, Regulation of hemoglobin synthesis during the development of the red cell, *N. Engl. J. Med.* **297**:1318, 1371, 1436.

Nienhuis, A., and Bunn, H., 1974, Hemoglobin switching in sheep and goats: Occurrence of Hbs A and C in the same red cell, *Science* **185**:946.

Nienhuis, A., Barker, J., and Anderson, W., 1977, Effect of erythropoietin on hemoglobin synthesis, *in Kidney Hormones,* Vol. II (J. Fisher, ed.), pp. 245–282, Academic Press, New York.

Nienhuis, A., Axelrod, D., Barker, J., Benz, E., Jr., Croissant, R., Miller, D., and Young, N., 1978, Regulation of the individual globin genes, *in Differentiation of Normal and Neoplastic Hematopoietic Cells* (B. Clarkson, P. Marks, and J. Till, eds.), Cold Spring Harbor Monograph Series, in press.

Nigon, V., and Godet, J., 1976, Genetic and morphogenetic factors and hemoglobin synthesis during higher vertebrate development: An approach to cell differentiation mechanisms, *Int. Rev. Cytol.* **46**:79.

Nute, P., Wood, W., Stamatoyannopoulos, G., Olweny, C., and Fialkow, P., 1976, The Kenya form of hereditary persistence of fetal hemoglobin: Structural studies and evidence for homogenous distribution of Hb F using fluorescent anti-Hb F antibodies, *Br. J. Haematol.* **32**:55.

Ogawa, M., Parmley, R., Bank, H., and Spicer, S., 1976, Human marrow erythropoiesis in culture. I. Characterization of methylcellulose colony assay, *Blood* **48**:407.

Olins, A., and Olins, D., 1974, Spheroid chromatin units ($\nu$ bodies), *Science* **183**:330.

Ottolenghi, S., Comi, P., Giglioni, B., Tolstoshev, P., Lanyon, W., Mitchell, G., Williamson, R., Russo, G., Musumeci, S., Schilliro, G., Tsistrakis, G., Charache, S., Wood, W., Clegg, J., and Weatherall, D., 1976, Delta-beta-thalassemia is due to a gene deletion, *Cell* **9**:71.

Pagnier, J., and Labie, D., 1975, Abnormal hemoglobin synthesis in some leukemic patients, *Biochemie* **57**:71.

Pagnier, J., Lopez, M., Mathiot, C., Habibi, B., Zamet, P., Baret, B., and Labie, D., 1977, An unusual case of leukemia with high fetal hemoglobin: Demonstration of abnormal hemoglobin synthesis localized in the red cell clone, *Blood* **50**:249.

Panet, A., and Cedar, H., 1977, Selective degradation of integrated murine leukemia proviral DNA by deoxyribonucleases, *Cell* **11**:933.

Papayannopoulou, T., Brice, M., and Stamatoyannopoulos, G., 1976, Stimulation of fetal hemoglobin synthesis in bone marrow cultures from adult individuals, *Proc. Natl. Acad. Sci. U.S.A.* **73**:2033.

Papayannopoulou, T., Nute, P., Stamatoyannopoulos, G., and McGuire, T., 1977a, Hemoglobin ontogenesis: Test of the gene excision, a hypothesis, *Science* **196**:1216.

Papayannopoulou, T., Brice, M., and Stamatoyannopoulos, G., 1977b, Hb F synthesis *in vitro:* Evidence for control at the level of primitive erythroid stem cells, *Proc. Natl. Acad. Sci. U.S.A.* **74**:2923.

Papayannopoulou, T., Bunn, F., and Stamatoyannopoulos, G., 1978a, Cellular distribution of Hb F in a clonal hematopoietic stem cell disorder: A patient with S/beta$^0$ thalassemia and chronic myelocytic leukemia, *N. Engl. J. Med.* **298**:72.

Papayannopoulou, T., Rosse, W., and Stamatoyannopoulos, G., 1978b, Fetal hemoglobin in paroxysmal nocturnal hemoglobinuvia, Evidence for random derivation of the Hb F containing erythrocytes (F-cells) from the PNH clone and from normal hemopoietic cell lines, *Blood*, in press.

Pataryas, H., and Stamatoyannopoulos, G., 1972, Hemoglobins in human fetuses: Evidence for adult hemoglobin production after the eleventh gestational week, *Blood* **39**:688.

Paul, J., 1976, Hemoglobin synthesis in cell differentiation, *Br. Med. Bull.* **32**:277.

Pembrey, M., Weatherall, D., and Clegg, J., 1973, Maternal synthesis of Hb F in pregnancy, *Lancet* **i**:1350.

Perrine, R., Brown, M., Clegg, J., Weatherall, D., and May, A., 1972, Benign sickle cell anemia, *Lancet* **ii**:1163.

Perry, R., 1976, Processing of RNA, *Annu. Rev. Biochem.* **45**:605.

Perry, R., and Kelley, D., 1976, Kinetics of formation of 5' terminal CAPS in mRNA, *Cell* **8**:433.

Piantadosi, C., Dickerman, H., and Spivak, J., 1976, Sequential activation of splenic nuclear RNA polymerases by erythropoietin, *J. Clin. Invest.* **57**:20.

Popovic, W., Brown, J., and Adamson, J., 1977, Influence of thyroid hormones on *in vitro* erythropoiesis. Mediation by a receptor with beta adrenergic properties, *J. Clin. Invest.* **60**:907.

Ramirez, F., Gambino, R., Maniatis, G., Rifkind, R., Marks, P., and Bank, A., 1975, Changes in globin messenger RNA content during erythroid cell differentiation, *J. Biol. Chem.* **250**:6054.

Ricco, G., Mazza, U., Turi, R., Pich, P., Camaschella, C., Saglio, G., and Bernini, L., 1976, Significance of a new type of human fetal hemoglobin carrying a replacement isoleucine $\rightarrow$ threonine at position 75 (E19) of the $\gamma$ chain, *Hum. Genet.* **32**:305.

Rosendaal, M., 1977, Age-dependent surface marker on haemopoietic stem cells, *Nature* **265**:147.

Ross, J., 1976, A precursor of globin messenger RNA, *J. Mol. Biol.* **106**:403.

Ross, J., Aviv, H., Schonick, E., and Leder, P., 1972, *In vitro* synthesis of DNA complementary to purified rabbit globin mRNA, *Proc. Natl. Acad. Sci. U.S.A.* **69**:254.

Schroeder, W., Huisman, T., Shelton, J., and Wilson, J., 1970, An improved method for quantitative determination of human fetal hemoglobin, *Anal. Biochem.* **35**:235.

Sforoniadou, K., Wood, W., Nute, P., and Stamatoyannopoulos, G., 1975, Globin chain synthesis in the Greek type ($^A$gamma) of hereditary persistence of fetal hemoglobin, *Br. J. Haematol.* **29**:137.

Shchory, M., and Weatherall, D., 1975, Hemoglobin synthesis in human fetal liver maintained in short-term culture, *Br. J. Haematol.* **30**:9.

Sheridan, B., Weatherall, D., Clegg, J., Pritchard, J., Wood, W., Callendar, S., Durrant, I., McWhirter, W., Ali, M., Partridge, J., and Thompson, E., 1976, The patterns of fetal hemoglobin production in leukemia, *Br. J. Haematol.* **32**:487.

Singer, J., and Adamson, J., 1976, Steroids and hematopoiesis. III. The response of granulocytic and erythroid-colony forming cells to steroids of different classes, *Blood* **48**:855.

Smith, D., Clegg, J., Weatherall, D., and Gilles, H., 1973, Hereditary persistence of hemoglobin associated with a gamma beta fusion variant, Hb Kenya, *Nature New Biol.* **246**:184.

Spivak, J., 1976, Effect of erythropoietin on chromosomal protein synthesis, *Blood* **47**:581.

Spohr, G., Dettori, G., and Manzari, V., 1976, Globin mRNA sequences in polyadenylated and nonpolyadenylated nuclear precursor messenger RNA from avian erythroblasts, *Cell* **8**:505.

Stamatoyannopoulos, G., Wood, W., Papayannopoulou, T., and Nute, P., 1975, A new form of hereditary persistence of fetal hemoglobin in blacks and its association with sickle cell trait, *Blood* **46**:683.

Stephenson, J., Axelrad, A., McLeod, D., and Shreeve, M., 1971, Induction of colonies of hemoglobin-synthesizing cells by erythropoietin *in vitro*, *Proc. Natl. Acad. Sci. U.S.A.* **68**:1542.

Strair, R., Skoultchi, A., and Shafritz, D., 1977, A characterization of globin mRNA sequences in the nucleus of duck immature red cells, *Cell* **12**:131.

Tepperman, A., Curtis, J., and McCulloch, E., 1974, Erythropoietic colonies in cultures of human marrow, *Blood* **44**:659.

Thurmon, T., Boyer, S., Crosby, E., Shepard, M., Noyes, A., and Stohlman, F., 1970, Hemoglobin switching in nonanemic sheep. III. Evidence for presumptive identity between the A→C factor and erythropoietin, *Blood* **36**:598.

VanVliet, G., and Huisman, T., 1964, Changes in the hemoglobin types of sheep as a response to anemia, *Biochem. J.* **93**:401.

Vaskov, V., and Efremov, G., 1967, Fourth hemoglobin type in sheep, *Nature* **216**:593.

Verma, I., Temple, G., Fann, H., and Baltimore, D., 1972, *In vitro* synthesis of DNA complementary erythrocyte 10S RNA, *Nature New Biol.* **235**:163.

Weatherall, D., and Clegg, J., 1972, *The Thalassemia Syndromes*, 2nd ed., Blackwell, Oxford, England.

Weatherall, D., and Clegg, J., 1975, Hereditary persistence of fetal hemoglobin, *Br. J. Haematol.* **29**:191.

Weatherall, D., Pembrey, M., and Pritchard, J., 1974, Fetal hemoglobin, *Clin. Haematol.* **3**:467.

Weatherall, D., Cartner, R., Clegg, J., Wood, W., MacRae, I., and MacKenzie, A., 1975, A form of hereditary persistence of fetal hemoglobin characterized by uneven cellular distribution of Hb F and the production of Hbs A and $A_2$ in homozygotes, *Br. J. Haematol.* **29**:205.

Weatherall, D., Clegg, J., and Wood, W., 1976, A model for the persistence or reactivation of fetal hemoglobin production, *Lancet* **ii**:660.

Weintraub, H., and Groudine, M., 1976, Chromosomal subunits in active genes have an altered conformation, *Science* **193**:848.

Weintraub, H., Worcel, A., and Alberts, B., 1976, A model for chromatin based upon two symmetrically paired half-nucleosomes, *Cell* **9**:409.

Weller, S., Aply, J., and Raper, A., 1966, Malformations associated with precocious synthesis of adult hemoglobin, *Lancet* **i**:777.

Wilson, M., Schroeder, W., and Graves, D., 1968, Postnatal change of Hbs F and $A_2$ in infants with Down's syndrome (G trisomy), *Pediatrics* **42**:349.

Wood, W., and Weatherall, D., 1973, Haemoglobin synthesis during human fetal development, *Nature* **244**:162.

Wood, W., Stamatoyannopoulos, G., Lim, G., and Nute, P., 1975, F cells in the adult: Normal adults and levels in individuals with hereditary and acquired elevations of Hb F, *Blood* **46**:671.

Wood, W., Pearce, K., Clegg, J., Weatherall, D., Robinson, J., Thorburn, G., and Dawes, G., 1976a, Switch from foetal to adult haemoglobin synthesis in normal and hypophysectomized sheep, *Nature* **264**:799.

Wood, W., Weatherall, D., and Clegg, J., 1976b, Interaction of heterocellular hereditary persistence of fetal hemoglobin with beta thalassemia and sickle cell anemia, *Nature* **264**:247.

Wood, W., Weatherall, D., Clegg, J., Hamblin, T., Edwards, J., and Barlow, A., 1977, Hetercellular hereditary persistence of fetal hemoglobin (heterocellular HPFH) and its interaction with beta thalassemia, *Br. J. Haematol.* **36**:461.

Wrightstone, R., Wilson, J., Miller, A., and Huisman, T., 1970, The structure of goat hemoglobins. IV. A third beta chain variant (beta[E]) with three apparent amino acid substitutions, *Arch. Biochem. Biophys.* **138**:451.

Zanjani, E., Mann, L., Burlington, H., Gordon, A., and Wasserman, L., 1974, Evidence for a physiologic role of erythropoietin in fetal erythropoiesis, *Blood* **44**:285.

5

# Mechanisms Underlying Marrow Toxicity from Chloramphenicol and Thiamphenicol

### Adel A. Yunis

## 5.1. Introduction

Despite the current availability of a large number of effective broad spectrum antimicrobials, chloramphenicol (CAP) continues to enjoy wide clinical use and thus remains the leading single cause of drug-induced aplastic anemia.

It is now established that CAP produces two types of hematologic toxicity (Yunis and Bloomberg, 1964; Yunis, 1969a,b, 1973a,b): (1) the common dose-dependent, reversible bone marrow suppression affecting primarily the erythroid precursors and occasionally involving the granulocytic and megakaryocytic elements, and (2) the rare complication characterized by pancytopenia, hypoplasia, or aplasia of the bone marrow, lack

---

ADEL A. YUNIS  •  Departments of Medicine and Biochemistry, University of Miami School of Medicine; Howard Hughes Laboratories for Hematological Research, Howard Hughes Medical Institute, Miami, Florida.

of dose–effect relationship, and, in most cases, a fatal outcome. Furthermore, current evidence supports the concept of a lack of relationship between these two types of toxicity.

Although many of the pathogenetic aspects of CAP toxicity remain uncertain, a great deal of progress has been made in. recent years, particularly in our understanding of the basic mechanisms underlying reversible bone marrow suppression. The advent of *in vitro* bone marrow culture techniques has served to facilitate the study of drug-induced direct bone marrow toxicity and various aspects of drug–cell interactions.

Because of its rarity, unpredictability, and lack of an experimental model, aplastic anemia from CAP has been much more difficult to investigate. Accordingly, progress in this area has been slow. The introduction into the European market of a CAP analog, thiamphenicol (TAP), which has thus far not been associated with aplastic anemia (Keiser, 1974), has reopened the question of structure–toxicity relationship in the CAP molecule and has raised several intriguing considerations regarding pathogenesis of CAP-induced aplastic anemia.

In this chapter an attempt is made to review the current status of knowledge of the pathogenetic aspects of the two types of toxicity from CAP and consider some of the structural and metabolic differences between CAP and TAP and their possible significance.


## 5.2. Historical Background

Hematologic toxicity from CAP became apparent soon after the drug became available in 1949 (Recinos *et al.*, 1949; Olshaker *et al.*, 1949; Volini *et al.*, 1950). Reversible selective erythroid suppression from CAP was first described by Lindau in 1952. The first case of aplastic anemia from CAP was reported by Rich *et al.* in 1950 in a patient who received four courses of the drug over an 80-day period. Death resulted from hemorrhage and infection 11 days from onset of symptoms. The subsequent appearance of many similar cases led to the withdrawal of CAP from the market. Upon its return with a warning on the label, the CAP sales dropped sharply in 1954 only to rise to a new high in 1958–1961 (Dameshek, 1960). A major contributor to this increase in CAP use was the erroneous belief, generated largely by description of reversible erythroid suppression by the drug, that one could prevent the occurrence of aplastic anemia by attention to dosage and duration of therapy, and by monitoring the blood counts.

Although in the individual case of aplastic anemia it is not possible to establish a causal relationship between aplasia and the drug, the cumulative evidence has left no doubt about the direct causation of aplastic anemia by CAP. Thus, in all series of drug-induced aplastic anemia reported in the literature, an association with CAP is the most frequent (Erslev and Wintrobe, 1962; Bithell and Wintrobe, 1967; Williams *et al.*, 1973).

## 5.3. Biochemistry and Pharmacology of Chloramphenicol

CAP (D(−)-threo-1-*p*-nitrophenyl-2-dichloroacetamido-1,3-propane-diol) (Rebstock *et al.*, 1949) was originally obtained from *Streptomyces venezuala,* an actinomycetes isolated by Burkholder in 1947. Chemical synthesis followed soon thereafter. The drug possesses the nitrobenzene moiety, a unique structural feature among antibiotics. It is relatively stable to heat and to wide pH variation (Goodman and Gilman, 1960). Only the D-stereoisomer is biologically active. An intact propanediol moiety appears critical for activity (Brock, 1961; Collins *et al.*, 1952; Rebstock *et al.*, 1949).

In the usual therapeutic concentrations CAP is primarily bacterio-static (Jackson, 1958). Concentrations in the range of 1–10 $\mu$g/ml are inhibitory to the gram-negative bacteria, *Aerobacter aerogenes, Escherichia coli, Klebsiella pneumoniae, Haemophilus pertussis, Salmonella typosa, Proteus, Neisseria, Brucella,* and *Vibrio cholerae* (Goodman and Gilman, 1960). Activity can also be demonstrated against richettsial organisms and the psitta-cosislymphogranuloma venereum group of viruses.

Bacterial resistance of CAP and its biochemical basis have been the subject of intensive studies. Several modes of inactivation of the CAP molecule occur in various bacteria—reduction of the nitro group (Smith and Worrel, 1950), hydrolysis of the amide linkage (Jackson, 1958), etc.—but there is no evidence that these are responsible for clinically important resistance to CAP. More recently conclusive evidence has been provided that inactivation of CAP occurs via enzymatic acetylation with acetyl-CoA as the acetyl donor (Okamoto and Suzuki, 1965; Suzuki and Okamoto, 1967; Shaw and Brodsky, 1968; Winshell and Shaw, 1969; Shaw, 1971):

Chloramphenicol + acetyl-S-CoA
$$\rightarrow \text{chloramphenicol-3-acetate} + \text{HS-CoA}$$

Chloramphenicol-3-acetate $\rightarrow$ chloramphenicol-1-acetate

Chloramphenicol 1-acetate + acetyl-S-CoA
$$\rightarrow \text{chloramphenicol-1,3-diacetate} + \text{HS-CoA}$$

Chloramphenicol acetate, which is formed very rapidly, is inactive as an antibiotic. The reaction is catalyzed by the enzyme acetyl transferase which is synthesized in all enteric bacteria carrying the R factor determinant for CAP resistance. This subject has been reviewed thoroughly by Shaw (1971).

## 5.4. Metabolism of Chloramphenicol

CAP is almost completely absorbed from the gastrointestinal tract. Serum levels of 20–40 $\mu$g/ml cal be obtained from an oral dose of 2 g and levels of 40–60 $\mu$g/ml from a dose of 4 g (Goodman and Gilman, 1960). The drug is concentrated largely in the kidneys, liver, and lungs as determined by microbiological assays (Glazko *et al.*, 1949) and by $^{14}$C-labeled CAP distribution (Yunis and Bloomberg, 1964). In the liver, the major site of degradation of CAP, the drug is conjugated to glucuronic acid, the glucuronide product being biologically inactive. About 90% of a given dose is excreted in the urine in 24 hr, 90% of which consists of the glucuronide conjugate and hydrolysis products and 10% of the biologically active form. The rat excretes CAP largely in the bile (Glazko *et al.*, 1952).

As might be expected, the serum half-life of active CAP is prolonged in liver disease while the half-life of the inactive conjugate is prolonged in renal insufficiency (Kunin *et al.*, 1959).

In contrast to man, lower animals are capable of eliminating the drug much more rapidly. Thus, it is impossible with equivalent doses to maintain similar blood levels in animals like the rabbit or the rat. For example, Weisberger *et al.* (1964a) used CAP in doses of 300–600 mg/kg intramuscularly in rabbits (equivalent to 21–42 g of the drug per day to a 70-kg man) to obtain serum drug levels of 5–20 $\mu$g/ml. Martelo *et al.* (1969) were able to obtain a serum CAP level of 32 $\mu$g/ml by giving rabbits 175 mg/kg intravenously in seven equal doses at hourly intervals. In studies in dogs serum CAP levels of 15–20 $\mu$g/ml were achieved by the daily oral administration of 150 mg/kg (Manyan and Yunis, 1970).

## 5.5. Pharmacology and Metabolism of Thiamphenicol

TAP differs from CAP by substitution of the *p*-nitro group with a methylsulfonyl moiety (Fig. 1). This alteration in structure has conferred on the molecule some distinct properties. In contrast to CAP, TAP does not undergo glucuronidation in the liver (Ferrari and Della Bella, 1974). Neither intact nor sonicated microsomal preparations can carry out glucuronidation of TAP, indicating that the enzyme itself (glucurosyl transfer-

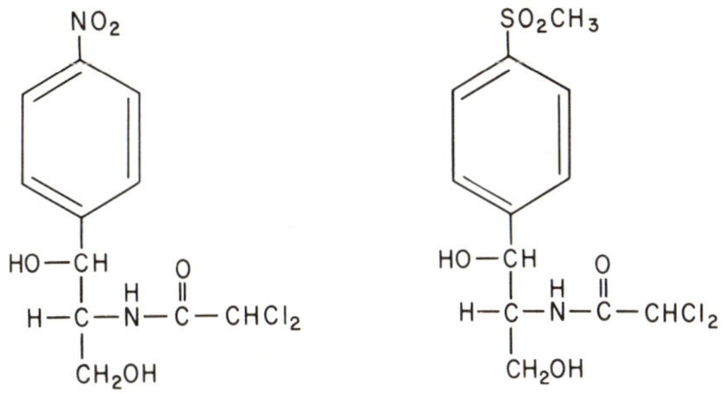

Fig. 1.   Structure of (left) chloramphenicol and (right) thiamphenicol.

ase) is inactive with TAP as a substrate. Furthermore, TAP does not inhibit the conjugation of CAP. Therefore, while CAP is excreted in the urine largely as the inactive glucuronide conjugate, 63% of a given TAP dose is excreted as the unchanged active compound (Cattebeni and Gazzaniga, 1974). The clinical pharmacological implications of these differences are clear; the excretion of active TAP in the urine renders this antibiotic more effective in urinary tract infections. Furthermore, while careful attention should be given to CAP dosage in patients with liver disease, with TAP renal clearance is of great importance in determining dosage (Tacquet *et al.*, 1974).

CAP and TAP have a similar antimicrobial spectrum. As with CAP, inactivation of TAP by bacteria is carried out by acetylation to the 1,3-diacetoxyl derivative, a reaction catalyzed by acetyl transferase, and requires CoA (Ferrari and Della Bella, 1974). The affinity of the enzyme is greater for CAP. It is of interest that there are present in the serum enzymes which are capable of hydrolyzing the acetylated derivative back to the free active form. As with CAP the acetylation accounts for bacterial resistance which is acquired through a stepwise mutation and is carried on an extrachromosomal DNA plasmid (Kayser and Wust, 1974).

## 5.6. Clinical Features of Chloramphenicol Toxicity

The current classification of hematologic toxicity from CAP into two types (Yunis and Bloomberg, 1964) in addition to its clinical and pathogenetic importance, carries considerable historical interest.

The devastating nature of CAP-induced aplastic anemia prompted many investigators to search for early signs of hematologic toxicity in the hope of providing a warning wherein discontinuation of the drug may avert the occurrence of irreversible bone marrow damage. In 1955 Krak-off *et al.* administered large doses of CAP to four patients with advanced cancer and noted reticulocytopenia and anemia which returned to pre-treatment levels upon discontinuation of the drug. It is of interest that a rechallenge with small doses of CAP failed to reproduce the hematologic changes. In 1958 Rubin *et al.* described early ferrokinetic changes indicative of suppressed erythropoiesis in patients on large CAP doses. These two early reports were soon followed by intensive studies on human volunteers all of which served to establish the common occurrence with large doses of CAP of an erythropoietic lesion characterized by (1) ferrokinetic changes consisting of increased plasma iron, increaed saturation of the iron binding globulin, delayed plasma clearance of $^{59}$Fe, and decreased iron utilization; (2) morphologic bone marrow changes consisting of vacuolization and maturation arrest in early erythroid cells and less frequently in granulocytic precursors (Rubin *et al.*, 1960; Rosenbach *et al.*, 1960; Saidi *et al.*, 1961; Jiji *et al.*, 1963; Gussof and Lee, 1966); and (3) reticulocytopenia and occasionally mild anemia, leukopenia, or thrombocytopenia. It is important to emphasize that this lesion is dose-dependent, can be produced virtually at will if large enough doses are given, and has always been reversible, with no known exceptions. A clear correlation of this lesion to CAP blood levels was nicely demonstrated in a double blind study by Scott *et al.* (1965); all patients developed evidence of bone marrow toxicity at drug levels of 35 $\mu$g/ml and in all subjects signs of toxicity disappeared after treatment was discontinued.

The most important question regarding reversible erythroid suppression from CAP has always centered around its possible relationship to bone marrow aplasia from the drug. This question was approached by Yunis and Bloomberg in 1964 by a detailed analysis of 95 reported cases of incidental CAP toxicity. Based on their analysis they classified hematologic toxicity into two types, the characteristics of which are summarized in Table I. As can be seen in this table, in addition to the foregoing characteristics, reversible erythroid suppression occurs concurrently with CAP administration and is associated with a normally cellular bone marrow. In contrast aplastic anemia is characterized by pancytopenia, an aplastic or hypoplastic bone marrow, a late clinical onset occurring 2 weeks to 5 months from the last dose, a lack of dose–effect relationship, and a fatal outcome relationship between these two toxicities is completely lacking. The erythropoietic lesion is a pharmacologic effect of CAP and should not be regarded as a warning of impending aplastic anemia. It will become clear from this review that current evidence has reinforced the validity of this classification and supports the concept of two separate unrelated bone marrow lesions induced by CAP.

**Table I.** Characteristics of Two Types of Hematologic Toxicity from Chloramphenicol

|  | Reversible toxicity | Bone marrow aplasia |
|---|---|---|
| Incidence | Common | Rare |
| Bone marrow cellularity | Cellular | Hypoplastic or aplastic |
| Relation to dose | Dose dependent | Not related to dose |
| Onset | Concurrent with drug therapy | Clinical onset 3 weeks to 5 months from last dose |
| Bone marrow changes | Maturation arrest—erythroid cells; cytoplasmic and/or nuclear vacuolization | Marrow aplasia, predominance of nonmyeloid elements |
| Peripheral blood changes | Reticulocytopenia, occasional leukopenia and/or thrombocytopenia, anemia if treatment is prolonged | Pancytopenia |
| Presenting symptoms | None. Pallor due to anemia (if treatment is prolonged) | Bleeding and/or infection |
| Outcome | Reversible | Usually fatal |

## 5.7. Pathogenesis

As has been pointed out earlier, a great deal of progress has been made in the past 10 years in our understanding of the biochemical mechanisms underlying reversible bone marrow suppression from CAP. On the other hand, the pathogenesis of CAP-induced aplastic anemia remains uncertain. Studies in this area have been very limited, primarily because of the rarity and unpredictability of this complication and the lack of an experimental model. The extensive use of TAP in Europe and the absence thus far of authenticated cases of aplastic anemia in association with this drug have raised some intriguing questions with important pathogenetic implications. Before considering these questions, it is pertinent to review briefly the metabolic effects of CAP and TAP in microorganisms versus mammalian cells.

### 5.7.1. Actions of CAP and TAP in Bacterial versus Mammalian Cells

In sensitive bacteria CAP is a potent and specific inhibitor of protein synthesis (Gale and Folkes, 1953; Wissman *et al.*, 1954; Hahn *et al.*, 1955). The mechanism of inhibition involves the stereospecific and reversible binding of CAP to the 50S ribosomal subunit (Wolfe and Hahn, 1965; Hazquez, 1966; Hurwitz and Braun, 1967) and a block in peptide bond formation, thus preventing the growth of the nascent polypeptide chain (Weber and Demoss, 1966; Das *et al.*, 1966; Cundliffe and McQuillen, 1967). Peptide bond formation is catalyzed by the enzyme peptidyl transferase (Monroe *et al.*, 1967), and integral part of the 50S ribosomal subunit, and involves the transfer of the growing peptide chain from a tRNA bond in the donor site to an aminoacyl-tRNA bond in the acceptor site on the same ribosome.

TAP is equally potent as an inhibitor of bacterial protein synthesis and exerts its effect by a similar mechanism. Competitive binding studies indicate that CAP and TAP share identical binding sites on the bacterial ribosome (Contreras *et al.*, 1974).

An entirely different situation exists with eukaryotic cells. In spite of early reports to the contrary (Weisberger *et al.*, 1963, 1964 b; Weisberger and Wolfe, 1964), it is now established that CAP does not bind to ribosomes of mammalian cells (Vazquez, 1964) and that ribosomal protein synthesis in these cells is resistant to CAP (Zelkowitz *et al.*, 1967, 1968). While most metabolic parameters in mammalian cells can be inhibited by inordinately high concentrations of CAP (Folette *et al.*, 1956; Erslev and Iossifides, 1962; Yunis and Harrington, 1960), only mitochondrial protein synthesis is sensitive to drug levels within therapeutic range (Roodyn *et al.*, 1961; Truman and Korner, 1962; Kroon, 1964; Garren and Crocco, 1967). Thus CAP concentrations of 10–20 $\mu$g/ml have been shown to inhibit protein synthesis in mitochondria of rat liver, beef heart, and adrenal. A similar degree of inhibition can be demonstrated by comparable concentrations of TAP (Yunis *et al.*, 1973, 1974; Yunis, 1973b; Nijhof and Kroon, 1974).

## 5.7.2. Pathogenesis of Reversible Erythroid Suppression from CAP

### 5.7.2.1. CAP and Mitochondrial Protein Synthesis

The virtually regular occurrence of reversible erythroid suppression from large doses of CAP and the excellent correlation with CAP blood levels strongly suggest a direct toxic effect of the drug on bone marrow cells which is likewise reversible. The discovery that mitochondrial protein synthesis is equisitely sensitive to CAP has led to a series of investigations aimed at establishing a relationship between this *in vitro* metabolic effect of the drug and its myelotoxicity.

In initial studies it was demonstrated that CAP in concentrations as low as 10 $\mu$g/ml caused profound inhibition of protein synthesis in mitochondria isolated from rabbits and human bone marrow cells (Martelo *et al.*, 1969). This inhibitory effect was not secondary to inhibition of mitochondrial respiration or oxidative phosphorylation since levels about 100 μg were required to inhibit these processes. Evidence relating this *in vitro* effect to myelotoxicity from CAP was derived from several lines of investigation. The first involved a comparative study with antibiotics not known to be myelotoxic. Among the antibiotics tested only tetracycline was equally inhibitory *in vitro,* but its effect could be reversed by high magnesium concentrations (Martelo *et al.*, 1969). Furthermore, whereas CAP inhibited bone mitochondrial protein synthesis *in vivo,* tetracycline was without effect. It was suggested from these observations that the avidity of tetracycline for the cations of metals and the high calcium and magnesium environment of the bone marrow may limit or prevent access of tetracycline to the target site of action, thereby protecting the bone marrow cells from its toxic action (Yunis *et al.*, 1970).

Another line of evidence relating bone marrow suppression to inhibition of mitochondrial protein synthesis was derived from hematologic and electromicroscopic correlation studies in patients receiving the drug (Yunis *et al.*, 1970; Smith *et al.*, 1970). In all patients an ultrastructural lesion was observed in marrow cell mitochondria characterized by condensation of the mitochondrial matrix without a change in matrical or overall mitochondrial volume. This lesion involved all marrow cell types and the extent of the changes correlated well with CAP blood levels and degree of elevation of serum iron concentrations. The mitochondrial ultrastructural changes were no longer demonstrable following discontinuation of CAP treatment. More severe ultrastructural alterations have recently been described in bone marrow cells from a seriously ill patient with staphylococcal pneumonia while under treatment with CAP (Skinnider and Gladially, 1976). It is of interest that in this study the well-documented vacuoles seen on light microscopy were shown to represent lipid droplets.

It is clear that CAP causes profound inhibition of mitochondrial protein synthesis *in vitro* and *in vivo.* It also produces an ultrastructural lesion in mitochondria, which, like clinical bone marrow suppression, occurs concurrently with drug therapy, is directly related to serum levels of CAP, and is likewise reversible. It is of interest in this regard that Manyan and co-workers demonstrated reversibility of the CAP effect at the mitochondrial level *in vitro* (D. R. Manyan and A. A. Yunis, unpublished); restoration of protein synthesis was observed after the drug was removed by mitochondrial washing.

Since the inhibition of mitochondrial protein synthesis by CAP is not tissue specific, one must account for the known vulnerability of erythroid cells to CAP through some additional mechanisms. The possibility exists that mitochondrial protein synthesis in erythroid cells is more sensitive to CAP, but this has not been investigated. On the other hand, there is evidence to suggest that the heme synthetic pathway may be one target for the CAP effect accounting for erythroid cell susceptibility. It is known that the inhibitory effect of CAP in mitochondria is directed primarily at the synthesis of structural or membranous proteins (Wheeldon and Lehninger, 1966; Neupert *et al.*, 1967; Beattie *et al.*, 1967). It is also known that the enzyme ferrochelatase (FC) which catalyzes the incorporation of iron into protoporhyrin, is intimately associated with the inner mitochondrial membrane (Jones and Jones, 1969; McKay *et al.*, 1969). This has raised the important question of whether this enzyme might be suppressed by CAP either by direct inhibition of FC synthesis or the synthesis of an FC-binding side on the inner mitochondrial membrane.

Manyan and co-workers have examined this possibility in dogs and their results can be summarized as follows (Manyan and Yunis, 1970; Manyan *et al.*, 1972): (1) The oral administration of CAP (100 mg/kg day) resulted in a drop in bone marrow FC activity to 5–35% of control levels. In contrast, the enzyme ALA synthetase, found in the soluble mitochondrial fraction, was not suppressed by CAP. (2) Accompanying the fall in FC activity, there was a rise in free erythrocyte protoporphyrin and accumulation of stainable iron in the bone marrow, findings consistent with a block in the last step of heme synthesis. (3) Reticulocytopenia developed in two of three dogs. All parameters returned to normal after the drug was discontinued. CAP did not affect FC activity *in vitro*. These results indicated an *in vivo* suppression of FC activity accompanied by a block in heme synthesis and depression in erythropoiesis. This action of CAP offers a reasonable biochemical explanation for the vulnerability of nucleated red cells to CAP. Suppression of FC activity adequately accounts for the appearance of ring sideroblasts commonly observed in bone marrow of patients receiving large doses of CAP.

Why a block in heme synthesis should result in maturation arrest in erythroid cells is not clear, however. It is likely that other important mitochondrial membranous proteins are involved. Suppression of synthesis of cytochrome $a + a_3$ and $b$ by CAP has been clearly shown, ultimately leading to suppressed mitochondrial respiration, compromised cellular synthetic processes and cessation of cell proliferation (Firkin and Linnane, 1969; Firkin, 1972). Inhibition of cellular proliferation by CAP can be demonstrated using a variety of *in vitro* culture systems, including HeLa cells (Firkin and Linnane, 1968) and bone marrow (Ratzan *et al.*, 1974). Therefore, while suppression of FC activity might explain the vulnerability of erythroid cells to CAP, the action of the drug on cytochrome synthesis should ultimately affect all proliferating cells. It is well known that reversible bone marrow suppression from CAP frequently involves all marrow elements.

To summarize, current evidence leaves little doubt that reversible bone marrow suppression from CAP results from inhibition of mitochondrial membranous protein synthesis, leading to suppressed mitochondrial respiration, and ultimately compromised cellular synthetic machinery and cessation of cell proliferation.

### 5.7.2.2. Effect of CAP on Bone Marrow Myeloid (CFU-C) and Erythroid (CFU-E) Colony Growth *in Vitro*

The *in vitro* bone marrow culture technique provides a potentially useful tool for the study of drug-induced direct toxicity and various aspects of drug–cell interactions. Using the bone marrow-in-agar culture system it has been shown that drugs which are capable of producing a dose-dependent granulocytopenia *in vivo*, e.g., CAP, TAP, and chlorpromazine, also cause reversible inhibition of human and murine CFU-C growth *in vitro* when used in concentrations within therapeutic range (Ratzan *et al.*, 1974; Yunis and Gross, 1975). Drugs that only rarely suppress marrow function unpredictably and without relationship to dose, e.g., phenylbutazone, diphenylhydantoin, have little or no effect on CFU-C growth. However, while CAP, TAP, and chlorpromazine consistently inhibit colony growth under defined *in vitro* conditions, they do not regularly produce granulocytopenia *in vivo*. This is undoubtedly due to the existence of *in vivo* modifying factors. Based on recent observations, Yunis has suggested (Yunis and Gross, 1975; Yunis, 1976) that the concentration of colony-stimulating factor (CSF) in the cell milieu *in vivo* may play an important role in determining the occurrence and/or degree of granulocytopenia from these drugs. Thus, in both murine and human bone marrow the degree of inhibition of colony growth by a given drug concentration is inversely proportional to the level of CSF in the medium. Both the total number of colonies inhibited as well as the percentage of inhibition are higher at the lower CSF levels. This is illustrated in Table II, which shows the effect of a fixed concentration of CAP on mouse and human CFU-C growth at three CSF levels. Almost complete protection from inhibition is observed at the level of 0.15. It was further shown that reversal of inhibition of CFU-C growth by CSF is directly related to CSF activity. CAP neither binds nor inactivates CSF; the mechanism of drug–CSF interaction remains unknown. A similar pattern of inhibition is shown with chlorpromazine (CPZ) (Fig. 2). Here the inhibition by 4 $\mu$g/ml CPZ is completely reversed by high CSF levels but reversal fails to occur at the CPZ concentration of 8 $\mu$g/ml.

**Table II.** Inhibition of CFU-C Growth by Cap and Reversal of Inhibition by High Levels of CSF

| CAP (μg/ml) | Mouse bone marrow CSF level | | | Human bone marrow CSF level | | |
|---|---|---|---|---|---|---|
| | 0.05 | 0.1 | 0.15 | 0.05 | 0.1 | 0.15 |
| 0 | 105 ± 5[a] | 140 ± 10 | 150 ± 8 | 62 ± 4 | 61 ± 7 | 60 ± 2 |
| 25 | 30 ± 3 | 100 ± 6 | 130 ± 11 | | | |
| 40 | | | | 26 ± 3 | 38 ± 9 | 54 ± 6 |
| 80 | | | | 10 ± 2 | 16 ± 2 | 38 ± 5 |

[a]Number of colonies ± SD.

While the relationship of *in vitro* findings to what occurs *in vivo* must be interpreted with caution, our observations do suglest that *in vivo* CSF levels may modulate the severity of drug-induced toxic neutropenia. For example, it is known that neutropenia in the course of CPZ treatment is often transient, with recovery occurring in the face of continued drug administration. This recovery could be the result of a rise in the level of CSF brought on by the drug challenge. Further studies are needed for a definitive conclusion.

The known vulnerability of erythroid cells to CAP and the results of studies on CFU-C have prompted similar studies on CFU-E growth (Yunis and Adamson, 1977). As in the case of CFU-C, CAP inhibits CFU-E growth in a sterospecific and concentration-dependent manner. However, an important difference appears to be the greater sensitivity of human CFU-E growth to CAP, complete inhibition being observed at the concentration of 10 μg/ml. Furthermore, the degree of inhibition was uninfluenced by the level of erythropoietin in the medium. This lack of reversal as observed in mouse marrow is illustrated in Fig. 3. This is in sharp

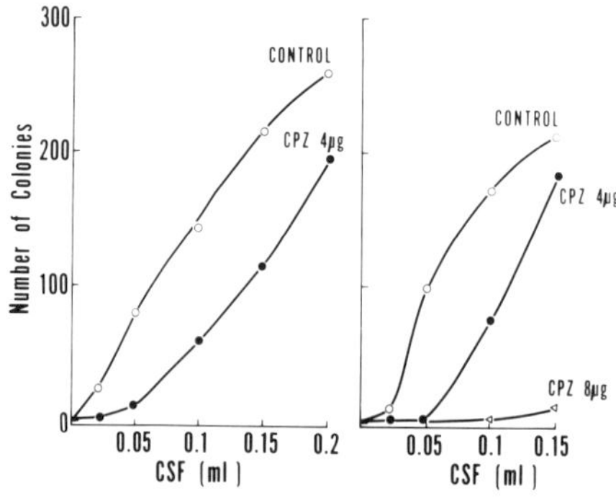


**Fig. 2.** The effect of CPZ (4 and 8 μg/ml) on mouse CFU-C growth and its relationship to CSF levels.

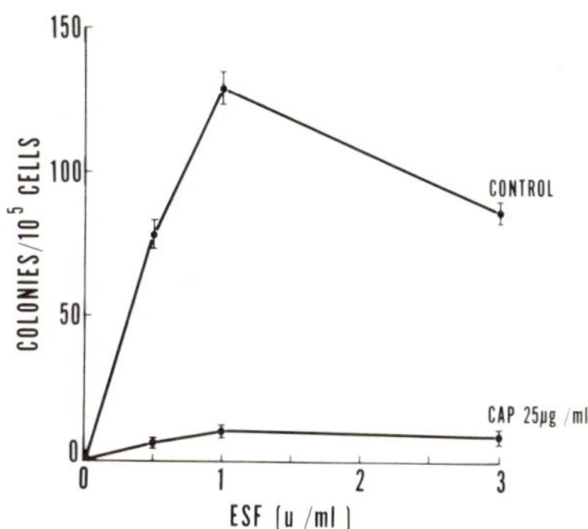


**Fig. 3.** The relationship of inhibition of mouse CFU-E growth by CAP to the level of ESF. No protection by ESF is observed. (Culture method as described by Stephenson *et al.*, 1971.)

contrast to what is observed with CFU-C growth and the protective effect of CSF. These results suggest that both the greater sensitivity of CFU-E to CAP and the lack of protection by ESF account for the known vulnerability to erythroid precursors to CAP *in vivo*.

## 5.7.3. Pathogenesis of CAP-Induced Aplastic Anemia

Bone marrow aplasia from CAP occurs rarely and unpredictably without any particular relationship to dose or duration of therapy, indicating individual predisposition as the major determining factor. On the basis of *in vitro* observations on DNA synthesis in bone marrow from patients who have recovered from CAP-induced aplastic anemia and from controls, we have postulated a genetic predisposition involving the pathway of DNA synthesis (Yunis and Harrington, 1960; Yunis and Arimura, 1963; Yunis and Bloomberg, 1964; Yunis, 1969a). Whereas CAP concentrations in the range 200–500 $\mu$g/ml are required to inhibit DNA synthesis in normal bone marrow, a drug concentration of 25–50 $\mu$g causes significant inhibition in marrow from previously afflicted subjects and some of their family members. Strong support for a genetically determined predisposition has been provided by one report describing the occurrence of CAP-induced aplastic anemia in identical twins (Nagao and Mauer, 1969).

A potential clue to the pathogenesis of CAP-induced aplastic anemia may be provided by TAP. This analog of CAP has been used extensively in Europe and has just been introduced into the market in the United Kingdom but is unavailable for clinical use in the United States. Whereas reversible bone marrow suppression in association with TAP treatment occurs as frequently as with CAP, there are to date no documented cases of aplastic anemia associated with TAP (Keiser, 1974). These clinical observations have reopened the question of structure toxicity relationship and suggest a major role for the *p*-nitro group in the causation of aplastic anemia. Accordingly, a detailed comparative metabolic study on CAP and TAP might provide a fruitful approach to this problem (Yunis *et al.*, 1973, 1974; Yunis, 1973a,b, 1974b, 1976).

## 5.7.4. Comparative Effects of CAP and TAP in Mammalian Cells; Common Effects Related to Reversible Marrow Suppression

As discussed earlier, CAP and TAP are equally potent as inhibitors of mitochondrial protein synthesis. The comparative effects of increasing concentrations of CAP and TAP on rat liver mitochondrial protein synthesis are shown in Fig. 4. The minimum inhibitory concentration for both drugs is about 1.6 $\mu$g/ml. As with CAP, the administration of TAP to dogs results in suppression of ferrochelatase activity and a block in the last step of heme synthesis (Yunis, 1973a, 1974b). In comparable concentrations TAP inhibits both CFU-C and CFU-E growth in a pattern very similar to that of CAP (Ratzan *et al.*, 1974). All these results are consistent with the fact that TAP produces dose-dependent reversible marrow suppression as readily as CAP and further supports the conclusion that this type of marrow toxicity is a consequence of mitochondrial injury.

## 5.7.5. Properties Distinct to CAP, Possible Relation to Aplastic Anemia

### 5.7.5.1. Effects on DNA Synthesis

Although CAP does not inhibit DNA synthesis when used in therapeutic levels (1–2 × 10⁻⁴ M), higher concentrations become progressively

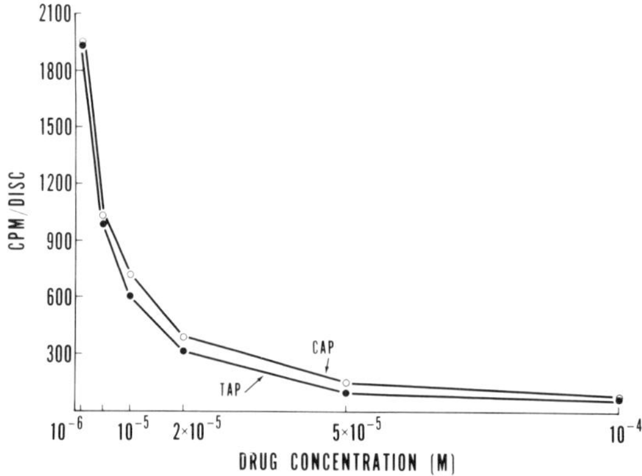


**Fig. 4.** Inhibition of rat liver mitochondrial protein synthesis as a function of CAP and TAP concentrations. (Experimental method as described by Yunis *et al.*, 1973.)

inhibitory (70% inhibition at $1.2 \times 10^{-3}$ M) (Yunis and Harrington, 1960; Yunis *et al.*, 1974; Yunis, 1973a,b). This has been demonstrated in rabbit, dog, and human marrow and in human lymphocyte cultures. The capacity to inhibit DNA synthesis at high concentrations appears to be a distinct property of CAP not shared by TAP. Furthermore, the inhibition is stereospecific as shown by the lack of effect of the L-threoisomer (Yunis, 1976) (Table III). This property of CAP may be related to the *p*-nitro group (Manyan *et al.*, 1975), since this is the only structural feature different from TAP. The nature of this relationship is not clear but may involve metabolic transformation of the *p*-nitro group to toxic products.

Recently Feeman and co-workers have confirmed and extended these observations (Freeman *et al.*, 1977). These authors found only slight inhibition of DNA synthesis by TAP. The inhibition by CAP was observed both under aerobic and anaerobic conditions and was not a result of an effect on the thymidine nucleotide pool. Freeman also believes that the *p*-nitro group of CAP is important for this metabolic effect. It is tempting to conclude from these studies that the *p*-nitro group, the capacity of CAP to inhibit DNA synthesis, and aplastic anemia from CAP are related, but the nature of this relationship remains uncertain.

### 5.7.5.2. Cellular and Mitochondrial Transport

An additional property that the *p*-nitro group confers on the CAP molecule and which may have pathogenetic importance in aplastic anemia concerns the cellular uptake and distribution of the drug. Studies in whole cells and isolated mitochondria (McLeod *et al.*, 1977; D. R. Manyan, T. F. McLeod, and A. A. Yunis, unpublished) have revealed sharp differences between CAP and TAP which can be summarized as follows: (1) CAP is taken up rapidly by whole cells, reaching maximal concentrations within 15 min with a cellular/extracellular ratio of 2–4. The uptake is little affected by temperature and is not influenced by metabolic inhibitors, indicating that it is neither active nor energy dependent. (2) The efflux of CAP is equally rapid and like influx is temperature independent. (3) In

**Table III.**   The Effect of CAP, Its L-Threoisomer, and TAP on the Incorporation of [$^{14}$C]Formate into DNA of Rabbit Bone Marrow

|  | Concentration | CPM/100 $\mu$g DNA |
|---|---|---|
| Control |  | $3300 \pm 150$ |
| CAP | $0.7 \times 10^{-3}$ M | $1800 \pm 120$ |
|  | $1.4 \times 10^{-3}$ M | $1250 \pm 70$ |
| L-threo-CAP | $0.7 \times 10^{-3}$ M | $3100 \pm 180$ |
|  | $1.4 \times 10^{-3}$ M | $2900 \pm 210$ |
| TAP | $0.7 \times 10^{-3}$ M | $3500 \pm 160$ |
|  | $1.4 \times 10^{-3}$ M | $3650 \pm 340$ |

contrast, the influx and efflux of TAP are comparatively slow at 37°C, with little or no movement occurring at 0°C. (4) A similar pattern of transport of CAP and TAP was demonstrated in isolated rat liver mitochondria. The influx and efflux of CAP across mitochondrial membranes were rapid and independent of both temperature and energy. The mitochondrial/extramitochondrial CAP ratio was consistently greater than 1. In contrast the uptake of TAP was considerably lower with I/E ratios consistently less than 1. Mitochondrial saturation was not observed with either drug (Fig. 5). This pattern of transport of CAP and TAP is most consistent with simple diffusion based on partitioning of the drugs in cellular and/or mitochondrial compartments. The greater uptake of CAP probably reflects its solubility in cell and mitochondrial lipid; the relatively stronger polarity of the methylsulfonyl moiety of TAP renders it less lipid soluble and thus more slowly diffusible across membranes.

The significance of the difference in transport between CAP and TAP in relation to metabolism and toxicity of the two drugs remains uncertain. It is of interest that at comparable blood levels more TAP is found in the urine per unit volume than CAP. The results of our studies which show a much slower intracellular influx of TAP offer a good physiologic explanation for this observation since diffusion of TAP across renal tubular cells would likewise be expected to be slower. This conclusion is corroborated by observations made directly on renal slices *in vitro* (T. F. McLeod and A. A. Yunis, unpublished).

As stated earlier, the degree of inhibition of mitochondrial protein synthesis by comparable concentrations of CAP and TAP is virtually identical. On the other hand, the observations that intramitochondrial

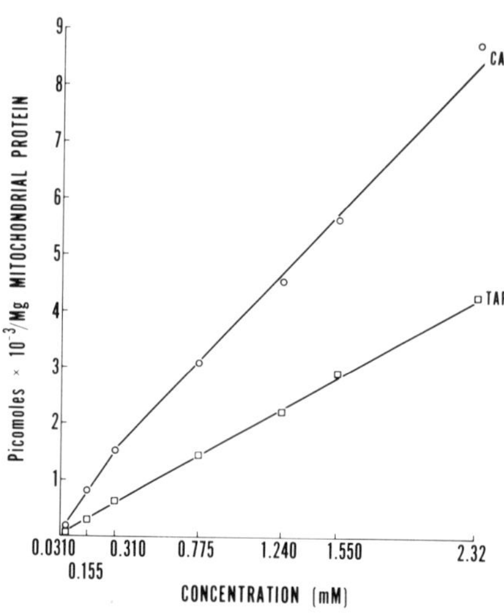


**Fig. 5.** The uptake of CAP and TAP by rat liver mitochondria as a function of drug concentration. The relationship of uptake to concentration is linear without evidence of saturation. Twice as much CAP as TAP was taken at all concentrations.

TAP concentrations reach only half those of CAP, suggest that TAP is a more potent inhibitor of mitochondrial protein synthesis. However, it is possible that the mitochondrial drug distribution is such that similar concentrations of CAP and TAP are attained at the mitochondrial ribosomal level. Whether the difference in the rate of influx of CAP and TAP accounts for the difference in their inhibitory capacity on DNA synthesis is undetermined. It is likely that both the inhibition of DNA synthesis and the rapid cellular uptake of CAP are a function of the structural property of the molecule.

### 5.7.5.3. Covalent Binding

An additional difference between CAP and TAP is in the extent of their intracellular covalent binding (Krishna, 1974; McLeod *et al.*, 1977; Yunis, 1976). When studied in whole cells there is a time-dependent covalent binding of CAP amounting to 4 pmol of drug/mg of cell protein at 30 min compared to only 1.5 pmol for TAP (McLeod *et al.*, 1977). Similarly, in isolated mitochondria the binding of CAP reaches a maximum of 8 pmol/mg mitochondrial protein in 30 min compared to 4 pmol of TAP (Yunis, 1976). The significance of covalent binding in relation to hematologic toxicity from CAP is uncertain.

To summarize, the fact that TAP, which has not been associated with aplastic anemia, differs from CAP only in substitution of the *p*-nitro group suggests that this structural feature of the CAP molecule is a major determining factor in the causation of aplastic anemia. Our studies also indicate that the *p*-nitro group somehow confers on the molecule the capacity to inhibit DNA synthesis, and to diffuse rapidly into nonpolar cell compartments. Whatever the relationship of these CAP properties to aplastic anemia, it is postulated that this complication results whenever the *p*-nitro group of CAP meets a favorable milieu in the predisposed host leading somehow to irreversible stem cell damage perhaps through its effects on DNA synthesis.

### 5.7.6. Possible Immunological Mechanisms in CAP-Induced Aplastic Anemia

In spite of the lack of experimental evidence for an immune mechanism in CAP-induced aplastic anemia, this possibility has never been excluded. CAP could conceivably act as a hapten by binding to some macromolecular component of bone marrow cells. The antigen thus produced may initiate the production of antibody by the host and subsequent antigen–antibody reaction resulting in bone marrow damage. Hamburger (1966) was able to produce CAP-specific antibody by coupling the reduced drug to albumin and using the product as the immunogen. There are no known reports describing the presence of anti-CAP antibody in sera of patients with CAP-induced aplastic anemia. However, the experiments of Hamburger suggest that CAP may act as a hapten *in vivo* by a similar mechanism involving reduction of the *p*-nitro group and covalent binding to macromolecules. It should be noted that according to this hypothesis, TAP, lacking the *p*-nitro group, would be incapable of undergoing a similar reaction. Schultz and Yunis (to be published) have confirmed the work of Hamburger and have shown that TAP can block the reaction between CAP and its antibody. Based on this observation a very sensitive radioimmunoassay for TAP and CAP has been devised by which drug levels as low as 1 $\mu$g/ml can be accurately measured.

A T-cell-mediated immune mechanism in aplastic anemia has recently been suggested from several reports based on improved CFU-C and/or CFU-E growth either by prior incubation of marrow cells with antithymocyte globulin or by selectively removing lymphocytes from the marrow cell population (Kagan *et al.*, 1976; Hoffman *et al.*, 1977). Inhibition of growth could be demonstrated by the readdition of the isolated lymphocytes. We have recently had the opportunity to carry out similar studies in two patients with CAP-induced aplastic anemia. In each case CFU-C growth was poor and did not improve after incubation of their marrow cells with antithymocyte globulin.

We have also coupled reduced CAP to human bone marrow extracts by the method of Hamberger. The product thus formed did not stimulate lymphocytes obtained from each of two patients who have partially recovered from CAP-induced aplastic anemia. Thus, our attempts to explore an immune mechanism for CAP-induced bone marrow aplasia have so far yielded negative results but further studies are needed before we can exclude the possibility.


## 5.8. Clinical Course of Chloramphenicol-Induced Aplastic Anemia

The clinical picture of CAP-induced aplastic anemia does not differ significantly from that of aplasia from other causes. The estimated incidence of bone marrow aplasia from CAP has undergone repeated revisions. Thus, earlier reports put the incidence at 1/60,000 to 1/200,000 (Leikin *et al.*, 1961; Smich *et al.*, 1964). However, based on the total sales of CAP in the state of California and all the cases of aplastic anemia in 1 year, an incidence of 1/24,000 to 1/40,000 has been estimated (Clarke, 1967). More recent data from Sweden, where a thorough and accurate reporting system has been in effect for years, place the incidence of aplastic anemia from CAP at 1/11,000 (Bottiger, 1974). Clearly the exact incidence cannot be determined with certainty, but it is generally accepted that the occurrence of aplastic anemia from CAP is uncommon or rare. The majority of reported cases have been females (ratio 2:1). The clinical manifestations begin several weeks to 5 months after the last dose (Yunis and Bloomberg, 1964). There is no constant relationship to total CAP dosage or duration of therapy. In the 61 cases analyzed by Yunis and Bloomberg (1964) the total CAP dose varied between 2 and 95 g.

The clinical onset may be insidious but is frequently explosive with fulminant infection or life-threatening hemorrhage out of proportion to the degree of thrombocytopenia. Physical examination in the uncomplicated case may reveal only pallor and some petechiae. There is no splenomegaly or lymphadenopathy. Characteristic laboratory findings are pancytopenia, a normochromic, normocytic anemia, and a hypoplastic or aplastic marrow. Occasionally, a cellular marrow aspirate may be obtained, but this is usually due to a patchy distribution of aplasia, as shown by multiple marrow punctures. The clinical course is progressively downhill, and the majority of patients succumb to their disease within 10 months from onset of symptoms. In the 49 fatal cases analyzed by Yunis and Bloomberg (1964), 63% of the deaths occurred in 7 months and all were dead within 18 months. Hemorrhage, frequently intracranial, and infection are the most frequent causes of death. Survival beyond 10 months is associated with improved outlook. A. Restrepo (1971, personal communication) studied a series of 57 cases of aplastic anemia of which 21 were thought to be due to CAP. Four of the 21 patients survived beyond 10 months and only 1 of the 4 died on further follow-up. The degree of neutropenia was the only index that seemed to have some correlation with prognosis. In a series of 101 cases of drug/induced aplastic anemia reviewed by Williams *et al.* (1973) survival correlated inversely with the percentage of nonmyeloid elements in the bone marrow.

The association of paroxysmal nocturnal hemoglobinuria (PNH) with aplastic anemia is well known (Lewis and Dacie, 1967). In four out of nine cases of drug-related aplastic anemia–PNH, the drug was thought to be CAP (Quagliani *et al.*, 1964). A number of cases of CAP-induced aplastic anemia have terminated in acute leukemia.

The occurrence of leukemia and/or PNH in the course of aplastic anemia from any cause indicates the emergence of a genetically altered stem cell clone. The potential leukemogenic effects of ionizing radiation in this regard are well known. It would appear that certain myelotoxic drugs including CAP may also have a leukemic potential (Brauer and Dameshek, 1967; Cohen and Creger, 1967; Fraumeni, 1967; R. J. Ratzan and A. A. Yunis, unpublished). The biochemical mechanisms involved remain in the realm of speculation.

## 5.9. Comments on Therapy

The principles of management of aplastic anemia from any cause are basically the same. In the absence of effective specific agents to stimulate hematopoiesis, treatment remains largely supportive and success depends to a large extent on the prevention and management of complications (Yunis, 1969b, 1973a, 1974a).

Retrospective studies directed at determining the efficacy of androgens in aplastic anemia have yielded variable results (Shahidi and Diamond, 1959; Sanchez-Medal *et al.*, 1969; Sanchez-Medal, 1971; Allen *et al.*, 1968; Williams *et al.*, 1973). A prospective study in a large number of patients is clearly required. In spite of the controversy surrounding the value of androgens, most hematologists, including the author, have witnessed gratifying hematologic remissions in the course of androgen therapy. Furthermore, such remissions can often be shown to be androgen dependent as evidenced by a relapse upon androgen withdrawal and a rise in hematologic values on reinstituting therapy. Based on the current concepts of the mechanism of action of androgens on erythropoiesis, only patients who have some residual erythropoietic activity, and hence a certain number of stem cells, would be expected to respond to androgens. The results of a study by Alexanian *et al.* (1972) seem to support this conclusion. Accordingly, androgens are more appropriately indicated in patients with mild to moderately severe aplastic anemia. Trial therapy should be continued for at least 6 months before it is deemed ineffective. Remission is usually heralded by a decrease in the transfusion requirement followed by a rise in hemoglobin and white cell count. The platelet count is the last to improve and in most cases never returns to normal. In the author's experience, most patients who recover have residual thrombocytopenia, often severe, but have very few hematologic manifestations. Therefore, attempts to raise the platelet count by continuing or raising the the dosage of androgen are unwarranted.

Bone marrow transplantation has recently emerged as a definitive treatment in certain selected cases of bone marrow aplasia. It is the treatment of choice in patients who have identical twin donors (Thomas *et al.*, 1975). Because of persistent serious problems associated with allogeneic marrow transplantation, among them fatal graft versus host disease, this form of treatment is reserved for patients with severe aplastic anemia where in the untreated mortality approaches 100%. Based on a prospective study conducted by the International Aplastic Anemia Group (Camita *et al.*, 1976) it is recommended that patients falling in this category and who have available a matched HLA donor should receive a marrow transplant as early as feasible. The improvement in survival observed thus far has been impressive.

In the absence of specific effective therapy, the prevention of drug-induced aplastic anemia is of utmost importance. Clearly all potential myelotoxic drugs should be used only where absolutely indicated. The danger of CAP should be especially emphasized. In this regard it is important to remember that there is no apparent relationship between reversible erythroid suppression from CAP and bone marrow aplasia from it. Therefore, the monitoring of blood counts as a preventive measure in patients receiving this drug is without proven value. The careful initial judgment of the physician concerning the need for the drug is the only sensible preventive approach.

The extensive clinical experience with TAP in Europe and the experimental studies which have been described suggest that this analog is a safer CAP substitute. However, TAP is as yet unavailable for clinical use in the United States.

## 5.10. Brief Summary

Chloramphenicol produces two types of hematologic toxicity: (1) common dose-dependent, reversible bone marrow suppression affecting primarily the erythroid precursors and occurring concurrently with drug administration, and (2) a rare complication characterized by marrow hypoplasia or aplasia, pancytopenia, a delayed clinical onset, a lack of dose–effect relationship, and, in most cases, a fatal outcome. Current evidence supports the concept of a lack of relationship between reversible erythroid suppression and aplastic anemia from CAP.

Both CAP and TAP exert their antimicrobial effect through inhibition of ribosomal protein synthesis by similar mechanisms. Both antibiotics are potent inhibitors of mitochondrial protein synthesis and through this metabolic effect they cause reversible suppression of bone marrow function. TAP differs in structure from CAP by substitution of the $p$-nitro group with a methylsulfonyl moiety. This structural feature confers on the molecule some properties distinct from those of CAP. Thus in contrast to CAP, TAP is not conjugated to the glucuronide form in the liver, but instead is excreted in the urine largely as the unaltered molecule. Perhaps most significant is that TAP has not to date been associated with any documented cases of aplastic anemia. The apparent absence of this serious hematologic complication from TAP renders this antibiotic of great potential importance among antimicrobial agents.

The pathogenesis of aplastic anemia from CAP remains uncertain. Since TAP has not been associated with aplastic anemia, this complication must somehow be related to the $p$-nitro group of CAP, a feature absent in the TAP molecule. Our comparative, metabolic studies indicate that the $p$-

nitro group also appears to confer on the CAP molecule the capacity to inhibit DNA synthesis and to diffuse rapidly into nonpolar cell compartments. However, the relationship of these CAP properties to aplastic anemia is not clear.

It is postulated that bone marrow aplasia results whenever the $p$-nitro group of CAP meets a favorable milieu in the predisposed host leading somehow to irreversible stem cell damage. This could be exerted through inhibition of DNA synthesis or conceivably by an immunological mechanism.

The clinical features of aplastic anemia from CAP and some of the current concepts in management have been outlined.


## References


Alexanian, R., Nadell, J., and Alfrey, C., 1972, Oxymetholone treatment for the anemia of bone marrow failure, *Blood* **40**:353.

Allen, D. M., Fine, M. H., and Necheles, T. E., 1968, Oxymetholone therapy in aplastic anemia, *Blood* **32**:83.

Beattie, D. S., Basford, R. E., and Koritz, S. B., 1967, The inner membrane as the site of the *in vitro* incorporation of L-$^{14}$C leucine into mitochondrial protein, *Biochemistry* **6**:3099.

Bithell, T. C., and Wintrobe, M. M., 1967, Drug-induced aplastic anemia, *Semin. Hematol.* **4**:194.

Bottiger, L. E., 1974, Drug-induced aplastic anemia in Sweden with special reference to chloramphenicol, *Postgrad. Med. J.* **50**:127.

Brauer, M. J., and Dameshek, W., 1967, Hypoplastic anemia and myeloblastic leukemia following chloramphenicol therapy, *N. Engl. J. Med.* **277**:103.

Brock, T. D., 1961, Chloramphenicol, *Bacteriol. Rev.* **25**:32.

Camita, B. M., Thomas, E. D., Nathan, D. G., Sautos, G., Gordon-Smith, E. C., Gale, R. P., Rappeport, J. M., and Storb, R., 1976, Severe aplastic anemia: A prospective study of the effect of early marrow transplantation on acute mortality, *Blood* **48**:63.

Cattabeni, F., and Gazzaniga, A., 1974, Identification of thiamphenicol excretion products in rat urine using gas-chromatography–mass-spectometry, *Postgrad. Med. J.* **50**:23.

Clarke, W. T. W., 1967, Fatal aplastic anemia and chloramphenicol. *Can. Med. Assoc. J.* **97**:815.

Cohen, T., and Creger, W. P., 1967, Acute myeloid leukemia following seven years of aplastic anemia induced by chloramphenicol, *Am. J. Med.* **43**:762.

Collins, R. J., Ellis, B., Hansen, S. B., MacKenzie, H. S., Moualin, R. J., Petrow, V., Stephenson, O., and Sturgeon, B., 1952, Structural requirements for antibiotic activity in the chloramphenicol series II, *J. Pharm. Pharmacol.* **4**:696.

Contreras, A., Barbacid, M., and Vazquez, D., 1974, Comparative aspects of the action of chloramphenicol and thiamphenicol on bacterial ribosomes, *Postgrad. Med. J.* **50**:50.

Cundliffe, E., and McQuillen, K., 1967, Bacterial protein synthesis: The effects of antibiotics, *J. Mol. Biol.* **30**:137.

Dameshek, W., 1960, Editorial, *JAMA* **174**:1853.

Das, H. K., Goldstein, A., and Kanner, L. C., 1966, Inhibition by chloramphenicol of the growth of nascent protein chains in *Escherichia coli, J. Mol. Pharmacol.* **2**:158.

Erslev, A. J., and Iossifides, I. A., 1962, *In vitro* action of chloramphenicol and chloramphenicol analogues on the metabolism of human immature red blood cells, *Acta Haematol.* **28**:1.

Ferrari, V., and Della Bella, D., 1974, Comparison of chloramphenicol and thiamphenicol metabolism, *Postgrad. Med. J.* **50**:17.

Firkin, F. C., 1972, Mitochondrial lesions in reversible erythropoietic depression due to chloramphenicol, *J. Clin. Invest.* **51**:2085.

Firkin, F. C., and Linnane, A. W., 1968, Differential effects of chloramphenicol on the growth and respiration of mammalian cells, *Biochem. Biophys, Res. Commun.* **32**:398.

Folette, J. H., Shugarman, P. M., Reynolds, J., Valentine, W. N., and Lawrence, J. S., 1956, The effect of chloramphenicol and other antibiotics on leukocyte respiration, *Blood* **11**:234.

Fraumeni, J. F., 1967, Bone marrow depression induced by chloramphenicol or phenylbutazone, *JAMA* **201**:150.

Freeman, K. B., Hasmukh, P., and Haldar, D., 1977, Inhibition of DNA synthesis in Erhlich ascites cells by chloramphenicol, *Mol. Pharmacol.* **13**:504.

Gale, E. F., and Folkes, J. B., 1953, The assimilation of amino acids by bacteria. XV. Actions of antibiotics on nucleic acid and protein synthesis in *Staphylococcus aureus, Biochem. J.* **53**:493.

Garren, L. D., and Crocco, M. R., 1967, Amino-acid incorporations by mitochondria of the adrenal cortex: The effect of chloramphenicol, *Biochem. Biophys. Res. Commun.* **26**:722.

Glazko, A. J., Wolf, L. M., Dill, W. A., and Bratton, A. C., 1949, Biochemical studies on chloramphenicol. II. Tissue distribution and excretion studies, *J. Pharmacol. Exp. Ther.* **96**:445.

Glazko, A. J., Dill, W. A., and Wolf, L. M., 1952, Observations on the metabolic disposition of chloramphenicol in the rat, *J. Pharmacol. Exp. Ther.* **104**:452.

Goodman, L. S., and Gilman, A., 1960, *The Pharmacological Basis of Therapeutics,* 2nd ed., p. 1394, MacMillan, New York.

Gussof, B. D., and Lee, S. L., 1966, Chloramphenicol-induced hematopoietic depression: A controlled comparison with tetracycline, *Am. J. Med. Sci.* **251**:8.

Hahn, F. E., Wissman, C. L., Jr., and Hopps, H. E., 1955, Mode of action of chloramphenicol. III. Action of chloramphenicol on bacterial energy metabolism, *J. Bacteriol.* **69**:215.

Hamburger, R. N., 1966, Chloramphenicol-specific antibody, *Science* **152**:203.

Hoffman, R., Zanjani, E., Lutton, J. D., Zalusky, R., and Wasserman, L. R., 1977, Suppression in aplastic anemia of erythroid-colony formation by lymphocytes, *N. Engl. J. Med.* **296**:10.

Hurwitz, C., and Braun, C. B., 1967, Measurement of binding of chloramphenicol by intact cells, *J. Bacteriol.* **93**:1677.

Jackson, G. G., 1958, Current concepts in therapy: Antibiotics. IX. Chloramphenicol, *N. Engl. J. Med.* **259**:1172.

Jiji, R. M., Gangarosa, E. J., and Dela Macorra, F., 1963, Chloramphenicol and its sulfamyl analogue, *Arch. Intern. Med.* **111**:70.

Jones, M. S., and Jones, O. T. G., 1969, The structural organization of haem synthesis in rat liver mitochondria, *Biochem. J.* **113**:507.

Kagan, W. A., Ascensao, J. A., Pahwa, R. N., Moore, M. A. S., and Good, R., 1976, Possible role of T lymphocytes in the pathogenesis of aplastic anemia, *Clin. Res.* **24**:440.

Kayser, F. H., and Wust, J., 1974, Resistance of gram-positive bacteria to chloramphenicol/thiamphenicol: Occurrence and genetic basis, *Postgrad. Med. J.* **50**:79.

Keiser, G., 1974. Co-operative study of patients treated with thiamphenicol. Comparative study of patients treated with chloramphenicol and thiamphenicol, *Postgrad. Med. J.* **50**:143.

Krakoff, I. H., Karnofsky, D. A., and Burchenal, J. H., 1955, Effects of large doses of chloramphenicol on human subjects, *N. Engl. J. Med.* **253**:7.

Krishna, G., 1974, Covalent binding of drugs to tissue macromolecules as a biochemical mechanism of drug toxicities with special emphasis on chloramphenicol and thiamphenicol, *Postgrad. Med. J.* **50**:73.

Kroon, A. M., 1964, Protein synthesis in heart mitochondria. II. A comparison of mitochondria from liver and heart with special reference to the role of oxidative phosphorylation. *Biochem. Biophys. Acta* **91**:145.

Kunin, C. M., Glazko, A. J., and Finland, M., 1959, Persistence of antibiotics in blood in patients with acute renal failure. II. Chloramphenicol and its metabolic products in the blood of patients with severe renal disease or hepatic cirrhosis, *J. Clin. Invest.* **38**:1498.

Leikin, S. L., Welch, H., and Quin, G., 1961, Aplastic anemia due to chloramphenicol, *Clin. Proc. Child. Hosp. (Wash.)* **17**:171.

Lewis, S. M., and Dacie, J. V., 1967, The aplastic anemia-paroxysmal nocturnal hemoglobinuria, *Br. J. Haematol.* **13**:236.

Lindau, W., 1952, Effect of chloromycetin upon erythropoiesis, *in Proceedings of the National Meeting of the American Federation for Clinical Research*, Abstract 72.

Manyan, D. R., and Yunis, A. A., 1970, The effect of chloramphenicol treatment on ferrochelatase activity in dogs, *Biochem. Biophys, Res. Commun.* **41**:926.

Manyan, D. R., Arimura, G. K., and Yunis, A. A.. 1972, Chloramphenicol-induced erythroid suppression and bone marrow ferrochelatase activity in dogs, *J. Lab. Clin. Med.* **79**:137.

Manyan, D. R., Arimura, G. K., and Yunis, A. A., 1975, Comparative metabolic effects of chloramphenicol analogues, *Mol. Pharmacol.* **11**:520.

Martelo, O. J., Manyan, D. R., Smith, U. S., and Yunis, A. A., 1969, Chloramphenicol and bone marrow mitochondria, *J. Lab. Clin. Med.* **74**:927.

McKay, R., Druyan, R., Getz, G. S., and Rabinowitz, M., 1969, Intramitochondrial localization of δ-aminolevulinate synthetase and ferrochelatase in rat liver, *Biochem. J.* **114**:455.

McLeod, T. F., Manyan, D. R., and Yunis, A. A., 1977, The cellular transport of chloramphenicol and thiamphenicol, *J. Lab. Clin. Med.* **90**:347.

Monroe, R. E., Maden, B. E. H., and Traut, R. R., 1967, The mechanism of peptide bone formation in protein synthesis, *in Genetic Elements Projections and Functions* (D. Shugar, ed.), p. 179, Academic Press, New York.

Nago, T., and Mauer, A. M., 1969, Concordance for drug-induced aplastic anemia in identical twins, *N. Engl. J. Med.* **281**:11.

Neupert, W., Brdiczka, D., and Bucher, T., 1967, Incorporation of amino acids into the outer and inner membrane of isolated rat liver mitochondria, *Biochem. Biophys, Res. Commun.* **27**:488.

Nijhof, W., and Kroon, A. M., 1974, The interference of CAP and TAP with the biogenesis of mitochondria in animal tissues: A possible clue to the toxic action, *Postgrad. Med. J.* **50**:53.

Okamoto, S., and Suzuki, Y., 1965, Chloramphenicol, dehydrostreptomycin, and kanamycin inactivating enzymes from multiple drug-resistant *Escherichia coli* carrying episome "R," *Nature* **208**:1301.

Olshaker, B., Ross, S., Recinos, A., and Twible, E., 1949, Aureomycin , *N. Engl. J. Med.* **241**:287.

Quagliani, K. M., Cartwright, G. E., and Wintrobe, M. M., 1964, Paroxysmal nocturnal hemoglobinuria following drug-induced aplastic anemia, *Ann. Intern. Med.* **61**:1045.

Ratzan, R. J., Moore, M. A. S., and Yunis, A. A., 1974, Effect of chloramphenicol on the *in vitro* colony forming cell, *Blood* **43**:363.

Rebstock, M. C., Crooks, H. M., Controulis, J., and Bartz, Q. R., 1949, Chloramphenicol. IV. Chemical Studies, *J. Am. Chem. Soc.* **71**:2458.

Recinos, A., Ross, S., and Olshaker, T. E., 1949, Chloromycetin in the treatment of pneumonia in infants and children (a preliminary report in 33 cases), *N. Engl. J. Med.* **241**:733.

Rich, M. L., Ritterhof, R. J., and Hoffman, R. J., 1950, A fatal case of aplastic anemia following chloramphenicol therapy, *Ann. Intern. Med.* **33**:1459.

Roodyn, D. B., Reis, P. J., and Work, T. S., 1961, Protein synthesis in mitochondria, *Biochem. J.* **80**:9.

Rosenbach, L., Caviles, A., and Mitus, W. J., 1960, Chloramphenicol toxicity: Reversible vacuolization of erythroid cells, *N. Engl. J. Med.* **263**:724.

Rubin, D., Weisberger, A. S., Botti, R. E., and Storaasli, J. P., 1958, Changes in iron metabolism in early chloramphenicol toxicity, *J. Clin. Invest.* **37**:1286.

Rubin, D., Weisberger, A. S., and Clark, D. R., 1960, Early detection of drug-induced erythropoietic depression, *J. Lab. Clin. Med.* **56**:453.

Saidi, P., Wallerstein, R. O., and Aggeler, P. M., 1961, Effect of chloramphenicol on erythropoiesis, *J. Lab. Clin. Med.* **57**:247.

Sanchez-Medal, L., 1971, The hemopoietic action of androstanes, *Prog. Hematol.* **7**:111.

Sanchez-Medal, L., Gormez-Leal, A., Duarte, L., and Guadalupe, M. G., 1969, Anabolic androgenic steroids in the treatment of acquired aplastic anemia, *Blood* **34**:283.

Scott, J. L., Finegold, S. M., Belthin, G. A., and Lawrence, J. S., 1965, A controlled double-blind study of the hematologic toxicity of chloramphenicol, *N. Engl. J. Med.* **272**:1137.

Shahidi, N. T., and Diamond, L. K., 1959, Testosterone-induced remission in aplastic anemia, *Am. J. Dis. Child.* **98**:293.

Shaw, W. V., 1971, Biochemical mechanisms of transferable drug resistance, *Adv. Pharmacol. Chemother.* **9**:13.

Shaw, W. V., and Brodsky, R. F., 1968, Characterization of chloramphenicol acetyltransferase from chloramphenicol-resistant *Staphylococcus aureus, J. Bacteriol.* **95**:28.

Skinnider, L. F., and Gladially, F. N., 1976, Chloramphenicol-induced mitochondrial and ultrastructural changes in hemopoietic cells, *Arch. Pathol. Lab. Med.* **100**:601.

Smick, K. M., Condit, P. K., Proctor, R. L., and Sutcher, V., 1964, Fatal aplastic anemia, an epidemiological study of its relationship to the drug chloramphenicol, *J. Chronic. Dis.* **17**:899.

Smith, G. N., and Worrel, C. S., 1950, The decomposition of chloromycetin by microorganisms, *Arch. Biochem.* **28**:232.

Smith, U., Smith, D., and Yunis, A. A., 1970, Chloramphenicol-related changes in mitochondria ultrastructure, *J. Cell Sci.* **7**:501.

Stephenson, J. R., Axelrad, A. A., McLeod, D. L., and Shreeve, M. M., 1971, Induction of colonies of hemoglobin synthesizing cells by erythropoietin *in vitro, Proc. Natl. Acad. Sci. U.S.A.* **68**:1542.

Suzuki, Y., and Okamoto, S., 1967, The enzymatic acetylation of chloramphenicol by the miltiple drug-resistant *Escherichia coli* carrying R factor, *J. Biol. Chem.* **242**:4722.

Tacquet, A., Cuvelier, D., Devulder, B., and Legros, J., 1974, Pharmacokinetic aspects of thiamphenicol in subjects with normal renal function and in patients with chronic renal insufficiency, with or without hemodialysis, *Postgrad. Med. J.* **50**:36.

Thomas, E. D., Storb, R., Clift, R. A., Fefer, A., Johnson, F. L., Neiman, P. E., Lerner, K. G., Glucksberg, H., and Bucknev, C. D., 1975, Bone marrow transplantation, *N. Engl. J. Med.* **292**:832.

Truman, D. E. S., and Korner, A., 1962, Initial stages in the incorporation of amino acids into protein in rat liver mitochondria, *Biochem J.* **85**:154.

Vazquez, D., 1964, Uptake and binding of chloramphenicol by sensitive and resistant organisms, *Nature* **203**:267.

Vazquez, D., 1966, Binding of chloramphenicol to ribosomes, *Biochem. Biophys. Acta.* **114**:277.

Volini, U. F., Greenspan, I., Ehrlich, I., Gonner, J. A., Felsenfeld, O., and Schwartz, S. O., 1950, Hematopoietic changes during administration of chloramphenicol, *JAMA* **142**:1333.

Weber, M. J., and Demoss, J. A., 1966, The inhibition by chloramphenicol of nascent protein formation in *E. coli, Proc. Natl. Acad. Sci. U.S.A.* **55**:1224.

Weisberger, A. S., and Wolfe, S., 1964, Effect of chloramphenicol on protein synthesis, *Fed. Proc.* **23**:976.

Weisberger, A. S., Armentrout, S., and Wolfe, S., 1963, Protein synthesis by reticulocyte ribosomes. I. Inhibition of polyuridilic acid-induced ribosomal protein synthesis by chloramphenicol. *Proc. Natl. Acad. Sci. U.S.A.* **50**:86.

Weisberger, A. S., Daniel, T. M., and Hoffman, A., 1964a, Suppression of antibody synthesis and prolongation of hemograph survival by chloramphenicol, *J. Exp. Med.* **120**:183.

Weisberger, A. S., Wolfe, S., and Armentrout, S., 1964b, Inhibition of protein synthesis in mammalian cell-free system by chloramphenicol, *J. Exp. Med.* **120**:161.

Wheeldon, L. W., and Lehninger, A. L., 1966, Energy linked synthesis and decay of membrane proteins in isolated rat liver mitochondria, *Biochemistry* **5**:3533.

Williams, D. M., Lynch, R. E., and Cartwright, G. E., 1973, Drug-induced aplastic anemia, *Semin. Hematol.* **10**:195.

Winshell, E., and Shaw, W. B., 1969, Kinetics of induction and purification of chloramphenicol acetyltransferase from chloramphenicol-resistant *Staphylococcus aureus*, *J. Bacteriol.* **98**:1248.

Wissman, C. L., Jr., Smadel, J. E., Hahn, F. E., and Hopps, H. E., 1954, Mode of action of chloramphenicol. I. Action of chloramphenicol on assimilation of ammonia and on synthesis of proteins and nucleic acids in *Escherichia coli*, *J. Bacteriol.* **67**:662.

Wolfe, A. D., and Hahn, F. E., 1965, Mode of action of chloramphenicol. IX. Effects of chloramphenicol upon a ribosomal amino acid polymerization system and its binding to bacterial ribosomes, *Biochem. Biophys. Acta.* **95**:146.

Yunis, A. A., 1969a, Drug-induced bone marrow injury, *Adv. Intern. Med.* **15**:347.

Yunis, A. A., 1969b, Aplastic anemia, *in Current Therapy* (H. Conn. ed.), p. 225, W. B. Saunders, Philadelphia.

Yunis, A. A., 1973a, Chloramphenicol toxicity, *in Blood Disorders Due to Drugs and Other Agents* (R. H. Girwood, ed.), p. 107, Excerpta Medica, Amsterdam.

Yunis, A. A., 1973b, Chloramphenicol-induced bone marrow suppression, *Semin. Hematol.* **X**:225.

Yunis, A. A., 1974a, Aplastic anemia, *in Current Therapy* (H. Conn, ed.), p. 234, W. B. Saunders, Philadelphia.

Yunis, A. A., 1974b, Effects of chloramphenicol on erythropoiesis, *in Proceedings of the Hahneman International Symposium on Drugs and Hematologic Reactions* (N. V. Dimitrov and J. H. Nodine, eds.), p. 133, Grune & Stratton, New York.

Yunis, A. A., 1976, Pathogenetic mechanisms in bone marrow suppression from chloramphenicol and thiamphenicol, Symposium on Aplastic Anemia, Kyoto, Japan.

Yunis, A. A., and Adamson, J. W., 1977, Differential *in vitro* sensitivity of marrow erythroid and granulocytic colony forming cells to chloramphenicol, *Am. J. Hematol.* **2**:355.

Yunis, A. A., Arimura, G. K., 1963, Biochemical predisposition to chloramphenicol-induced bone marrow aplasia, *Clin. Res.* **11**:201.

Yunis, A. A., and Bloomberg, G. R., 1964, Chloramphenicol toxicity: Clinical features and pathogenesis, *Prog. Hematol.* **4**:138.

Yunis, A. A., and Gross, M. A., 1975, Drug induced inhibitions of mycloid colony growth: Protective effect of colony stimulating factor, *J. Lab. Clin. Med.* **86**:499.

Yunis, A. A., and Harrington, W. J., 1960, Patterns of inhibition by chloramphenicol of nucleic acid synthesis in human bone marrow and leukemic leukocytes, *J. Lab. Clin. Med.* **56**:831.

Yunis, A. A., Smith, U. S., and Restrepo, A., 1970, Reversible bone marrow suppression from chloramphenicol, *Arch. Intern. Ned.* **126**:272.

Yunis, A. A., Manyan, D. R., and Arimura, G. K., 1973, Comparative effect of chloramphenicol and thiamphenicol on DNA and mitochondrial protein synthesis in mammalian cells, *J. Lab. Clin. Med.* **81**:713.

Yunis, A. A., Manyan, D. R., and Arimura, G. K., 1974, Comparative metabolic effects of chloramphenicol and thiamphenicol in mammalian cells, *Postgrad. Med. J.* **50**:50.

Zelkowitz, L., Tchou, H., Arimura, G. K., and Yunis, A. A., 1967, Chloramphenicol and protein synthesis in mammalian cell free system, *Clin. Res.* **15**:67.

Zelkowitz, L., Arimura, G. K., and Yunis, A. A., 1968, Chloramphenicol and protein synthesis in mammalian cells, *J. Lab. Clin. Med.* **71**:596.

# Morphologic and Functional Observations on Bone Marrow Megakaryocytes

## Martha E. Fedorko

## 6.1. Some Historical Observations on Megakaryocytes

Investigators have been fascinated for over 70 years by the megakaryocyte, a cell which is partly distinguished by its large size. Megakaryocytes were named and recognized as a cell type apart from osteoclasts by Howell (1890). However, it remained for James Homer Wright (1906) to describe the true nature of these cells as progenitors of platelets. With the use of Romanofsky stains Wright was able to accomplish his now classic morphologic observations. He identified the different regions of the cell by their staining properties and their characteristic granulation which he cited as being similar to that of blood platelets. He maintained that megakaryocytes lose their cytoplasm and interpreted their morphologic appearance to indicate that loss of cytoplasm was accomplished by detachment of buds

MARTHA E. FEDORKO  •  Rockefeller University, New York, New York.

or fragments from pseudopods. He correlated the appearance of blood platelets in mammals with the appearance of megakaryocytes to strengthen his argument.

The progenitor role of megakaryocytes extends both to morphologic and functional spheres, in that there are marked similarities between megakaryocytes and platelets. We will try to illustrate these points in the description of megakaryocyte morphology and function presented here.

## 6.2. Some Unique Properties of Megakaryocytes—Cell Size and Polyploidy

Some of the major unique properties of megakaryocytes which set them apart from other cell types and which stimulated early investigative curiosity were their large size and nuclear configuration. The early work of Japa (1943) defined the size limits of human megakaryocytes as between 30 and 100 $\mu$m. Whether megakaryocytes had individual nuclei or whether the nucleus was lobulated was left open to question. This author stated that in the acetocarmine preparations there was evidence for both types of structure. Our electron micrographs give evidence in some instances for interconnecting nuclear strands much like those present in the polymorphonuclear leukocyte. Electron microscopy cannot settle easily and unequivocally that plurinuclearity does or does not exist; this problem apparently still remains unsolved (de Leval and Paulus 1971), but uninuclearity is favored.

Japa's schematic drawings give evidence for the fact that cell size was proportional to the number of nuclear lobes present. In normal individuals, according to Japa's classification, the majority of megakaryocytes (35%) were classified as degenerating, but next in order of frequency were those with 8, 4, and 16 "nuclear units." Evidence presented by Odell and Jackson (1968, 1970) illustrated that megakaryocyte size was directly proportional to the ploidy classes and maturation stages within the megakaryocyte series. The most accurate estimations on DNA content of megakaryocytes has been accomplished by cytophotometric and fluorometric determinations of DNA values in individual megakaryocyte nuclei. For further discussion of the aspects on megakaryocyte ploidy the reader is referred to reviews by others on the subject (de Leval and Paulus, 1971).

## 6.3. Statement of the Problem Handicapping Megakaryocyte Studies

The kinetic aspects of megakaryocytopoiesis have been studied (Ebbe, 1965) but to date morphologic studies have been drawn from relatively small populations of cells (0.2% in normal marrow). Analysis of such small cell numbers at both the scanning and transmission electron microscope level would, indeed, be very difficult. In the past megakaryocytes were studied in tissue block or by some adaptation of the smear method for light microscopy and autoradiography. The former was handicapped by the small cell numbers available, the latter by possible cell loss during the preparation. We felt that concentrations of isolated megakaryocyte populations would make morphologic studies easier and more definitive. In addition, with the conventional preparations the preservation of these cells could be variable. There was some indication from the work by Ardlie (1972) that inhibitors of platelet function helped to preserve platelets. This phenomenon was also probably applicable to megakaryocytes.

## 6.4. Newer Advances in Cell Separation Procedures

Previous work by others has illustrated the comparative advantages of working with a homogeneous population of leukocytes (Hirsch, 1956; Cohn and Benson, 1965). We had been making some observations on megakaryocytes in mixed cell suspensions of marrow in explant culture and desired to apply some of the methodology used with other cell types in the study of megakaryocytes. About the time we directed our interest toward megakaryocytes newer techniques were being developed which could apply to numerous cell systems to isolate relatively homogeneous populations or subclasses of cells (Pretlow *et al.* 1975; Harwood, 1974). It therefore seemed feasible that some of these methods could be used to obtain a substantially enriched population of megakaryocytes.

### 6.4.1. Cell Separative Procedures

Cell separative procedures could be divided into (1) obtaining and disaggregating the tissue and (2) sedimentation procedures to separate out a particular cell population. The first procedure implies selection of a proper animal species to give adequate cell yield and involved freeing megakaryocytes from their positions often near the endothelial cells lining the sinusoids to form a single cell population. In our case this was accomplished by using guinea pig marrow, mincing, and vigorous pipetting through a wide bore pipet in the presence of a low calcium and magnesium solution. The latter procedure might have an effect on disrupting the junctions of the sinusoidal lining cells. This method, when compared to various enzymatic digestions, proved to be the most effective.

### 6.4.2. Summary of Cell Sedimentation Techniques

The sedimentation techniques used to separate populations of cells may be summarized as follows: (1) Differential sedimentation which involves centrifuging out the largest cells to the bottom in the absence of a gradient. (2) Isopycnic gradient centrifugation which involves separation of cells according to their different densities. Centrifugation is accomplished in a continuous, preferably linear density gradient which is of sufficient force to bring all cells to locations in the gradient equal to their own densities. (3) Velocity, rate zonal, or isokinetic gradient centrifugation which separates cells that differ with respect to rates of sedimentation. The velocity of the sedimenting cell is a function of volume, gravitational force, and effective mass and is an inverse function of the viscosity of the gradient.

Without any prior experimental trials if one had to predict the optimal method for separating megakaryocytes, it might appear to be method (3), velocity sedimentation, because of the large size of the megakaryocyte. However, the results of experimental trials proved to be contrary to what was expected.

## 6.5. Model Systems to Isolate Megakaryocytes

There now exist several protocols for the isolation of megakaryocytes. Two methods employ separations from mouse marrow (Nakeff and Maat, 1974; Nakeff and Flaek, 1976) and one uses separation from guinea pig marrow (Levine and Fedorko, 1976). Our preliminary results showed a moderately good yield of mouse bone marrow megakaryocytes and an excellent yield from guinea pigs.

### 6.5.1. Factors Affecting Yield and Preservation of Megakaryocytes

The method we currently use to isolate guinea pig megakaryocytes has been described in detail (Levine and Fedorko, 1976). Marrow from several different animal species was studied but marrow of two femora from guinea pigs gave the largest yield of megakaryocytes ($2.76 \times 10^6$ cells). This yield was approximately twice that obtained from rats and mice. The presence of citrate, absence of calcium and magnesium, as well as the addition of adenosine and theophylline significantly improved the yield from paired femoral marrow of drug-treated and control specimens. Not only was the yield of megakaryocytes increased from drug-treated guinea pig marrow but the morphologic preservation was also markedly improved. It was noted that in poorly preserved specimens there was loss of cytoplasmic granules probably by fusion to components of the demarcation membrane system (DMS) and subsequent degranulation. The resulting morphology showed that there was marked dilatation of the vacuolar system in these megakaryocytes. Apparently known inhibitors of platelet aggregation in the presence of a low calcium environment were effective in preserving megakaryocyte structure.

## 6.5.2. Combined Methods for Guinea Pig Marrow Megakaryocytes

Equilibrium density centrifugation followed by velocity sedimentation (Fig. 1) produced approximately a 100-fold enrichment. Histograms of megakaryocyte size before and after concentration showed that the distribution of the immature, intermediate, and mature megakaryocytes was approximately the same (Levine and Fedorko, 1976). An example of the megakaryocyte preparation is shown in Fig. 2.

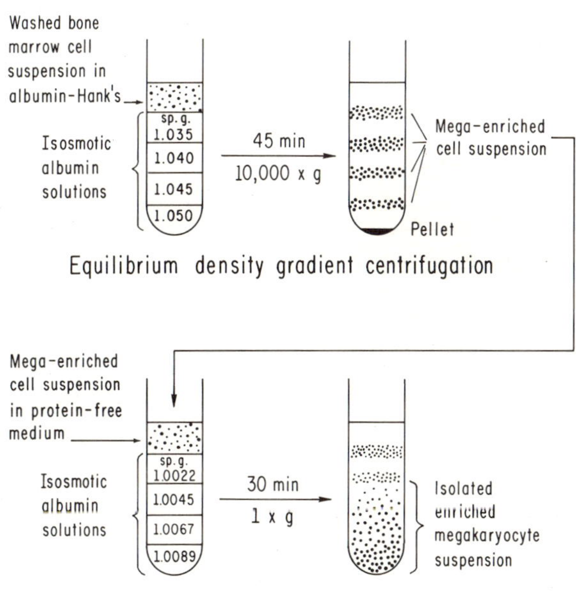


**Fig. 1.** Diagram of procedure to obtain a concentrated megakaryocyte preparation from guinea pig marrow.

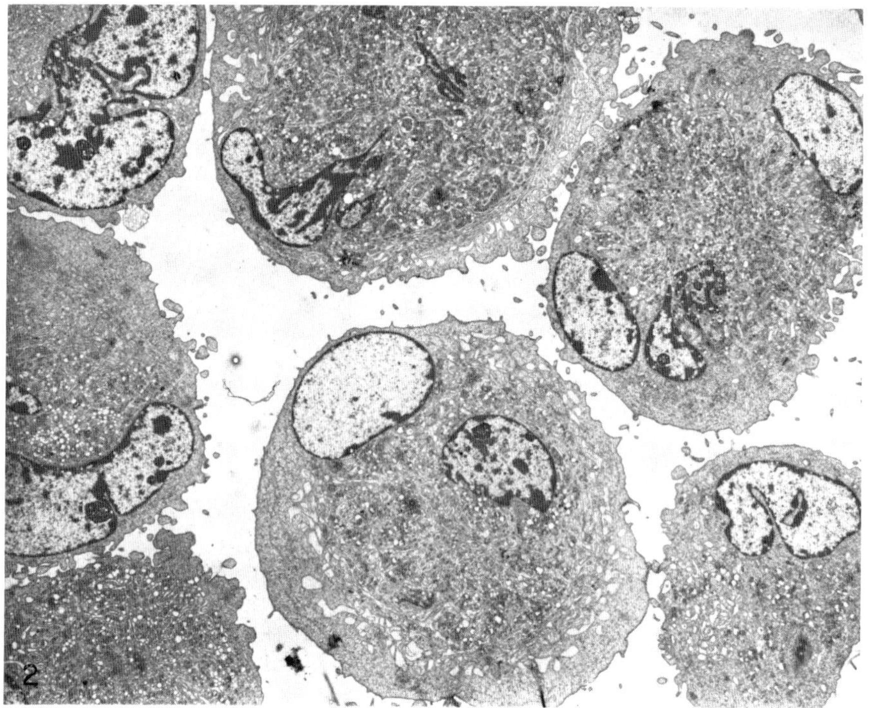

**Fig. 2.** Appearance of megakaryocyte preparation obtained after density centrifugation and velocity sedimentation.

### 6.5.3. Methods in Use with Mouse Bone Marrow Megakaryocytes

Nakeff's first method (Nakeff and Maat, 1974) employed a gradient of 0.5–2% bovine albumin through which mouse megakaryocytes sedimented at unit gravity for 30–45 min in the cold. The cell suspensions containing megakaryocytes were enriched from 0.03% to as high as 1% in certain fractions. In addition to this separation which is based on cell volume and uses velocity sedimentation, Nakeff and his co-workers (Nakeff and Flaek, 1976) more recently employed albumin density gradient separations which rely on the cellular density of megakaryocytes to achieve cell separation. Discontinuous gradients of albumin solutions ranging from 16 to 38% were employed for the separation at $1000 \times g$ for 30 min. Greater than 15-fold enrichment was obtained from mouse bone marrow by this method.

## 6.6. Studies on Megakaryocyte Maturation

The maturation of megakaryocytes has been studied by several investigators (Bessis, 1956; Feinendegen *et al.*, 1962; Breton-Gorius, 1973). Others have interpreted the results of their kinetic studies based on the light microscopic appearance of various maturation stages of the megakaryocyte (Ebbe, 1965.) In general the studies have been performed on megakaryocytes *en bloc* or on smears where their members would be limited and the very immature, rather small cells would not be recognized. The method of isolation of megakaryocytes afforded the advantage of obtaining large numbers of these cells and a cell population which was first separated on the basis of cell density. This presented the possibility that if the immature cells possessed an increased density, they would appear in the isolated cell preparation. Furthermore, when cells were isolated in suspension they were likely to assume a configuration and peripheral cell membrane profile which was common to members of the series. This was true in discriminating between the monocytic and granulocytic series and proved also true for megakaryocytes.

In evaluation of megakaryocyte maturation it was of interest to determine whether there were features of maturation found in other marrow cell lines. The general rule appears to be that blasts are moderately large cells with a good complement of polyribosomes. One step further along in maturation the cell is larger, and usually has a great period of synthetic activity that results in synthesis of distinctive cell components. However, the uniqueness of the megakaryocyte might lead to some degree of variance from the maturation schemes of other cell types. Odell and Jackson (1968, 1970) studied the relation of size to the labeling index of the megakaryocyte. From these studies it was evident, first, that due to the ploidy which megakaryocytes possess there might be overlap in their size at the different maturation stages. Second, megakaryocytes normally develop an intricate membrane system, the demarcation membrane system (DMS), which eventually surrounds prospective platelets. Many of the biologic aspects of membrane synthesis are unknown. Third, the cell eventually sheds its cytoplasm in the form of platelets.

### 6.6.1. Ultrastructure of Maturing Megakaryocytes

#### 6.6.1.1. Megakaryoblast

In the isolated guinea pig megakaryocyte population the megakaryoblast has several distinctive morphologic characteristics. The blast (as

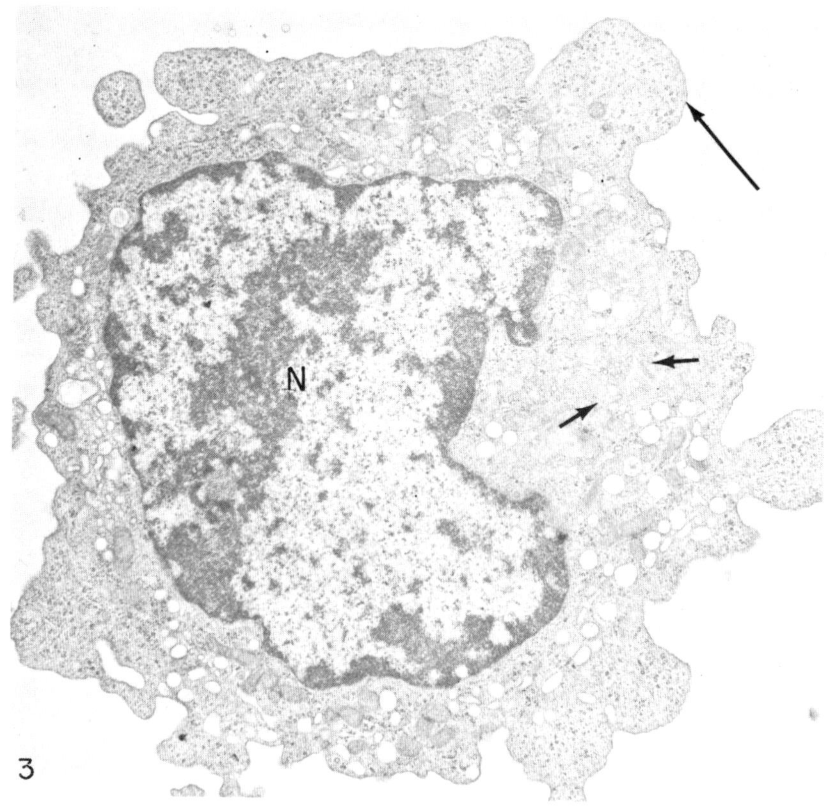



**Fig. 3.** Ultrastructural appearance of an isolated guinea pig megakaryoblast. Note the characteristic configuration of the cell membrane which shows bleblike protrusions (long arrows). The nucleus (N) is minimally indented, has moderate margination of nuclear chromatin, and prominent nucleoli. The peripheral cytoplasm is filled with polyribosomes. The midcytoplasmic zone is filled with vacuolar and mitochondria. A few scattered elements of the Golgi complex are found in the nuclear hof area (short arrows). ×13,832 (reduced 10% for reproduction).

identified in this population) ranges in size from about 8 to 10 $\mu$m. Cells of this maturation stage as well as more mature cells are often found in close proximity to endothelial cells. The cell margin is distinctive, with bleblike protrusions. (Fig. 3). The peripheral margin of the cytoplasm contains many polyribosomes. The midzone of the cell contains mitochondria, clear vacuoles up to 0.25 $\mu$m in size, and scattered strips of rough endoplasmic reticulum. Characteristic components of the Golgi complex, vesicles, vacuoles, and lamellae, occupy the perinuclear area. The nucleus may be large with few minor indentations at its peripheral margin. Often the nucleus is bilobed; both types of nuclei show moderate margination of chromatin and numerous nucleoli.

### 6.6.1.2. Immunohistochemical Studies on Megakaryoblasts

Immunohistochemical procedures were employed to confirm the morphologic finding on the identity of the megakaryoblast. Rabbit anti-guinea pig platelet antiserum which formed an immunoprecipitation line with washed platelet extracts was used in the indirect antibody labeling method employing goat anti-rabbit globulin conjugated with ferritin and the peroxidase bridging reaction (Willingham *et al.*, 1971). In both experiments there is surface membrane labeling of immature megakaryocytes and presumed blasts, as well as the more mature members of the series (Figs. 4 and 5). Labeled megakaryoblasts show the morphologic features described earlier. Leukocyte elements of the marrow do not label, nor is there labeling of megakaryocytes when normal rabbit serum is substituted for specific antiplatelet antisera. These findings are interpreted to correlate with our morphologic identification of the megakaryoblast.

### 6.6.1.3. Intermediate Megakaryocyte, Stage I

The next maturation stage, designated intermediate stage I (probably equivalent to the promegakaryocyte of others), ranges in size from about 10 to 15 $\mu$m (Fig. 6). The peripheral cell surface has the characteristic protrusions which are also found in the blast forms. The peripheral margins of cytoplasm are filled with abundant polyribosomes. The nucleus is lobulated with minimal margination of nuclear chromatin and prominent nucleoli. The outstanding morphologic feature of this stage of maturation is that the unique internal demarcation membrane system (DMS) characteristic of these cells begins to form. Earlier studies by MacPherson (1972) have suggested that this system of membrane starts forming in one area of the cell cytoplasm in conjunction with the appearance of a polar peripheral tuft of cell membrane (Fig. 7). The distribution of this peripheral cell membrane system varies with the additives in the suspending medium. Behnke (1968) has demonstrated that the DMS was a derivative of the cell membrane. In the system using guinea pig megakaryocytes we found it difficult to demonstrate this with the usual methodology. However, tannic acid added to the fixative produces an electron-dense complex which is easily demonstrated in the DMS (Fedorko and Levine, 1976), and helps in distinguishing the DMS from other intracellular components. During the early stages of formation the DMS may

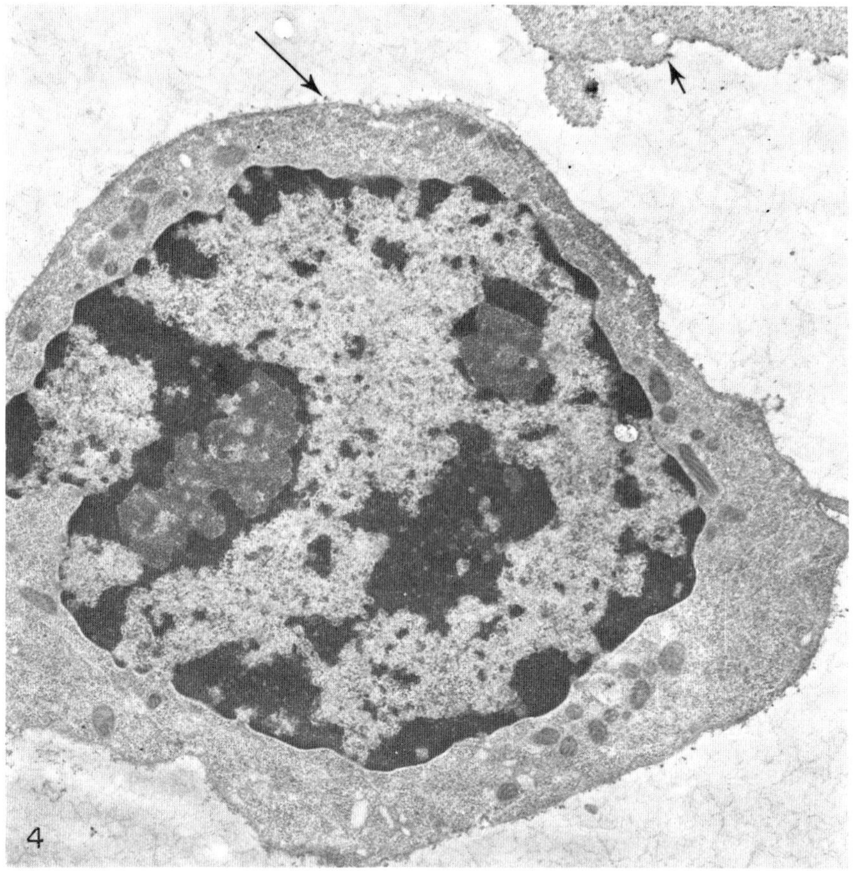

**Fig. 4.** Electron microscope appearance of membrane surface labeling of the megakaryoblast with specific anti-guinea pig platelet antiserum used in the peroxidase bridging reaction. The electron-dense deposit of peroxidatic activity on the cell surface (long arrow) indicates the localization of antiplatelet antibody on the surface of the immature cell. The cell margin at the upper right shows surface membrane label on more mature megakaryocyte (short arrow).

become rather extensively distributed through the central zones of the cell. There is minimal cytoplasmic granule formation near the Golgi complex, but any significant number of characteristic cytoplasmic granules are not present. Mitochondria are distributed in a zone at the margin of the lobulated cell nucleus. Scattered strips of rough endoplasmic reticulum are found in the peripheral zones of the cell.

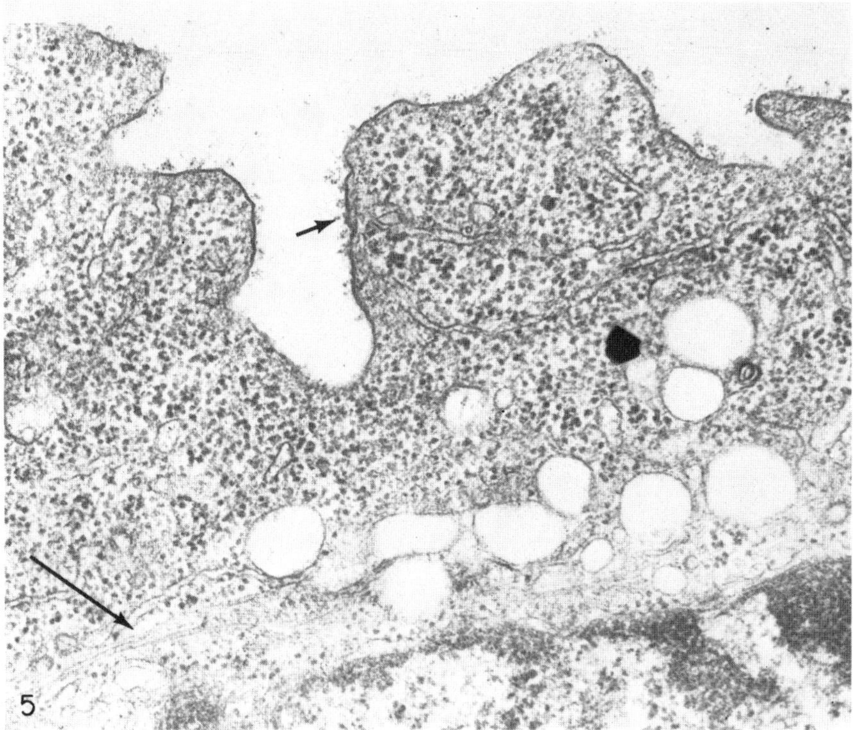

**Fig. 5.** Membrane surface labeling of a guinea pig megakaryoblast with rabbit antiplatelet antiserum in the indirect immunohistochemical method employing ferritin-labeled antibody. Shown is the peripheral cell membrane with ferritin localized on its surface (short arrow). The presence of ferritin indicates antiplatelet antibody. The portion of the megakaryoblast shown has bundles of microtubules in the perinuclear zone (long arrow). ×39,000 (reduced 10% for reproduction).

### 6.6.1.4. Intermediate Megakaryocyte, Stage II

The next maturation stage (intermediate stage II or megakaryocyte; Fig. 8) has all the components the cell will ever possess but not in their final destined arrangement. The size of these cells ranges from 12 to 30 μm. The cell margin can show the distinctive irregularity seen in the younger forms. The nucleus is multilobulated with moderate margination of the chromatin and nuclear pores appear prominent. The DMS is extensive and often appears as short moderately dilated or narrow channels. Cytoplasmic granules with their characteristic nucleoid core are prominent and mitochondria are randomly distributed throughout the

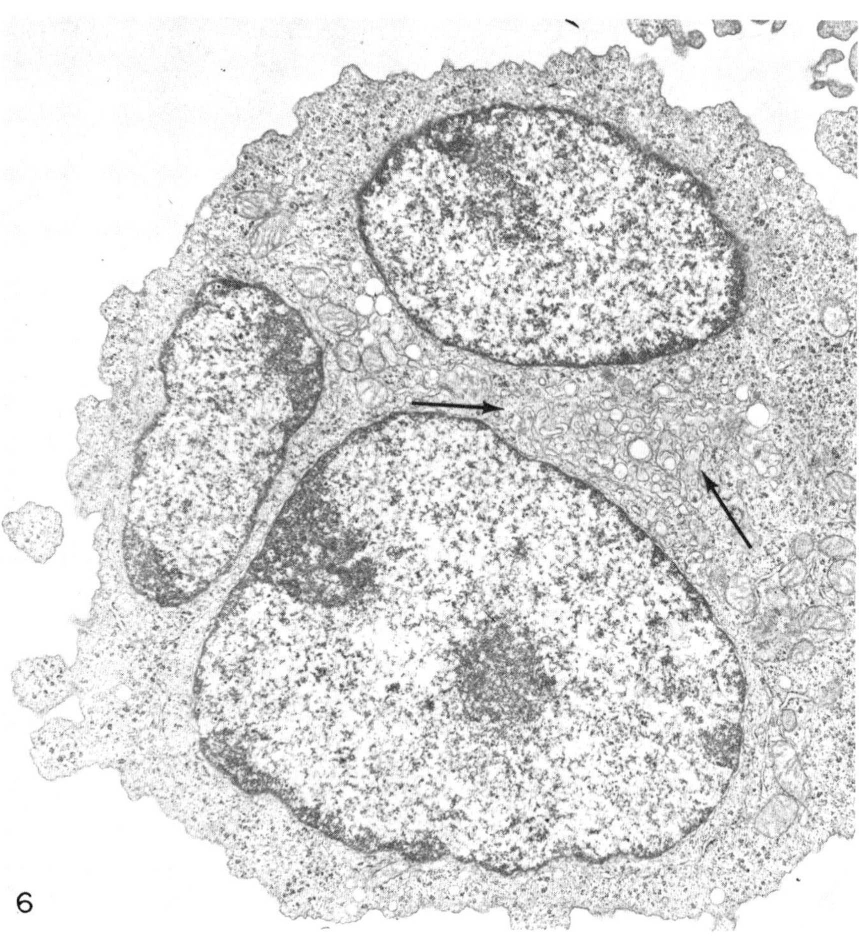

**Fig. 6.** Ultrastructural appearance of intermediate stage I megakaryocyte (promegakaryoblast) from a guinea pig. The peripheral cell membrane has the characteristic irregularity described in Fig. 3. The peripheral zone of cytoplasm contains many polyribosomes in clusters. The midzone of the cytoplasm shows short strips of endoplasmic reticulum and numerous mitochondria. The central areas of the cell contain an intricate network of membranes, the primordia of the demarcation membrane system (DMS) (arrows). Cytoplasmic granules are rare. The lobulated nucleus has characteristic features of immaturity, i.e., minimal margination of chromatin around the nuclear membrane and prominent nucleoli. ×13,780 (reduced 10% for reproduction).

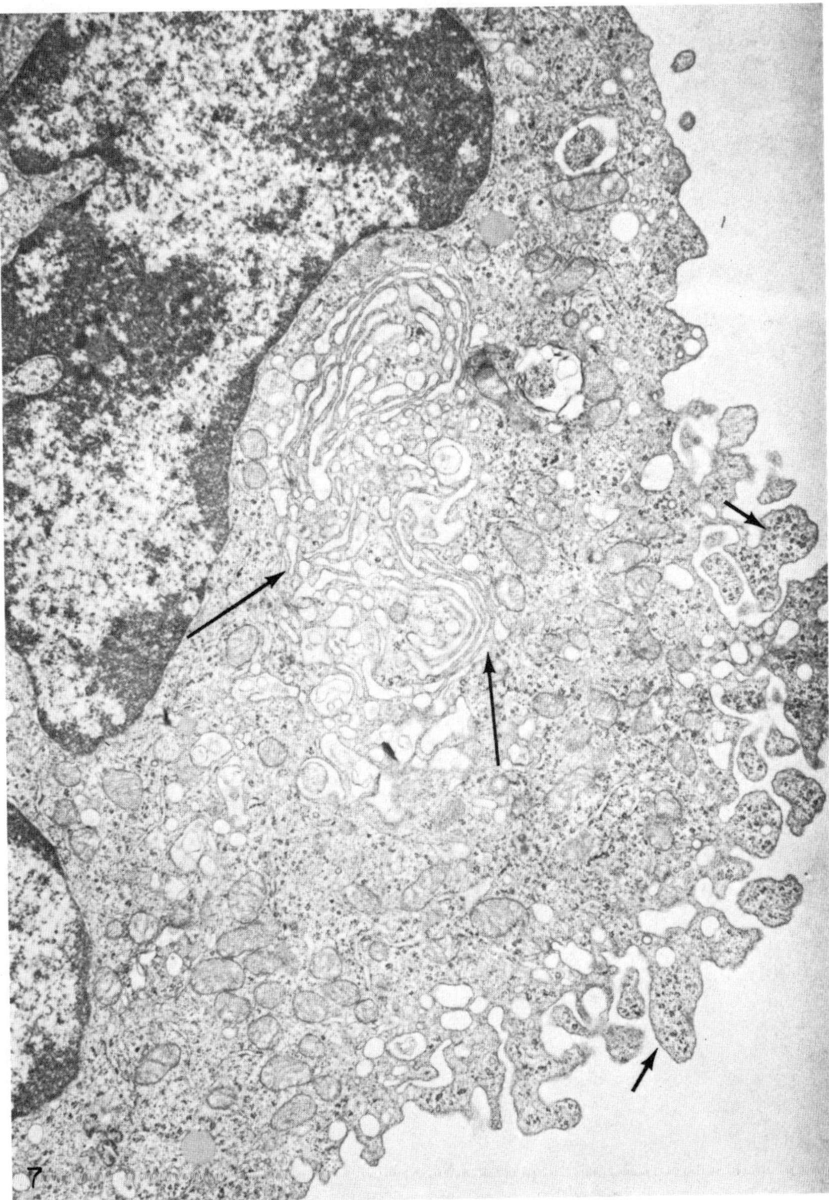

**Fig. 7.** Electron microscope configuration of intermediate type I guinea pig megakaryocyte (promegakaryoblast) which was isolated without any additives except citrate. Shown is the localized area of protrusions (short arrow) distal to the developing internal network of the DMS (long arrows). In the midzone of the cytoplasm are found mitochondria and vacuolar elements. ×15,600 (reduced 10% for reproduction).

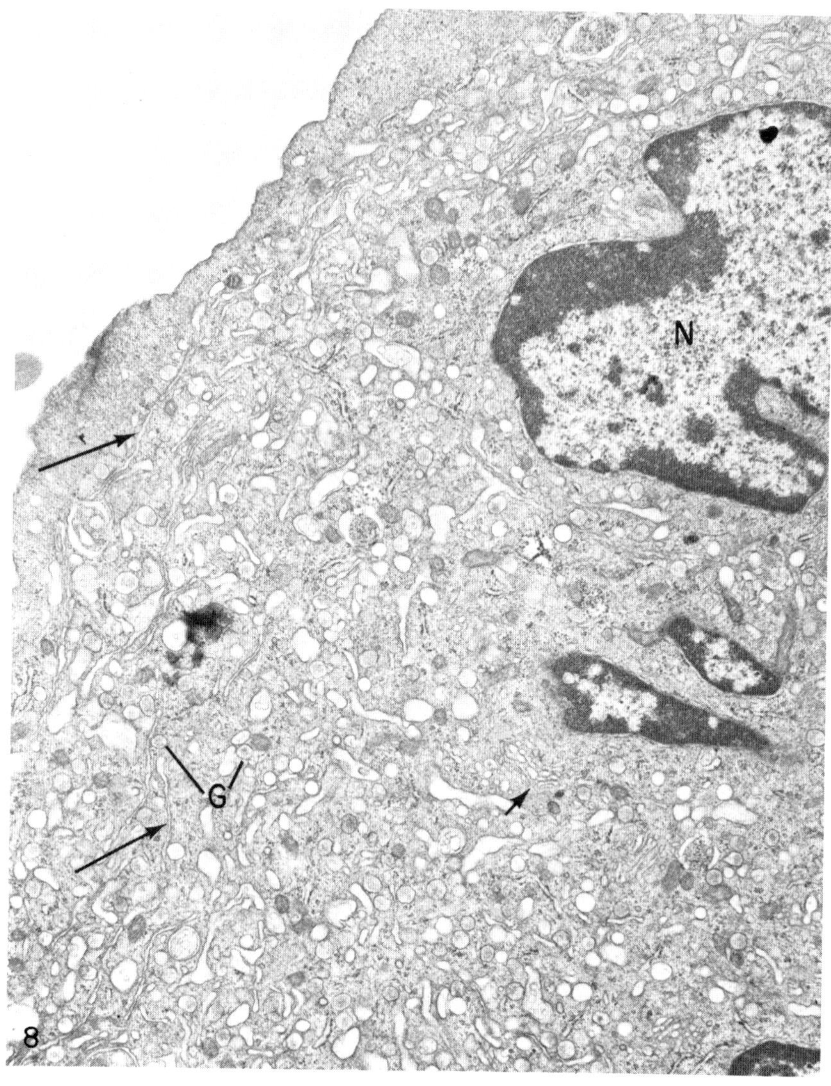

**Fig. 8.**  Electron microscope appearance of a guinea pig megakaryocyte, intermediate (stage II). Shown is the multilobulated appearance of the nucleus (N). At the margin of one of the nuclear lobes is one portion of the characteristically multifocal Golgi complex (short arrow), random distribution of cytoplasmic granules (G), and abundant short profiles of the DMS (long arrows). ×15,600 (reduced 10% for reproduction).

cytoplasm. Most often strips of rough endoplasmic reticulum are scattered in the cytoplasm but occasionally are segregated into areas which show the membranes in stacks. The Golgi complex is multifocal, situated at the margins of the nucleus, and composed of vesicles, vacuoles, and lamellae. Occasionally a dense core may be found in a budding Golgi vacuole which has the diameter of a cytoplasmic granule. Tubules which may be found around the nucleus in more immature forms tend to be distributed in random fashion throughout the cytoplasm, and polyribosomes are not prominent.

### 6.6.1.5. Mature Megakaryocyte

The mature megakaryocyte, which can be up to 60 $\mu$m in size, has a cell margin characteristic of this entire cell series. The peripheral margin is irregular and the peripheral cytoplasm is devoid of organelles except ribosomes and filaments. This cell has a well-developed DMS which outlines prospective platelets. There is a full complement of cytoplasmic granules. These platelet fields extend to the margin of the nucleus (Fig. 9). Higher magnification of the platelet fields shows the wide extent of the DMS surrounding cytoplasm, mitochondria, and granules with the characteristic nucleoid (Fig. 10). The nucleus shows many lobulations and heavy margination of nuclear chromatin and prominent nuclear pores.

### 6.6.1.6. Platelet-Shedding Megakaryocyte

The megakaryocyte in the process of shedding platelets is characterized in part by its nucleus which is convoluted and has its lobes compactly stacked. There is marked margination of the nuclear chromatin, with prominent nuclear pores situated in the areas of dense chromatin. Variable amounts of cytoplasm are present, depending on the degree of platelet shedding that has already taken place (Fig. 11).

### 6.6.2. Observations on Platelet Formation

The mechanism of platelet shedding has been a vaguely defined process. Various theories have been proposed to explain the phenomenon (Pisciotta *et al.*, 1953; Thiery and Bessis, 1956; Behnke, 1969). Platelet shedding can probably occur in a relatively short span of time, and only a fraction of the normal megakaryocyte population is poised to release platelets at any one time. It then became a problem to locate enough cells at the proper stage of maturation for study. For this reason marrows from normal mice, from mice that were bled, and from mice that received high or low doses of vincristine (Rak, 1972) were studied. Marrow from four

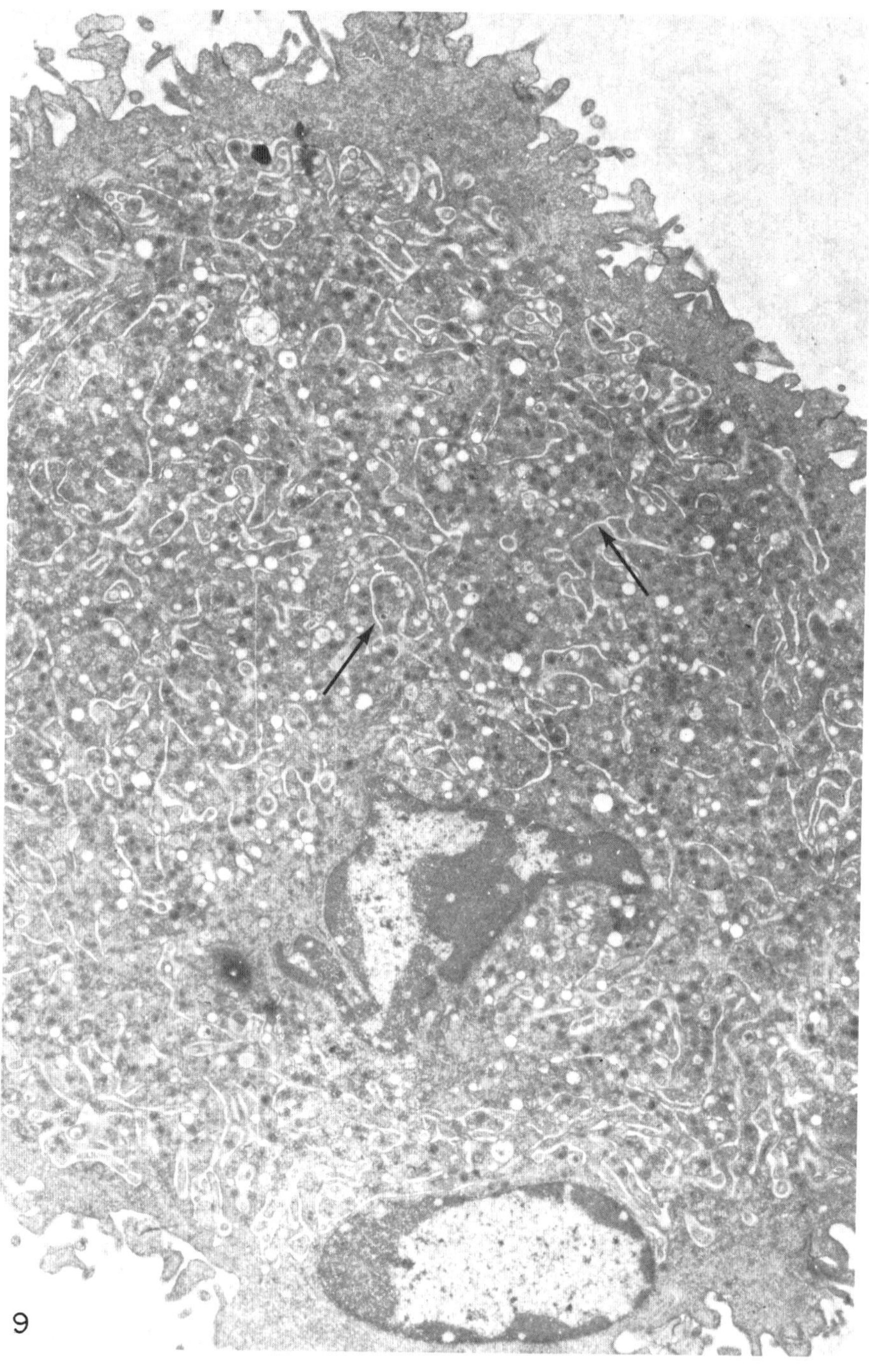

9

**Fig. 9.** Electron microscopic appearance of a mature megakaryocyte. Shown is the irregular cell membrane and peripheral rim of cytoplasm devoid of many organelles. The midzone of the cell is divided into platelet fields by the DMS (arrows). ×6,950 (reduced 10% for reproduction).

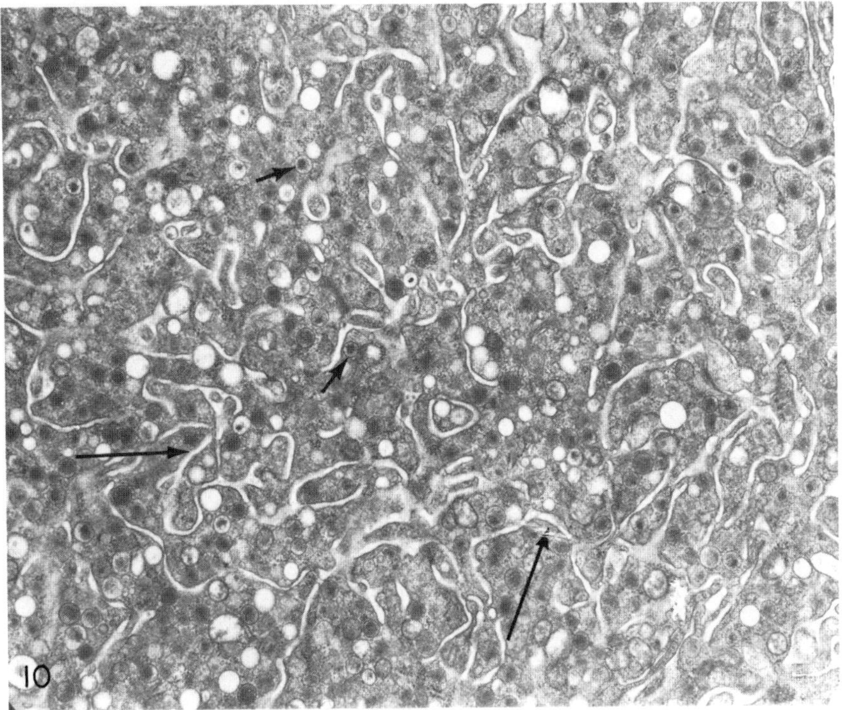

**Fig. 10.** Higher power magnification of the platelet fields of a mature megakaryocyte. Shown are the profiles of the DMS outlining prospective platelets (long arrows) and the characteristic cytoplasmic granules (short arrows). ×18,500 (reduced 3% for reproduction).

mice in each group was sampled. The method of fixation was as follows: removal of the femur, which was cleaned of adherent muscles; the prompt immersion of the femur in glutaraldehyde; the opening of the marrow cavity; removal of the marrow tissue; and then cutting of the tissue into 1- to 2-mm³ blocks. These procedures were accomplished in the presence of fixative and fixation was performed as described previously (Levine and Fedorko, 1976). Thick alkaline azure-stained sections were obtained from Epon-embedded marrow and the appropriate cells were identified mainly by their characteristic configuration and staining of their nuclei. Approximately 150 mouse megakaryocytes in the platelet-shedding phase of maturation were located and studied.

Once again the close proximity of these cells to the marrow vascular endothelium was noted. These mature megakaryocytes were often found protruding through the endothelial wall into or in close proximity to the marrow vascular sinus.

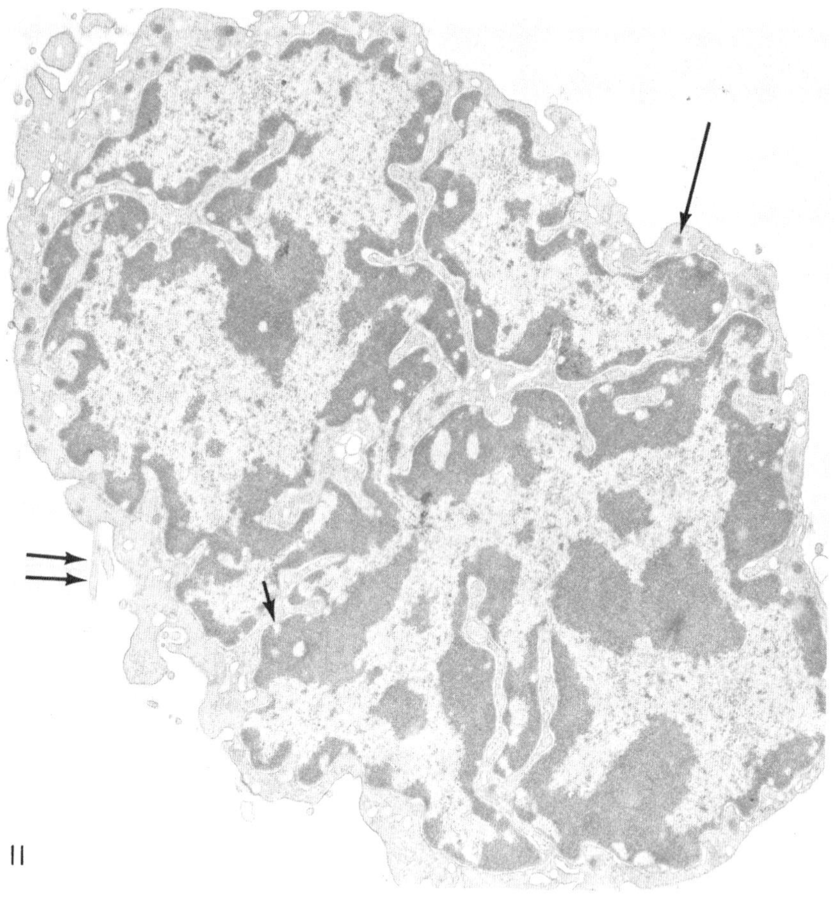



**Fig. 11.**  Electron microscopic appearance of a postplatelet-producing megakaryocyte. Shown is the large extremely convoluted nucleus with pronounced margination of the nuclear chromatin and prominent nuclear pores (short arrow). There is a narrow peripheral rim of cytoplasm containing a few cytoplasmic granules (long arrow) and vacuoles. The cell membrane is somewhat irregular, with a localized area of finger-like protrusion (double arrow). ×13,260 (reduced 10% for reproduction).

The characteristic appearance of a mature megakaryocyte is shown in Fig. 12. This appearance may be modified by the method of fixation used, but the appearance of the mature megakaryocyte differs from the one in the process of shedding platelets under the conditions of fixation. In mature megakaryocytes platelet fields are well demarcated but there is a peripheral rim of cytoplasm which is devoid of many organelles. In this

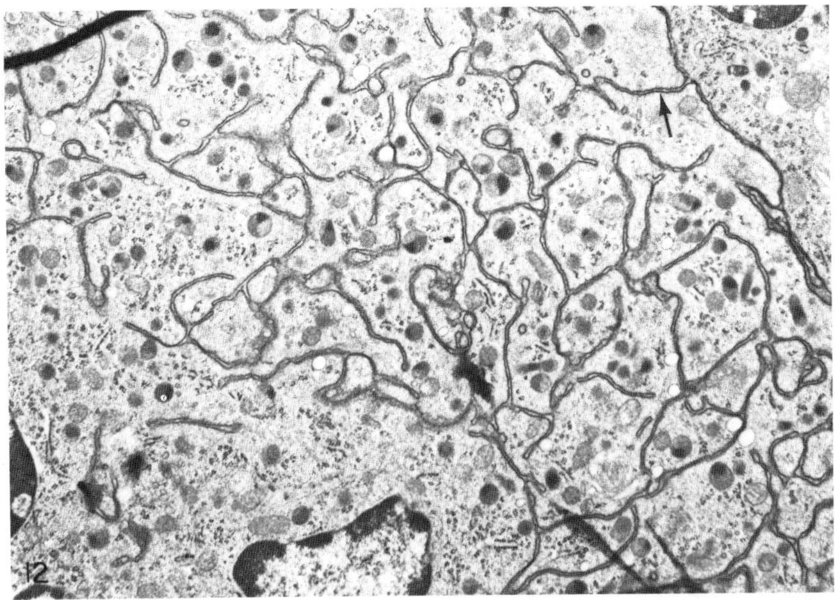

**Fig. 12.**   Electron microscope appearance of mature megakaryocyte with its prominent platelet fields. With the method of fixation employed (rapid immersion in glutaraldehyde) the outermost zone is relatively devoid of organelles except polyribosomes, but there is one profile of the DMS (arrow) which extends to the outer surface. ×16,050 (reduced 10% for reproduction).

rim there may be a rare to occasional profile of DMS which extends to the peripheral cell margin. This distinguishes the mature megakaryocyte from the one which is shedding platelets. In the latter cell platelet fields extend to the cell margin, and the DMS becomes dilated so that the appearance of individual platelets becomes more suggestive. In the mouse which has been bled prior to bone marrow study, there is occasionally seen a prospective platelet in a megakaryocyte platelet field attached to a narrow stalk of cytoplasm (Fig. 13). This finding is more frequently seen in animals treated with the vinca alkaloids (Fig. 14) and is rarely seen in guinea pig megakaryocytes (Fig. 15). The possibility exists that this mode of platelet formation exists normally and what is seen in cells treated with certain drugs *in vivo* is an exaggeration or a modification of a normal process. The other fact suggested by this finding is that contraction or constriction is an important part of the process of platelet formation. Further studies would be needed to demonstrate microfilaments (elements of the contractile system) in the stalk. In general, however, platelet

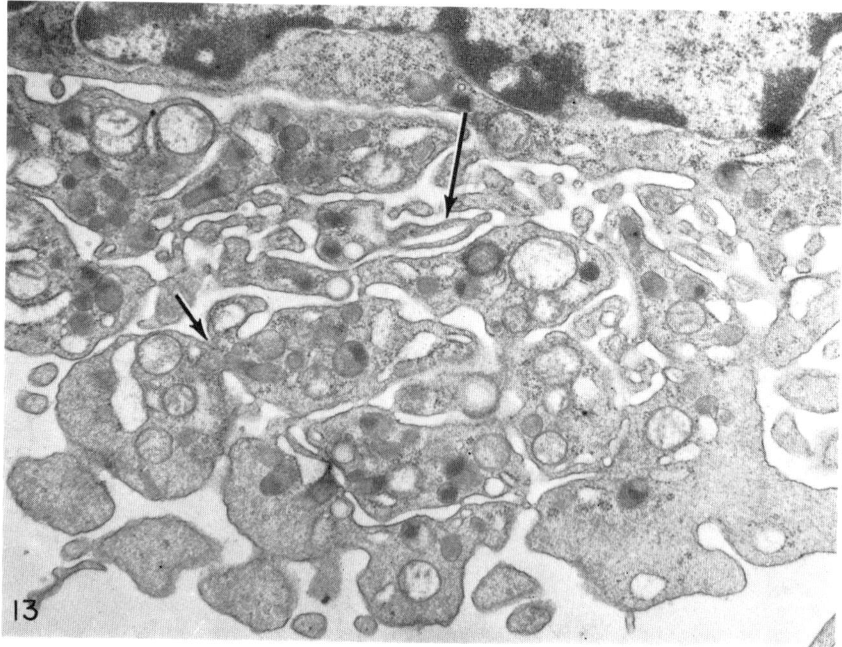

**Fig. 13.** Electron microscope appearance of mature mouse megakaryocyte from an animal which was bled 4 hr earlier. Shown are the discrete platelet profiles formed by dilatations in the DMS. The prospective platelets are attached to the main body of the cell by a narrow constriction (short arrow) or by longer stalks (long arrow). ×19,500 (reduced 10% for reproduction).

shedding was often encountered in vascular sinuses of the species studied and was accomplished by fragmentation of the cell cytoplasm. These findings are on the whole in agreement with observations of Behnke (1969).

## 6.6.3. Survival of Megakaryocytes in Tissue Culture

The *in vitro* survival and maturation of megakaryocytes has been studied in marrow from two animals, guinea pigs and mice. In the guinea pig a concentrated megakaryocyte preparation was obtained as described previously (Levine and Fedorko, 1976) and plated at a concentration of $0.5 \times 10^5$ cells/ml (Levine, 1976a). Megakaryocytes had good viability until 72 hr in culture. These cultured cells showed evidence of maturation by

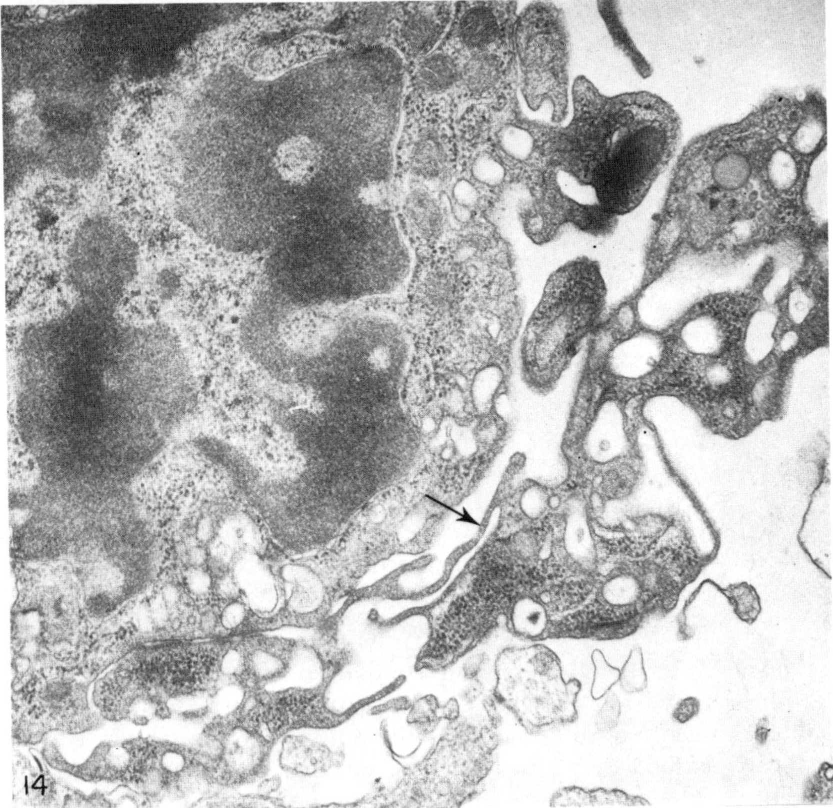

**Fig. 14.** Electron microscopic appearance of a mature mouse megakaryocyte obtained from a mouse treated with vinca alkaloids *in vivo* and in the process of shedding platelets. Shown is an area of cytoplasm apparently detaching from the cell proper (arrow) but attached by a narrow stalk. ×15,600 (reduced 10% for reproduction).

decrease in ribosomal content, increase in cytoplasmic granules, and development of platelet demarcating channels.

In another experimental system (M. Fedorko, in preparation) survival of mouse megakaryocytes was noted. This system employed tissue culture of mouse marrow explants from Imferon-treated mice. Under the conditions of culture megakaryocyte survival was good up to 3 days. Immature megakaryocytes were more prominent than intermediate stage II megakaryocytes. No megakaryocytes with well-developed platelet fields were present. Immature megakaryocytes (blasts) had the distinctive morphologic characteristics described for the guinea pig megakaryocytoblast,

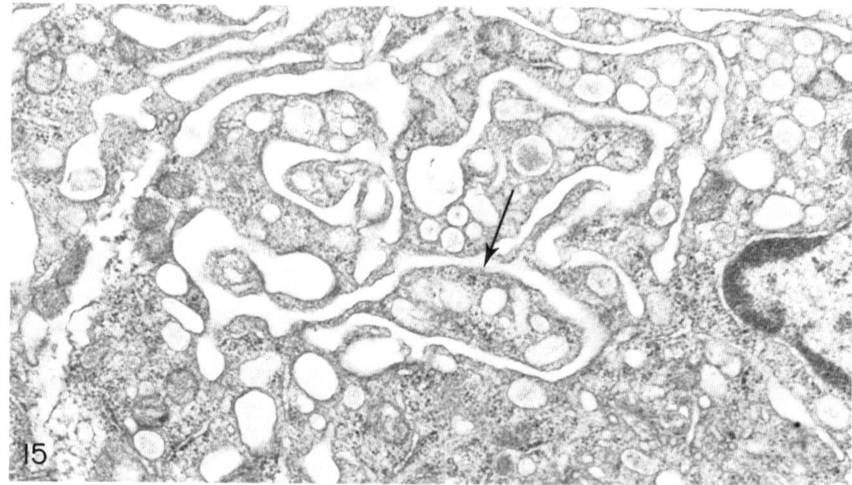

**Fig. 15.** Electron microscope appearance of platelet fields of mature guinea pig mega-karyocyte. Shown is the configuration of a prospective platelet (arrow) which is attached to the remainder of the cytoplasm by a narrow stalk. ×23,400 (reduced 10% for reproduction).

i.e., bleblike peripheral membrane configuration, immature features of the nucleus, and a prominent complement of polyribosomes. Another feature distinctive of this stage of maturation *in vitro* was the presence of multivesicular bodies, the formation of which may be due to tissue culture conditions. In this culture system there were present immature mega-karyocytes with a distinctive morphology not seen in normal marrow (Fig. 16). These cells were 15 $\mu$m in size, had a large nucleus with the character-istics of immaturity described previously, and no appreciable profiles of the demarcation membrane system or cytoplasmic granules, but promi-nent content of rough endoplasmic reticulum distributed in stacks. Nor-mally, rough endoplasmic reticulum is scattered throughout the cyto-plasm with some prominence around the nucleus. From what is known about granule formation in other cell types, granule protein content is synthesized in the rough endoplasmic reticulum, transported to the Golgi complex, and then transported to granules (Caro and Palade, 1964; Fedorko and Hirsch, 1966). It may be postulated that this is also true in the production of the megakaryocyte granules. However, the separate maturation phase described here is not noted in normal marrow prepara-tions. The appearance of this maturation stage *in vitro* may represent a relative maturation arrest produced by conditions of tissue culture.

In the marrow explant system there is other evidence for distorted megakaryocyte maturation. In cells with moderate amounts of DMS this

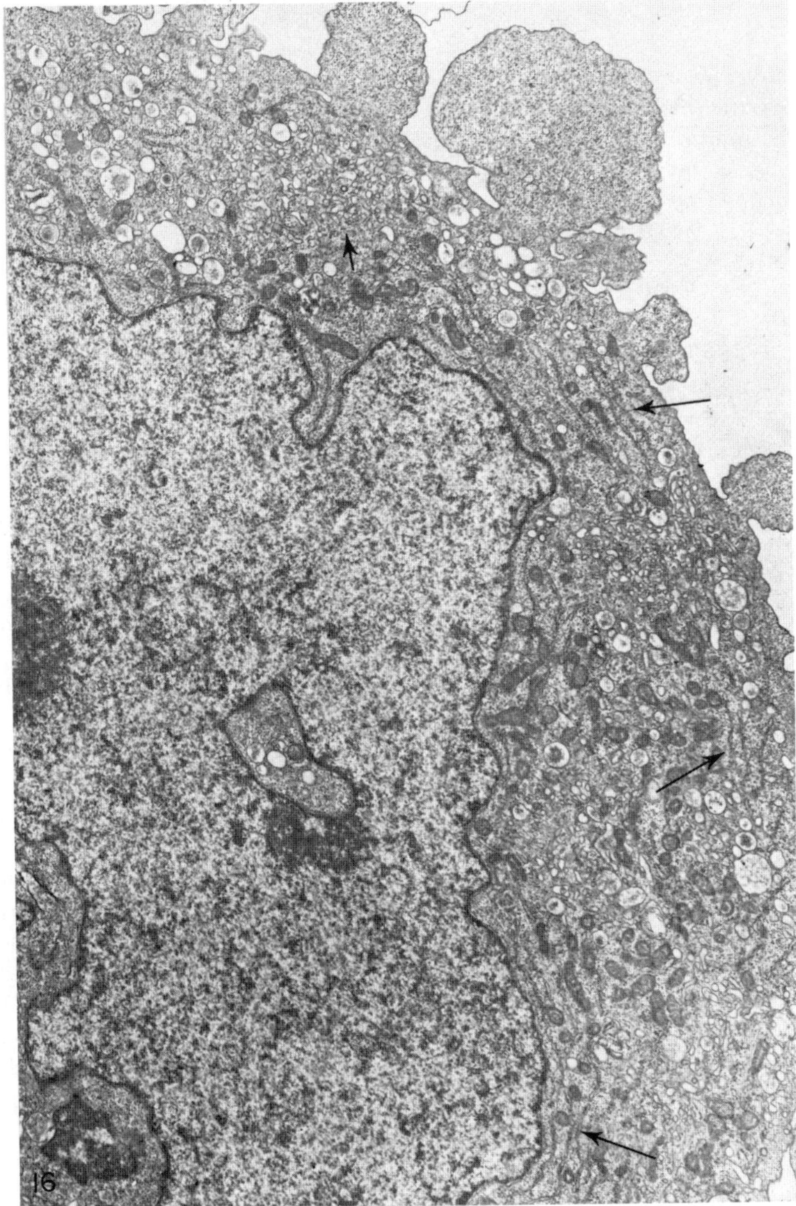

**Fig. 16.** Electron microscope appearance of a mouse megakaryocyte precursor after 3 days culture in an explant tissue culture system. The cell is 15 $\mu$m in size. The nucleus is also large with signs of immaturity—very little marginated chromatin at the nuclear membrane and prominent nucleoli. Stacks of rough endoplasmic reticulum (long arrows) are scattered in the cytoplasm and there is focal accumulation of DMS (short arrows). Mitochondria and a few vacuoles are found throughout the cytoplasm. The peripheral cell margin shows the characteristic blebs which contain many polyribosomes. $\times$15,600 (reduced 15% for reproduction).

membrane system appears to develop in a canalicular fashion rather than from the ordered platelet fields seen normally. It may therefore be concluded that mouse megakaryocytes survive in culture and show some degree of maturation. However, in the absence of any poietins which might be needed for cell maturation no evidence for significant platelet production has been obtained.

## 6.6.4. Features of the Cytoskeleton in Megakaryocytes

### 6.6.4.1. Tubulin

With the advent of fixation in warm (37°C) glutaraldehyde followed by osmium the presence and distribution of microtubules could be studied at the ultrastructural level. A marginal bundle of approximately ten microtubules has been described in platelets (diameter 2 $\mu$m). Several authors have also described their presence in megakaryocytes (Schulz and Schiller, 1968; Behnke, 1969). Microtubules have been observed to converge on centrioles and have been observed circling around the nucleus in our preparations of immature megakaryocytes. They are distributed throughout the platelet fields of more mature megakaryocytes in no ordered arrangement. More insight into the distribution and content of tubulin can be obtained with the use of drugs known to react with tubulin. White (1968) has reported on the effects of vinca alkaloids on platelet microtubules and noted the production of cytoplasmic inclusions. It is now known that the vinca alkaloids interact with binding sites on tubulin, precipitate tubulin, and result in inhibition of microtubule assembly (Wilson, 1975). In our laboratory Levine (1975) has studied the occurrence and structure of these alkaloid induced inclusions in cultured guinea pig megakaryocytes and Fedorko (unpublished) has noted these inclusions in cultured mouse megakaryocytes. Their fine structure has been described in detail elsewhere (Levine, 1976b), and is illustrated in Fig. 17. For the purposes of discussion here their prominence in megakaryocytes *in vitro* gave some indication of the large intracellular pool of tubulin in these cells.

### 6.6.4.2. Microfilaments

The contractile protein in platelets (Behnke *et al.*, 1971; Zucker-Franklin and Grusky, 1972) and megakaryocytes is known as thrombosthenin and is composed of actenoid and myosinoid elements, about 15% of platelet protein (Bettex-Galland and Luscher, 1965). Nachman *et al.*

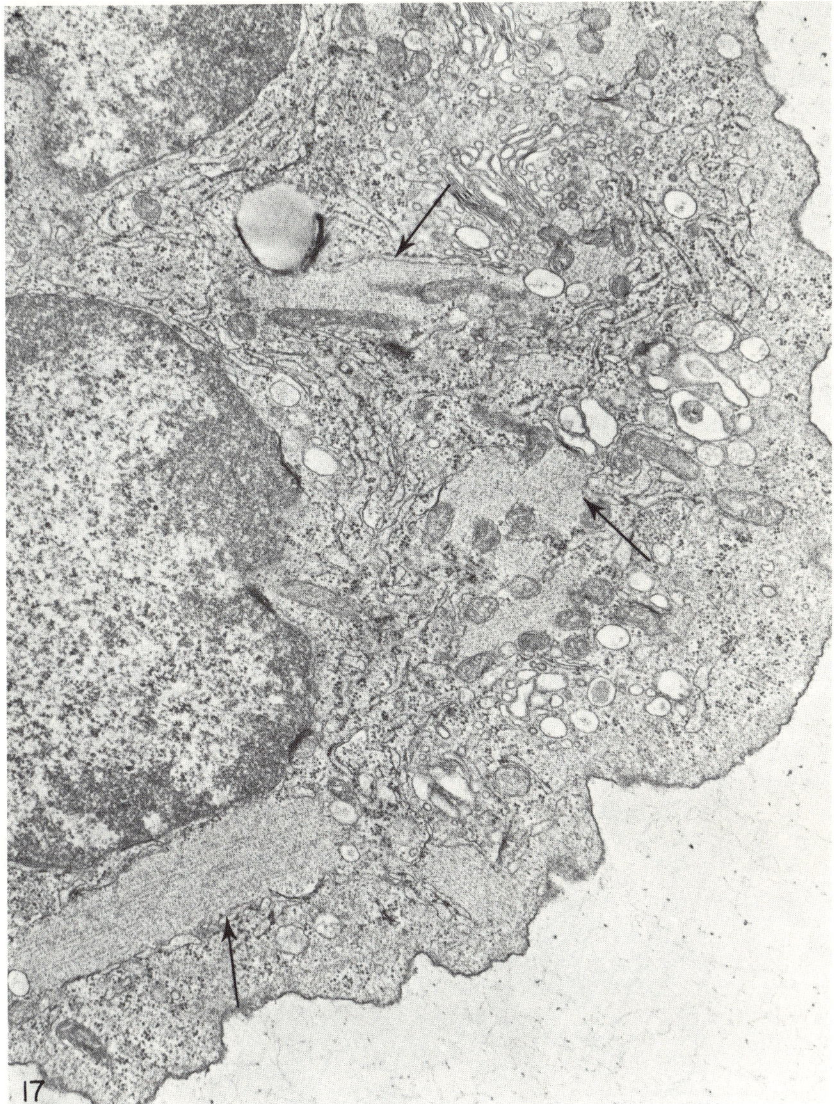

**Fig. 17.** Electron microscope appearance of guinea pig megakaryocyte exposed to vincristine $1 \times 10^{-8}$ M for longer than 15 min *in vitro*. This cell is immature, at the megakaryoblast stage of maturation. The most remarkable feature found in the cytoplasm is the presence of the characteristic crystalloids (arrows) indicating the presence of the tubulin–drug complex. $\times 23,400$ (reduced 10% for reproduction). (Courtesy of R. Levine.)

(1967) observed intense fluorescence in megakaryocytes fixed with acetone and exposed to antibody prepared to partially purified thrombosthenin. Filaments between 50 and 120 Å, some of which were decorated with heavy meromyosin, have been identified in megakaryocytes (Behnke and Emmersen, 1972). We have studied the filament system in a variety of experimental conditions in megakaryocytes by two methods: (1) extracting megakaryocytes with glycerol and (2) special uranyl staining of routinely fixed speciments (E. Wang, personal communication). When this methodology is employed it is readily observed that in immature megakaryocytes with bilobed nuclei abundant filaments extend from the perinuclear zone to the cell margin. In the more mature cells with evidence of cytoplasmic granule formation and moderately well-developed DMS, there is a peripheral rim of microfilaments beneath the cell membrane (Fig. 18). A heretofore glycerol-nonextractable submembranous deposit is located beneath the leaflets of the DMS in a discontinuous layer (Fig. 19). The true nature of these structures remains to be clarified. There now exists new methodology in immunohistochemistry at the light and ultra-

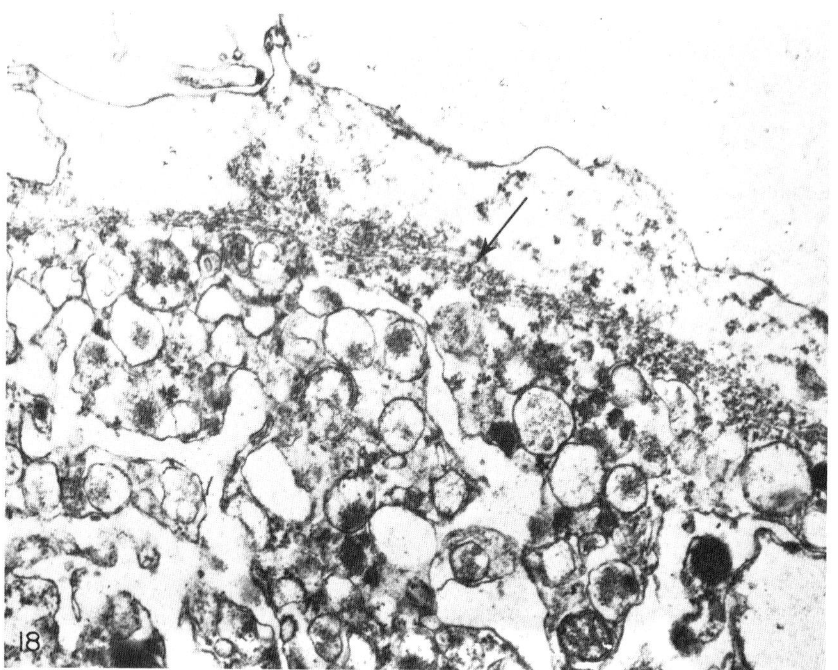

**Fig. 18.**  Ultrastructure of guinea pig megakaryocyte extracted with buffered glycerol. A prominent band of microfilaments (arrow) is seen in a margin beneath the cell membrane.

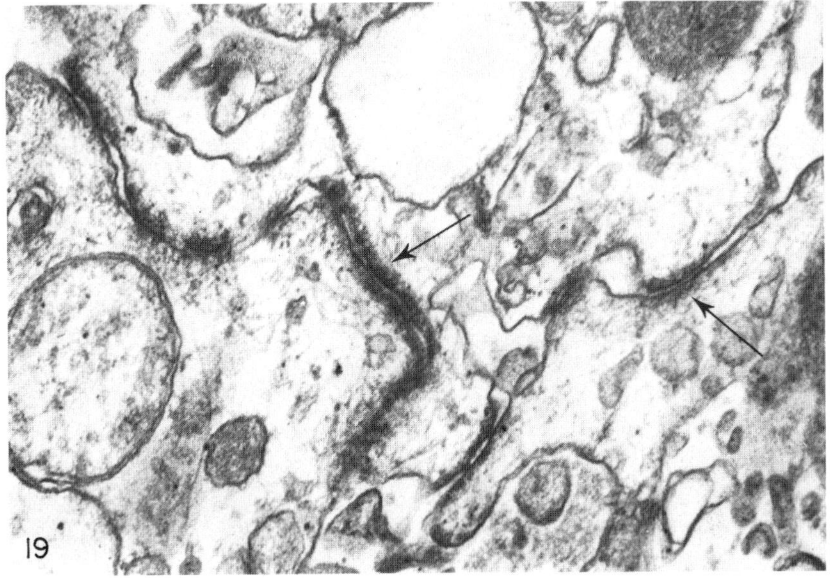

**Fig. 19.** Ultrastructural appearance of a guinea pig megakaryocyte exposed to buffered glycerol and then processed for electron microscopy. Shown is the discontinuous deposit of electron-dense components (arrow) beneath the membrane of the DMS. ×58,500 (reduced 10% for reproduction).

structural levels which will enable more detailed investigations of the contractile system.

In two experimental situations this filamentous network appears to be rearranged in moderately mature megakaryocytes. After exposure to cytochalasin there is dilatation of the DMS and the cytoplasm becomes a network of narrow extensions which show apparently disconnected accumulations of filamentous material, so-called thin (60 Å) and thick filaments (100 Å) (Fig. 20). In relation to the response of aggregators of platelets (epinephrine, etc.) there is also rearrangement of microfilaments of megakaryocytes (illustrated in the following section.)

## 6.7. Functional Capacity of Megakaryocytes

### 6.7.1. Uptake and Release of Serotonin

Intermediate stage II and mature megakaryocytes with platelet fields possess many of the structural features that are common to platelets, i.e., the demarcation membrane system, the structural analog of the open canalicular system in platelets, and cytoplasmic granules. It became of

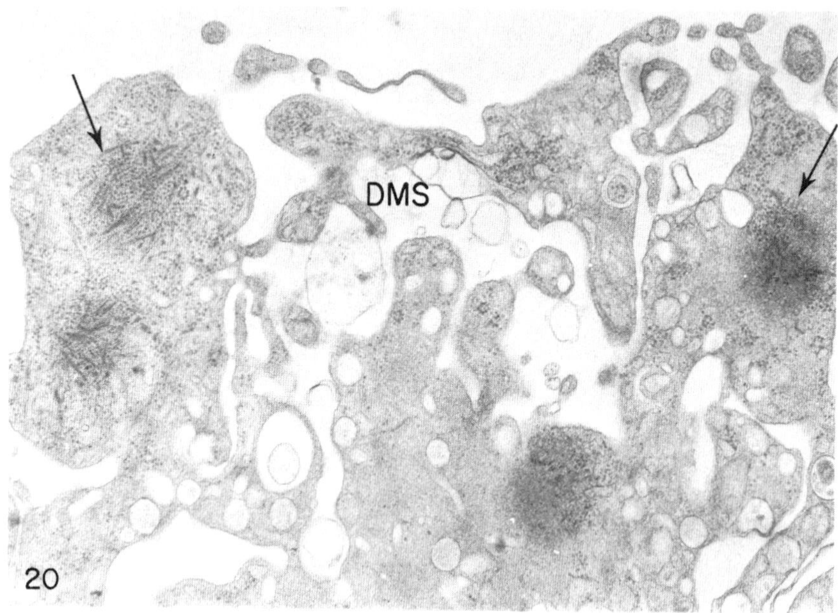


**Fig. 20.** Electron microscope appearance of guinea pig megakaryocyte exposed to 3 μg/ml cytochalasin B for 4 hr. Shown are the protrusions of the cytoplasm and marked dilatation of the DMS. Within the cytoplasm are centrally located accumulations of microfilamentous elements (arrows). ×23,296 (reduced 10% for reproduction).

interest to demonstrate whether megakaryocytes would have the functional capacity that platelets possess—to concentrate serotonin (Fedorko, 1977a). The conventional methods used to demonstrate this capability in platelets were unsuccessful. The use of a filter cell wash system which circumvented repeated centrifugations enabled us to demonstrate that uptake of radiolabeled serotonin by megakaryocytes was linear within the first 30 min and tapered off between 30 and 60 min (Fig. 21). Incorporation of serotonin was inhibited by cold, 2 $\mu$M reserpine, and 20 $\mu$M imiprimine (see Table I).

The effect of certain agents—ADP, thrombin, and epinephrine—has been demonstrated to produce aggregation of platelets (Holmsen, 1974). Similarly, isolated megakaryocytes which were previously loaded with [$^3$H]serotonin released significant amounts of isotope when exposed to ADP, thrombin, epinephrine, and ionophore A23187 (Table II). In contrast to what was true of platelets, protein in the suspending solution appeared to exert a protective effect on serotonin loss (see Table III) produced by ADP.

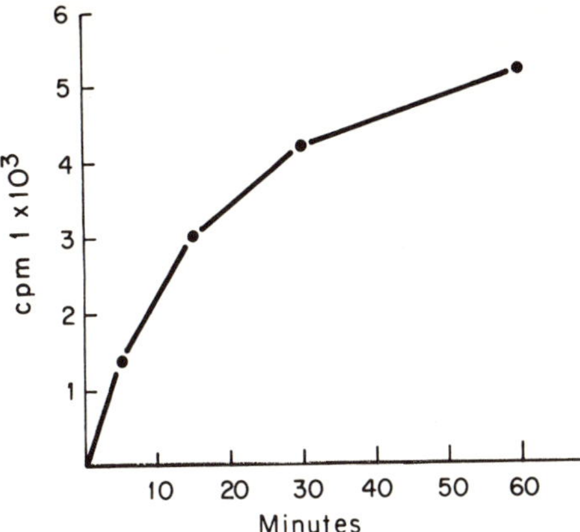


**Fig. 21.** Uptake of 0.5 $\mu$M [³H]serotonin [5-hydroxy(G-3H)tryptamine creatinine sulfate, 0.5 $\mu$M] by isolated guinea pig megakaryocytes. Points represent an average of two determinations.

**Table I.** Effect of Temperature and Chemical Agents[a] on Incorporation of [³H]Serotonin[b] Isolated Guinea Pig Megakaryocytes

| Variable | Cell content (cpm) | Inhibition of uptake (%) |
|---|---|---|
| Temperature, 37°C | $2 \times 10^4$ | 79 |
| 4°C | $5 \times 10^3$ | |
| Temperature, 37°C | $2.9 \times 10^3$ | |
| 4°C | $1.2 \times 10^3$ | 59 |
| | $1.1 \times 10^3$ | |
| No reserpine | $6.7 \times 10^3$ | |
| Reserpine, 2 $\mu$M | $2.4 \times 10^3$ | 64 |
| No reserpine | $2.9 \times 10^3$ | |
| Reserpine, 2 $\mu$M | $1.4 \times 10^3$ | 41 |
| | $1.9 \times 10^3$ | |
| No imiprimine | $6.7 \times 10^3$ | 82 |
| Imiprimine, 20 $\mu$M | $1.2 \times 10^3$ | |
| No imiprimine | $2.9 \times 10^3$ | |
| Imiprimine 20 $\mu$M | $1.4 \times 10^3$ | 52 |
| | $1.4 \times 10^3$ | |

[a]In preparations with drugs and control specimens incubations were carried out at 37°C.
[b]Cell preparation was incubated in serotonin (0.5 $\mu$M) and variable for 30 min.

**Table II.**  Effect of Various Agents on [³H]Serotonin Release by Guinea Pig Megakaryocytes

| Additive | Number of determinations | [³H]Serotonin release (%, mean) |
|---|---|---|
| ADP | | |
| $1 \times 10^{-3}$ M | 7 | 63 |
| $1 \times 10^{-4}$ M | 4 | 46 |
| $1 \times 10^{-5}$ M | 4 | 45 |
| Thrombin | | |
| 100 units/ml | 4 | 80 |
| 10 units/ml | 9 | 43 |
| 1 unit/ml | 4 | 32 |
| Epinephrine | | |
| $1 \times 10^{-3}$ M | 7 | 68 |
| $1 \times 10^{-4}$ M | 4 | 48 |
| $1 \times 10^{-5}$ M | 4 | 42 |
| Ionophore A23187 | | |
| 12 $\mu$M | 6 | 75 |
| 1.6 $\mu$M | 3 | 63 |
| Dimethyl sulfoxide 1.2% | 2 | 0 |

In conjunction with the kinetic studies on serotonin release produced by these triggering agents morphologic studies were performed to illustrate surface changes in megakaryocyte contour by scanning microscopy and internal changes by electron microscopy. The normal configuration of a guinea pig megakaryocyte isolated without any additives showed a round cell with a localized zone of protrusion (Fig. 22a). When exposed to the various triggering agents there was a marked change in megakaryo-

**Table III.**  Effect of Albumin Solution[a] on [³H]Serotonin Release by Isolated Guinea Pig Megakaryocytes

| Additive to cell preparations | Uptake (cpm) | ³H release (%) |
|---|---|---|
| | | $5.4 \times 10^3$ |
| [³H]Serotonin, ADP $1 \times 10^{-3}$ M | $1.0 \times 10^3$ | 80 |
| [³H]Serotonin, albumin, ADP $1 \times 10^{-3}$ M | $5.0 \times 10^3$ | 0 |
| [³H]Serotonin | $2.7 \times 10^3$ | |
| [³H]Serotonin, ADP $1 \times 10^{-3}$ M | $1.2 \times 10^3$ | 56 |
| [³H]Serotonin, albumin | $2.6 \times 10^3$ | |
| [³H]Serotonin, albumin, ADP $1 \times 10^{-3}$ M | $2.9 \times 10^3$ | 0 |

[a] Isolated megakaryocytes were washed once and incubated for 30 min with 0.5 $\mu$M [³H]serotonin; then either albumin (final concentration 20%) of specific gravity 1.3430, or ADP, or both were added.

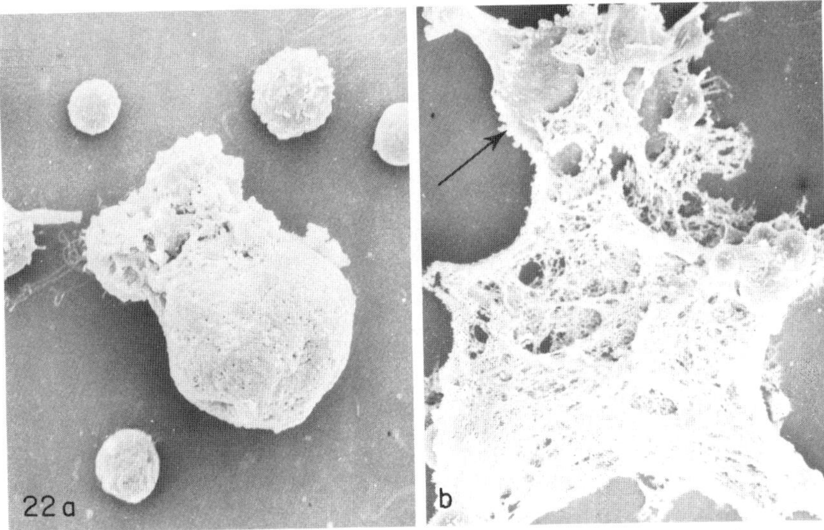

**Fig. 22.** Scanning electron microscopic appearance of guinea pig megakaryocytes isolated with no chemical additives: (a) after normal isolation procedures; (b) after exposure to 10 units thrombin for 15 min. Shown in b is the dramatic increase in surface area of the cell, with formation of pseudopods with a weblike appearance. The nucleus (arrow) is located at one pole of the cell. ×2000 (reduced 10% for reproduction).

cyte configuration demonstrated by scanning microscopy (Fig. 22b). The surface area of the cell increased, the nucleus relocated at one pole of the cell, and the cytoplasm formed pseudopods with a weblike arrangement. The ultrastructure of the normal megakaryocyte showed that the localized zone of protrusion formed distal to a band of microfilaments (Fig. 23). Electron micrographs of megakaryoctyes exposed to triggering agents showed marked changes with the appearance of peripheral blebs and prominent rearrangement of an underlying zone of contractile filaments (Figs. 24 and 25). Degranulation was more difficult to evaluate, but on the whole diminished granule content and dilatation of the DMS gave presumptive evidence for degranulation. Although these described changes were illustrated here after exposure to ADP, similar changes were obtained after exposure to epinephrine, thrombin, and calcium ionophore.

## 6.7.2. Uptake of Particles and Macromolecules by Megakaryocytes

During isolation of megakaryocytes it was noted that often an autologous erythrocyte was within, not on, a megakaryocyte. Examination at the

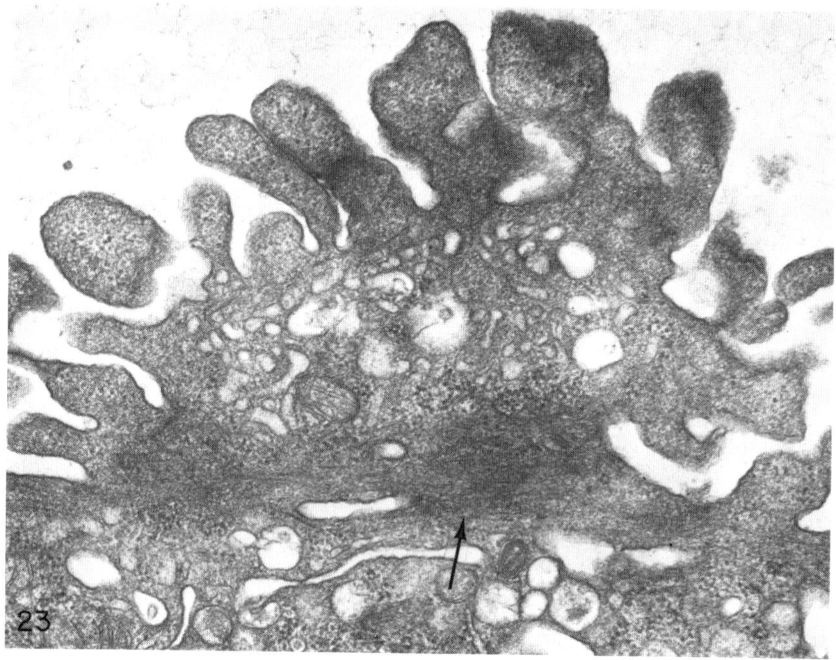

**Fig. 23.** Electron microscopic appearance of area of protrusion in normal guinea pig megakaryocyte illustrated in Fig. 22a. Shown are the peripheral protrusions of the cell membrane, and the underlying zone of contractile filaments (arrow). ×35,100 (reduced 10% for reproduction).

ultrastructural level showed that erythrocytes as well as leukocytes could be found within megakaryocytes (Fedorko, 1977b). The structure of the vacuole wall was such that it showed linear arrangement of finger-like projections which was quite different from that seen with other phagocytes. Incorporation of tannic acid into the fixative showed that precipitates of a presumed tannic acid–protein complex occurred around the red cell; this indicated that the erythrocyte rested in an open vacuole. Similarly, when megakaryocytes were incubated with *Micrococcus lysodeikticus* and latex particles 1.1–7 $\mu$m in size there was extensive uptake of these particles and they rested in open vacuoles (Figs. 26–28). Therefore, it appears, as in the case with platelets, that the particles are actually trapped within preformed elements of the demarcating membrane system.

The technique of rosette formation was able to detect the type of receptor present on cells exposed to either IgG, IgM, and complement-coated (C3b and C3d) erythrocytes. The system which contained C3b formed rosettes. One may conclude, therefore, that in contrast to macro-

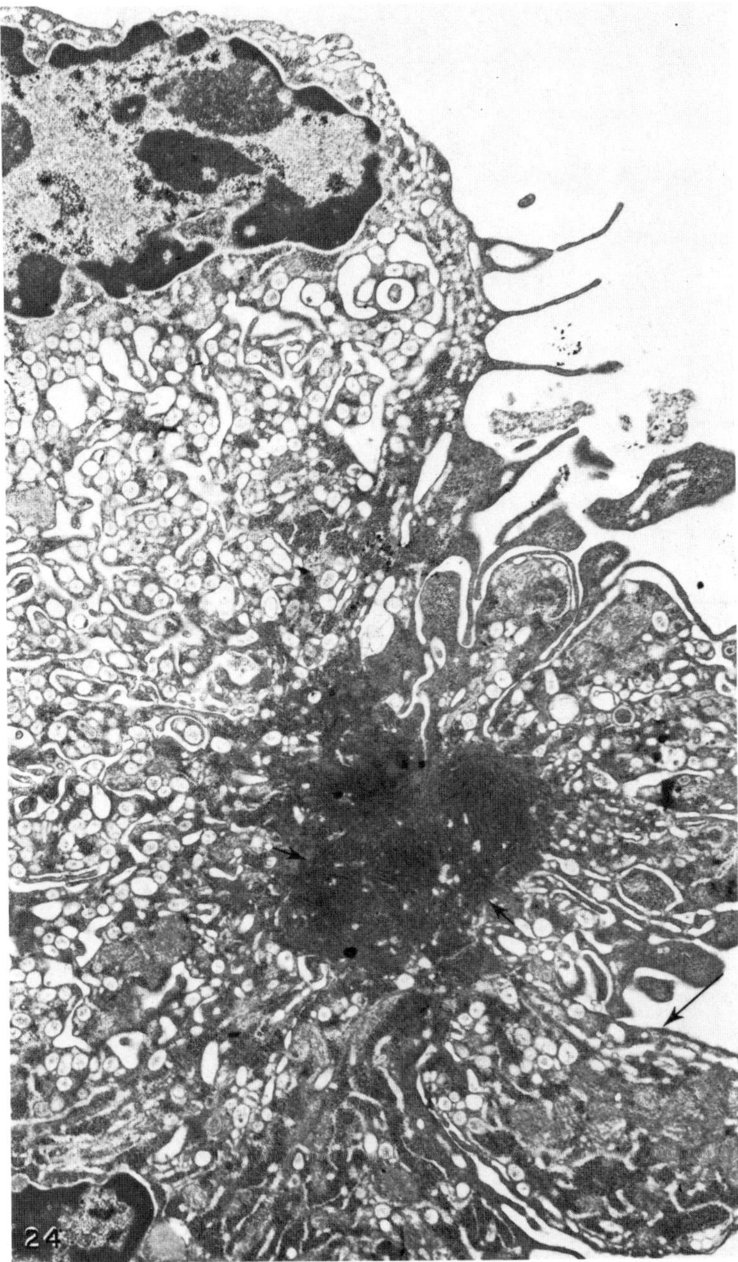

**Fig. 24.** Electron microscopic appearance of isolated guinea pig megakaryocyte exposed to $1 \times 10^{-3}$ M ADP for 30 min. Shown is the eccentric location of the nucleus, the dramatic changes in the cell membrane, with the formation of bulbous protrusions (long arrow). More centrally placed to these protrusions is a large mass of filaments (short arrow). $\times 15,600$ (reduced 20% for reproduction).

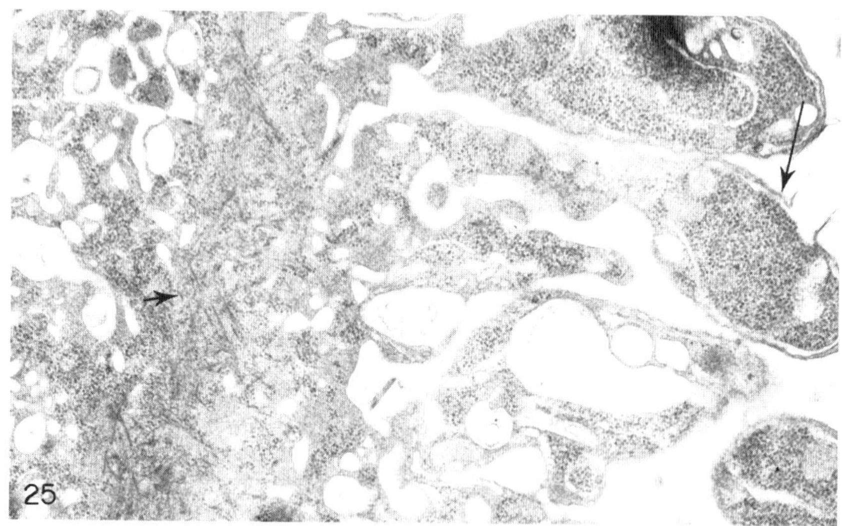

**Fig. 25.** Shown are the ultrastructural changes in the peripheral portion of isolated guinea pig megakaryocyte exposed to $1 \times 10^{-4}$ M epinephrine for 10 min. The peripheral bulbous protrusions (long arrow) which contain a peripheral rim of endoplasmic reticulum and a more proximal zone of filaments (short arrow) are evident. ×23,400 (reduced 10% for reproduction).

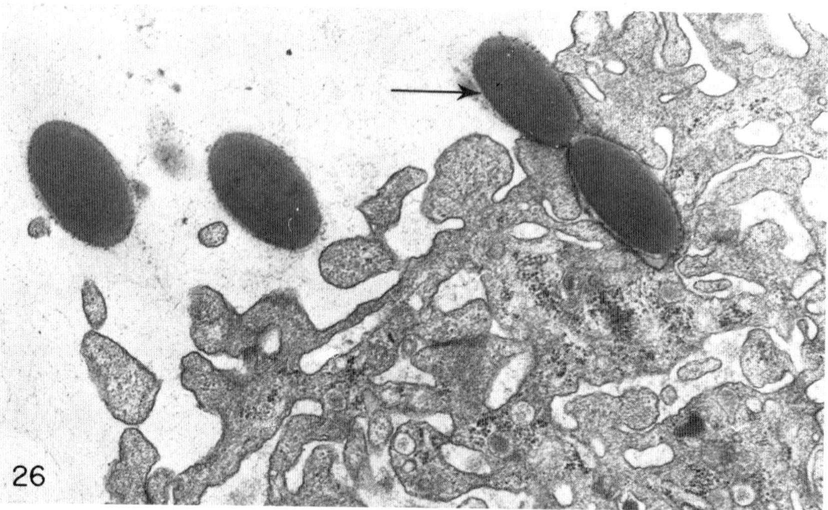

**Fig. 26.** Ultrastructural appearance of guinea pig megakaryocyte in the early phases of uptake of polystyrene latex particles 1.1 $\mu$m in size. Shown is a doublet being taken into the channels of the DMS (arrow). Note that the cell margin is irregular and one of the protrusions has apparently rotated laterally to incorporate the particles into preexisting channels. ×19,500 (reduced 10% for reproduction).

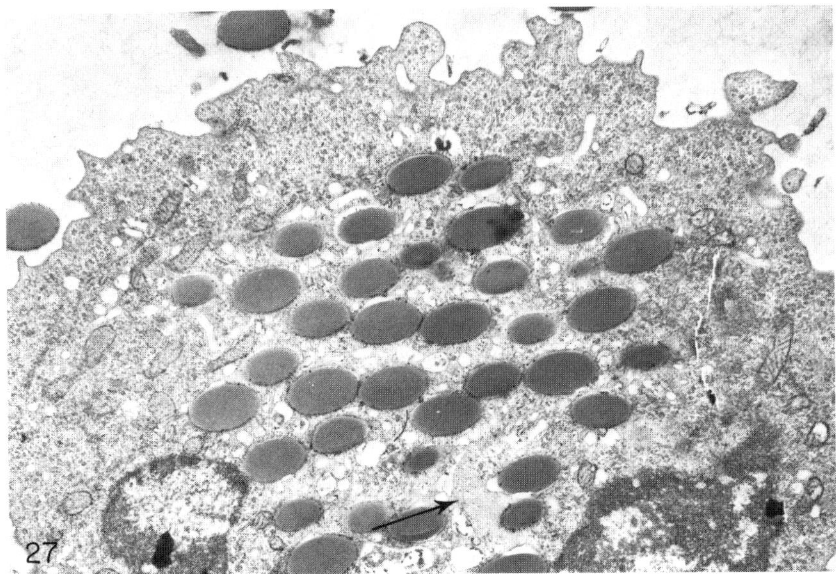

**Fig. 27.** Ultrastructural appearance of guinea pig megakaryocyte which has taken up latex particles into the cytoplasm. Around some particles the areas of the cytoplasm show a zone of filamentous network (arrow). $\times$13,910 (reduced 10% for reproduction).

phages the megakaryocyte is a nonprofessional phagocyte. The function of the C3b receptor is unknown.

When megakaryocytes were exposed to horseradish peroxidase 0.1 mg/ml for 2 hr *in vitro* there was significant uptake of the macromolecule (Fig. 29). Therefore, like many other cell types megakaryocytes possess the ability to pinocytose macromolecules.

### 6.7.3. Effect of Antiplatelet Antiserum on Megakaryocytes

Exposure of megakaryocytes to rabbit antiplatelet antiserum in the presence of complement produced significant cell lysis and release of serotonin.

## 6.8. Thesis We Wish to Develop

There are several morphologic similarities between megakaryocytes and platelets and this is quite understandable owing to the progenitor role

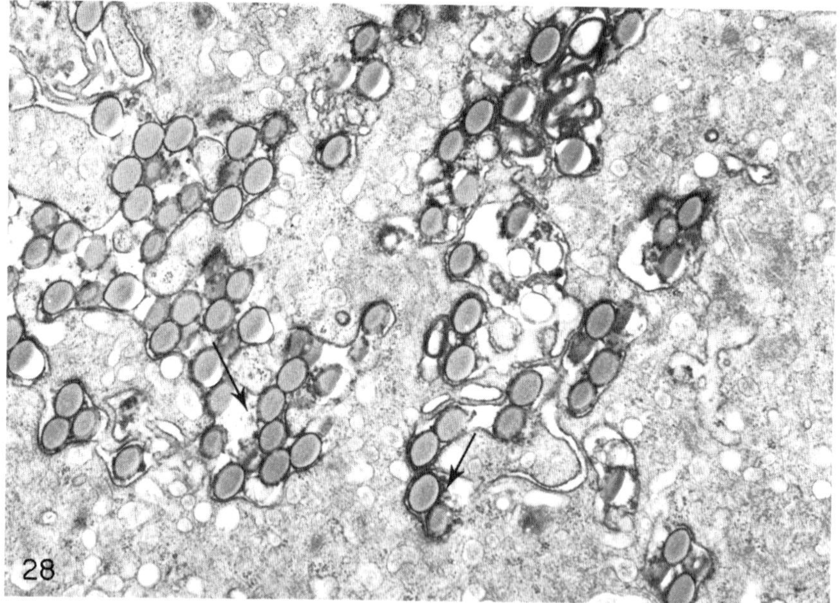

**Fig. 28.** Electron microscopic appearance of isolated guinea pig megakaryocyte which had taken up latex particles and was then exposed to fixative containing tannic acid. Note the electron-dense deposit of a presumed tannic acid–protein complex (arrows) within the open vacuoles. ×17,550 (reduced 10% for reproduction).

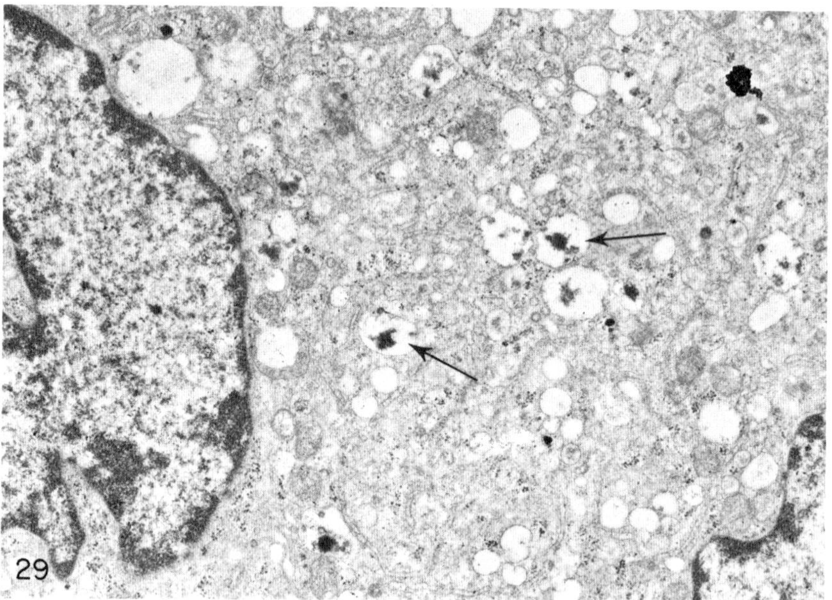

**Fig. 29.** Ultrastructural appearance of guinea pig megakaryocyte which was exposed to 1 mg/ml peroxidase *in vitro*. Shown are vacuoles which contain the electron-dense reaction product of peroxidase (arrows). ×17,550 (reduced 10% for reproduction).

of megakaryocytes. The description of the functional capacity of the megakaryocyte is noteworthy in a major respect. It is demonstrated here that megakaryocytes can take up serotonin, release it under appropriate conditions after exposure to specific platelet-releasing agents, take up particles, and respond to specific antiplatelet antiserum by cell lysis. These functions have been well documented in platelets (Born and Mills, 1969; Hovig, 1974; Mustard and Packham, 1970; White, 1971, 1972, 1974) and it is noteworthy that megakaryocytes possess the same capability.

ACKNOWLEDGMENTS

The author acknowledges the permission of the *Journal of Cell Biology* to reproduce Figs. 1, 2, 9, and 10, and *Laboratory Investigation* to reproduce Figs. 21 through 26, 28, and 29.

The technical assistance of Ms. P. Wiesenthal is also gratefully acknowledged.

# References

Ardlie, N., 1972, Studies on the mechanism of adenosine diphosphate-induced platelet aggregation, Ph.D. Thesis, McMaster University, Hamilton, Ontario xx:1.

Behnke, O., 1968, Electron microscope study of the megacaryocyte of the rat bone marrow, *J. Ultrastruct. Res.* **24**:412.

Behnke, O., 1969, An electron microscope study of the rat megacaryocyte. II. Some aspects of platelet release and microtubules, *J. Ultrastruct. Res.* **26**:111.

Behnke, O., and Emmersen, J., 1972, Structural identification of thrombosthenin in rat megakaryocytes, *Scand. J. Haematol.* **9**:130.

Behnke, O., Kristensen, B., and Nielsen, L., 1971, Electron microscopical observations on actinoid and myosinoid filaments in blood platelets, *J. Ultrastruct. Res.* **37**:351.

Bessis, M., 1956, *Cytology of the Blood and Blood-Forming Organs,* p. 448, Grune & Stratton, New York.

Bettex-Galland, M., and Luscher, E., 1965, Thrombosthenin, the contractile protein from blood platelets and its relation to other contractile proteins, *Adv. Protein Chem.* **20**:1.

Born, G., and Mills, D., 1969, Potentiation of the inhibitory effect of adenosine on platelet aggregation by drugs that prevent its uptake, *J. Physiol. (London)* **202**:41.

Breton-Gorius, J., 1973, Aspects ultrastructuraux de la maturation des mégacaryocytes humains normaux, *Nouv. Rev. Fr. Hematol.* **13**:504.

Caro, L., and Palade, G., 1964, Protein synthesis, storage, and discharge in the pancreatic exocrine cell, *J. Cell Biol.* **20**:473.

Cohn, Z., and Benson, B., 1965, The differentiation of mononuclear phagocytes. Morphology, cytochemistry and biochemistry, *J. Exp. Med.* **121**:153.

de Leval, M., and Paulus, J., 1971, Normal megakaryocyte maturation, *in Platelet Kinetics* (J. Paulus, ed.) p. 183, North-Holland, Amsterdam.

Ebbe, S., 1965, Megakaryocytopoiesis in the rat, *Blood* **26**:20.

Fedorko, M., 1977a, The functional capacity of guinea pig megakaryocytes. I. Uptake of $^3$H-serotonin by megakaryocytes and their physiologic and morphologic response to stimuli for the platelet release reaction, *Lab. Invest.* **36**:310.

Fedorko, M., 1977b, The functional capacity of guinea pig megakaryocytes. II. The uptake of particles and macromolecules and the effect of rabbit antiguinea pig platelet antiserum, *Lab. Invest.* **36**:321.

Fedorko, M., and Hirsch, J., 1966, Cytoplasmic granule formation in myelocytes, *J. Cell Biol.* **29**:307.

Fedorko, M., and Levine, R., 1976, Tannic acid effect on membrane of cell surface origin in guinea pig megakaryocytes and platelets, *J. Histochem. Cytochem.* **24**:601.

Feinendegen, G., Odartchenko, N., Cottier, H., and Bond, V., 1962, Kinetics of megakaryocyte proliferation, *Proc. Soc. Exp. Biol. Med.* **111**:177.

Harwood, R., 1974, Cell separation by gradient centrifugation, *Int. Rev. Cytol.* **38**:369.

Hirsch, J., 1956, Phagocytin: A bactericidal substance from polymorphonuclear leucocytes, *J. Exp. Med.* **103**:589.

Holmsen, H., 1974, Are platelet shape change, aggregation and release reaction tangible manifestations of one basic platelet function? *in Platelets* (M. Baldini and S. Ebbe, eds.), p. 207, Grune & Stratton, New York.

Hovig, T., 1974, The ultrastructural basis of platelet function, *in Platelets* (M. Baldini and S. Ebbe, eds.), p. 221, Grune & Stratton, New York.

Howell, W., 1890, Observations upon the occurrence, structure, and function of the giant cells of the marrow, *J. Morphol.* **4**:117.

Japa, J., 1943, A study of the morphology and development of the megakaryocytes, *Br. J. Exp. Pathol.* **24**:73.

Levine, R., 1976a, *In vitro* culture of isolated guinea pig megakaryocytes (Abstract), *Blood* **46**:1030.

Levine, R., 1976b, Macrotubule-ribosome complexes induced by vincristine, colchicine, and phodophyllotopin (Abstract), *J. Cell Biol.* **70**(pt. 2):210a.

Levine, R., and Fedorko, M., 1976, Isolation of intact megakaryocytes from guinea pig femoral marrow, *J. Cell Biol.* **69**:159.

MacPherson, G., 1972, Origin and development of the demarcation system in megakaryocytes of rat bone marrow, *J. Ultrastruct. Res.* **40**:167.

Mustard, J., and Packham, M., 1970, Factors influencing platelet function: Adhesion, release, and aggregation, *Pharmacol. Rev.* **22**:97.

Nachman, R., Marcus, A., and Safier, L., 1967, Platelet thrombosthenin: Subcellular localization and function, *J. Clin. Invest.* **46**:1380.

Nakeff, A., and Flaek, D., 1976, Separation of megakaryocytes from mouse bone marrow by density gradient centrifugation, *Blood* **48**:133.

Nakeff, A., and Maat, B., 1974, Separation of megakaryocytes from mouse bone marrow by velocity sedimentation, *Blood* **43**:591.

Odell, T., and Jackson, C., 1968, Polyploidy and maturation of megakaryocytes, *Blood* **32**::102.

Odell, T., and Jackson, C., 1970, Megakaryocytopoiesis, *in Hemapoietic Cellular Proliferation* (F. Stohlman, ed.), p. 278, Grune & Stratton, New York.

Pisciotta, A., Stefanini, M., and Dameschek, W., 1953, Studies on platelets. X. Morphologic characteristics of megakaryocytes by phase contrast microscopy in normals and in patients with idiopathic thrombocytopenic purpura, *Blood* **8**:703.

Pretlow, T., Weir, E., and Zellergren, J., 1975, Problems connected with the separation of different kinds of cells, *Int. Rev. Exp. Pathol.* **14**:91.

Rak, K., 1972, Effect of vincristine on platelet production in mice, *Br. J. Haematol.* **22**:617.

Schulz, H., and Schiller, K., 1968, Mikrotubuli and filamente in prospektiven plättachenfeldern der megakaryocyten, *Z. Zellforsch.* **87**:389.

Thiery, J., and Bessis, M., 1956, Mécanisme de la plaquettogenèse étude *in vitro* par la microcinématographie, *Rev. Hematol.* **11**:162.

White, J., 1968, Effects of colchicine and vinca alkaloids on human platelets. II. Changes in the dense tubular system and formation of an unusual inclusion in incubated cells, *Am. J. Pathol.* **53**:447.

White, J., 1971, Platelet morphology, *in The Circulating Platelet* (S. A. Johnson, ed.), p. 45, Academic Press, New York.

White, J., 1972, Uptake of latex particles by blood platelets, *Am. J. Pathol.* **69**:439.

Willingham, M., Spicer, S., and Graber, C., 1971, Immunocytologic labeling of calf and human lymphocyte surface antigens, *Lab. Invest.* **25**:211.

Wilson, L., 1975, Microtubules as drug receptors: Pharmacologic properties of microtubule protein in the biology of cytoplasmic microtubules, *Ann. N.Y. Acad. Sci.* **253**:213.

Wright, J., 1906, The origin and nature of the blood plates, *Boston Med. Surg. J.* **154**:643.

Zucker-Franklin, D., and Grusky, G., 1972, The actin and myosin filaments of human and bovine blood platelets, *J. Clin. Invest.* **51**:419.

# Mechanisms of Heparin Therapy

## Robert D. Rosenberg

## 7.1. Introduction

A variety of substances present in normal blood oppose the action of thrombin and other serine proteases of the hemostatic mechanism. Indeed, early in this century, several investigators recognized that thrombin gradually lost activity when added to defibrinated plasma or serum (Contejean, 1895; Seegers *et al.*, 1964; Morowitz, 1968). On this basis, they suspected that a specific inactivator of this enzyme, antithrombin, must be present in plasma under normal physiological conditions. In 1916 McLean isolated heparin from the liver, as well as the heart, and demonstrated its potent anticoagulant action. Confusion about its inhibitory effects on purified procoagulants was resolved in 1939 by Brinkhous *et al.*, who showed that heparin was effective as an anticoagulant only in the presence of a plasma component which they termed heparin cofactor. In the 1950s the work of Waugh and co-workers (Waugh and Fitzgerald, 1956) and Monkhouse *et al.* (1955) indicated that plasma antithrombin activity and plasma heparin cofactor activity are intimately related. These investigators suggested that heparin acts to accelerate, by 50- to 100-fold, the rate at which antithrombin neutralizes thrombin. In 1968, this

ROBERT D. ROSENBERG  •  Sidney Farber Cancer Institute, Harvard Medical School, Beth Israel Hospital, Boston, Massachusetts.

hypothesis was substantiated by Abildgaard, who obtained small amounts of a purified human plasma protein that functions in both capacities. We subsequently confirmed this observation (Rosenberg and Damus, 1973).

Our own investigations, summarized in the following, provided a detailed mechanistic analysis of the interaction of thrombin with this inhibitor and its mucopolysaccharide cofactor (Rosenberg and Damus, 1973). Our knowledge of the biochemical basis of this event suggested to us that this inhibitory mechanism might possess an extraordinarily broad range of activity. Indeed, we have subsequently demonstrated that antithrombin inactivates virtually all of the serine proteases of the coagulation–fibrinolytic system and that heparin dramatically accelerates the neutralization of each of these enzymes (Rosenberg *et al.*, 1975; Damus *et al.*, 1973; Stead *et al.*, 1976a,b). Furthermore, we have utilized antithrombin's affinity for heparin to fractionate preparations of this mucopolysaccharide. Surprisingly, we have found that only a small portion of the material is responsible for virtually all of the anticoagulant activity (Lam *et al.*, 1976). In this chapter, we shall outline these recent advances and consider their physiologic as well as pharmacologic implications.

## 7.2. The Properties of Human Antithrombin

Human antithrombin can be isolated from plasma in purified form by a variety of procedures which utilize Sephadex G-200 gel filtration, DEAE–Sephadex or DEAE–cellulose fractionation, isoelectric focusing, and affinity chromatography with heparin bound to an insoluble matrix such as Sepharose 4B. The final product is physically homogeneous as judged by various electrophoretic and immunoelectrophoretic techniques (Rosenberg and Damus, 1973, 1976).

To determine that this single protein possesses both antithrombin and heparin cofactor activity, we studied the inactivation of purified human thrombin in the presence and absence of heparin (Fig. 1). If thrombin is added to buffer with or without heparin, no loss in enzymatic activity is noted. If thrombin is incubated for varying periods of time with antithrombin, a slow, progressive decline in the enzyme's activity becomes apparent ("antithrombin effect"). If thrombin is incubated with a mixture of heparin and antithrombin, its enzymatic activity is inhibited almost instantaneously ("heparin cofactor effect"). From the final concentrations of enzyme and inhibitor present in these and other experiments, we can estimate that the equivalence point of this interaction occurs at a 1:1 molar ratio of enzyme to inhibitor. The stoichiometry is similar in the presence or absence of heparin (Rosenberg and Damus, 1973).

To determine whether this inhibitor is responsible for most of the

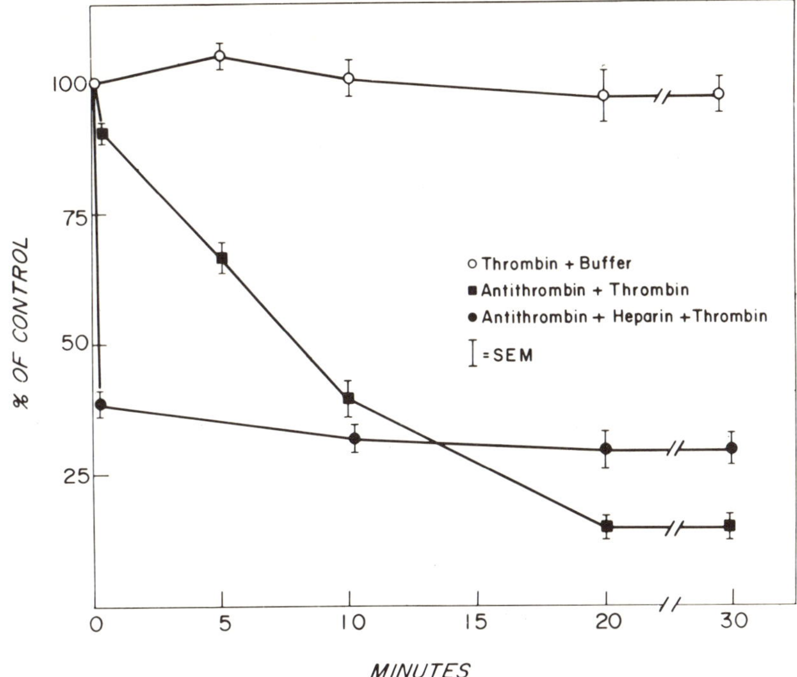


**Fig. 1.** Inhibition of thrombin by antithrombin in the presence and absence of heparin. Final concentration of enzyme and inhibitor was 0.162 and 0.164 absorbance units/ml, respectively. Final concentration of added heparin was 12 units/ml. Esterolytic activity of thrombin was measured with tosyl-L-lysine methyl ester (Cyclo Chemical Company, Los Angeles) by continuously recording uptake of 0.01 M NaOH in a pH stat fitted with automatic buret and chart recorder. Buffer was 0.005 M Tris-HCl in 0.15 M NaCl (pH 8.3). All protein preparations were extensively dialyzed against this assay buffer. Concentration of substrate was 0.015 M, and reaction velocity at $37° \pm 0.1°C$ was recorded for the first 3 min. Plots of thrombin concentration versus reaction velocity were linear, with remarkably constant slope and intercept. (Adapted from Rosenberg and Damus, 1973.)

antithrombin and heparin cofactor activities normally present in plasma, we immunoprecipitated this component from defibrinated plasma and measured the residual activities. Thus a γ-globulin fraction from antisera directed against the inhibitor or a γ-globulin fraction from normal rabbit serum was mixed in ratios of 1:2, 1:1, 2:1, and 3:1 with defibrinated plasma. The mixtures were maintained at 37°C for 1 hr and at 4°C for 16 hr. They were centrifuged and the supernatants were assayed for antithrombin as well as heparin cofactor activities. The data shown in Table I reveal that both activities decline in parallel fashion as the concentration of γ-globulin is increased and that less than 10% of either activity remains at the highest level of added γ-globulin (Rosenberg and Damus, 1973).

**Table I.**  Immunoprecipitation of Antithrombin from Pooled Defibrinated
Human Plasma

|  | Ratio of $\gamma$-globulin directed against the inhibitor to pooled defibrinated human plasma | | | |
|---|---|---|---|---|
|  | 1:2 | 1:1 | 2:1 | 3:1 |
| Antithrombin activity in supernate (%) | 43 | 24 | 23 | 10 |
| Heparin cofactor activity in supernate (%) | 43 | 32 | 24 | 8 |

## 7.3. The Synthesis and Structure of Heparin-like Molecules

Heparin is a mucopolysaccharide of molecular weight 5000–30,000. This natural product is found in a variety of organs including heart, lungs, intestines, etc. The biosynthesis of this component has been studied with cell-free systems derived from transplantable mouse mastocytomas (Lindahl *et al.*, 1977). Initially, the heparin molecule is formed as an alternating copolymer of *N*-acetylglucosamine and glucuronic acid (Silbert *et al.*, 1975). Thereafter, the polymer is modified by a multistep process which takes place to a varying extent within different segments of the polysaccharide chain. Thus heparin, the biosynthetic end product, has a complex primary structure.

This series of postsynthetic modifications can be broadly divided into three major areas (Fig. 2). Within each stage of the process, the pertinent enzyme is presented with a product from the preceding step and only if this macromolecule has the appropriate structure will it be further transformed.

First, glucosamine residues are variably deacetylated and the exposed amino groups serve as acceptors of sulfate residues in a transfer reaction with PAPS. Second, glucuronic acid residues are variably epimerized to iduronic acid. Third, the glucosamine and iduronic acid residues are *O*-sulfated to a major extent.

The ultimate structure of the mucopolysaccharide is depicted in Fig. 3. It is important to note that this represents only one of many possible arrangements of hexosamine and uronic acid residues that exist within the polysaccharide chain of heparin.

The mucopolysaccharide, itself, is coupled to a polypeptide (or polypeptides) via a linkage region which consists of a galactose–galactose–xylose–serine sequence (Lindahl and Roden, 1972). Little is known of the structure of this protein core.

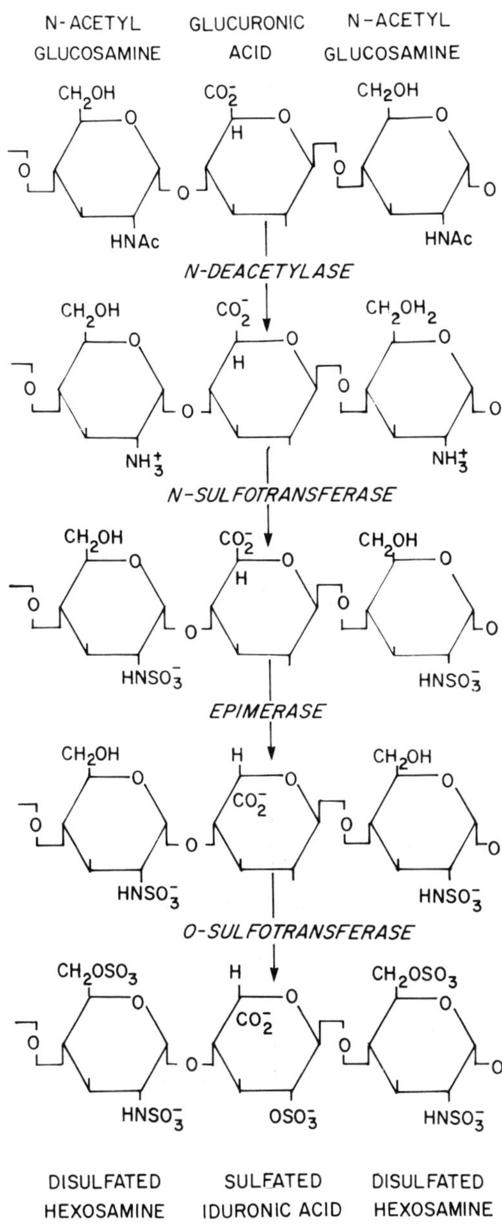



**Fig. 2.** Biosynthesis of heparin.

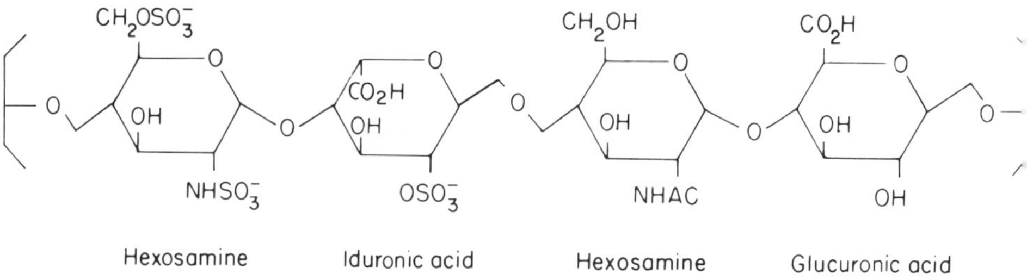

**Fig. 3.** Structure of heparin.

Heparan sulfate, a substance homologous to heparin, is a mucopolysaccharide of molecular weight 50,000–100,000. This macromolecule is present in ubiquitous fashion as a major component of cell surfaces including those of the endothelium and the platelet (Buonassisi, 1973; Horner, 1975). It has been suggested that this substance is also formed as a copolymer of $N$-acetylglucosamine and glucuronic acid. However, at the site of mucopolysaccharide synthesis, low levels of the deacetylase enzyme are present and this results in a high frequency of $N$-acetylglucosamine residues within the polysaccharide chain of heparan sulfate. The preservation of these structures prevents neighboring segments of the macromolecule from continuing through the series of reactions involving $N$-sulfation, uronic acid epimerization, and $O$-sulfation. Thus heparan sulfate differs quantitatively from heparin in that it possesses more $N$-acetyl groups, more glucuronic acid moieties, and fewer $N$- or $O$-sulfated residues. However, current evidence suggests that heparin-like regions exist within the structure of the heparan sulfate molecule. Furthermore, this highly charged macromolecule is coupled to a protein core in a fashion similar to that of heparin.

Considerable effort has been expended in defining the linear sequence, three-dimensional configuration, and biologic behavior of heparin-like macromolecules (Silva and Dietrich, 1975; Taylor *et al.*, 1973; Nieduszynski and Atkins, 1973). It has been widely appreciated that preparations of heparin have potent anticoagulant properties whereas fractions of heparan sulfate exhibit only small amounts of the activity (Teien *et al.*, 1976). Other mucopolysaccharides are unable to act as anticoagulants (Teien *et al.*, 1976). However, the precise relationship between the structure of heparin-like components and their anticoagulant properties remains elusive.

Heparin preparations exhibit considerable polydispersity in molecular size (Laurent, 1961), variations in the ratio of glucuronic acid to iduronic acid (Hovingh and Linker, 1970), alterations in the amount of ester and $N$-sulfation (Danishefsky *et al.*, 1969), as well as differing extents of *N*-acetylation (Ehrlich and Stivala, 1973). Changes in each of these parameters correlate only to a limited degree with heparin's anticoagulant potency. Thus, it has been tacitly assumed that this mucopolysaccharide may exhibit a variety of alternative structures each equally capable of activating antithrombin.

We considered the possibility that heparin preparations were grossly impure and that only a small fraction of the molecules were responsible for its distinctive biologic properties. In this case, attempts to relate the structure of the bulk material to anticoagulant potency would be futile.

Numerous investigators have fractionated heparin preparations by gel filtration, ion exchange chromatography, or electrophoresis without observing any substantial increase in purity (Ehrlich and Stivala, 1973; Cifonelli and King, 1973). Therefore, we decided to utilize a biologic approach to fractionation and attempted to employ specific affinity for antithrombin as the means for obtaining highly active preparations of the mucopolysaccharide (Lam *et al.*, 1976).

Samples containing 100 $\mu$g of antithrombin or 10 $\mu$g of heparin were examined separately by sucrose density gradient centrifugation. As shown in Fig. 4 (upper and middle panels), single, narrow, nonoverlapping peaks of either protein or heparin were observed. When both components were mixed together at the final concentrations and solvent conditions previously employed, two major alterations in the pattern of component distribution were apparent (Fig. 4, lowest panel). First, the profile of the antithrombin concentration revealed a significant degree of polydispersity with large amounts of protein present at high sedimentation velocities (fractions 1–12). In addition, a shift in the sedimentation velocity of the antithrombin peak to a slightly higher value was noted. Second, heparin is no longer present as a discrete peak but is distributed throughout the density gradient. Approximately one-third of this component is located under the antithrombin peak, suggesting that it has been drawn into this region because of strong interactions with the inhibitor. Approximately two-thirds of the heparin is present at its original position in the density gradient and therefore does not appear to be forming a stable complex with antithrombin. This is significant since a two- to threefold molar excess of the inhibitor was present in the original reaction mixture. Thus, heparin bound to the inhibitor might represent an active species while heparin unable to complex with antithrombin could signify a chemically similar but inactive form of the mucopolysaccharide (Lam *et al.*, 1976).

To validate this hypothesis, it was essential to quantitate the anticoagulant activity of each of these heparin species. Thus, fractions were collected either from areas of the density gradient free of protein (fractions 20–28) or from regions in which heparin was bound to antithrombin (fractions 4–18). Heparin fractions unable to bind to antithrombin were

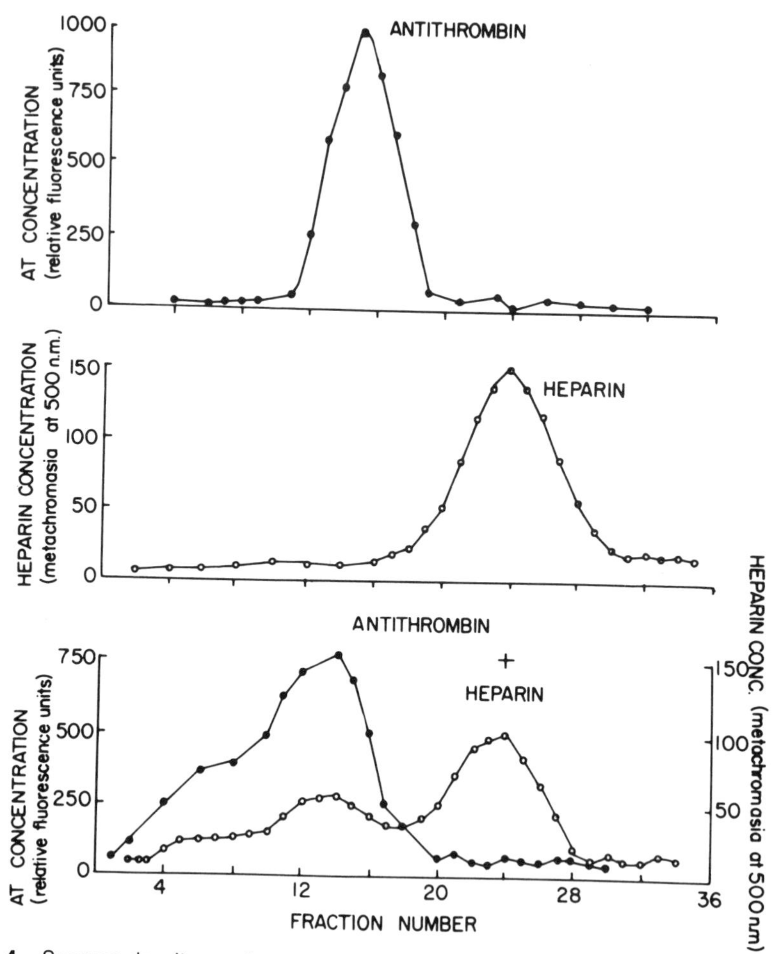



**Fig. 4.** Sucrose density gradient centrifugation of antithrombin and heparin. Heparin and/or antithrombin were utilized at final concentrations of 33.3 and 333 $\mu$m/ml, respectively. Each component had previously been extensively dialyzed against 0.15 M NaCl in 0.01 M sodium phosphate (pH 7.5). Approximately 300 $\mu$l of these solutions was overlayed on 4.7 ml of 10–15% (w/v) sucrose density gradients in which the solvent was 0.15 M NaCl in 0.01 M sodium phosphate (pH 7.5). After centrifugation at 224,000 × $g$ for 20 hr, 4°C, the bottom of each tube was punctured and fractions of ≈ 120 $\mu$l were collected for analyses. AT = antithrombin. (Adapted from Lam *et al.*, 1976.)

assayed for anticoagulant activity as well as mucopolysaccharide content. The average specific activity (anticoagulant activity per milligram of heparin) obtained during three separate experiments was 38 units/mg. Heparin which had bound to antithrombin was freed of protein and analyzed in a similar fashion. The average specific activity of these samples was 367 units/mg. This is considerably higher than the specific activity of the unfractionated heparin (155 units/mg). Fractionation of these two heparin forms was uniquely dependent on the presence of antithrombin. Attempts to duplicate this isolation procedure with bovine serum albumin, a plasma protein similar in size to antithrombin, were unsuccessful. Indeed, heparin does not interact with this plasma component, as judged by sucrose density gradient centrifugation (Lam *et al.*, 1976).

Thus, our data show that the heparin preparation examined consisted of two distinct forms which differ greatly in their ability to bind to and activate antithrombin. The first form constituted approximately two-thirds of the chemical mass of the unfractionated heparin and did not bind to antithrombin under the conditions of these experiments. This fraction was responsible for only about 15% of the total anticoagulant activity of the original material and was termed "relatively inactive" heparin. The relatively low anticoagulant potency appears not to be an intrinsic property of this molecular species. The second form, comprising one-third of the remaining chemical mass of unfractionated heparin, bound tightly to antithrombin, contained approximately 85% of the total anticoagulant activity of the original material, and was termed "active" heparin. The heparin utilized in these studies was indistinguishable from other preparations of the mucopolysaccharide. Indeed, we have recently analyzed heparin obtained from a variety of sources and have obtained virtually identical data. Our results have been confirmed by Lindhal and his co-workers (Hook *et al.*, 1976).

Thus far, no attempt has been made to fractionate heparan sulfate via its affinity for antithrombin. However, trace amounts of material with significant anticoagulant potency may well be hidden within the relatively inactive heparan sulfate bulk species. The structure of this postulated component may be similar to that of the active form of heparin.

At the present time, we have only fragmentary knowledge of the specific features which distinguish the biologically active form from the relatively inactive heparin species. We have ascertained that both species contain the two types of uronic acid as well as glucosamine and that molecular weight is not a critical parameter (Rosenberg and Jordan, 1977). Furthermore, we have demonstrated that the most active form of heparin possesses additional glucuronic acid moieties. An appropriate spacing of these residues in close approximation to iduronic acid groups seems to represent a key structural element responsible for the molecule's anticoagulant potency (Rosenberg *et al.*, 1978).

## 7.4. Heparin's Mechanism of Anticoagulant Action

In order to study the neutralization of thrombin by heparin and its cofactor, reaction mixtures were examined by gel electrophoresis and an enzyme–inhibitor complex was observed (Rosenberg and Damus, 1973). This interaction product was stable after treatment at 100°C with varying combination of denaturing agents. These findings suggested that complex formation could be analyzed by serially denaturing samples and following the molecular weights of the resultant species by sodium dodecyl sulfate gel electrophoresis (Rosenberg and Damus, 1973).

Antithrombin and thrombin migrate as single bands in this electrophoretic system with apparent molecular weights of 62,300 and 33,800, respectively. When these proteins are incubated together, both bands disappear over 5 min as enzyme activity is neutralized and a complex of 88,700 mol. wt. is formed (Fig. 5). If heparin is added to the system, complex formation is virtually instantaneous (Fig. 6). The molecular weight of this complex is identical to the molecular weight obtained in the absence of heparin. These observations demonstrate that antithrombin neutralizes the activity of thrombin by formation of a 1:1 enzyme–inhibitor complex and that heparin acts by dramatically accelerating the rate of formation of the complex (Rosenberg and Damus, 1973).

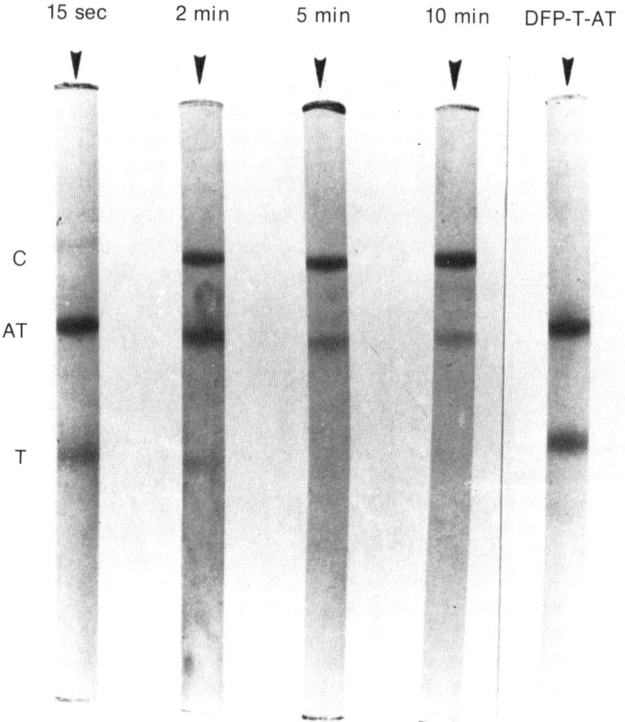


**Fig. 5.** SDS-acrylamide gel electrophoretic analysis of thrombin–antithrombin and DFP-treated thrombin–antithrombin interactions. C, Complex; AT, antithrombin; T, thrombin. (Adapted from Rosenberg and Damus, 1973.)

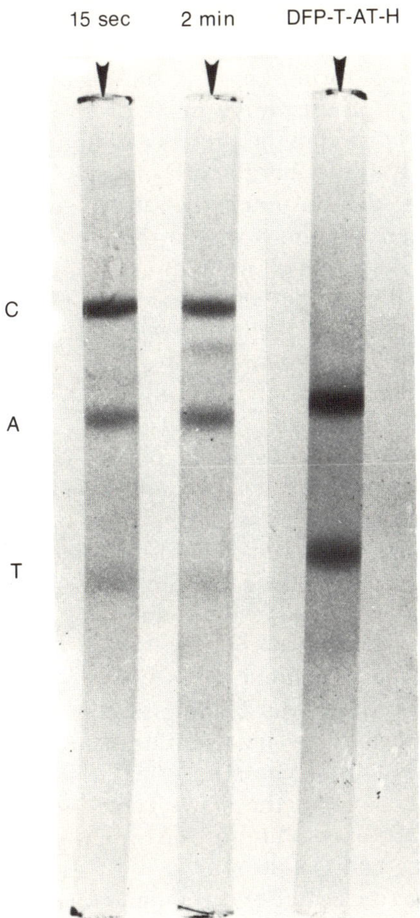


**Fig. 6.** SDS-acrylamide gel electrophoretic analysis of thrombin–antithrombin–heparin and DFP-treated thrombin–antithrombin–heparin interactions. C, Complex; AT, antithrombin; T, thrombin. (Adapted from Rosenberg and Damus, 1973.)

In a highly specific fashion, diisopropylphorofluoridate (DFP) allyl-phosphorylates a unique serine residue in thrombin. This moiety, in concert with several other amino acid residues in its immediate neighborhood, is responsible for the ability of thrombin to scission peptide bonds. Using the native enzyme and this specific modification, we have shown that the active center serine of thrombin is necessary for interaction with antithrombin in the presence or absence of heparin (Rosenberg and Damus, 1973).

First, thrombin's active serine center is essential for the formation of a remarkably stable enzyme–inhibitor complex. Mixtures of thrombin and inhibitor as well as DIP–thrombin (DFP-treated thrombin) and inhibitor were examined by sodium dodecyl sulfate gel electrophoresis. As expected, the inhibitor forms an undissociable complex with native enzyme. No interaction product was observed with DFP-treated protease. Similar results were obtained in the presence of optimal concentrations of heparin (Figs. 5 and 6) (Rosenberg and Damus, 1973).

Second, we have demonstrated that modified thrombin does not compete with native enzyme for a site on the inhibitor. In these experiments, after the DIP–thrombin was admixed with the antithrombin, native enzyme was added. Whether the activity of the native enzyme is preserved depends on the competition between DIP–thrombin and native thrombin for inhibitor. In the presence and absence of heparin, we established that less than 25% of the DIP–thrombin binds to the inhibitor site occupied by the native enzyme. Therefore, residues other than those constituting the enzyme's active center probably are of minimal importance in initiating the customary enzyme–inhibitor complex (Rosenberg and Damus, 1973).

Third, it was shown that interaction of the inhibitor with thrombin is greatly reduced if the active serine residue is blocked. To this end, the inhibitor was filtered, with and without heparin, through columns of thrombin–Sepharose, DIP–thrombin–Sepharose, and ethanolamine–Sepharose. Whereas the inhibitor is almost completely adsorbed by the thrombin–Sepharose column, the binding of this protein to the DIP–thrombin–Sepharose column is equivalent to that observed with the control ethanolamine–Sepharose column. Thus, with three independent methods, we have shown that the active center serine of thrombin is required for its interaction with antithrombin in the presence or absence of heparin (Rosenberg and Damus, 1973).

Since the active serine center of thrombin is known to have a remarkably narrow specificity for unique arginine–X bonds, we suspected that antithrombin utilized this residue as a reactive site. Therefore, we treated the inhibitor with 1,2-cyclohexanedione in order to modify arginine residues and were able to demonstrate an almost complete destruction of heparin cofactor as well as antithrombin activity. The apparent specificity of this chemical modification was shown by amino acid analysis, which indicated that 21% of the inhibitor's arginine residues had been altered. However, the absorbance spectrum of the modified inhibitor suggested that some lysine modification may also have occurred (Rosenberg and Damus, 1973).

The minor degree of lysine modification induced by 1,2-cyclohexanedione has been shown to have minimal effect on the activity of protease inhibitors with lysine–x reactive sites. But antithrombin is unlike all other protease inhibitors, since heparin dramatically accelerates its action. In view of the acidic nature of heparin, it seems likely that lysine residues of the antithrombin might function as a binding site for this highly charged species. Thus, alteration of lysine residues might be expected to affect the activity of the inhibitor independently of reactive site modification (Rosenberg and Damus, 1973).

Indeed, treatment of the inhibitor with $O$-methylisourea virtually abolishes heparin cofactor activity with only a minimal effect upon antithrombin activity. Under the conditions utilized, this chemical has been shown to guanidinate the $\epsilon$-amino groups of lysine. Amino acid analysis confirmed the specificity of this modification and demonstrated that 63% of the inhibitor's lysyl groups had been guanidinated (Rosenberg and Damus, 1973).

The physical interaction of heparin with guanidinated inhibitor was examined in order to determine whether a loss of heparin cofactor activity was due to a reduced ability of the modified protein to bind the mucopolysaccharide. Both native and modified inhibitor were mixed with heparin–Sepharose, the solutions were centrifuged, and the amount of inhibitor present in the supernatant was determined by immunological techniques. Under conditions in which 63% of the native inhibitor adsorbed to this matrix, no significant amount of the guanidinated inhibitor was bound (Rosenberg and Damus, 1973).

Of course, one might question whether guanidinated $\epsilon$-amino lysyl groups are at the binding site and are thus directly involved in the interaction with heparin, or whether the inhibition of heparin binding results from the modification of $\epsilon$-amino lysyl groups located elsewhere in the molecule with a resultant change in the conformation of the inhibitor. Since the guanidinated inhibitor loses little, if any, antithrombin activity, and can still form a stable complex with thrombin, a major conformational alteration seems unlikely. But in an attempt to determine whether heparin binds directly to lysine residues, a 100-fold molar excess of heparin was mixed with inhibitor and the solution was subsequently exposed to 0.3 M $O$-methylisourea for 62 hr. Approximately 65% of the inhibitor's heparin cofactor function was protected against activity loss. The protection afforded by heparin against inactivation by $O$-methylisourea suggests that lysyl groups on the inhibitor are directly involved in heparin binding (Rosenberg and Damus, 1973).

Since the guanidinated inhibitor retains its antithrombin activity, modification of reactive site arginine residue(s) by 1,2-cyclohexanedione seems certain. However, the inhibition of heparin cofactor activity by this agent might be ascribed to altered lysine residues of the heparin binding site. As indicated earlier heparin can protect this binding site against lysine modification for up to 62 hr under the appropriate conditions. Utilizing the protective effects of heparin under identical solvent conditions, we have studied the inactivation of the inhibitor by 2,3-butanedione, an alternate reagent of specificity identical with 1,2-cyclohexanedione, and were able to show that heparin cofactor activity virtually disappeared within 6 hr. Therefore, arginine residues are of critical importance for heparin cofactor function. This conclusion is strengthened by the known specificity of the thrombin active site for arginine–X bonds as well as by the demonstration that this active site is required for the formation of a protease–protease inhibitor complex in the presence of heparin (Rosenberg and Damus, 1973).

Whether one or more arginine residues are necessary for inhibitor function and whether the same residues are critical for both antithrombin and heparin cofactor activity remain to be determined. However, in a fashion analogous to other protease inhibitors, we suspect that a unique arginine residue forms the reactive site of antithrombin. Furthermore, we believe that the simplest and most attractive hypothesis of inhibitor function would require this reactive site to be employed for both antithrombin and heparin cofactor action.

We have been able to further analyze the interactions of low-molecular-weight forms of heparin with antithrombin by utilizing "highly active" and "relatively inactive" forms of the mucopolysaccharide. The two species differed in their anticoagulant activity by $\approx 100$-fold but exhibited virtually identical molecular weights of $\approx 6000$. These components had been isolated from heparin preparations by affinity techniques similar to those outlined in the section on mucopolysaccharide structure.*

We have examined the binding of these two heparin forms to antithrombin. Initially, we employed isotopically labeled heparins and have been able to demonstrate that the stoichiometry of the mucopolysaccharide antithrombin interaction is 1:1. Subsequently, we noted that binding of either heparin form to antithrombin resulted in an enhancement of the protein's intrinsic fluorescence at 330 nm. This optical phenomenon was employed to obtain equilibrium constants for the interaction of antithrombin with the "highly active" and "relatively inactive" heparin forms of $8 \times 10^{-8}$ and approximately $10^{-5}$, respectively. In the case of "highly active" heparin, plots of bound heparin/free heparin versus the free heparin concentration (Scatchard plot) were linear with correlation coefficients that averaged .99. Thus the binding of heparin to antithrombin can be described as a simple 1:1 molecular interaction. Furthermore, the anticoagulant potency of heparin species correlates to some degree with their ability to bind to antithrombin (Rosenberg and Jordan, 1977).

We have also studied the neutralization of thrombin by antithrombin in the presence and absence of the "highly active" form of heparin. Dilute reaction mixtures were utilized so that the rapid rate of enzyme inactivation could be slowed to permit monitoring of this interaction with standard manual techniques. The radioactive substrate benzoyl arginine ethyl

---

*In a communication soon to be published, we demonstrate that the "active" material can itself be subdivided into several different forms, the most active of which is termed "highly active" heparin.

ester was employed to assay the resultant low concentrations of enzyme. When thrombin and antithrombin were mixed at final concentrations of $1.0 \times 10^{-7}$ and $1.0 \times 10^{-7}$ M, respectively, only $\approx 15\%$ loss of enzymatic activity was observed over the ensuing 10 min. If the "highly active" form of heparin is added to the reaction mixture at a final concentration of $5 \times 10^{-9}$ M, the rate of enzyme neutralization increases dramatically. Indeed, inactivation of thrombin is complete after 1.5 min of incubation. Further increase in the concentration of added heparin results in a more rapid neutralization of enzyme. When the level of added heparin is $2 \times 10^{-8}$ or greater, the rate of inactivation becomes too rapid to monitor, unless the levels of thrombin and antithrombin are decreased significantly (Rosenberg and Jordan, 1977).

Thus, the "highly active" form of heparin acts as a catalyst in this reaction. Relatively small amounts of this mucopolysaccharide are able to accelerate dramatically the interaction of considerably larger amounts of thrombin and antithrombin (Rosenberg and Jordan, 1977). The ability of heparin to function in this fashion might be explicable if it were to be displaced from the protease inhibitor during formation of the thrombin–antithrombin complex. Then, the mucopolysaccharide would be available to bind to free inhibitor and cyclically promote subsequent rounds of thrombin–antithrombin interactions.

To partially establish the validity of this mechanism, we have sought direct evidence for this displacement of mucopolysaccharide. This has been accomplished by utilizing isotopically labeled heparin in conjunction with a technique for separating free mucopolysaccharide from mucopolysaccharide bound to inhibitor. The addition of thrombin to the preformed heparin–antithrombin complex results in the release of mucopolysaccharide. The displacement of heparin is proportional to the amount of thrombin added. Complete liberation of mucopolysaccharide occurs when the molar concentration of added thrombin is equal to the molar concentration of the heparin–antithrombin complex (Rosenberg and Jordan, 1977).

On the basis of these data, it would appear that antithrombin neutralizes the activity of thrombin by complex formation via a reactive site (arginine)–active center (serine) interaction. If small amounts of heparin were added to the system, it would preferentially bind to the lysyl residues on antithrombin. The resulting heparin–antithrombin complex rapidly inactivates thrombin. This is most probably due to a heparin-dependent conformational alteration of the inhibitor which renders the reactive site arginine more accessible to the active serine center of thrombin. Once thrombin–antithrombin complex formation has occurred, heparin is released and is again available for binding to free inhibitor. Thus the mucopolysaccharide is capable of catalyzing numerous subsequent rounds of thrombin–antithrombin complex formation (Fig. 7).

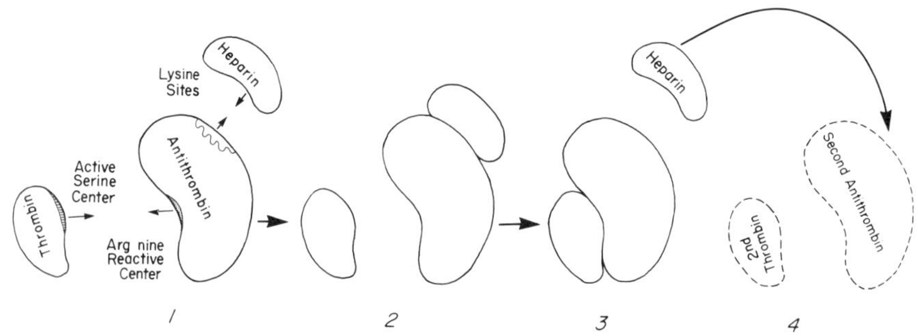



**Fig. 7.**  Mechanism of heparin action.

## 7.5. The General Nature of Heparin's Anticoagulant Action

The formation of thrombin is the end result of either of two pathways of sequential reactions in which minute quantities of abundant plasma zymogens are converted into their active serine protease counterparts (Davie and Ratnoff, 1964; Nemerson and Pitlick, 1972; Gladner and Laki, 1958). Within the first pathway, injury to the endothelial cell layer exposes collagen or other subintimal components that facilitate the conversion of factor XII to factor XIIa. In concert with this transformation, prekallikrein is converted to an active protease, kallikrein. This latter enzyme appears to be capable of accelerating the production of factor XIIa from its precursor zymogen. Factor XIIa subsequently converts factor XI to factor XIa with the help of a cofactor, high-molecular-weight kininogen. Factor XIa, in turn, proteolyzes factor IX to form factor IXa. Factor IXa together with a cofactor (factor VIII) and a lipid surface (platelets) converts factor X to its active species (factor Xa). Within the second pathway, subtle alterations in the endothelium expose tissue factor, which activates factor VII. This molecular species can also catalyze the formation of factor Xa from its precursor zymogen. Once factor Xa has been generated, the presence of platelets and another cofactor (factor V) ensures a very rapid conversion of prothrombin to thrombin. Finally, thrombin proteolyzes fibrinogen to yield fibrin which polymerizes to form the clot. This resultant fibrin meshwork is cross-linked via transpeptidation reactions.

There is excellent evidence that activation of coagulation system zymogens can occur in two ways. On the one hand, prekallikrein, factor XI, factor IX, factor X, and prothrombin are transformed to potent enzymatic species (serine proteases) by scission of peptide bonds (Colman *et al.*, 1971; Davie *et al.*, 1975; Blomback *et al.*, 1967). On the other hand, factor VII appears to be converted to its active form by a conformation-dependent transition which exposes appropriate secondary binding sites or a serine active center, or both (Nemerson, 1976). Factor XII may be activated in either fashion. Thus, collagen can induce a conformational change in this protein which results in a dramatically increased procoagulant activity, and kallikrein, trypsin, etc., may cleave the precursor zymogen to produce activated enzymatic forms of factor XII (Cochrane *et al.*, 1973).

Clot dissolution is achieved, in part, through the fibrinolytic mechanism. During this process a cascade of proteolytic reactions initiated by factor XIIa as well as tissue enzyme culminates in the conversion of plasminogen to plasmin. This enzyme is able to hydrolyze fibrin and thus resolve the clot. This function of plasmin is known to depend on the serine active center of the protein (Summaria *et al.*, 1967).

Since we had demonstrated that the thrombin–antithrombin complex occurs via an arginine–serine interaction, it seemed reasonable to us that this inhibitor would neutralize all serine proteases of the coagulation–fibrinolytic system in a similar fashion. We were particularly encouraged in this belief since other investigators utilizing coagulation assays had shown that the activity of factor Xa was neutralized by antithrombin and that this inactivation occurred far more rapidly in the presence of heparin (Biggs *et al.*, 1970; Seegers *et al.*, 1964; Yin *et al.*, 1971). We repeated these experiments with purified human factor Xa and antithrombin. Our data demonstrated that, as in the case of thrombin, the inhibition of factor Xa activity is due to 1:1 complex formation between enzyme and inhibitor. Heparin dramatically accelerates the rate of this complex formation but does not alter the reaction stoichiometry (Harpel and Rosenberg, 1976).

Thus we predicted that coagulation factors IXa, XIa, and XIIa, as well as plasmin would be neutralized by antithrombin in a similar yet heretofore unsuspected fashion (Rosenberg *et al.*, 1975; Damus *et al.*, 1973; Stead *et al.*, 1976b; Highsmith and Rosenberg, 1974). To this end we isolated human factor IXa in an electrophoretically homogeneous form and examined its interaction with antithrombin in the presence and absence of heparin (Rosenberg *et al.*, 1975). To demonstrate that factor IXa activity is inactivated by antithrombin, we mixed the enzyme and inhibitor and assayed the resulting solution sequentially. A time-dependent decay of factor IXa activity was observed with only 43% of the original activity remaining after 30 min of incubation with the inhibitor. No significant reduction of activity was observed when buffer was substituted for the antithrombin. To show that heparin accelerated the factor IXa–antithrombin interaction, the inhibitor was incubated with the mucopolysaccharide before adding the enzyme, and the resulting solution was immediately assayed. However, the presence of heparin required a modification of the standard procedure for quantitation of factor IXa activity. The measurement of this enzyme's proteolytic activity is completely dependent on the extent to which factor IXa can trigger terminal zymogen–serine protease transitions of the coagulation cascade. Heparin inhibits these events instantaneously via its interaction with antithrombin. Therefore, a valid determination of factor IXa activity requires that this mucopolysaccharide be neutralized before assay. This was accomplished by adding protamine sulfate to incubation mixtures before the factor IXa activity of these solutions was quantitated. Utilizing this assay technique, heparin-dependent neutralization of factor IXa by antithrombin was observed to be virtually instantaneous. Furthermore, the interaction of enzyme and inhibitor was also directly monitored by sodium dodecyl sulfate gel electrophoresis. In this system antithrombin and factor IXa migrated as single components with apparent molecular weights of 65,500 ± 200 and 40,000 ± 100, respectively. When these proteins were incubated together, the enzyme band gradually disappeared while the inhibitor band significantly decreased in intensity. Simultaneously, a new species emerged, with an apparent molecular weight of 89,700 ± 300 (Fig. 7). The interaction of antithrombin and factor IXa was also studied in the presence of heparin (2.16 units/ml). The protein concentrations, conditions of incubation, and analytic methods were identical with those described above. Gel 5 of Fig. 8 reveals that formation of the new molecular species was complete within 15 sec. The apparent molecular weight of this component was identical to that obtained in the absence of heparin. This new species represents a 1:1 stoichiometric complex of enzyme and inhibitor. Thus heparin dramatically accelerates the rate of formation of the factor IXa–antithrombin complex without affecting its stoichiometry (Fig. 8) (Rosenberg *et al.*, 1975).

To ascertain whether antithrombin inactivates factor XIa, we incubated antithrombin with partially purified human factor XIa and sequentially measured residual factor XIa activity as a function of time. As shown in Fig. 8, factor XIa activity declines progressively. However, no significant reduction of this activity is observed when buffer is substituted for antithrombin. To test whether heparin accelerates the interaction between factor XIa and antithrombin, we utilized DEAE–cellulose in order to remove heparin and antithrombin–heparin complexes from the incubation mixtures prior to assay of factor XIa activity. Thus antithrombin, heparin, and factor XIa were incubated together for 1, 3, or 5 min, and DEAE–cellulose was subsequently added. The solutions were centrifuged for 30 sec to remove the chromatographic matrix as well as bound heparin and the respective supernatants were assayed. Factor XIa activity was found to be virtually absent from all incubation mixtures (Fig. 9) (Damus *et al.*, 1973).

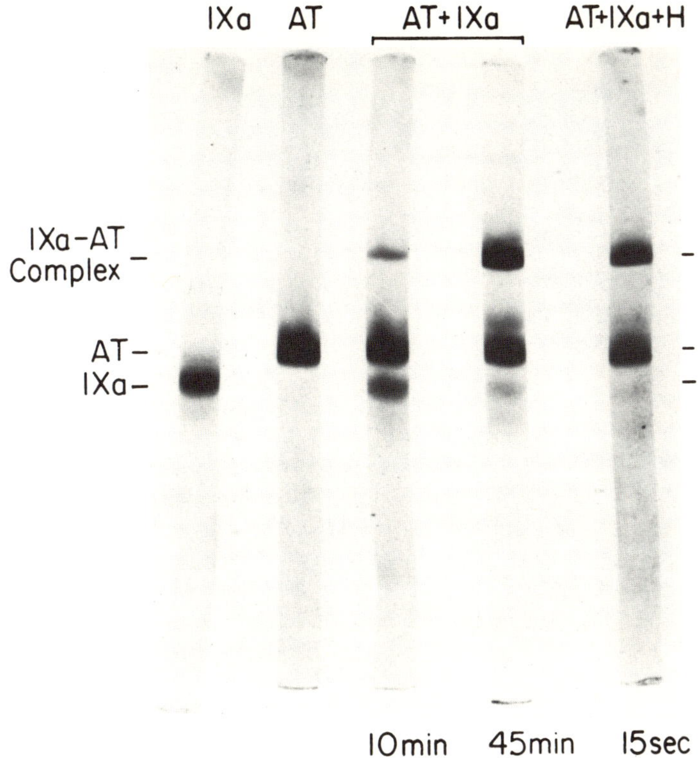



**Fig. 8.** Sodium dodecyl sulfate gel electrophoretic analysis of human factor IXa–human antithrombin interactions in the presence and absence of heparin. At the time indicated, aliquots were removed, denatured in the absence of reducing agents, and examined by the SDS gel electrophoresis. Gel 1 represents factor IXa (IXa); gel 2 shows antithrombin (AT); gels 3 and 4 depict the interaction of enzyme and inhibitor after 10 and 45 min of incubation, respectively; gel 5 reveals the extent of this interaction after 15 sec of incubation in the presence of heparin (H). (Adapted from Rosenberg, *et al.*, 1975.)

The activation of factor XII occurs via fragmentation of this zymogen into a diverse spectrum of enzymatically potent species with molecular weights varying from 28,000 to 80,000 (Kaplan and Austen, 1971; Bagdasarian *et al.*, 1973; Revak *et al.*, 1974). We purified human factor XII by a variety of column chromatographic techniques. The final product was homogeneous as judged by standard electrophoretic methods (Stead *et al.*, 1976a,b). Subsequently, this preparation was incubated with trace quantities of proteolytic enzymes, which resulted in the generation of enzymatically potent fragments of molecular weight 28,000 (factor XIIa$_{\text{LMW}}$). Alternatively, the zymogen was permitted to surface activate

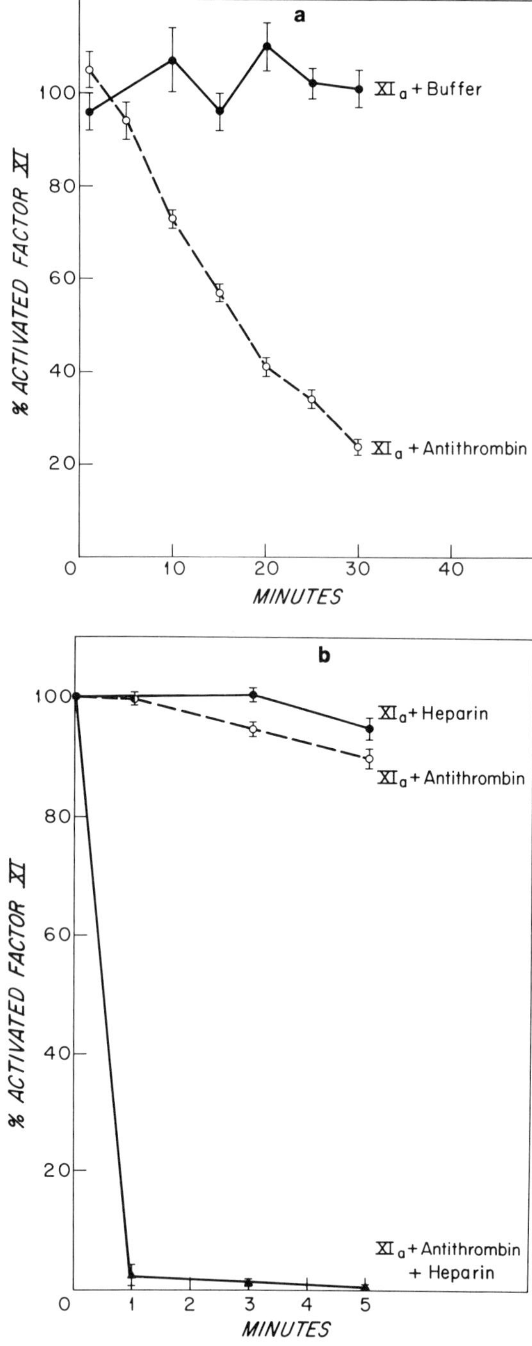



**Fig. 9.** (a) Inhibition of factor XIa by antithrombin. Factor XIa was incubated with buffer or antithrombin. —●— Factor XIa + buffer; —○— factor XIa + antithrombin. (b) Inhibition of factor XIa by antithrombin and heparin. —○— Factor XIa + heparin; —●— factor XIa + antithrombin; —▲— factor XIa + heparin + antithrombin. (Adapted from Damus *et al.,* 1973.)

which yielded an enzymatically potent fragment of molecular weight 75,000 (factor XIIa$_{HMW}$). Fragments generated by either method of activation exhibited procoagulant factor XIIa activity as well as kinin-generating activity. The large fragment was homogeneous by sodium dodecyl sulfate gel electrophoresis as well as by disc gel electrophoresis. The small fragments were homogeneous by sodium dodecyl sulfate gel electrophoresis, but showed microheterogeneity upon disc gel electrophoretic analysis (Stead *et al.*, 1976a,b).

When either the large or the small fragments of factor XIIa were incubated with autithrombin, a slow progressive decline in both procoagulant as well as the kinin-generating activity was noted. In the presence of heparin, the neutralization of both activities was virtually instantaneous. Since heparin does not affect the measurement of kinin generation, the mucopolysaccharide was not removed from incubation mixtures before bioassay. However, since it was important to eliminate the mucopolysaccharide from the incubation mixtures before quantitating factor XIIa procoagulant activity, we used a combination of the methods previously utilized to study the inactivation of factor IXa and factor XIa (see earlier).

The interactions of these two forms of factor XIIa with antithrombin in the presence and absence of heparin were also examined by sodium dodecyl sulfate gel electrophoresis. Factor XIIa$_{LMW}$ stains poorly in this electrophoretic system. Therefore we utilized $^{125}$I-labeled factor XIIa$_{LMW}$ to facilitate the analysis of enzyme–inhibitor interactions. Antithrombin and factor XIIa$_{LMW}$ migrate as single components with apparent molecular weights of $58,000 \pm 2000$ (stained gel) and $28,000 \pm 1500$, respectively. When these proteins are incubated together, the isotopically labeled band gradually waned, exhibiting a 50% reduction after 15 min. Simultaneously, a new component is evident with an apparent molecular weight of $85,000 \pm 3000$ (Fig. 10, upper panel). The interaction of antithrombin and factor XIIa$_{LMW}$ has also been studied in the presence of heparin (10 units/ml). The protein concentrations, conditions of incubation, and analytic methods were identical to those described earlier. The lower panel of Fig. 10 reveals that complex formation was complete within 30 sec. The apparent molecular weight of this complex was identical to that obtained in the absence of heparin (Stead *et al.*, 1976a,b).

Thus in the absence of heparin, factor XIIa$_{LMW}$ is progressively inactivated by complex formation with antithrombin. The apparent molecular weight of this interaction product suggested that it represents a 1:1 stoichiometric complex of the two reactants. In the presence of heparin, the formation of this complex was instantaneous. However, no change in the 1:1 stoichiometry of the reaction was noted. Identical results were obtained when factor XIIa$_{HMW}$ was analyzed. The two forms of factor XIIa utilized in this study differ greatly in their characteristics and enzymatic potencies. Therefore it is reasonable to assume that other

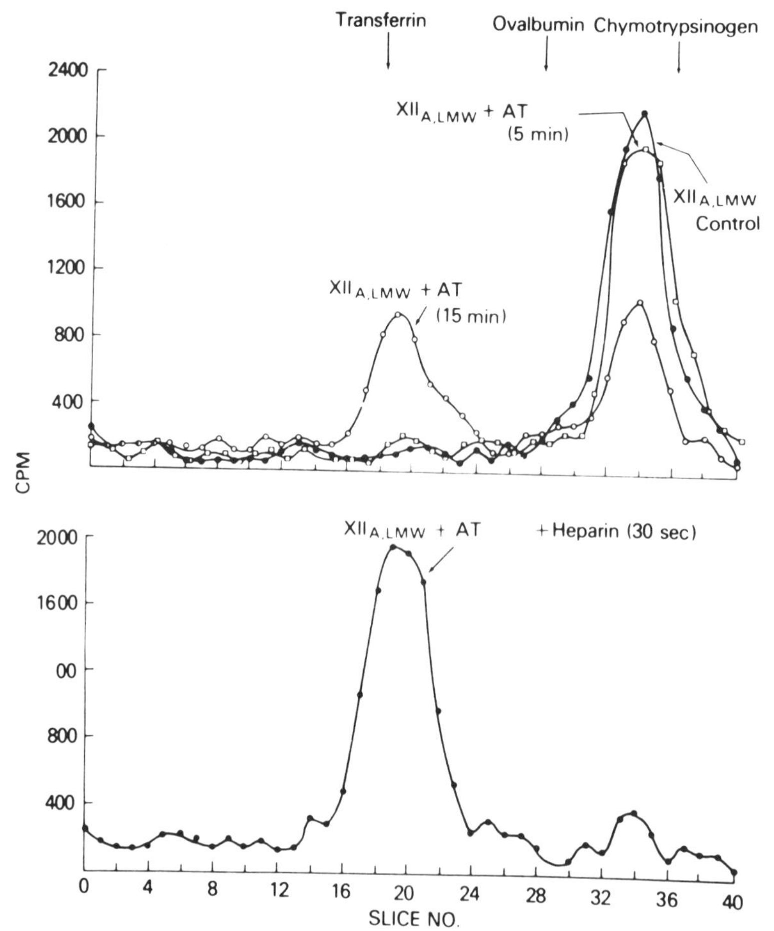


**Fig. 10.** Reduced SDS gel electrophoretic analysis of factor XIIa$_{LMW}$–antithrombin interactions in the presence and absence of heparin. Factor XIIa$_{LMW}$ radiolabeled with $^{125}$I was mixed with buffer, antithrombin, or heparin and antithrombin for varying periods of time prior to electrophoretic analysis. After completion of the separation, gels were sliced into 1.2-mm segments and counted for $^{125}$I. The direction of protein migration is from right (cathode) to left (anode). (Adapted from Stead *et al.*, 1976b.)

serine protease types derived from this zymogen will be inactivated by antithrombin and heparin in similar fashion (Stead *et al.*, 1976a,b).

Therefore, factors XIIa, XIa, Xa, and IXa and thrombin are slowly but progressively inactivated by antithrombin in the absence of heparin and virtually instantaneously neutralized by the inhibitor in the presence of this mucopolysaccharide. These observations have recently been confirmed by a variety of laboratories (Kurachi *et al.*, 1976; Chan *et al.*, 1977;

Summaria *et al.*, 1977). The only possible exception to this generalized mechanism of heparin action is factor VIIa. Preliminary, but inconclusive, reports from other laboratories suggest that interaction of factor VIIa (factor VII–tissue factor complex) and antithrombin is minimal in the presence or absence of heparin (Godal *et al.*, 1974). This may be due to the conformation-dependent activation of this zymogen rather than the generation of a discrete serine protease via peptide bond scission.

As a logical extension of this pattern of inhibitor specificity, we have also attempted to determine whether serine proteases, generated in systems separate from but linked to the hemostatic mechanism, would be neutralized in an analogous manner. As examples of these studies, we shall consider the interactions of this inhibitor and its acidic mucopolysaccharide cofactor with the fibrinolytic system, the kinin-generating mechanism, and a critical serine protease bound to the surface of the macrophage.

Plasmin is the enzyme end product of the fibrinolytic system. To study the interaction of antithrombin with this serine protease, we isolated its zymogen from human plasma and activated this component to plasmin by the addition of small quantities of urokinase. When antithrombin was incubated with plasmin for 15–30 min, 90–100% of the enzyme was inactivated. Furthermore, the presence of heparin dramatically accelerated the rate of this inactivation of plasmin by antithrombin with nearly complete inhibition occurring within 30 sec of incubation. Sodium dodecyl sulfate gel electrophoresis has also been used to monitor this enzyme–inhibitor interaction. These studies have revealed that antithrombin functions as a potent antiplasmin by forming an undissociable complex that is stable in the presence of denaturing or reducing agents, or both. The molecular weight of this complex when compared with that of the enzyme and inhibitor indicates a 1:1 stoichiometric combination of plasmin and antithrombin. Heparin dramatically increases the rate of formation of this complex without affecting the dissociability or stoichiometry (Highsmith and Rosenberg, 1974). Several other inhibitors of plasmin activity are known to exist in the blood. Indeed $\alpha_2$-macroglobulin was for many years believed to be the most potent inactivator of plasmin. In a collaborative effort with the laboratory of Dr. P. Harpel, we have demonstrated that antithrombin in the presence of heparin neutralizes the activity of plasmin slightly faster than $\alpha_2$-macroglobulin. However, a new inhibitor has recently been isolated (Moroi and Aoki, 1976). It appears to be the most rapidly acting plasmin inactivator and therefore the principal physiologic antagonist of the fibrinolytic system. These new observations suggest that heparin-activated antithrombin will be unable to compete effectively for plasmin until $\alpha_2$-antiplasmin is consumed.

The interaction of antithrombin and heparin with purified human kallikrein has also been investigated. The enzymatic potency of kallikrein can be quantitated either by measuring its esterolytic activity with the small-molecular-weight substrate TAMe or by determining bradykinin release from kininogen by a radioimmunoassay. With both assay techniques, one can demonstrate that in the absence of heparin, antithrombin slowly neutralizes the activity of human kallikrein. In the presence of heparin, the inhibitory process is accelerated only 1.5- to 2-fold (Rosenberg *et al.*, 1976). This is a unique example of an interaction in which a serine protease is neutralized by antithrombin, but where heparin does not dramatically accelerate complex formation. It would appear that additional specificity is required on the part of a serine protease if heparin is to catalyze its instantaneous inactivation by this inhibitor.

Antithrombin may be an important modulator of serine proteases present on cell surfaces. In collaboration with H. Remold we have shown that antithrombin is capable of greatly increasing the potency of macrophage inhibitory factor (MIF) by neutralizing the activity of a unique serine protease bound to the macrophage surface. However, if heparin is added to this system, the inactivation of the enzyme by antithrombin is prevented (Remold and Rosenberg, 1975). This phenomenon appears to be due to the electrostatic repulsion of the highly negatively charged heparin–antithrombin complex from the similarly charged macrophage surface. It may explain the known effects of heparin on delayed hypersensitivity reactions.

## 7.6. Pharmacologic Implications

### 7.6.1. Possible Side Effects of Commercial Preparations of Heparin

As we have noted in preceding sections of this chapter, heparin preparations currently in clinical usage are quite heterogeneous. Indeed, only 20–30% of the bulk mucopolysaccharide has any appreciable ability to bind to and activate antithrombin.

The "inactive" mucopolysaccharide species present in all heparin preparations may be responsible for undesirable side effects of this medication. It has been known for some time that heparin can induce platelets to undergo release reactions *in vitro* (Eika, 1972). Recently, clinical studies have revealed that substantial numbers of patients who are being given this drug experience significant reductions in their platelet count (Bell, 1976). These observations suggest that heparin infusions may activate platelets, cause their deposition within the vasculature, and thus produce systemic thrombocytopenia. If such is the case, perhaps heparin species, incapable of binding to antithrombin, are available in plasma for interactions with platelets and are responsible for these unwanted phenomena.

## 7.6.2. Clinical Assay of Heparin Function

It has been shown that heparin can be employed in certain groups of presurgical patients for prophylaxis against the development of venous thrombosis and its sequela (Kakkar *et al.*, 1971). In addition, this drug can be utilized to treat established venous thrombotic disease and dramatically reduce the incidence of pulmonary embolism (Hirsh and Genton, 1975). In order to extend the prophylactic usage of this anticoagulant to other groups of patients and improve the therapy of established thrombotic disease, we must consider the inadequacies of the present assay utilized for monitoring drug administration as well as the identification of clinical states that may be refractory to heparinization.

From the foregoing review of heparin's function, it should be obvious that optimal dosage of this anticoagulant is dependent on a knowledge of the concentrations and relative distributions of the serine proteases which this mucopolysaccharide is instrumental in neutralizing. Thus, the dosage of heparin required for an individual patient should be adjusted according to the procoagulant stimulus with which this drug must deal. Therefore, a patient with activation of the early clotting factors (factors XIIa and XIa), whose concentrations in plasma are low, may require only a minimal dosage of heparin in order to assure prophylaxis against thrombosis. On the other hand, an individual with activation of the clotting mechanism so extensive as to have produced factor Xa or thrombin, whose concentrations in the plasma are considerable, may require a significantly greater dosage to achieve the same degree of protection.

Present assays attempt to regulate heparin therapy by determining the degree to which plasma from a heparinized patient inhibits the *in vitro* addition of an arbitrary amount of either thrombin or factor Xa, or else the extent to which this plasma prevents *in vitro* generation of an arbitrary amount of serine proteases during kaolin activation (activated partial thromboplastin time) (Blomback *et al.*, 1959; Yin *et al.*, 1973; Marder, 1970). In either case, no attempt is made to judge the effect of the heparin-activated plasma antithrombin in inhibiting the serine proteases of the coagulation cascade generated within the patient's circulatory system. In effect, it is as if one were to treat a diabetic patient by measuring the amount of injected insulin present in his circulatory system rather than the resultant reduction in blood glucose levels. This critique of present methodology is pertinent to situations in which either standard dosages of heparin are employed after thrombus formation or low dosages are administered prior to clot development.

Several groups of investigators are establishing methods for the direct or indirect measurement of *in vivo* levels of the serine proteases active in coagulation. With the advent of more sophisticated assay procedures, it may become apparent that certain patients are refractory to heparinization. For example, Nossel *et al.* (1971) have measured fibrino-peptide A levels in individuals with pulmonary embolism who were treated with this drug. In most of these patients, heparin administration results in an immediate reduction of fibrinopeptide A levels. This is consistent with the half-life of this small molecular species and suggests that thrombin's action has been instantaneously suppressed. In some individuals, however, fibrinopeptide A evolution remained elevated during the first 30 min after injection of 10,000 units of heparin. We interpret these data to indicate that this group of patients are resistant to heparin therapy despite the fact that samples of their blood are incoagulable as judged by clinical assay procedures (partial thromboplastin time, whole blood clotting time, etc.).

Based on our knowledge of the biochemistry of heparin, one can suggest a variety of molecular explanations for these refractory states. The simplest mechanisms would involve a more rapid clearance of heparin, grossly reduced concentrations of antithrombin, or an increase in the levels of the molecular species other than antithrombin which interact with heparin. These phenomena are unlikely to play a significant role in the genesis of these refractory states since the blood must have been grossly incoagulable immediately after drug administration. The more likely explanation is that these refractory states are due to various local events that might permit *in vivo* clotting but whose effects are not measurable by currently employed assay techniques. This paradoxical state could be caused by the sequestration of thrombin such that it is inaccessible to heparin action or by localized reductions in the level of anticoagulant. For example, we have demonstrated that a serine protease similar to activated intermediates of the coagulation cascade is present on the macrophage membrane (Remold and Rosenberg, 1975). This enzyme is neutralized by antithrombin but, when heparin is added to the inhibitor, the inactivation is prevented. This phenomenon is due to the exclusion of the negatively charged heparin–antithrombin complex from the similarly charged macrophage surface. In an analogous manner, thrombin may be adsorbed to damaged endothelium or platelet membrane in such a way as to render it inaccessible to heparin–antithrombin neutralization yet capable of local thrombus formation. An alternate mechanism for generating a refractory state would involve a decrease in the local availability of heparin. This could occur by local release of large quantities of platelet factor 4 which directly neutralize heparin. This phenomenon could be due to altered local blood flow properties or restricted surface abnormalities which induce platelet release reactions. The local anticoagulant function of heparin might be exhausted and fibrin deposition could occur, as evidenced by the fibrinopeptide A release. The systemic levels of this drug as judged by the activated partial thromboplastin time, the whole blood clotting time, and the factor Xa inhibition assays would be unaffected.

## 7.7. Physiologic Implications

This newly acquired knowledge of the structure and function of heparin may have important physiologic implications. The significance of *in vitro* inhibitor heparin interactions to *in vivo* modulation of the coagulation system remains speculative. The data outlined herein have demonstrated that this acidic mucopolysaccharide, in conjunction with antithrombin, inhibits in an instantaneous fashion virtually all of the enzymatic steps of the coagulation system. This is to be contrasted with the relatively slow neutralization of many of these enzymes by other circulating plasma inhibitors.

To examine the possible relevance of this inhibitory mechanism to normal physiological processes, let us consider the sequela of congenital antithrombin deficiency *vis-à-vis* the plasma levels of this inhibitor and examine the probable *in vivo* location of heparin-like material.

Congenital reductions in antithrombin levels are uniquely associated with fatal thrombotic complications. The first report of this syndrome in 1965 described several generations of a family with recurrent venous thromboembolism in conjunction with a plasma antithrombin concentration that averaged 40% of normal (Egeberg, 1965). Other families were subsequently reported to exhibit venous and arterial thrombotic episodes in association with partial deficiencies of antithrombin (Shapiro *et al.*, 1973; Grunberg *et al.*, 1975).

The data presented earlier indicate that the *in vitro* addition of antithrombin to serine proteases of the coagulation mechanism results in the neutralization of their proteolytic activity only after many minutes have passed. Thus, the production of potent serine proteases should trigger clot development long before inhibition by antithrombin has occurred, and it is surprising that modest reductions in plasma concentrations of this molecular species result in such striking thrombotic phenomena.

The discrepancy between clinical observations of inhibitor deficiency and *in vitro* kinetics of serine protease–antithrombin interaction could be resolved if heparin-like material were shown to activate this component *in vivo*. Under these conditions, plasma antithrombin would almost instantaneously inactivate serine proteases, and a reduction in its concentration would have profound pathophysiological effects.

Heparin has not only been isolated from various organs but is also thought to be present in mast cells. More importantly, heparan sulfate, which possesses some anticoagulant properties, has been found on a variety of cell surfaces including those of the endothelium (Buonassisi, 1973) and the platelet (Horner, 1975). How much of the "highly active" hemostatically potent fraction of heparin is present at these locales remains to be determined. However, the availability of heparin-like components would permit antithrombin to be selectively activated at blood–surface interfaces where enzymes of the hemostatic mechanism are generated. Thus, the plasma protease inhibitor would be critically placed to neutralize these enzymes and thereby protect natural surfaces against thrombus formation.

Furthermore, the catalytic nature of heparin would ensure the continual regeneration of the nonthrombogenic properties of these natural surfaces. Once the antithrombin bound to platelet surface or vessel wall mucopolysaccharide has complexed with enzyme, the enzyme–inhibitor complex would be liberated into the circulation. The heparin-like material would again be available to recruit free antithrombin and thereby continually renew the ability of the surface to resist the attack of serine proteases of the hemostatic mechanism. Alterations of this protective barrier could be responsible for early arterial or venous prethrombotic lesions in man.

ACKNOWLEDGMENTS

This work was supported by the National Institutes of Health Grants HL19131, HL20079, and HL21602, as well as by the American Heart Association Grant 75-952.

The author is a recipient of an American Heart Established Investigatorship Award.

# References

Abildgaard, U., 1968, Highly purified antithrombin III with heparin cofactor activity prepared by disc electrophoresis, *Scand. J. Clin. Lab. Invest.* **21**:89–91.

Bagdasarian, A., Lahiri, B., and Coleman, R. W., 1973, Origin of the high molecular weight activator of prekallikrein, *J. Biol. Chem.* **248**:7742–7747.

Bell, W. R., 1976, Thrombocytopenia occurring during heparin therapy, *N. Engl. J. Med.* **295**:276–277.

Biggs, R., Denson, K. W. E., Akman, N., Barrett, R., and Hadden, M., 1970, Antithrombin III, Antifactor Xa and heparin, *Br. J. Haematol.* **19**:283–305.

Blomback, B., Blomback, M., Olsson, P., *et al.*, 1959, Determination of heparin level of the blood: Some observations on heparin elimination and correlation between heparin level and clotting time after intravenous injection, *Acta Chir. Scand. (Suppl.)* **245**:259–264.

Blomback, B., Blomback, M., Hessel, B., and Iwanaga, S., 1967, Structure of *N*-terminal fragments of fibrinogen and specificity of thrombin, *Nature* **215**:1445–1448.

Brinkhous, K. M., Smith, H. P., Warner, E. D., *et al.*, 1939, The inhibition of blood clotting: An unidentified substance which acts in conjunction with heparin to prevent the conversion of prothrombin into thrombin, *Am. J. Physiol.* **125**:683–687.

Buonassisi, V., 1973, Sulfated mucopolysaccharide synthesis and secretion in endothelial cell cultures, *Exp. Cell Res.* **76**:363–368.

Cifonelli, J. A., and King, J., 1973, Structural studies on heparins with unusually high *N*-acetylglucosamine contents, *Biochim. Biophys. Acta* **320**:331–341.

Cleland, R. C., Cleland, M. C., and Lipsky, J. J., 1968, Ionic polysaccharides. I. Adsorption and fractionation of polyelectrolytes on (diethylamino) ethyl cellulose, *J. Am. Chem. Soc.* **90**:3141–3146.

Chan, J., Burrowes, C., Habel, F., Movat, H., 1977, *Biochem. Biophys. Res. Commun.* **74**:150–158.

Cochrane, C. G., Revak, S. D., and Wuepper, K. D., 1973, Activation of Hageman factor in solid and fluid phases, *J. Exp. Med.* **138**:1564–1583.

Colman, R. W., Girey, G. J. D., Zacest, R., *et al.*, 1971, The human plasma kallikrein-kinin system, *Prog. Hematol.* **7**:255–298.

Contejean, C., 1895, Recherches sur les injections intraveineuses de peptone et leur influence sur la coagulabilité du sang chez le chien, *Arch. Physiol. Norm. Pathol.* **7**:45–53.

Damus, P. S., Hicks, M., and Rosenberg, R. D., 1973, A generalized view of heparin's anticoagulant action, *Nature* **246**:355–357.

Danishefsky, I., Steiner, H., Bella, A., and Friedlander, A., 1969, Investigations on the chemistry of heparin, *J. Biol. Chem.* **244**:1741–1745.

Davie, E. W., and Ratnoff, O. D., 1964, Waterfall sequence for intrinsic blood clotting, *Science* **145**:1310–1312.

Davie, E. W., Fujikawa, K., Legaz, M. E., *et al.*, 1975, Role of proteases in blood coagulation, *in Proteases and Biologic Control* (E. Reich, D. Rifkin, E. Shaw, eds.), p. 65, Cold Spring Harbor Laboratory, New York.

Egeberg, O., 1965, Inherited antithrombin deficiency causing thrombophilia, *Thromb. Diath. Haemorrh.* **13**:516–530.

Ehrlich, J., and Stivala, S. S., 1973, Chemistry and pharmacology of heparin, *J. Pharm. Sci.* **62**:517–544.

Eika, C., 1972, On the mechanism of platelet aggregation induced by heparin and polybrene, *Scand. J. Haematol.* **9**:248–257.

Fearnley, G. R., 1969, Fibrinolysis, *in Recent Advances in Blood Coagulation* (L. Poller, ed.), pp. 229–261, Little Brown, Boston.

Gladner, J. A., and Laki, K., 1958, The active site of thrombin, *J. Am. Chem. Soc.* **80**:1263–1264.

Godal, H. C., Ryah, M., and Laake, K., 1974, Progressive inactivation of purified factor VII by heparin and antithrombin III, *Thromb. Res.* **5**:773–776.

Grunberg, J., Smallridge, R., and Rosenberg, R. D., 1975, Inherited antithrombin III deficiency causing mesenteric venous infarction, *Ann. Surg.* **181**:791–794.

Harpel, P. C., and Rosenberg, R. D., 1976, *in Progress in Hemostasis*, Vol. 3 (T. Speat, ed.), Grune & Stratton, New York.

Highsmith, R. F., and Rosenberg, R. D., 1974, The inhibition of human plasmin by human antithrombin-heparin cofactor, *J. Biol. Chem.* **249**:4335–4338.

Hirsh, J., and Genton, E., 1975, Low-dose heparin prophylaxis for venous thromboembolism, *in Prophylactic Therapy of Deep Vein Thrombosis and Pulmonary*

*Embolism* (J. Frantantoni and S. Wessler, eds.), pp. 183–206, DHEW Publ. No. (NIH) 76-866, Washington, D.C.

Horner, A. A., 1975, Demonstration of endogenous heparin in rat blood, *in Heparin: Structure, Function and Clinical Implications* (R. A. Bradshaw and S. Wessler, eds.), p. 85, Plenum Press, New York.

Höök, M., Bjork, I., Hopwood, J., Lindahl, U., 1976, Anticoagulant activity of heparin: Separation of high-activity and low-activity species by affinity chromatography on immobilized AT, *FEBS Lett.* **66**:90–93.

Hovingh, P., and Linker, A., 1970, The enzymatic degradation of heparin and heparitin sulfate, *J. Biol. Chem.* **245**:6170–6175.

Kakkar, V. V., Nicolaides, A. N., Field, E. S., and Flute, P. T., 1971, Low doses of heparin in prevention of deep-vein thrombosis, *Lancet* **2**:669–677.

Kaplan, A. P., and Austen, K. F., 1970, Prealbumin activator of prekallikrein, *J. Immunol.* **105**:802–811.

Kaplan, A. P., and Austen, K. F., 1971, A prealbumin activator of prekallikrein, *J. Exp. Med.* **133**:696–712.

Kaplan, A. P., Sphagg, J., and Austen, K. F., 1971, The bradykinin-forming system in man, *in Biochemistry of the Acute Allergic Reaction—Second International Symposium* (K. F. Austen and E. L. Becker, eds.), pp. 279–298, Blackwell, Oxford.

Kurachi, K., Fujikawa, K., Schmier, G., and Davie, E. W., 1976, *Biochemistry* **15**:373–377.

Lam, L. H., Silbert, J. E., and Rosenberg, R. D., 1976, The separation of active and inactive forms of heparin, *Biochem. Biophys. Res. Commun.* **69**:570–577.

Laurent, T. C., 1961, Studies on fractionated heparin, *Arch. Biochem. Biophys.* **92**:224–231.

Lindahl, U., and Roden, L., 1972, *in The Glycoproteins* 2nd ed. (R. Gottschall, ed.), Elsevier, Amsterdam.

Lindahl, U., Höök, M., Backstrom, G., Jacobsson, I., Riesenfeld, J., Malmstrom, A., Roden, L., and Feingold, D. S., 1977, Structure and biosynthesis of heparin-like polysaccharides, *Fed. Proc.* **36**:19–24.

Marder, V. J., 1970, A simple technique for the measurement of plasma heparin concentration during anticoagulant therapy, *Thromb. Diath. Haemorrh.* **24**:230–239.

McClean, J., 1916, The thromboplastic action of cephalin, *Am. J. Physiol.* **41**:250–257.

Monkhouse, F. C., France, E. S., and Seegers, W. H., 1955, Studies on the antithrombin and heparin cofactor activities of a fraction adsorbed from plasma by aluminum hydroxide, *Circ. Res.* **3**:397–402.

Moroi, M., and Aoki, N., 1976, Isolation and characterization of $\alpha_2$-plasmin inhibitor from human plasma, *J. Biol. Chem.* **251**:5956–5965.

Morowitz, P., 1968, *The Chemistry of Blood Coagulation*, C. C. Thomas, Springfield, Illinois.

Nemerson, Y., 1976, Biological control of factor VII, *Thromb. Haemostasis* **35**:96–100.

Nemerson, Y., and Pitlick, F. A., 1972, The tissue factor pathway of blood coagulation, *Prog. Hemostasis Thromb.* **1**:1–37.

Nieduszynski, J. A., and Atkins, E. D. T., 1973, Conformation of the mucopolysaccharides—X-ray fibre diffraction of heparin, *Biochemistry* **135**:729–733.

Nossel, H. L., Younger, L. R., Wilner, G. D., Procupez, T., Canfield, R. E., and Butler, V. P., 1971, A radioimmunoassay for human fibrinopeptide A, *Proc. Natl. Acad. Sci. U.S.A.* **68**:2350–2353.

Remold, H. G., and Rosenberg, R. D., 1975, Enhancement of migration inhibitory factor (MIF) by plasma esterase inhibitor, *J. Biol. Chem.* **250**:6608–6613.

Revak, S. D., Cochrane, C. G., Johnston, A. R., and Hugli, T. E., 1974, Structural changes accompanying enzymatic activation of human Hageman factor, *J. Clin. Invest.* **54**:619–627.

Rosenberg, R. D., 1973, Heparin action, *Circulation* **XLIX**:603–605.

Rosenberg, R. D., 1977, Biological actions of heparin, *Semin. Hematol.* **14**:427–440.

Rosenberg, R. D., and Damus, P. S., 1973, The purification and mechanism of action of human antithrombin-heparin cofactor, *J. Biol. Chem.* **248**:6490–6505.

Rosenberg, R. D., and Damus, P. S., 1976, The purification and properties of human antithrombin-heparin cofactor, *in Methods in Enzymology* Vol. 45, Academic Press, New York.

Rosenberg, R. D., and Jordan, R. E., 1977, *Chemistry and Biology of Thrombosis,* Ann Arbor Science Publications, Ann Arbor, Michigan.

Rosenberg, J. S., McKenna, P., and Rosenberg, R. D., 1975, Inhibition of human factor IXa by human antithrombin-heparin cofactor, *J. Biol. Chem.* **250**:8883–8888.

Rosenberg, R. D., Lahiri, B., Talmo, R. G., Mitchell, B., Bagdasarian, A., and Coleman, R. F., 1976, Antithrombin III: An inhibitor of human plasma kallikrein, *Arch. Biochem. Biophys.* **175**:737–747.

Rosenberg, R. D., Armand, G., and Lam, L. H., 1978, Structure–function relationships of heparin species, *Proc. Natl. Acad. Sci. U.S.A.,* in press.

Rosenberg, R. D., and Damus, P. S., 1973, The purification and mechanism of action of human antithrombin-heparin cofactor, *J. Biol. Chem.* **248**:6490–6505.

Seegers, W. H., Cole, E. R., Harmision, C. R., *et al.,* 1964, Neutralization of autoprothrombin C activity with antithrombin, *Can. J. Biochem.* **42**:359–364.

Shapiro, S. S., Prager, D., and Martinez, J., 1973, Inherited antithrombin III deficiency associated with multiple thromboembolic phenomena, presented at the 16th Annual Meeting of the American Society of Hematology, Chicago, p. 63.

Silbert, J. E., Kleinman, H. K., and Silbert, C. K., 1975, Heparin and heparin-like substances of cells, *Adv. Exp. Med. Biol.* **52**:51–60.

Silva, M. E., and Dietrich, C. P., 1975, Structure of heparin, *J. Biol. Chem.* **250**:6841–6846.

Stead, N., Kaplan, A. P., and Rosenberg, R. D., 1976a, The inhibition of activated factor XII by antithrombin-heparin cofactor, *J. Biol. Chem.* **251**:6481–6488.

Stead, N., Kaplan, A., and Rosenberg, R. D., 1976b, Inhibition of factor XIIa with antithrombin, *Clin. Res.* **24**:321A.

Summaria, L., Boreisha, I. G., Arzadon, L., and Robbins, K., 1977, Activation of human glu-plasinogen to glu-plasmin by urokinase in presence of plasmin inhibitors, *J. Biol. Chem.* **252**:3945.

Summaria, L., Hsieh, B., Groskopf, W. R., Robbins, K. C., and Barlow, G. H., 1967, The isolation and characterization of the *S*-carboxymethyl beta (light) chain derivative of human plasmin: The localization of the active site on the beta (light) chain, *J. Biol. Chem.* **242**:5046–5052.

Taylor, R. L., Shively, J. T., Conrad, H. E., and Cifonelli, J. A., 1973, Uronic acid composition of heparins and heparan sulfates, *Biochemistry* **12**:3633–3636.

Teien, A. N., Abildgaard, U., and Höök, M., 1976, Anticoagulant effect of heparan sulfate and dermatan sulfate, *Thromb. Res.* **8**:855–867.

Waugh, D. F., and Fitgerald, M. A., 1956, Quantitative aspects of antithrombin and heparin in plasma, *Am. J. Physiol.* **184**:627–639.

Yin, E. T., Wessler, S., and Stoll, P. J., 1971, Rabbit plasma inhibitor of the activated species of blood coagulation factor X: Purification and some properties, *J. Biol. Chem.* **246**:3694–3702.

Yin, E. T., Wessler, S., and Butler, J. V., 1973, Plasma heparin: A unique, practical submicrogram-sensitive assay, *J. Lab. Clin. Med.* **81**:298–310.

# Factors Thought to Contribute to the Regulation of Egress of Cells from Marrow

Marshall A. Lichtman, Jack K. Chamberlain, and Patricia A. Santillo

## 8.1. Introduction

In the mid-nineteenth century scientists learned that the marrow was the site of blood cell development. Since that seminal observation, three fundamental questions regarding the marrow have remained incompletely understood. First, what selective pressures led to the cavity of bone evolving as the site of blood cell production in the adult? Second, in part a corollary to the first, what local factors in the marrow environment contribute to the support and regulation of hematopoietic cell proliferation and differentiation? Third, what factors determine the retention of immature cells and the selective delivery of mature cells, i.e., the delivery of cells prepared for their functional role, subserved in the blood and tissues?

MARSHALL A. LICHTMAN, JACK K. CHAMBERLAIN, and PATRICIA A. SANTILLO • Departments of Medicine and of Radiation Biology and Biophysics, University of Rochester School of Medicine, Rochester, New York 14642.

In this chapter we discuss the last of the three questions, confining our review to those factors that have been hypothesized as contributing to the control of cell egress from marrow.

## 8.2. Evidence for Discriminatory Release of Marrow Cells

The quantitative evaluation of discriminatory release of blood cells begins with a consideration of the ratio of marrow cells of a specific morphologic age to blood cells of the same age. Thus, the marrow-to-blood ratio of myeloblasts per kilogram of body weight compared to the marrow-to-blood ratio of neutrophils per kilogram of body weight can be used as an index of whether undifferentiated or differentiated cells are released more readily (lower marrow-to-blood ratio) from marrow. The numerator and denominator of this ratio may be influenced by factors that make interpretation difficult. For example, selective differences in circulation time, sequestration by the spleen, or death in the circulation could bias the denominator of the ratio. Also, the prevalence of immature cells outside of the marrow is difficult to ascertain. The quantity of cells in or entering the tissues influences these calculations. The marrow-to-blood ratio of neutrophils is a falsely high estimate of the marrow-to-extramedullary ratio since the tissue neutrophils are neglected. These factors make the marrow-to-blood ratio a semiquantitative estimate of the relationship of intramedullary to extramedullary cells. In most cases the factors noted act to minimize the differences between the high marrow-to-blood ratio of immature cells and the lower marrow-to-blood ratio of mature cells.

Table I shows the marrow-to-blood (M/B) ratios that can be derived from data in the literature regarding the prevalence of hematopoietic cells

**Table I.** Distribution of Hematopoietic Cells in Marrow and Blood[a]

| | Red cells | | Granulocytes | | |
|---|---|---|---|---|---|
| | Nucleated | Reticulocytes | Immature | Mature | Megakaryocytes |
| Marrow | $3 \times 10^9$ | $6 \times 10^9$ | $5 \times 10^9$ | $6 \times 10^9$ | $6 \times 10^6$ |
| Blood | ~0 | $3 \times 10^9$ | $<5 \times 10^5$ | $0.6 \times 10^9$ | $2 \times 10^2$ |
| M/B ratio | $\infty$ | 2:1 | >10,000:1 | 10:1 | 30,000:1 |

[a]Data represent number of cells per kilogram of body weight. The number of marrow red cells and granulocytes was taken from the studies of Donohue *et al.* (1958), the number of marrow megakaryocytes from Harker (1968), and the number of blood megakaryocytes from Kaufman *et al.* (1965). The marrow/blood ratio does not consider the pool of extravascular neutrophils in the tissues. This pool, estimated by some to represent as much as 100-fold the blood neutrophil pool, would markedly reduce the marrow-to-extramedullary ratio of mature granulocytes.

in marrow and blood. A marked reduction in the ratio is present when reticulocytes (M/B ratio $\cong$ 2:1) are compared to nucleated red cells (M/B ratio $\cong$ $\infty$) or when immature granulocytes (M/B ratio > 10,000:1) are compared to mature granulocytes (M/B ratio < 10:1). Megakaryocytes, although found in the right heart blood in low concentrations in subjects without hematopoietic disease, have a very low extramedullary prevalence compared to their numbers in marrow (M/B $\cong$ 30,000:1). The marrow-to-blood ratio of platelets cannot be calculated since there are no data regarding the number of free platelets in the hematopoietic spaces. It is probable that few if any detached platelets are normally present in the hematopoietic compartment, making such considerations meaningless. These ratios, despite the limitations that must be placed on the inferences drawn from them, provide strong support for the discriminatory release of differentiated, functional cells and the retention in marrow of incompletely differentiated cells.

## 8.3. Factors Governing Release of Hematopoietic Cells

Four factors have been considered to play a role in the regulation of marrow cell egress (Lichtman *et al.*, 1977b; Sabin, 1928). One factor is the anatomical organization of the marrow. In particular, the localization of developing hematopoietic cells in the extravascular spaces of marrow makes their entry into the venous circulation a mandatory requirement for egress. A second factor is the developmental change that occurs in the nucleus and cytoplasm of maturing cells. These alterations allow translocation of terminally differentiated cells from the hematopoietic compartment to the efferent vascular channels of marrow. The third factor in the regulation of the release of marrow cells is the role of cell-releasing substances, a putative set of chemicals that facilitate the rate of release of specific morphologic cell types. Such chemicals are presumably responsible for the selective acceleration of the release of reticulocytes, neutrophils, eosinophils, or other hematopoietic cells depending on bodily needs. The fourth factor relates to the vascular and neural structures in marrow. There is limited knowledge of the functional importance of nerve fibers in the marrow. Also, the precise regulation of blood flow in the circulation of marrow has resisted detailed study. In a global sense, the flow of blood through marrow vascular channels could influence the total delivery of new cells since these cells exit in the efferent blood of bone. The regulation of flow may be mediated by vasoactive compounds, neural regulation, or other factors that may influence the blood supply at the arteriolar level or the patency of smaller presinus or postsinus vessels.

Neurogenic influences may exist independent of vasoregulatory fibers since some myelinated and nonmyelinated nerves course through marrow unassociated with the adventitia of arteries. In nervous tissues, studies have identified a regulatory role for free, nonsynaptic nerve endings.

### 8.3.1. Marrow Ultrastructure

The marrow may be considered to have two major parts, its vascular channels and the hematopoietic compartment, positioned in the intersinusoidal spaces. These two compartments, vascular and hematopoietic, are linked anatomically by the reticular cells that compose the adventitial surface of the marrow vascular sinuses and whose cytoplasmic processes extend from the abluminal surface of the sinus wall into the hematopoietic compartment, forming a latticework on which hematopoietic cells reside.

The anatomy of the vascular compartment of marrow has been studied by histologic examination, injection preparation of vessels, and vital microscopy (Bränemark, 1959; Brookes and Harrison, 1957; De Bruyn *et al.*, 1966, 1970). The fine structure of the vascular sinuses and hematopoietic compartment of marrow have been studied intensively by transmission and scanning electron microscopy (Campbell, 1967, 1972; De Bruyn *et al.*, 1966, 1971, 1975; Leblond, 1975; Pease, 1956; Tanaka, 1969; Tavassoli, 1974a; Trubowitz and Masek, 1970; Watanabe, 1966; Weiss, 1961, 1967, 1970; Weiss and Chen, 1975; Zamboni and Pease, 1961).

### 8.3.1.1. Arterial Blood Supply

The major supply of blood to marrow is derived from the nutrient artery (see Fig. 1). This artery enters the marrow through the nutrient canal in an angulated fashion, bifurcates to ascend and descend in the marrow cavity as the central artery, and gives off branches, the radial arteries which arborize toward the cortex. The radial (or medullary) arteries become fine arterioles and penetrate the endosteum of the diaphysis spreading into an intracortical arborization. These cortical vessels reach capillary size and are contained within the haversian canals and canals of Volkmann. These vessels communicate also with periosteal capillaries which are fed from arteries external to bone. The intracortical vessels communicate also with the sinuses of marrow. The sinuses are the vessels that are in intimate contact with hematopoietic cells of marrow. Hematopoietic cells must enter the sinuses to reach the systemic circulation. Rarely, the radial or medullary artery may terminate directly in the marrow sinuses (De Bruyn *et al.*, 1970; Irino *et al.*, 1975; Weiss and Chen,

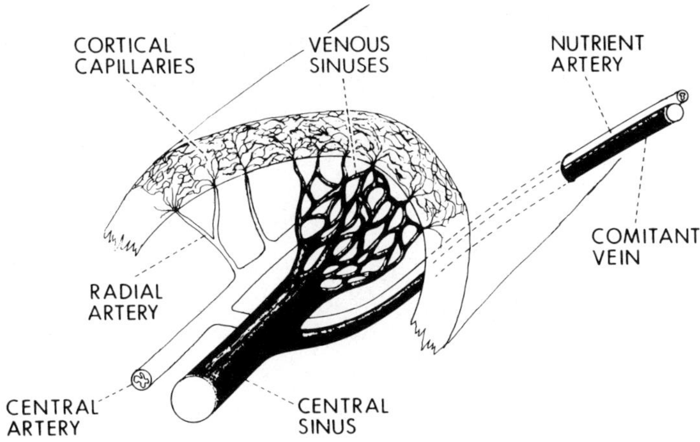



**Fig. 1.** A schematic representation of the circulation of the marrow. The nutrient artery, central arteries, and radial arteries feed the cortical capillaries. The cortical capillaries anastomose with the marrow sinuses which drain into the large central sinus. The central sinus enters the comitant vein by which the marrow effluent enters the systemic venous circulation. An interesting feature of the circulation of marrow is the transit of nearly all arterial blood through cortical capillaries before entering the marrow sinuses. Not shown are the arterial communications from muscular arteries that feed the periosteum and penetrate the cortex to anastomose with intracortical vessels.

1975). The importance of this direct source of blood to the marrow sinuses is disputed. Most evidence indicates that this is a minor route for blood entering marrow sinuses.

The transit of arterial blood through the cortex of bone before entering the marrow sinuses is a vascular pattern that suggests a functional relationship between cortex and marrow. The haversian canals have been suggested as a source of hematopoietic stem cells for the regeneration of marrow parenchyma after experimental injury (Maloney and Patt, 1969). Thus, the intracortical circulation may permit reconstitution of the marrow stem cell pool, at least under circumstances of extreme injury. The cortex may provide other cells or chemicals to the marrow through these channels. These chemicals may be important for the regulation of cell proliferation, cell release, or other features of marrow function.

### 8.3.1.2. Vascular Sinuses

The sinuses of marrow begin at the endosteal surface and are fed primarily from intracortical capillaries. These vessels course through the medullary cavity of bone, anastomose, and eventually drain into a large central venous sinus (Fig. 2). The size of the marrow sinuses varies in

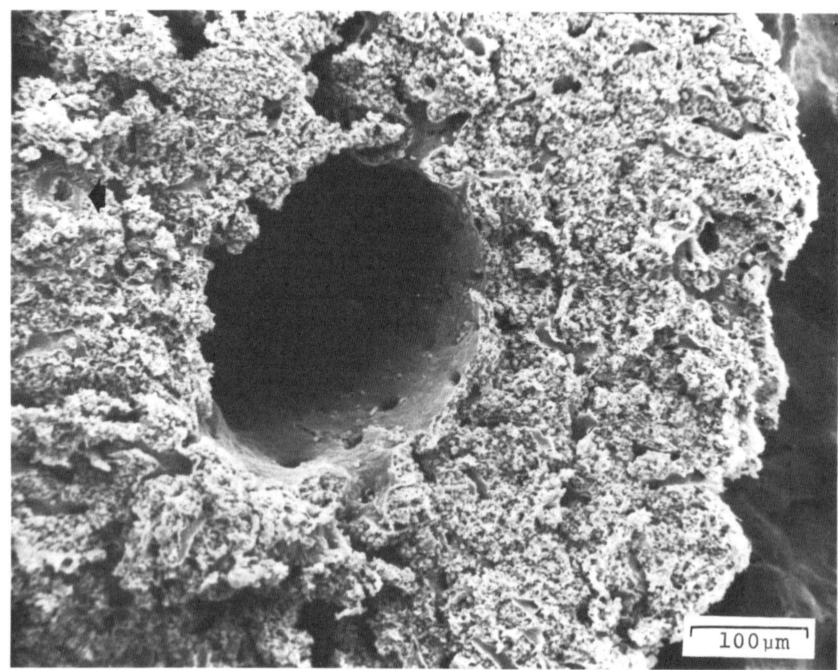



**Fig. 2.**  A scanning electron micrograph of a cross section of rat femoral marrow. The bony cortex has been removed. An enormous central sinus is present. The orifices of collecting sinuses can be seen in the wall of the central sinus. The arrow indicates a central artery. At this enlargement, the individual marrow sinuses and intersinal hematopoietic cells are difficult to define.

diameter from 10 to 30 $\mu$m (Fig. 3). As they approach the central sinus they may coalesce and form somewhat larger collecting sinuses before entering the central sinus (De Bruyn *et al.*, 1970).

*8.3.1.2a. Endothelium.*  The luminal surface of the vascular sinus is composed of endothelial lining cells that are a type of squamous epithelium with a mosaic pattern when examined *enface* using stains to bring out the sites of union of two cells (Campbell, 1967; De Bruyn *et al.*, 1970, 1971; Watanabe, 1966; Weiss, 1961, 1965, 1967; Zamboni and Pease, 1961). In cross section (Fig. 4) the cell junctions are distinct and often are overlapping or interdigitating. The endothelial cell cytoplasm forms a complete covering for the inner surface of the sinus. Thus, holes in the endothelium must develop *pari passu* with cell migration. Large gaps are not seen in well-fixed transmission micrographs. Small gaps (0.5–2.0 $\mu$m

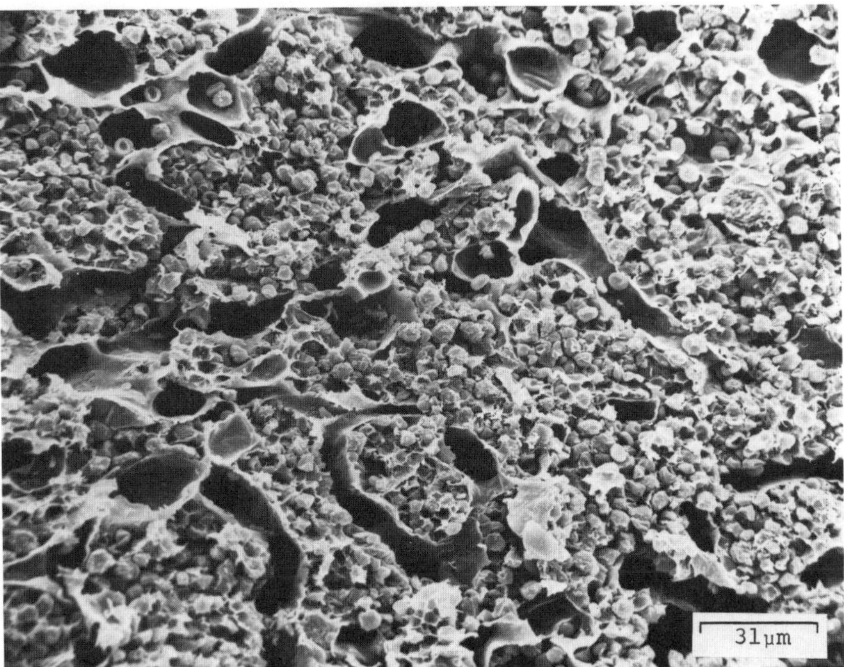

**Fig. 3.** A scanning electron micrograph of rat femoral marrow. The hematopoietic cells are grouped between the interlacing network of vascular sinuses. Many cells are dislodged when the marrow is transected and separate spaces are present where cells had been.

in diameter) are frequent in scanning micrographs of the luminal surface of sinus walls and can be seen occasionally in transmission micrographs. These may be artifacts, induced during the preparation of marrow, or may be sites where cells in passage were lost during the rigors of preparation. Marked attenuation, short of discontinuity, may be seen in transmission micrographs (Fig. 5). At these sites, endothelial cell cytoplasm has thinned to a diameter that approaches a double membrane in thickness. In some cases these attenuated areas may provide a locus minoris resistentiae for cell penetration. Studies have not established that such thinning is an absolute prerequisite to egress. Microvacuolization is a prominent feature of the cytoplasm of marrow sinus endothelial cells (De Bruyn *et al.*, 1975). Pinocytotic vacuoles of varying size may be seen throughout the endothelial cell cytoplasm. This process permits exposure of the hematopoietic environment to materials that traverse the endothelial cell from the sinus blood.

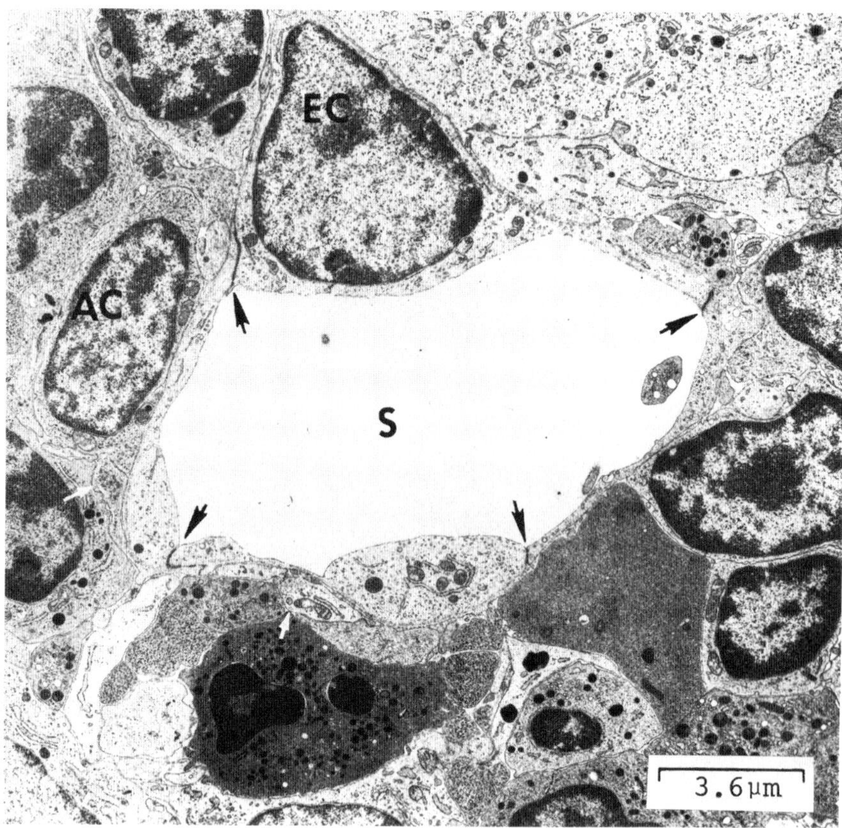



**Fig. 4.** A transmission electron micrograph of mouse femoral marrow. The cross section of a sinus is shown (the lumen labeled S). The junctions of endothelial cells are indicated by the dark arrows. The endothelial cell cytoplasm forms a complete covering for the sinus lumen. The nucleus and body of an endothelial cell is indicated by EC. The abluminal surface of the sinus is formed by adventitial reticular cells. A cell body and nucleus is indicated by AC. An incomplete covering of the abluminal surface of the sinus is formed by the cytoplasmic processes of adventitial reticular cells. Such a process is indicated by the single light arrow.

*8.3.1.2b. Adventitia.* The abluminal or adventitial surface of the vascular sinus is composed of reticular cells (Watanabe, 1966; Weiss, 1965, 1967; Weiss and Chen, 1975). They are connective tissue cells that relate both to the sinus wall on their luminal side and to the hematopoietic cells on their abluminal side (Weiss and Chen, 1975). The reticular cell bodies are largely contiguous to the sinus (Fig. 6). Their extensive cytoplasmic

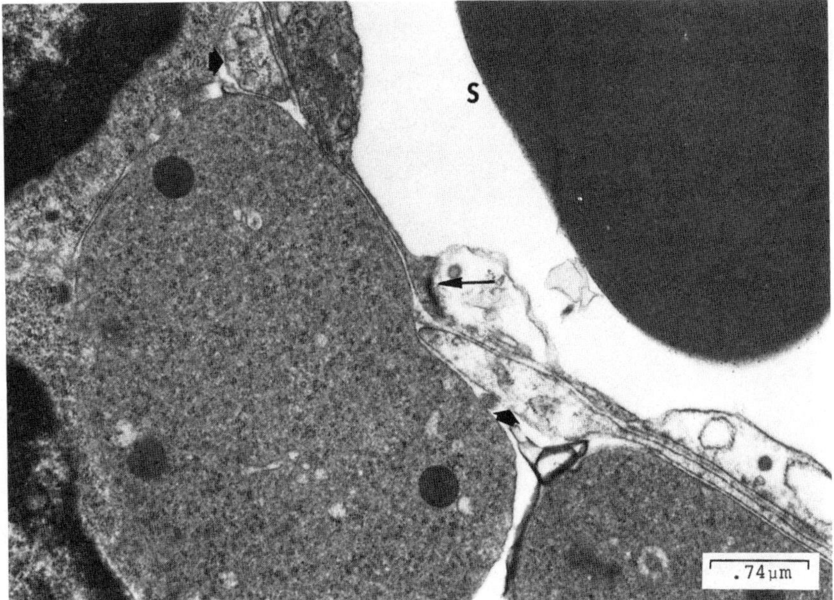


**Fig. 5.** Transmission electron micrograph of a portion of a sinus from mouse marrow. The sinus lumen is indicated by the S. The long arrow indicates an endothelial cell junction. A markedly attenuated portion of endothelial cell cytoplasm is present above the arrow. Abutting this attenuated site is a reticulocyte. The blunt arrows point to adventitial reticular cell cytoplasmic processes that contribute to the abluminal side of the sinus wall. The interruption in the reticular cell cytoplasm is exemplified in this micrograph. Cell egress seems to occur most frequently where adventitial reticular cell cytoplasm is interrupted and may be preceded by endothelial cell attenuation.

processes envelope the outer wall of the sinus to form an adventitial sheath. This covering is heavily interrupted, and has been estimated to cover about 65% of the adventitial surface of the sinus (Chamberlain *et al.*, 1975b; Weiss, 1970).

The reticular cells are related most closely to fibroblasts. These cells are neither phagocytic nor capable of developing into hematopoietic cells. They synthesize reticular fibers that provide much if not all of the physical support for hematopoietic cells. There is little precise information about their function. It is possible that they are vital elements for the normal physiology of marrow. Their intimate association with developing hematopoietic cells has raised interest in as yet poorly understood cell–cell interactions (Weiss and Chen, 1975). The reticular cell could be the source of humoral regulators of cell proliferation.

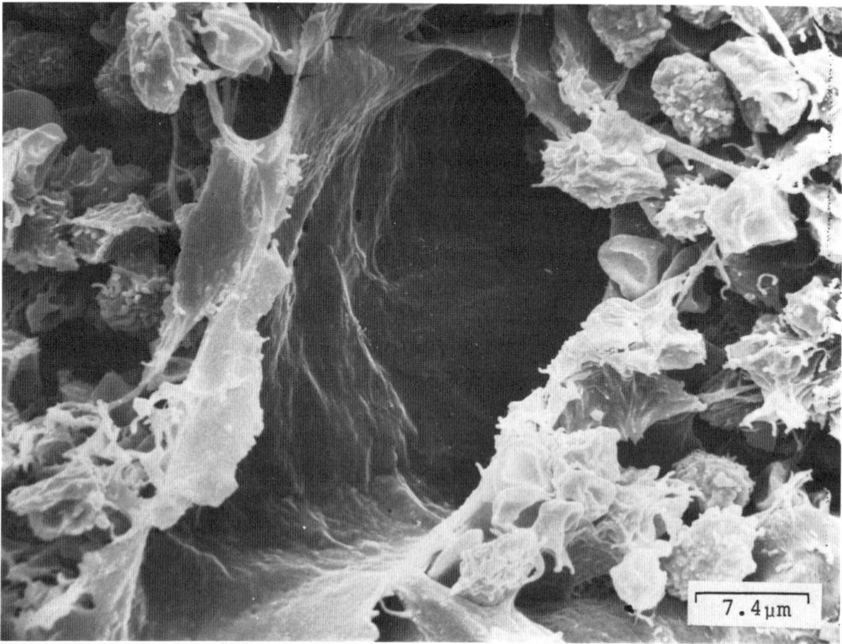



**Fig. 6.** A scanning electron micrograph of a marrow sinus. Hematopoietic cells are present in the spaces outside the sinus. A reticular cell body is indicated by the arrow on the left side of the sinus. Reticular processes can be seen in the hematopoietic compartment extending from reticular cells.

### 8.3.1.3. Venous Drainage

Arterial blood can enter the marrow from several sources, principally the central artery, but arteries from neighboring muscles that feed the periosteum of the diaphysis and the metaphysis can also provide arterial blood to marrow. Likewise, efferent blood from the marrow sinuses is drained principally by the large central sinus which empties into the comitant vein that exits through the nutrient foramen to join the systemic venous circulation (Fig. 7). The central sinus may have other large branches that penetrate the cortex as emissary veins. These veins are in essence accessory comitant veins but do not leave the cortex through the nutrient foramen. The cortical capillaries of bone may also communicate with venules outside the periosteum. The physiologic significance, if any, of this complex interconnecting arterial and venous system is not known. The presumption is that most if not all hematopoietic cells that mature and are delivered to the circulation through the wall of the vascular

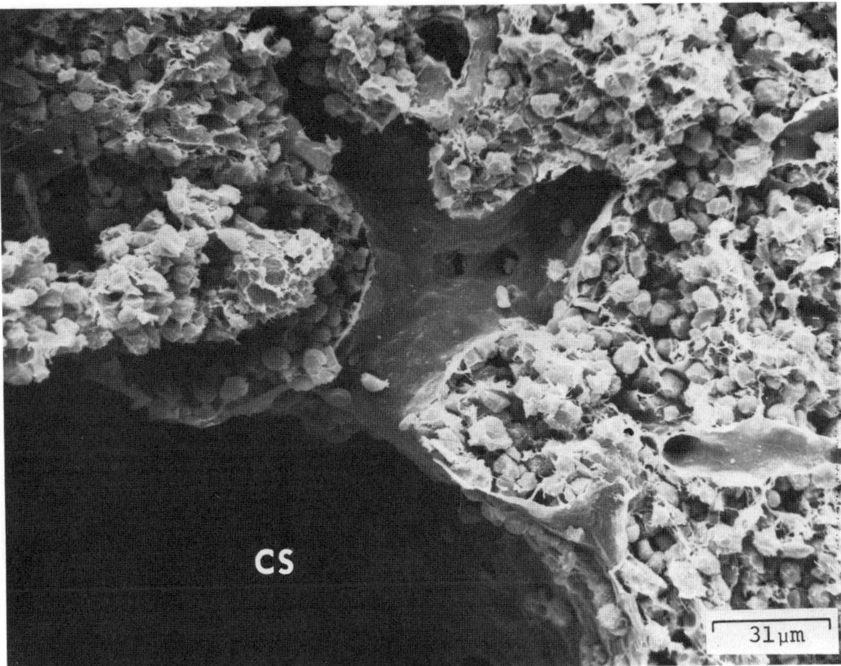


**Fig. 7.** A scanning electron micrograph of rat femoral marrow in which a collecting sinus can be observed entering the central sinus (CS). The orifice of smaller sinuses can be seen entering the collecting sinus.

sinuses drain into the central sinus of marrow and from there into the systemic circulation.

### 8.3.1.4. Hematopoietic Compartment

The parenchyma of marrow is composed of developing erythrocytes, granulocytes, and megakaryocytes. These cells are densely packed and supported by an interlacing network of reticular cell processes.

*8.3.1.4a. Reticular Cell Networks.* The cytoplasmic processes of reticular cells extend into the hematopoietic compartment as well as over the outer surface of the sinus wall (Fig. 8). Their processes form a continuous bridgework between sinuses and form an arbor on which hematopoietic cells rest. Some of the processes seem to partially enwrap over hematopoietic cells. Other more cylindrical, blunt processes terminate against

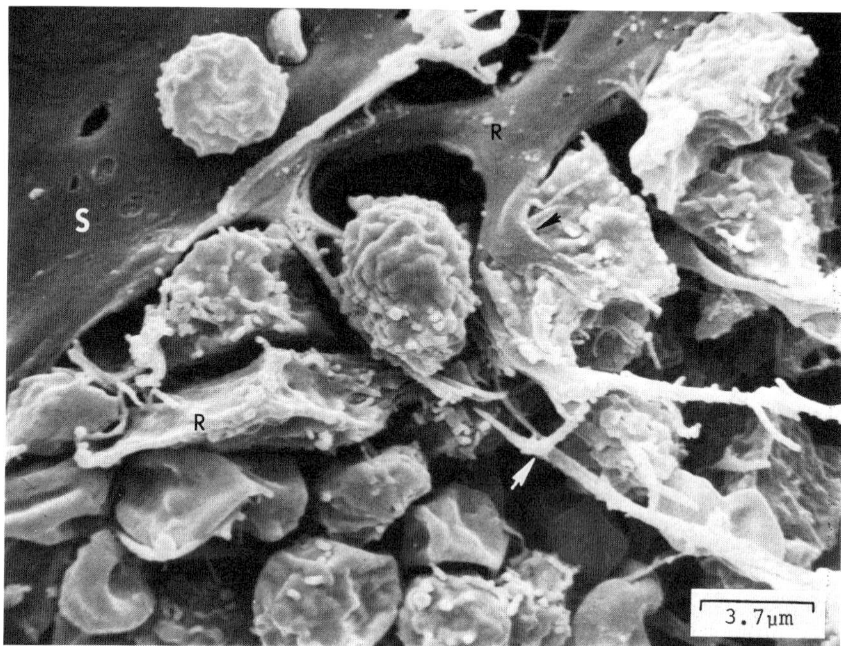

**Fig. 8.** A scanning electron micrograph of the interface between the sinus lumen (S) and the hematopoietic compartment. Reticular cell bodies (R) and processes (R) can be seen extending into the hematopoietic cells. Broad reticular cell processes may partially enwrap cells or narrower processes may branch against developing blood cells (arrows). Small defects may be seen in the endothelial surface of the sinus. These may be artifacts, places where cells were in the process of migration at the time of preparation of the femur, or may represent actual small losses in continuity. A protrusion of a cell in transit is also present in the sinus.

hematopoietic cells. These anatomical relationships have suggested that a functional as well as structural relationship may exist between reticular cell processes and hematopoietic cells (Weiss and Chen, 1975). The reticular cell process could act as an anchor for immature hematopoietic cells, reducing the possibility of their discharge from the marrow.

*8.3.1.4b. Specific Location of Hematopoietic Cells.* The hematopoietic cells in marrow may not be distributed randomly. Careful quantitative studies of the position of developing blood cells have not been made. There is little evidence for a specific localization of granulocytic or histiocytic cells. Some evidence has been garnered that developing erythroblasts may organize themselves in groups around a centrally placed histiocyte. This organization has been referred to as erythroblastic islets (Ben-Ishay and Joffey, 1972; Bessis, 1958; Bessis and Breton-Gorius, 1962; Pease, 1956). The histiocyte may serve to sustain erythroid proliferation and maturation in some way. The rings of erythroblasts may move centrifugally in relation to the central histiocyte as they mature. Inspection of random sections of marrow does not provide convincing evidence of this being a steadfast relationship. It is difficult to be certain of the proportion of marrow erythroblasts that are in islet structures.

Considerable evidence has accrued to indicate that megakaryocytes are preferentially placed adjacent to marrow sinuses (Fig. 9) (Becker and De Bruyn, 1976; Behnke, 1969; Keyserlingk and Albrecht, 1968; Lichtman *et al.*, 1977a; Weiss, 1967; Wright, 1910). All platelet-forming megakaryocytes may reside on the edge of a marrow sinus and release platelets directly into the sinus. The proximate relationship of megakaryocytes to sinuses (Fig. 10) would obviate the requirement for platelets to have a substantial amount of motility and chemotaxis which would otherwise be required if they had to find their way to and penetrate the sinus wall in the process of egress.

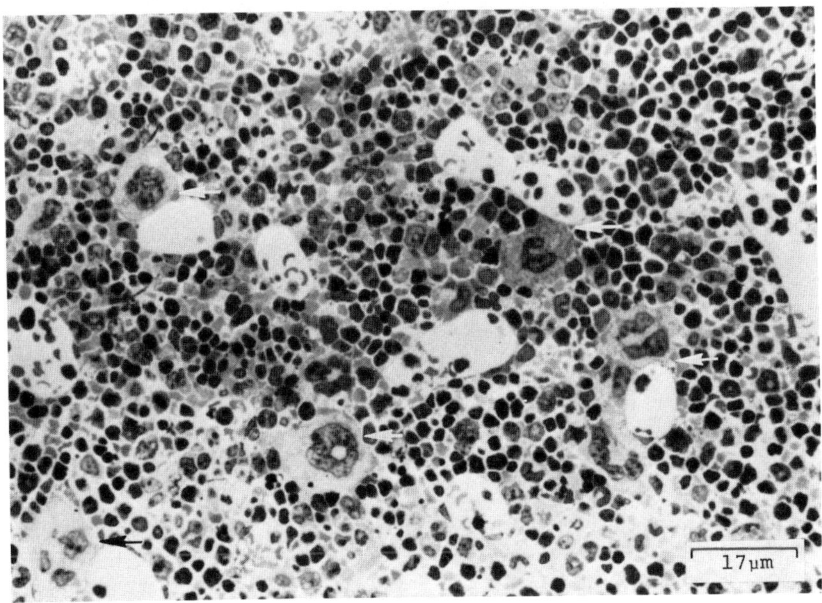



**Fig. 9.** Light micrograph of a cross section of mouse femoral marrow. Four of five (white arrows) megakaryocytes are abutting on sinus endothelium. Quantitative evidence for this long-observed relationship between megakaryocyte and sinus wall has been presented (Lichtman *et al.*, 1977a).

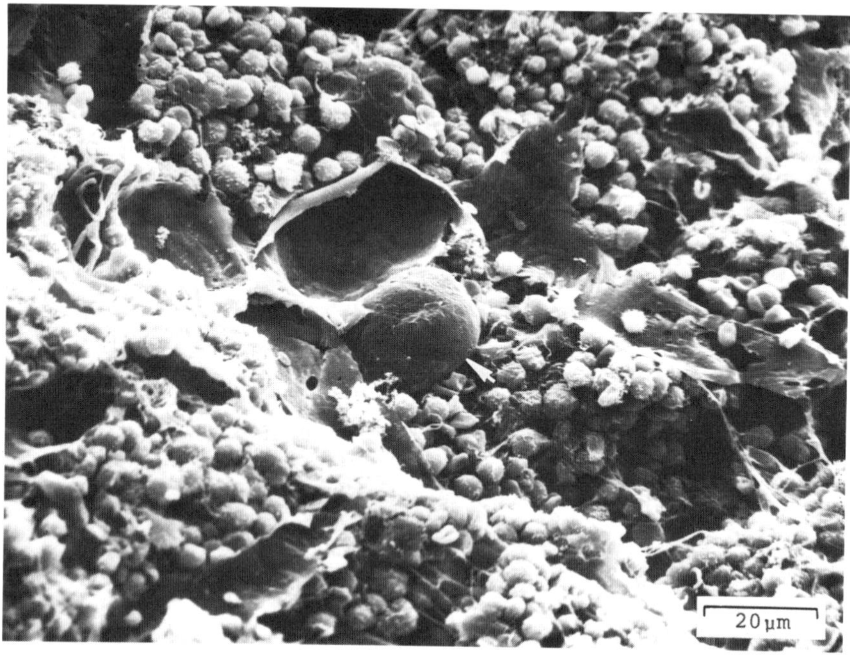

**Fig. 10.** A scanning electron micrograph of the exposed transected surface of rat femur. A megakaryocyte is shown (arrow) abutting a sinus wall.

Granulocytes do not appear to have special loci in the hematopoietic compartment. Histiocytes may have a slight predisposition to a perisinal position, although this has not been quantified.

*8.3.1.4c. Fat Cells.* Large cells with a compressed nucleus and an enormous amount of cytoplasm distended by fat are present in the marrow (Tavassoli, 1974b, 1976). The prevalence of fat cells is a function of the bone being examined and the species under study. Fat cells, however, are present even in red marrow. The fat cell in extramedullary tissue is closely related to the fibroblast. In marrow the exact origin of the fat cell is not certain; however, the adventitial reticular cell of marrow may be the cell that becomes engorged with fat (Weiss and Chen, 1975). The marrow fat cells differ from other adipocytes in that they are preserved longer during fasting.

*8.3.1.4d. Macrophages.* The marrow macrophage is presumably derived from the monocyte which itself is an offspring of an early granulocytic precursor, probably a cell that is somewhere between the committed granulocyte stem cell (colony-forming unit in culture) and the myeloblast. Its special role in marrow is at least threefold. First, it is part of the erythroblastic islet serving as a nursing cell for that structure (Bessis, 1973). Second, it is responsible for ingesting and degrading erythroblast nuclei (Ben-Ishay and Joffey, 1971) and in this sense contributes to the process of reticulocyte egress since enucleation favors the egress of red cells (Boström, 1948; Tavassoli and Crosby, 1973; Tavassoli, 1974a). The nucleus could act as a physical hindrance to egress through a narrow barrier. The marrow macrophage is also capable of ingesting damaged erythroblasts (Ben-Ishay, 1974) and erythrocytes (Luk and Simon, 1974; Tavassoli, 1974a) (Fig. 11). Third, the macrophage is a source of colony-stimulating activity, a mandatory requirement for granulocyte proliferation and maturation *in vitro*. Thus, it could be a source of a vital granulopoietin. The *in vivo* significance of this monokine is not established.

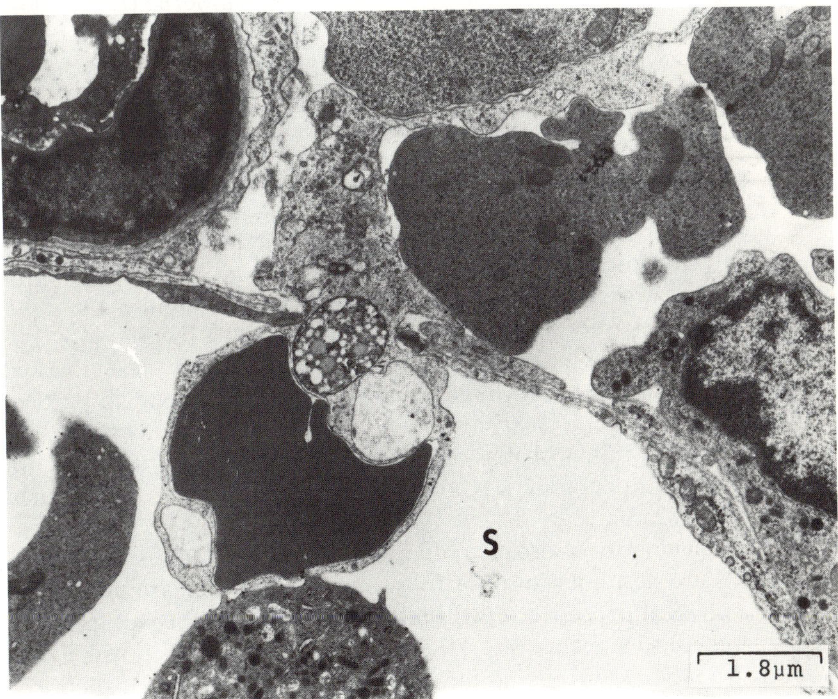


**Fig. 11.** The cytoplasmic process of a mouse marrow macrophage is shown extending from the hematopoietic compartment through the sinus wall. An engulfed red cell is in the intraluminal (S) portion of the cytoplasmic process. Degenerating material in large vacuoles is also evident.

## 8.3.2. Biophysical Properties of Developing Hematopoietic Cells

During maturation of blood cells in the marrow, well-known and striking morphologic changes occur that coincide with the achievement of functional capability. The erythroid cell begins as a poorly differentiated blast cell and eventually becomes an anucleate discoid sack of hemoglobin. The granulocytic cell, also a poorly differentiated blast cell initially, becomes a cell engorged with specific (and nonspecific) granules, with a segmented nucleus. The megakaryocyte begins as a blast cell and by endomitosis becomes a multinucleate giant cell capable of producing platelets by cytoplasmic shedding.

In addition to these changes, evident by light microscopy, the cell changes in its ability to deform, move, and undergo directed movement. Directed movement or chemotaxis requires a sensing mechanism to convert random to goal-directed motility. The development of deformability, motility, and chemotaxis may be essential for normal and regulated marrow egress of cells. The structural changes that underlie the development of motility in hematopoietic cells cannot be seen with the light microscope, but can be appreciated by physiologic studies of developing hematopoietic cells.

### 8.3.2.1. Cell Motility

Since egress of cells across the marrow sinus wall involves translocation in spatial terms, motility of the cell is required. Active motility is not a feature of immature hematopoietic cells. Their limited motility may contribute to their retention in marrow since some probing by pseudopods is probably required to initiate penetration of the sinus wall. A marked increase in motility occurs with maturation of the granulocyte, in particular. These cells become actively ameboid at the later stages of their development and this probably contributes to their ability to search out the sinus wall and penetrate it (Giordano and Lichtman, 1973; Lichtman and Weed, 1972a,b).

The reticulocyte is also a motile cell (Bessis, 1973). Its peripheral movements are desultory and not fully ameboid but they are noticeable. Since the physical process of egress may initially involve probes (pseudopods) of reticulocyte cytoplasm (De Bruyn *et al.*, 1971) it is possible that the abortive motility of reticulocytes is an important feature for their exit from the marrow (Bessis, 1973).

The megakaryocyte also develops the ability to form pseudopods from its peripheral cytoplasm (Fig. 12) (Thiery and Bessis, 1956). In effect the megakaryocyte positioned next to the sinus wall can thrust out a projection of peripheral cytoplasm in a manner analogous to a reticulo-

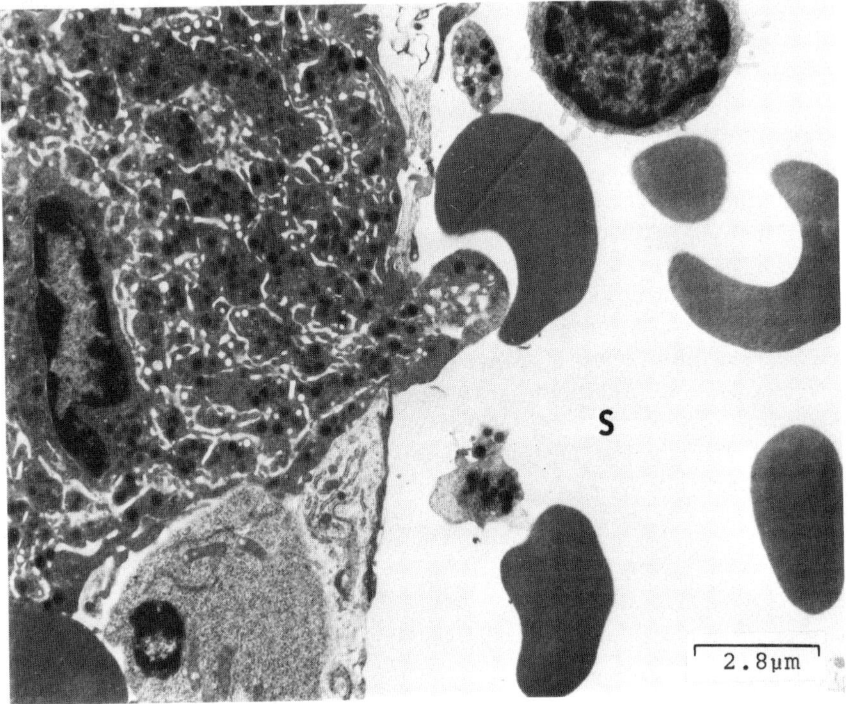

**Fig. 12.** A transmission electron micrograph of mouse marrow. A megakaryocyte is sending out a pseudopod into a sinus lumen (S).

cyte or granulocyte. This projection appears to be a pseudopod, anatomically (Behnke, 1969; Keyserlingk and Albrecht, 1968; Lichtman *et al.*, 1977a).

The factors that underlie pseudopod formation have been the subject of intensive study (Jahn and Bovee, 1969). It is probable that the mechanism of cell movement involves contractile proteins analogous to muscle actin and myosin (Pollard and Weihing, 1974). These proteins have been identified in granulocytes, monocytes, erythrocytes, and megakaryocytes. The differences in the character of the movement of reticulocytes, granulocytes, and megakaryocytes are probably a function of the amount, type, and organization of contractile proteins in these cell types.

### 8.3.2.2. Cell Deformability

The ability of cells to deform seems to be related to their ability to move. Highly ameboid cells seem to be most easily deformable under artificial circumstances. Deformability of hematopoietic cells of different stages of maturation has been examined by their ability to be filtered through micropore membranes (Lichtman, 1973; Lichtman and Kearney, 1976), to penetrate micropore membranes actively (Giordano and Lichtman, 1973; Lichtman and Kearney, 1976), and to be aspirated into glass microcapillary tubes (Leblond *et al.*, 1971a,b; Lichtman, 1970, 1973; Lichtman and Weed, 1972a,b). These studies of granulocytes and erythrocytes have shown that these cells become more easily deformable as they become more mature. In the case of the erythroblast a marked increase in the ability to enter small diameter pores is present following enucleation. The mature granulocyte is capable of entering a 3-$\mu$m-pore-diameter capillary tube or penetrating a 1- to 3-$\mu$m filter during ameboid movement, whereas immature granulocytes cannot penetrate these size channels *in vitro*. This alteration in the biophysical character of maturing cells may play an important role in marrow egress since most cells undergo marked deformation during migration through pores in the marrow sinus wall.

### 8.3.2.3. Cell Chemotaxis

Like motility, chemotaxis of granulocytes is a feature of mature rather than immature cells (Giordano and Lichtman, 1973). Since motility is meager in immature cells, it is not possible to be sure whether the receptors for chemoattractants are present on immature cells by tests that require physiologic effects. Chemotaxis may be important because it may underlie the ability of mature marrow cells to accelerate their release in response to periods of increased demand for cells. This aspect of cell release may be most important for granulocytes and monocytes, highly motile cells capable of increased directed movement in a chemotactic gradient. Whether marrow reticulocytes can respond to a chemoattractant is unknown. Platelet release may be accelerated by the more rapid penetration of megakaryocyte pseudopods through the sinus wall, a reaction that could be facilitated by a chemoattractant for megakaryocyte peripheral cytoplasm.

### 8.3.3. Cell Releasing Factors

Evidence has been garnered that marrow cells can have their release accelerated by chemicals referred to as releasing factors (Boggs, 1966; Dornfest, 1970; Schultz *et al.*, 1973). Accelerated cell release could operate to facilitate cell delivery in two ways. First, a rapid release of reticulocytes and neutrophils from the marrow could increase their circulating pools rapidly since two-thirds of the reticulocytes are in the marrow and 90% of the neutrophils outside the tissues are in the marrow. There may be a small proportion of free platelets in the marrow (Aster, 1967; Odell and Murphy, 1974). If megakaryocyte cytoplasm is considered as a platelet pool, blood platelet counts could be increased rapidly without the production of new cells. With the exception of neutrophils, rapid release of marrow differentiated cells would produce a quantitatively trivial effect on the circulating pool. Second, the later stages of marrow transit time can be shortened by delivering newly produced cells into the circulation without a period of residence in a marrow pool of terminally differentiated cells. Accelerated release has an abbreviated effect unless increased production of cells ensues. This is especially true in the case of cells with a very short circulatory sojourn or tissue survival time. Most physiologic studies have been directed at understanding the response of marrow granulocytes to periods of increased needs. Less is known about the role of releasing factors in the delivery of red cells and platelets.

### 8.3.3.1. Physiologic Evidence

*In vivo* experiments indicate that accelerated release of marrow neutrophils occurs in response to neutropenia (Boggs *et al.*, 1966). *In vitro* experiments have also shown that reduced granulocyte counts in plasma can increase the release of marrow cells as judged by the elution of cells from isolated perfused femurs (Dornfest *et al.*, 1962a,b; Dornfest, 1970; Gordon *et al.*, 1960, 1964; Katz *et al.*, 1966; Lapin *et al.*, 1969). The release of marrow neutrophils in response to neutropenia appears to be mediated by a chemical releasing factor that is distinctive from endotoxin. It is possible that each cell type—reticulocytes, eosinophils, neutrophils, basophils, monocytes, and platelets—has a factor that may act to accelerate its release, specifically. Also, releasing factor for granulocytes appears to be chemically distinct from the factors responsible for the selective increase in the proliferation and maturation of each cell type (Broxmeyer *et al.*, 1974; Chikkappa *et al.*, 1977; Rothstein *et al.*, 1971). Some overlap in the effect of releasing factors may occur. Neutrophilia and reticulocytosis or neutrophilia and thrombocytosis occur in some reactive processes, e.g., hemolytic anemia or inflammation. To the extent that increased rate of release contributes to the increased cell counts, the releasing factor may work nonspecifically, for instance, by decreasing the barrier presented by the marrow sinus wall. This would favor release of any cell type. Alternatively, several specific releasing factors could play a role in these occurrences. The site of elaboration of releasing factors, the physiologic systems that control their concentrations in the marrow, and the specific nature of their interaction with cells have not been defined.

Cell releasing factors could affect egress rate in several ways. They could function as a specific chemoattractant, accelerating movement of differentiated cells into the marrow sinus. Also, they could act on the sinus wall or other stromal structures to reduce the impediment to egress. For example, a reduction in adventitial cell covering on the abluminal surface of the sinus may facilitate penetration of the endothelial cell by differentiated hematopoietic cells (Chamberlain *et al.*, 1975a; Weiss, 1970). They could also act on the endothelial cell to reduce the thickness of its cytoplasm, accounting for the very thin areas that develop, through which cells may migrate. Alternatively, a releasing factor could provide a molecular bridge to attach the migrating cell to the abluminal surface of the sinus endothelial cell, initiating a reaction that leads to the development of a migration channel.

### 8.3.3.2. Candidate Factors

Convincing evidence for a releasing factor for granulocytes has been obtained in studies of rats perfused with neutropenic plasma and in neutropenic dogs. These studies established that neutrophilia-inducing activity was not the result of endotoxemia and did not result from demargination of neutrophils. The neutrophilia was the result of release of new cells from marrow (Boggs *et al.*, 1966; Gordon *et al.*, 1960, 1964). These studies have provided support for a neutrophilia-inducing factor that acts by enhancing release of preformed neutrophils from the marrow.

Evidence has also been gathered to implicate plasma complement in marrow granulocyte release (Alpers *et al.*, 1972; Rother, 1972). It is not known whether complement acts to maintain the steady state blood concentration of neutrophils or whether it superimposes itself to perturb the steady state and thus contribute to neutrophilia. Complement factors are known to be chemoattractants for mature but not immature granulocytes (Giordano and Lichtman, 1973) and they could call forth differentiated cells, selectively. Glucocorticoid hormones and androgenic steroids also can induce release of marrow mature granulocytes (Bishop *et al.*, 1968; Deinard and Page, 1974; Vogel *et al.*, 1967). Their physiologic role is unclear.

Endotoxin also may facilitate granulocyte egress (Boggs *et al.*, 1968; Weiss, 1970). This effect could be related to an activation of complement by endotoxin. Endotoxin may result in accelerated granulocyte egress by reducing adventitial cell cover on the abluminal surface of the sinus wall also (Weiss, 1970).

Studies have implicated erythropoietin as a releasing factor for reticulocytes, in addition to its established role in stimulating proliferation of erythroid cells (Chamberlain *et al.*, 1975a,b; Fisher *et al.*, 1965; Gordon *et al.*, 1962). Thus, in the case of erythroid cells, the same chemical may be able to induce proliferation and accelerated release. The effect of erythropoietin on red cell release has not been fully elucidated. The administration of the hormone has been shown to reduce the adventitial cell cover of the sinus wall and may facilitate access of the reticulocyte to the endothelial cell. The reduction of adventitial reticular cell cover does not explain selectivity of release since such a change might facilitate egress of any cell type. Thus, it cannot be considered established that reduction in adventitial cell cover is a significant factor in accelerating the rate of egress. If it is, another factor probably contributes to a specific cell's egress.

### 8.3.4. Control of Blood Flow in Marrow

Several laboratories have examined the physiologic controls that may be exerted on blood flow to bone (Drinker *et al.*, 1922; Michelson, 1967, 1968). There is evidence that autonomic and autoregulatory mechanisms control blood flow through bone and presumably marrow. There is little firm evidence for the relationship of flow to cell release. There probably is a relationship between blood supply and the level of hematopoiesis. In studies of the histogenesis of marrow after experimental injury, restoration of hematopoiesis is dependent on the antecedent restoration of a sinusoidal circulation.

In a global sense, blood flow is required to deliver all hematopoietic cells from marrow to the systemic venous circulation. There is no evidence that blood flow can determine selective release of cells. Specific hematopoietic cells are not positioned adjacent to specific sinuses; thus recruitment of sinuses would not increase the delivery of cells in a specific manner. Since recruitment of cells is selective (i.e., if neutrophils are needed, their release is accelerated more or less specifically), an increase in flow of blood could not explain this aspect of marrow cell release.

### 8.3.5. Neural Structures in Marrow

Marrow has extensive networks of myelinated and nonmyelinated nerve fibers (Calvo and Forteza-Vila, 1970; Fliedner *et al.*, 1956, 1970) (Fig. 13). The main nerve to marrow follows the nutrient artery and its branches and the nerve innervates the muscular wall of these vessels. Nerves are evident also at the place where radial arteries branch toward the marrow periphery. Many nerve fibers appear to be independent of blood vessels. Some small branches make contact with sinuses while other branches continue in close contact to blood cell precursors. Nerves have been found to terminate within the hematopoietic compartment. The possible function of these neural networks within the hematopoietic compartment is not known. Contrary evidence has also been reported in

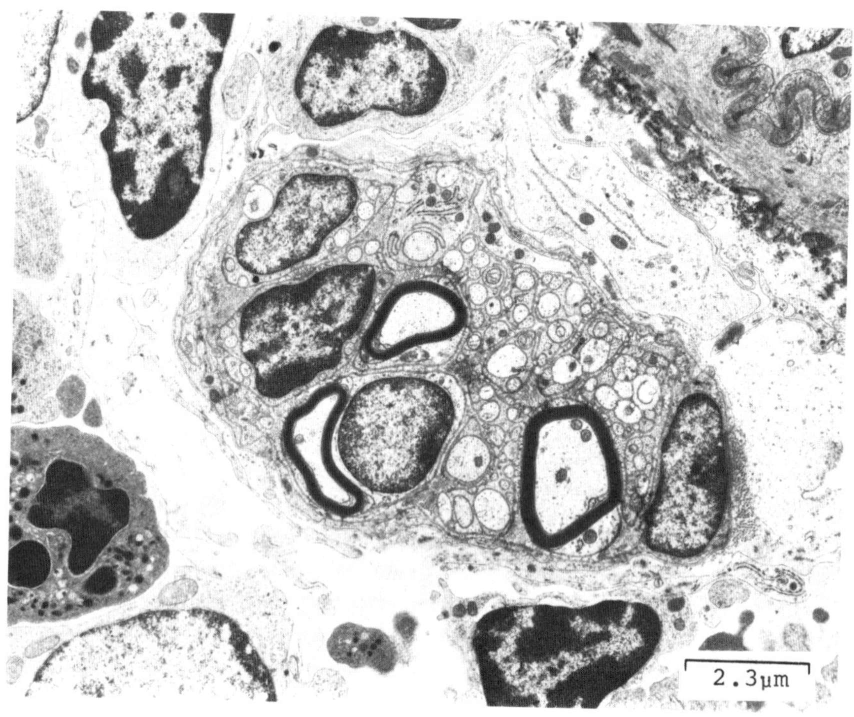



**Fig. 13.**  A transmission electron micrograph of a nerve in the hematopoietic compartment of mouse marrow. The nerve contains myelinated and poorly myelinated axons.
Schwann cells are present in the nerve bundle. A portion of an artery is present in the
upper right corner. Nerve fibers are present in its adventitia. Nerves in the hematopoietic
compartment unassociated with the adventitia may subserve a role other than
vasoregulation.

which free nerve endings in the hematopoietic compartment have not
been found (Miller and McCuskey, 1973). The presence of substantial
numbers of myelinated and nonmyelinated nerve fibers in the parenchyma of marrow unassociated with vessels, suggests that neural or neuro-
humoral influences may play a role additional to vasomotor control in
hematopoietic tissue. This is in keeping with recent evidence that several
central nervous system regions have free nerve terminals (nonsynaptic)
and that neurohumors may actually bathe these neural cells regulating
their threshold of responsivity.

## 8.4. The Anatomical Process of Release

The process of cell egress from the hematopoietic compartment to
the vascular sinus has been observed directly by both transmission and

scanning electron microscopy. Characteristic features of egress have been confirmed in several laboratories (Campbell, 1972; Chamberlain *et al.*, 1975a,b; De Bruyn *et al.*, 1971; Lichtman *et al.*, 1977b; Weiss, 1967, 1970). First, cell migration occurs through channels that develop at the time of cell transit and do not preexist. This conclusion is reached largely from two observations. First, very few breaks in endothelial continuity are seen in the sinus wall of well-fixed preparations of animal marrow by transmission electron microscopy. Moreover, mature cells abutting the sinus ready for egress are pressed against intact endothelium. In some cases small pseudopods of cells can be seen entering sinus endothelial cell cytoplasm without having broken through the luminal portion of the plasma membrane of the endothelial cell. Thus, it has been concluded that migrating cells make the hole that develops in the endothelial cell cytoplasm. Second, the diameter of migration channels is almost always much narrower than the spherical diameter of the cell, requiring substantial deformation of the cell during transit. The lateral pressure the marked deformation of the migrating cell exerts on the endothelial cell cytoplasm, as in a balloon so deformed, maintains continuity of the endothelial wall. This may prevent free communication from sinus to hematopoietic compartment, microhemorrhage, and platelet aggregation, or other injurious effects. Third, cell transit appears to be through the cytoplasm and not the intercellular junction of sinus endothelial cells. The presence of an endothelial cell junction next to a migrating cell occurs with a frequency that appears to exceed chance although a careful quantitative study of this has not been made. This association may be the result of cell egress occurring at the most peripheral part of endothelial cell cytoplasm where it is thin and less of a barrier rather than the result of the parajunctional cytoplasm having a specific character leading to egress at that site. Fourth, mature cells but not immature cells are found in the process of egress. Fifth, propulsion is presumably required for the cells to translocate across the sinus wall.

Adventitial reticular cell cytoplasm is absent at the site of penetration of the abluminal surface of the endothelial cell and the sinus wall may become attenuated at the site of cell egress. Dynamic studies of egress have not been made and static observations may be misinterpreted. For example, it is not known whether adventitial cell cover must be absent at the point of egress or whether the migrating cell can penetrate the reticular cell cytoplasm. Also, marked attenuation of the endothelial cell cytoplasm, as shown in Fig. 5, has not been established as being invariably necessary for cell penetration of the sinus.

It is not known how the exiting cell initiates egress. For example, does the pressure of pseudopod formation against the abluminal side of the endothelial cell wall lead to penetration into the sinus? Is there greater specificity in this process involving specific enzymes or sugars on the surface of the migrating cell in order for a migration pore to develop? Are there retaining structures in the hematopoietic compartment that are detached as the cell matures?

## 8.4.1. Erythrocytes

Passage of reticulocytes through the sinus wall usually occurs after enucleation of the erythroblast (Fig. 14). Occasionally, reticulocyte egress occurs simultaneously with enucleation, the nucleus apparently being removed in part by the resistance it meets at the site of the migration channel. Enucleation during egress is an infrequent event since most reticulocytes in the hematopoietic compartment are anucleate prior to their entry into the sinus (Fig. 15). Marked deformation usually occurs during reticulocyte egress and the location of egress is often at the periphery of an endothelial cell, near the cell junction.

## 8.4.2. Granulocytes, Monocytes, Lymphocytes

The shape of granulocytes, monocytes, and lymphocytes in egress through the sinus wall is similar to that of reticulocytes. Marked deformation of the cells occurs as they penetrate the cytoplasm of the endothelial cell to enter the sinus lumen (Fig. 16). Moreover, their egress also occurs

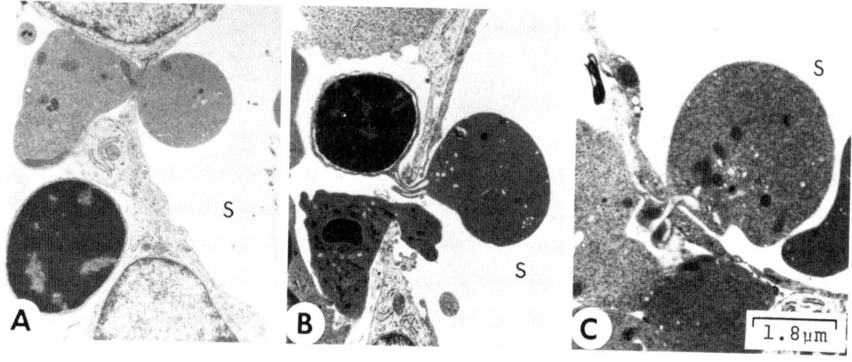


**Fig. 14.** A composite of three transmission electron micrographs of reticulocytes in egress. In each case the migration channel is very narrow and marked deformation of the cell occurs. (A) The reticulocyte is in egress just below an interdigitating endothelial junction. An erythroblast nucleus has been left in the perisinal space to be engulfed by a macrophage. (B) The reticulocyte in egress largely in the sinus lumen is still attached to its nucleus by a slender cytoplasmic filament. A granulocyte is in egress through the same migration channel. Most red cells in egress appear to have been completely enucleated in the hematopoietic compartment prior to exit. (C) A reticulocyte that has largely entered into the sinus lumen.

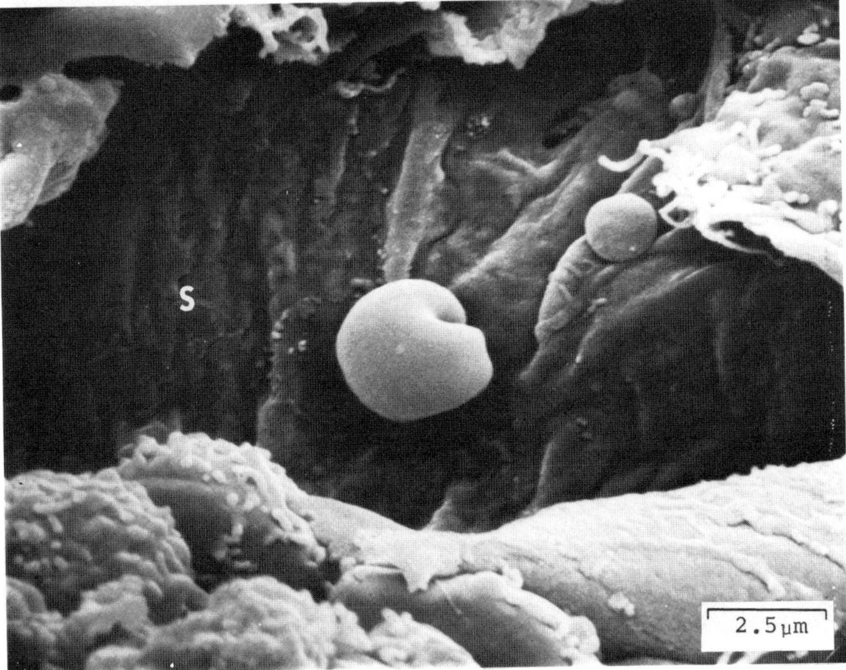


**Fig. 15.** A scanning electron micrograph of a marrow sinus. Two reticulocytes in different phases of egress are present. The smooth surface and the folds in the cell near the migration pore are characteristic of emigrating red cells.

frequently adjacent to junction of endothelial cells. The nucleus of the granulocyte, usually segmented, does not require marked deformation to traverse the migration pore, whereas the nuclei of monocytes and lymphocytes require more deformation to traverse the narrow migration pores in the sinus wall (Figs. 17 and 18). Little is known of the changes in nuclear deformability with cell maturation.

## 8.4.3. Platelets

The release of platelets into the vascular sinus occurs principally by the penetration of megakaryocyte periphery through the sinus wall (Becker and De Bruyn, 1976; Behnke, 1969; Lichtman *et al.*, 1977a). This is facilitated by the parasinusoidal position of the megakaryocyte. Peripheral cytoplasm probes the endothelial cell and small pseudopods may enter the abluminal surface of the endothelial cell and eventually penetrate it (Fig. 19). Large pseudopods of megakaryocte cytoplasm enter the

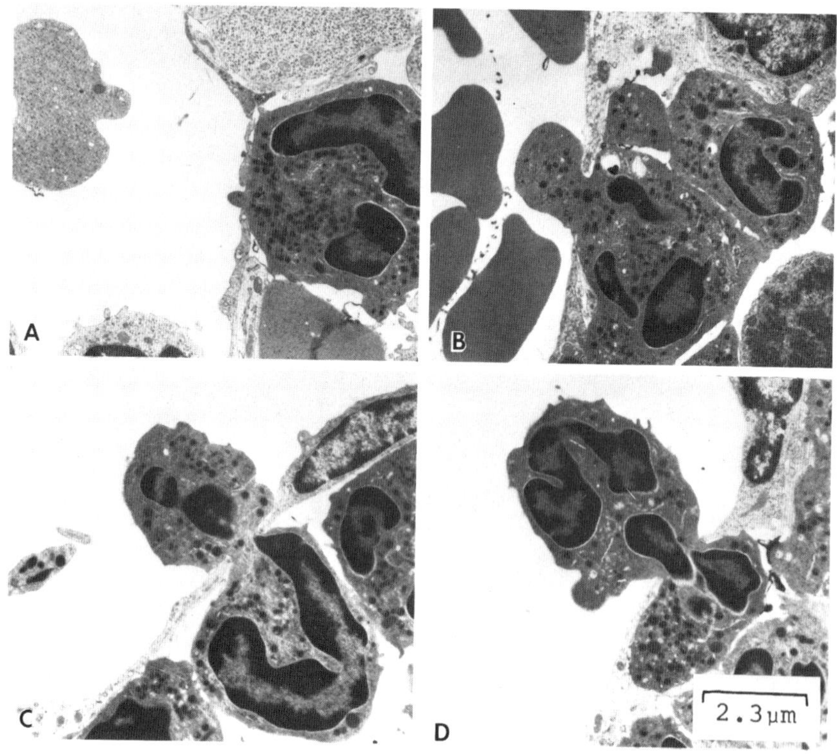



**Fig. 16.** A composite of four transmission electron micrographs of different granulocytes in egress. In each case a different proportion of the granulocyte has entered the sinus; however, the migration pore remains very narrow in relation to the spherical diameter of the cell. (A–D) Granulocytes in egress with increasing proportions of the cell in the sinus lumen.

sinus and become detached (Fig. 20). Little is known of the mechanism that detaches the pseudopod of platelets from the body of the megakaryocyte before the whole cell enters the sinus. These packets of platelets are presumably fragmented further in the circulation. The ability of megakaryocytes to form pseudopods has been observed *in vitro* (Thiery and Bessis, 1956). The presence of cytoplasmic pseudopods *in vivo* has been confirmed by many laboratories.

The presence of specialized organelles (contractile proteins) in the periphery of megakaryocyte cytoplasm probably endows it with ameboid movement. Observations of marrow by electron microscopy suggest that a pseudopod of megakaryocyte cytoplasm breaks off before the entire cell traverses the sinus wall (Fig. 21). Whole megakaryocytes or megakaryo-

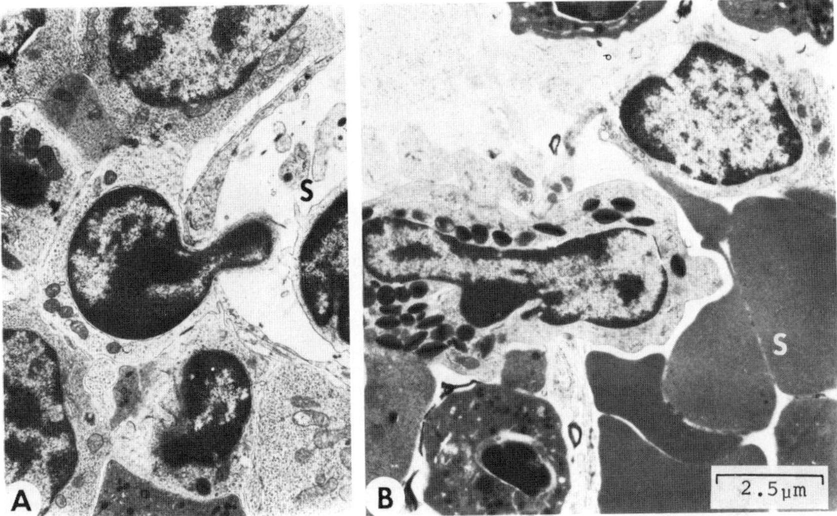

**Fig. 17.**   (A) A lymphocyte in egress. The nucleus is undergoing marked deformation as it enters the sinus (S). (B) An eosinophil traversing the sinus wall with one-third of the cell in the lumen of the sinus (S).

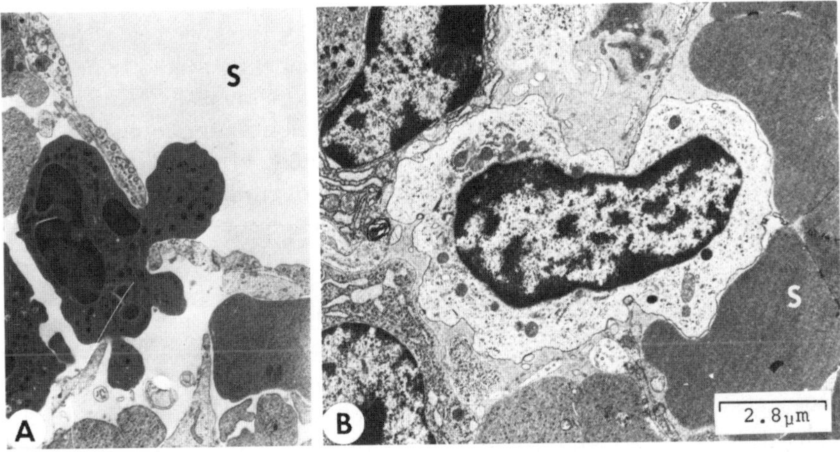

**Fig. 18.**   (A) A granulocyte in egress into the sinus (S). (B) A monocyte entering the sinus lumen (S).

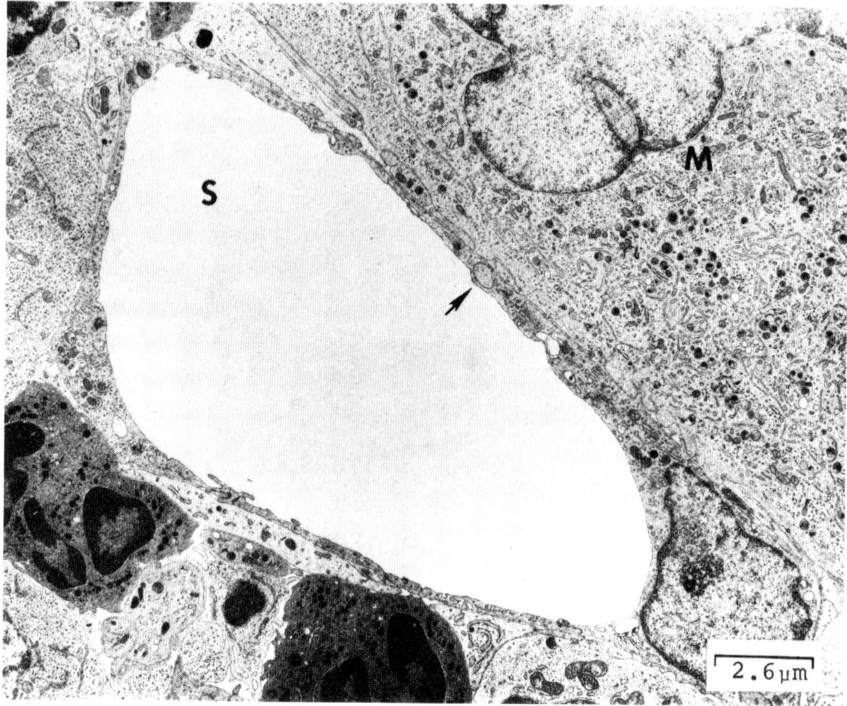

**Fig. 19.**   A megakaryocyte is shown adjacent to a marrow sinus (S). A bud of megakaryo-cyte cytoplasm (arrow) is invaginating the endothelial cell.

cyte nuclei are rarely seen in the sinuses of immersion-fixed bones. The fate of residual, "exhausted" megakaryocytes is unclear. A very small number of megakaryocytes enters the circulation. In general, however, after platelet production occurs by detachment of pseudopods, most exhausted megakaryocytes are presumably degraded in marrow. No direct evidence about the nature of this process has been presented.

## 8.5.  Release of Immature Cells in Healthy Subjects

The system that retains immature cells and megakaryocytes in the marrow is imperfect. In cell concentrates of blood one may find occasional immature granulocytes and megakaryocyte nuclei or whole megakaryo-cytes (Efrati and Rozenszajn, 1960). Nucleated red cells are very rarely

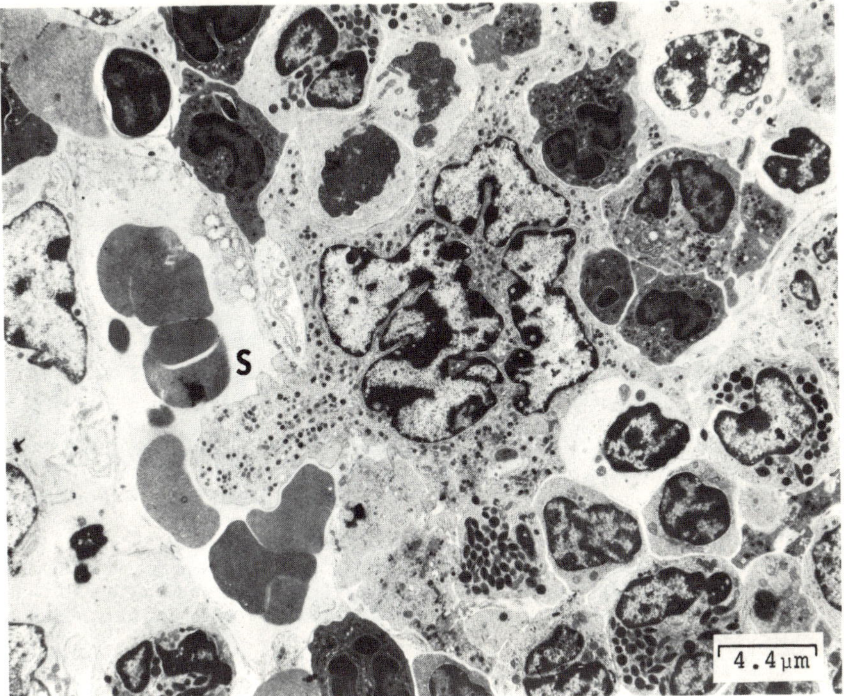

**Fig. 20.** A large pseudopod of a megakaryocyte's cytoplasm is in the sinus (S). The pseudopod is as large or larger than the red cells in the sinus.

seen. The absence of rare circulating erythroblasts may relate in part to splenic sequestration and enucleation of the late normoblast after release (Simpson and Kling, 1967). It is probable that very few nucleated red cells escape the marrow in any case. This is supported by the rarity of finding nucleated red cells in transit through the sinus wall or in the sinuses in marrow even after erythropoietin administration. Escaped immature cells may be trapped in organs like the spleen where they may mature and reenter the circulation. This is probably not a quantitatively important pathway since splenectomized individuals do not have large numbers of immature cells in the blood and because immature blood cells are very rare in spleen and other tissues in healthy individuals. The precise explanation for the small percentage of immature granulocytes in the blood is unknown. The late myelocyte and metamyelocyte have developed the capacity to move, respond to chemoattractants, and deform, albeit less well than the mature neutrophil, and thus may occasionally exit marrow

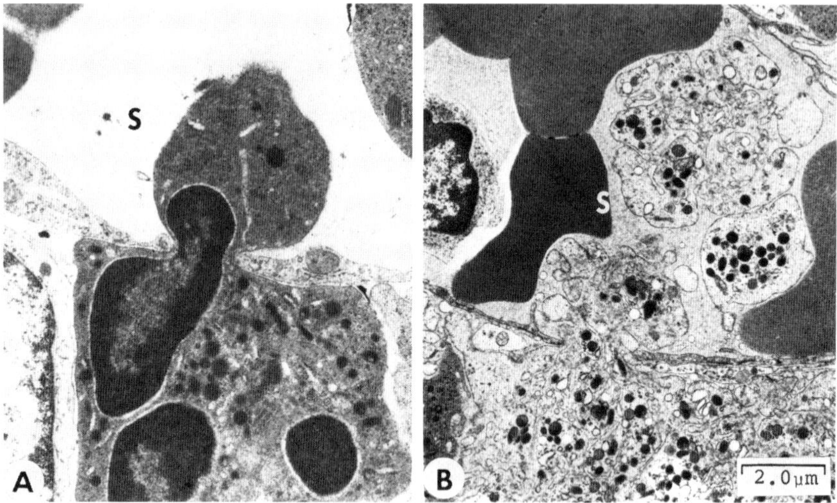

**Fig. 21.** The similarity of granulocyte egress (A) to platelet egress (B). The peripheral cytoplasm of the megakaryocyte protrudes a pseudopod into the sinus in a manner similar to the granulocyte or reticulocyte. Large packets of cytoplasm are detached. Note that the platelet packets are the size of red cells. Further demarcation and fragmentation takes place in the circulation.

by normal mechanisms. Alternatively, the sinus wall may undergo cyclic minor breakdowns, thereby allowing less mature cells to emerge. One may find in micrographs of marrow occasional degenerating megakaryocytes that project into the sinus lumen as though they have broken through a sinus wall. This may account for their presence in the venous circulation.

## 8.6. Release of Immature Cells in Pathological States

The exact mechanisms for the development of striking increases of immature cells in the blood under a variety of circumstances are not fully known. Increased circulating nucleated erythroid cells occur when there is intense stimulation to erythropoiesis such as during hypoxic states or hemolytic anemias. A similar slight increase in the proportion of immature granulocytes may occur when there is stimulation of granulopoiesis.

When cancers have metastasized to marrow, in the presence of hematopoietic malignancies, and in circumstances in which increased collagen is deposited in marrow, the prevalence of immature cells increases in the circulation. It has been hypothesized that damage to the architecture of marrow with a breakdown of the integrity of sinus walls allows cells to enter the circulation less discriminantly. Animal studies of transplantable leukemia have indicated that the extent of sinusoidal wall damage is correlated with the appearance of leukemic blast cells in the circulation (Chen *et al.*, 1972). Even in the circumstance in which the marrow is replaced by leukemic cells, a difference exists in the ratio of immature to mature cells in the marrow and blood. Blood tends to have a higher proportion of differentiated cells than marrow.

It is probable also that in some pathological states such as leukemia, the ability of undifferentiated cells to penetrate the sinus wall is greater than is that of their normal immature counterparts. Technical difficulties in the preparation of human marrow for quantitative analysis of its cytoarchitecture has slowed the progress toward a better understanding of the loss of full discrimination in the release of cells in pathological states.

## 8.7. Summary

The overall interactions of the four major factors that contribute to marrow cell egress are depicted in Fig. 22. A schematic of the hematopoietic compartment and a penetrating marrow sinus is shown. The complete endothelial lining of the marrow sinus and the extravascular position of hematopoietic cells contribute to the retention of cells in the marrow. The reticular cells forming the interrupted adventititial cover of the marrow sinus also send processes into the hematopoietic compartment. These processes may anchor hematopoietic cells. Immature cells are stimulated by cytopoietins to undergo proliferation and differentiation that adapt the cell so that it can penetrate the sinus wall. The rate of penetration may be governed by releasing factors that accelerate directed motility and reduce the adventitial cell covering of the sinus wall. Neural and vascular factors, poorly understood, may also facilitate egress.

ACKNOWLEDGMENT

The authors thank Joanne Lichtman for her invaluable assistance in the preparation of the bibliography. This work was supported by U.S. Public Health Service Grants HL 18208, and by a contract with the U.S. Energy Research and Development Administration at the University of Rochester Biomedical and Environmental Research Project and has been assigned Report No. UR-3490-1193.

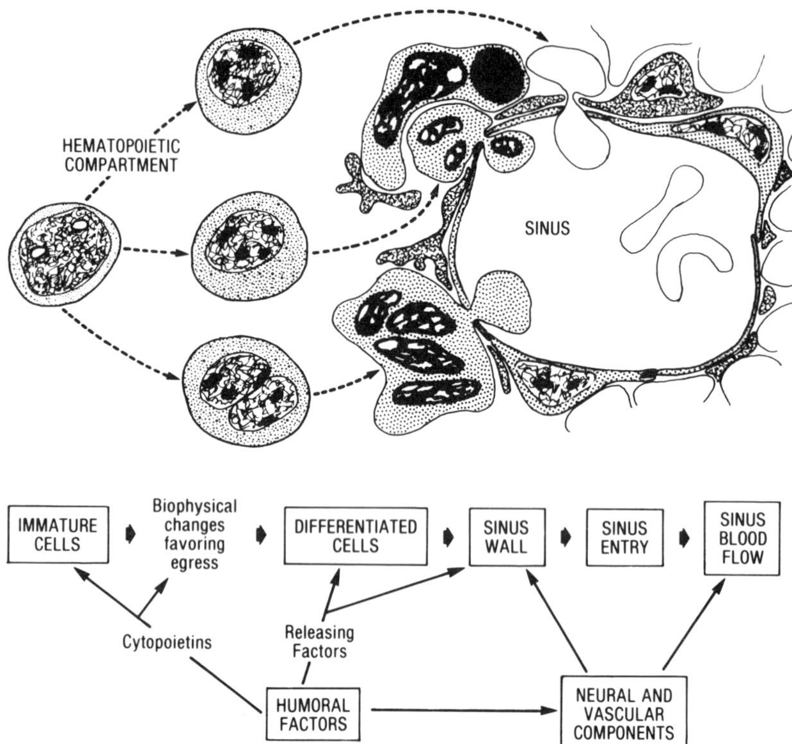



**Fig. 22.** A schematic diagram of the factors that may be involved in controlling the release of marrow cells. The central relationship between the hematopoietic compartment and marrow sinus is depicted. The drawing highlights the similarity of the egress process for the three major hematopoietic cells: reticulocytes in the top pathway, granulocytes and monocytes in the center pathway, and platelets in the lower pathway. Immature cells undergo biophysical changes under the influence of cytopoietins that favor egress. In the case of the reticulocyte, enucleation precedes egress. This is shown by the solid black inclusion in the perisinal macrophage representing nucleophagocytosis antecedent to digestion of the erythroblast nucleus. The cytoplasmic protrusion of the megakaryocyte presumably detaches itself from the cell and will further fragment into platelets in the circulation.

# References


Alpers, C. A., Colten, H. R., Rosen, F. S., Rabson, A. R., Mac Nab, G. M., and Gear, J. S. S., 1972, Homozygous deficiency of C3 in a patient with repeated infection, *Lancet* **ii:**1179.

Aster, R. H., 1967, Studies of the mechanism of "hypersplenic" thrombocytopenia in rats, *J. Lab. Clin. Med.* **70:**736.

Becker, R. P., and De Bruyn, P. P. H., 1976, The transmural passage of blood cells into myeloid sinusoids and the entry of platelets into the sinusoidal circulation: A scanning electron microscopic investigation, *Am. J. Anat.* **145**:183.

Behnke, O., 1969, An electron microscope study of the rat megakaryocyte. II. Some aspects of platelet release and microtubules, *J. Ultrastruct. Res.* **26**:111.

Ben-Ishay, Z., 1974, Reticular cells in erythroid islands: Their erythroblastophagocytic function, *J. Reticuloendothel. Soc.* **16**:340.

Ben-Ishay, Z., and Joffey, J. M., 1971, Reticular cells of erythroid islands of rat bone marrow in hypoxia and rebound, *J. Reticuloendothel. Soc.* **10**:482.

Ben-Ishay, Z., and Joffey, J. M., 1972, Ultrastructural studies of erythroblastic islands of rat bone marrow, *Lab. Invest.* **26**:637.

Bessis, M., 1958, L'îlot érythroblastique, unité fonctionnelle de la moelle osseuse, *Rev. Hématol.* **13**:8.

Bessis, M., 1973, The erythrocytic series, *in Living Blood Cells and Their Ultrastructure* (M. Bessis, ed.), Chapter II, pp. 85–180, Springer-Verlag, Berlin.

Bessis, M., and Breton-Gorius, J., 1962, Iron metabolism in the marrow as seen by electron microscopy: A critical review, *Blood* **19**:635.

Bishop, C. R., Athens, J. W., Boggs, D. R., Warner, H. R., Cartwright, G. E., and Wintrobe, M. M., 1968, Leukokinetic studies. XIII. A non-steady state kinetic evaluation of the mechanism of cortisone-induced granulocytosis, *J. Clin. Invest.* **47**:249.

Boggs, D. R., 1966, Homeostatic regulatory mechanisms of hematopoiesis, *Annu. Rev. Physiol.* **28**:39.

Boggs, D. R., Cartwright, G. E., and Wintrobe, M. M., 1966, Neutrophilia-inducing activity in plasma of dogs recovering from drug-induced myelotoxicity, *Am. J. Physiol.* **211**:51.

Boggs, D. R., Marsh, J. C., Chervenick, P. A., Cartwright, G. E., and Wintrobe, M. M., 1968, Neutrophil releasing activity in plasma of normal human subjects injected with endotoxin, *Proc. Soc. Exp. Biol. Med.* **127**:689.

Boström, L., 1948, Are non-nucleated erythrocytes formed by budding off of cytoplasm from normoblast, *Acta Med. Scand.* **81**:303.

Bränemark, P.-I., 1959, Vital microscopy of bone marrow, *Scand. J. Clin. Lab. Invest.* **11**(Suppl. 38):1.

Brookes, M., and Harrison, R. G., 1957, The vascularization of the rabbit femur and tibiofibula, *J. Anat.* **91**:61.

Broxmeyer, H., Van Zant, G., Zucali, J. R., LoBue, J., and Gordon, A. S., 1974, Mechanisms of leukocyte production and release. XII. A comparative assay of the leukocytosis-inducing factor (LIF) and the colony-stimulating factor (CSF), *Proc. Exp. Biol. Med.* **145**:1262.

Calvo, W., and Forteza-Vila, J., 1970, Schwann cells of the bone marrow, *Blood* **36**:180.

Campbell, F. R., 1967, Fine structure of the bone marrow of the chicken and the pigeon, *J. Morphol.* **123**:405.

Campbell, F. R., 1972, Ultrastructural studies of transmural migration of blood cells in the bone marrow of rats, mice and guinea pigs, *Am. J. Anat.* **135**:521.

Chamberlain, J. K., Leblond, P. F., and Weed, R. I., 1975a, Reduction of adventitial cell cover: An early direct effect of erythropoietin on bone marrow ultrastructure, *Blood Cells* **1**:655.

Chamberlain, J. K., Weiss, L., and Weed, R. I., 1975b, Bone marrow sinus cell packing: A determinant of cell release, *Blood* **46**:91.

Chen, L.-T., Handler, E. E., Handler, E. S., and Weiss, L., 1972, An electron microscopic study of the bone marrow of the rat in experimental myelogenous leukemia, *Blood* **39**:99.

Chikkappa, G., Chanana, A. D., Chandra, P., Commerford, S. L., and Cronkite, E. P., 1977, Granulocytopoiesis: Studies on leukocyte-inducing and colony-stimulating factors, *Proc. Soc. Exp. Biol. Med.* **154**:192.

De Bruyn, P. P. H., Thomas, T. B., and Michelson, S., 1966, Fine structure of the vascular components of guinea pig bone marrow, *Anat. Rec.* **154**:499.

De Bruyn, P. P. H., Breen, P. C., and Thomas, T. B., 1970, The microcirculation of the bone marrow, *Anat. Rec.* **168**:55.

De Bruyn, P. P. H., Michelson, S., and Thomas, T. B., 1971, The migration of blood cells of the bone marrow through the sinusoidal wall, *J. Morphol.* **133**:417.

De Bruyn, P. P. H., Michelson, S., and Becker, R. P., 1975, Endocytosis, transfer tubules and lysosomal activity in myeloid sinusoidal endothelium, *J. Ultrastruct. Res.* **53**:133.

Deinard, A. S., and Page, A. R., 1974, A study of steroid-induced granulocytosis in a patient with chronic benign neutropenia of childhood, *Br. J. Haematol.* **28**:333.

Donohue, D. M., Reiff, R. H., Hanson, M. L., Betson, Y., and Finch, C. A., 1958, Quantitative measurement of the erythrocytic and granulocytic cells of the marrow and blood, *J. Clin. Invest.* **37**:1571.

Dornfest, B. S., 1970, Perfusion techniques. A tool in elucidating blood cell release phenomena, *in Regulation of Hematopoiesis*, Vol. I, *Red Cell Production* (A. S. Gordon, ed.), pp. 237–267, Appleton-Century-Crofts, New York.

Dornfest, B. S., LoBue, J., Handler, E. S., Gordon, A. S., and Quastler, H., 1962a, Mechanisms of leukocyte production and release. I. Factors influencing leukocyte release from isolated perfused rat femora, *Acta Haematol.* **28**:42.

Dornfest, B. S., LoBue, J., Handler, E. S., Gordon, A. S., and Quastler, H., 1962b, Mechanisms of leukocyte production and release. II. Factors influencing leukocyte release from isolated perfused rat legs, *J. Lab. Clin. Med.* **60**:777.

Drinker, C. D., Drinker, K. R., and Lund, C. C., 1922, The circulation in the mammalian bone marrow, *Am. J. Physiol.* **62**:1.

Efrati, P., and Rozenszajn, L., 1960, The morphology of buffy coat in normal human adults, *Blood* **16**:1012.

Fisher, J. W., Lajtha, G., Buttoo, A. S., and Porteous, D. D., 1965, Direct effects of erythropoietin on the bone marrow of the isolated perfused hind limbs of rabbits, *Br. J. Haematol.* **11**:342.

Fliedner, T. M., Sandkühler, S., and Stodtmeister, R., 1956, Untersuchungen über die Gefässarchitektonik des Knochenmarkes der Ratte, *Z. Zellforsch.* **45**:328.

Fliedner, T. M., Calvo, W., Haas, R., Forteza, J., and Bohne, F., 1970, Morphologic and cytokinetic aspects of bone marrow stroma, *in Hematopoietic Cellular Proliferation* (F. Stohlman, Jr., ed.), pp. 67–86, Grune & Stratton, New York.

Giordano, G. F., and Lichtman, M. A., 1973, Marrow cell egress: The central interaction of barrier pore size and cell maturation, *J. Clin. Invest.* **52**:1154.

Gordon, A. S., Neri, R. O., Siegel, C. D., Dornfest, B. S., Handler, E. S., LoBue, J., and Eisler, M., 1960, Evidence for a leukocytosis inducing factor, *Acta Haematol.* **23**:323.

Gordon, A. S., LoBue, J., Dorfest, B. S., and Cooper, G. W., 1962, Reticulocyte and leukocyte release from isolated perfused rat legs and femurs, *in Erythropoiesis* (L. O. Jacobson and M. Doyle, eds.), pp. 321–327, Grune & Stratton, New York.

Gordon, A. S., Handler, E. S., Siegel, Ch. D., Dornfest, B. S., and LoBue, J., 1964, Plasma factors influencing leukocyte release in rats, *Ann. N.Y. Acad. Sci.* **113**:766.

Harker, L. A., 1968, Megakaryocyte quantitation, *J. Clin. Invest.* **47**:452.

Irino, S., Ono, T., Watanabe, K., Toyota, K., Unot, J., Takasugi, N., and Murakami, T., 1975, SEM studies on microvascular architecture, sinus wall, and transmural passage of blood cells in the bone marrow by a new method of infection replica and noncoated specimens, *in Scanning Electron Microscopy, Proceedings of the Eighth Annual Meeting* (O. Johari and I. Corvin, eds.), pp. 268–274, ITT Research Institute, Chicago.

Jahn, T. L., and Bovee, E. C., 1969, Protoplasmic movements within cells, *Physiol. Rev.* **49**:793.

Katz, R., Gordon, A. S., and Lapin, D. M., 1966, Mechanisms of leukocyte production and release. VI. Studies on the purification of the leukocytosis-inducing factor (LIF), *J. Reticuloendothel. Soc.* **3**:103.

Kaufman, R. M., Airo, R., Pollack, S., and Crosby, W. H., 1965, Circulating megakaryocytes and platelet release in the lung, *Blood* **26**:720.

Keyserlingk, D. G., and Albrecht, M., 1968, Über die pseudopodien von megakaryocyten und ihre bedeutung für die freisetzung von thrombocyten, *Z. Zellforsch.* **89**:320.

Lapin, D. M., LoBue, J., Gordon, A. S., Zanjani, E. D., and Schultz, E. F., 1969, Mechanisms of leukocyte production and release. IX. Kinetics of leukocyte release in leukocytapheresed rats, *Proc. Soc. Exp. Biol. Med.* **131**:756.

Leblond, P. F., La Celle, P. L., and Weed, R. I., 1971a, Rhéologie des érythroblastes et des érythrocytes dans la sphérocytose congénitale, *Nouv. Rev. Fr. Hematol.* **11**:537.

Leblond, P. F., La Celle, P. L., and Weed, R. I., 1971b, Cellular deformability: A possible determinant of the normal release of maturing erythrocytes from the bone marrow, *Blood* **37**:40.

Leblond, P. F., Chamberlain, J. K., and Weed, R. I., 1975, Scanning electron microscopy of erythropoietin-stimulated bone marrow, *Blood Cells* **1**:639.

Lichtman, M. A., 1970, Cellular deformability during maturation of the myeloblast: Possible role in marrow egress, *N. Engl. J. Med.* **283**:943.

Lichtman, M. A., 1973, Rheology of leukocytes, leukocyte suspensions and blood in leukemia, *J. Clin. Invest.* **52**:350.

Lichtman, M. A., and Kearney, E. A., 1976, The filterability of normal and leukemic human leukocytes, *Blood Cells* **2**:491.

Lichtman, M. A., and Weed, R. I., 1972a, Alteration of the cell periphery during granulocyte maturation: Relationship to cell function, *Blood* **39**:301.

Lichtman, M. A., and Weed, R. I., 1972b, Peripheral cytoplasmic characteristics of leukocytes in monocytic leukemia: Relationship to clinical manifestations, *Blood* **40**:52.

Lichtman, M. A., Chamberlain, J. K., Simon, W., and Santillo, P. A., 1977a, The parasinusoidal location of megakaryocytes in marrow: A determinant of platelet release and a physiologic version of vascular invasion and metastasis, *Trans. Assoc. Am. Physicians* **90**:313.

Lichtman, M. A., Chamberlain, J. K., Weed, R. I., Pincus, A., and Santillo, P. A., 1977b, The regulation of the release of granulocytes from normal marrow, *in The Granulocytes: Function and Clinical Utilization,* pp. 53–75, Alan R. Liss, New York.

Luk, S. C., and Simon, G. T., 1974, Phagocytosis of colloidal carbon and heterologous red blood cells in the bone marrow of rats and rabbits, *Am. J. Pathol.* **77**:423.

Maloney, M. A., and Patt, H. M., 1969, Origin of repopulating cells after localized bone marrow depletion, *Science* **165**:71.

Michelson, K., 1967, Pressure relationships in the bone marrow vascular bed, *Acta Physiol. Scand.* **71**:16.

Michelsen, K., 1968, Hemodynamics of the bone marrow circulation, *Acta Physiol. Scand.* **73**:264.

Miller, M. L., and McCuskey, R. S., 1973, Innervation of bone marrow in the rabbit, *Scand. J. Haematol.* **10**:17.

Odell, T. T., Jr., and Murphy, J. R., 1974, Effects of degree of thrombocytopenia on thrombopoietic response, *Blood* **44**:147.

Pease, D. C., 1956, Electron microscopic study of the red bone marrow, *Blood* **11**:501.

Pollard, T. D., and Weihing, R. R., 1974, Actin and myosin in cell movement, *CRC Crit. Rev. Biochem.* **2**:1.

Rother, K., 1972, Leucocyte mobilizing factor: A new biological activity derived from the third component of complement, *Eur. J. Immunol.* **2**:550.

Rothstein, G., Christensen, R. D., Hügl, E. H., and Athens, J. W., 1971, The relation of diffusible granulopoietic stimulator (DGS) to neutropenia and neutrophil releasing factor (NRF), *Blood* **38**:820.

Sabin, F. R., 1928, Bone marrow, *Physiol. Rev.* **8**:191.

Schultz, E. F., Lapin, D. M., and LoBue, J., 1973, Humoral regulation of neutrophil production and release, *in Humoral Control of Growth and Differentiation,* Vol. I (J. LoBue and A. S. Gordon, eds.), pp. 51–64, Academic Press, New York.

Simpson, C. F., and Kling, J. M., 1967, Mechanism of denucleation in circulating erythroblasts, *J. Cell Biol.* **35**:237.

Tanaka, Y., 1969, An electron microscopic study of nonphagocytic reticulum cells in human bone marrow. I. Cells with intracytoplasmic fibrils, *Acta Haematol. Jap.* **32**:275.

Tavassoli, M., 1974a, Bone marrow erythroclasia: The function of perisinal macrophages relative to the uptake of erythroid cells, *J. Reticuloendothel. Soc.* **15**:163.

Tavassoli, M., 1974b, Marrow adipose cells: Ultrastructural and histochemical characterization, *Arch. Pathol.* **98**:189.

Tavassoli, M., 1976, Marrow adipose cells: Histochemical identification of labile and stable components, *Arch. Pathol. Lab. Med.* **100**:16.

Tavassoli, M., and Crosby, W. H., 1973, Fate of the nucleus of marrow erythroblasts, *Science* **173**:912.

Thiery, J.-P., and Bessis, M., 1956, Mécanisme de la plaquettogenèse. Etude in vitro par la microcinématographie, *Rev. Hematol.* **11**:162.

Trubowitz, S., and Masek, B., 1970, The structural organization of the human marrow matrix in thin sections, *Am. J. Clin. Pathol.* **53**:908.

Vogel, M. J., Yankee, R. A., Kimball, H. R., Wolff, S. M., and Perry, S., 1967, The effect of etiocholanolone on granulocyte kinetics, *Blood* **30**:474.

Watanabe, Y., 1966, An electron microscopic study on the reticulo-endothelial system in the bone marrow, *Tohoku J. Exp. Med.* **89**:167.

Weiss, L., 1961, An electron microscopic study of the vascular sinuses of the bone marrow of the rabbit, *Bull. Johns Hopkins Hosp.* **108**:171.

Weiss, L., 1965, The structure of bone marrow. Functional interrelationship of vascular and hematopoietic compartments in experimental hemolytic anemia, *J. Morphol.* **117**:467.

Weiss, L., 1967, The histopathology of bone marrow, *Clin. Orthop.* **52**:13.

Weiss, L., 1970, Transmural cellular passage in the vascular sinuses of rat bone marrow, *Blood* **36**:189.

Weiss, L., and Chen, L.-T., 1975, The organization of hematopoietic cords and vascular sinuses in bone marrow, *Blood Cells* **1**:617.

Wright, J. H., 1910, The histogenesis of the blood platelets, *J. Morphol.* **21**:263.

Zamboni, L., and Pease, D. C., 1961, The vascular bed of the red bone marrow, *J. Ultrastruct. Res.* **5**:65.

# Structure and Function of Thymosin and Other Thymic Factors

## Teresa L. K. Low and Allan L. Goldstein

## 9.1. Introduction

At the turn of the century, Beard (1899, 1900) reported that the thymus gland was the source of the leukocytes that migrated out to create "new centers for growth, for increase and for useful work for themselves and for the body." He also postulated that the thymus was the parent source of all the lymphoid structure. In the decades that followed, studies on the immunological function of the thymus yielded two sets of contradictory observations. On the one hand, it was suggested that the thymus did not participate in immune reactions. This thought was based on the findings that the normal thymus did not form antibodies (Fagraeus, 1948a) or respond to antigenic stimulation (Fagraeus, 1948b). Furthermore, in most studies no significant influence of adult thymectomy on antibody forma-tion was observed (Hammar, 1938; Harris *et al.*, 1948; Maclean *et al.*,

TERESA L. K. LOW and ALLAN L. GOLDSTEIN • Department of Biochemistry, The George Washington University Medical Center, Washington, D.C. 20037.

1956). On the other hand, it was observed that the thymus underwent rapid involution in acute infections and that benign thymomas and "immunologic paralysis" occurred to patients with acquired agammaglobulinemia (Good and Varco, 1955), thus implying that the thymus may be involved in the control of lymphoid system and immune responses.

However, it was not until 1961 that the contribution of the thymus to the ontogenesis and maintenance of the lymphoid system was fully recognized. The dramatic demonstrations were made by Miller (1961) and Archer and Pierce (1961). They found that neonatal thymectomy, in contrast to adult thymectomy, in mice and in rabbits was associated with severe depletion in the lymphocyte population and serious immunological defects in the mature animal. These authors thus established that the thymus was necessary for the normal development of the immune response. The impact of their observations was so great that subsequent studies led to the rapid development of the field of cellular immunology and helped to define the properties of the thymic-dependent lymphocytes (T cells). It is now understood that functions under thymic control in mammals include primary transplant and tumor immunity, as well as viral, mycobacterial, fungal, and protozoal immunity. It is also well recognized that subpopulations of T cells (e.g., helper cells, suppressor cells, killer cells) may also influence the activity of B cell populations that produce antibodies (Gershon, 1975).

The endocrine function of the thymus has been the subject of many intensive as well as extensive investigations ever since the results of the *in vivo* effect of thymic extracts (Roberts and White, 1949; Gregoire and Duchateau, 1956; Comsa, 1956; Metcalf, 1956; Duplan *et al.*, 1962; Nakamoto, 1957; DeSomer *et al.*, 1963; Jankovic *et al.*, 1965; Klein *et al.*, 1965, 1966) and the effect of thymus grafts in cell-impermeable Millipore diffusion chambers (Levey *et al.*, 1963a,b; Osoba and Miller, 1964; Trench *et al.*, 1966) were disseminated. These reports also prompted our research on thymosin. Our studies were initiated in 1964 in the laboratory of Dr. Abraham White at the Albert Einstein College of Medicine. In order to establish the endocrine role of the thymus, we have isolated and are characterizing the thymic factors which act in lieu of an intact thymus gland to reconstitute thymectomized animals or enhance immunological competence in normal animals. These studies led to the isolation and identification of a lymphocytopoietic factor in rat and mouse thymus extracts (Klein *et al.*, 1965, 1966). Later, a stable form of the biologically active fraction was prepared from calf thymus which was termed thymosin (Goldstein *et al.*, 1966).

In this chapter, we shall first review the basic concept of the endocrine role of the thymus. Then we shall focus our attention primarily on the recent advances in our knowledge of the chemistry and biology of thymosin. Studies in our laboratory within the past 2 years have lent support to the hypothesis that thymosin consists of a family of biologically active polypeptide components. Ongoing studies suggest that these peptides may act in concert, sequentially, or separately on pre-T and T cell populations to maintain normal immunological reactivity. Lastly, the potential clinical application of thymosin and its relationship to aging will be discussed.

## 9.2. Endocrine Role of Thymus

The thymus gland is a bilobed lymphoid organ located immediately beneath the breastbone in the chest. In 160 A.D. Galen observed that the thymus grows rapidly during fetal life and during the first year after birth and then undergoes gradual involution with advancing age (cf. Duckworth, 1962). Although the thymus has probably been known since the day of Herophilos and Erasistratos (cf. Andreasen, 1947), until the last decade its function and physiological role were unknown.

### 9.2.1. Physiological Effects of Thymectomy

In 1845, Restelli initiated studies of experimental thymectomy in sheep, dogs, and calves in order to investigate the nature of thymus function. His studies reached no definitive conclusions regarding the physiological role of the thymus. Only 6 of 98 animals survived the immediate operation and all died within 23 days postoperatively as a consequence of infections. In fact, the early research on the effects of extirpation of the thymus gland yielded a large body of striking but conflicting results. This was owing largely to the following factors: (1) incomplete surgical thymectomy, (2) lack of knowledge of species variations in the anatomy of the thymus, and (3) failure to acknowledge the species differences in the state of development and function of lymphoid structures at birth. However, a number of these studies did suggest a possible role of the thymus in influencing skeletal growth (Comsa, 1938), gonadal development (Comsa, 1944; Gregoire, 1945), and maintenance of muscle tone (Abelous and Billard, 1896). It is also impressive to note the large number of deaths in thymectomized animals from apparent infections recorded in the earlier literature. These deaths were probably due partly to inadequate facilities for housing experimental animals and were perhaps partly related to the then unrecognized role of the thymus in host immunity.

The modern era of thymology began with the reports that neonatal thymectomy in the mouse (Miller, 1961) and in the rabbit (Archer and Pierce, 1961) results in failure of normal postnatal growth, lymphoid tissue development and maturation, and development of parameters of immunological competence. It has now been established that in many animals, including rabbits (Good *et al.*, 1962), rats (Jankovic *et al.*, 1962), guinea pigs (Fichtelius *et al.*, 1961), hamsters (Sherman and Dameshek, 1963), opposums (Miller *et al.*, 1965), dogs (Tilney *et al.*, 1965), and in the human (DiGeorge, 1968), removal or failure of the thymus to develop in the newborn will produce a diminished population of lymphocytes in lymphoid tissue, as well as in the blood. In addition, host immunological competence either fails to develop normally or is markedly depressed.

## 9.2.2. Reconstitution of Immune Functions with Crude and Purified Thymic Extracts

The effects of neonatal and adult thymectomy and the resulting physiological and biochemical alterations and deficiencies have been studied extensively and have helped to establish that the thymus has an endocrine role. This approach has established the major role of thymus in the development of the lymphoid system and immunological function. Another approach to demonstrate the endocrine role of the thymus has relied on reconstitution experiments with cell-free thymus extracts.

Beginning as early as 1896 with the report by Abelous and Billard describing restoration of muscle tone in thymectomized frogs given crude thymic extracts, and continuing today, many investigators have attempted to isolate putative thymic hormones and have examined effects of a variety of thymic extracts in both normal and thymectomized animals (cf. Goldstein and White, 1970, 1971; Trainin, 1974; White and Goldstein, 1968; Goldstein *et al.*, 1970).

Prior to 1961, thymic extracts have been reported to stimulate such diverse processes as calcium and phosphorus metabolism (Eskelund and Plum, 1953; Schwartz *et al.*, 1953), gonadal growth (Rowntree *et al.*, 1934), and glucose metabolism (Bomskov and Sladovic, 1940). Thymic extracts were also found to modify animal growth and development (Goslar, 1958; Nowinski, 1930, 1933; Rowntree *et al.*, 1934) and influence muscle metabolism and myasthenia gravis (Adler, 1937; Thurner, 1924; Torda and Wolff, 1947; Wolf and Erb, 1970). In 1940, Bomskov and Sladovic reported that only extracts from normal thymus produced lymphocytosis in rats, guinea pigs, and pigeons. Telkkä and Teir (1955) observed a rise in thymic lymphoid mitotic activity that was induced by thymus extracts. Comsa (1957a) described the lymphopoietic effect of a purified thymic extract given to thyroidectomized guinea pigs. A most important finding of Comsa's during this period was the demonstration of a direct influence of thymic extract on lymphoid tissue (Comsa, 1940, 1956), and that some of the effects of thymectomy in guinea pigs (Comsa, 1955) could be corrected by thymic extract treatment.

In 1949, Roberts and White reported that partially purified fractions from rat thymus were effective in producing lymphoid tissue hypertrophy and lymphocytosis in rats. This lymphopoietic activity of crude thymic extracts was subsequently supported in 1956 by Gregoire and Duchateau in their studies with implantation of thymus epithelium and by Metcalf (1956) in his study with cell-free thymic extracts. Of major importance was the finding that irradiated, cortically depleted implants of pig and rabbit thymuses caused hyperplasia of regional lymph nodes (Gregoire and Duchateau, 1956), suggesting the production of a hormonal factor from thymus epithelial cells capable of activating lymphoid cells.

In the period between 1961 and 1966, experiments in this field were primarily confined to thymectomy restoration by thymus tissue enclosed in cell-impermeable Millipore chambers (Osoba and Miller, 1964; Aisenberg and Wilkes, 1965; Schaller and Stevenson, 1967; MacGillivray *et al.*, 1964; Levey *et al.*, 1963a,b).

Later, experimentation using cell-free products of the thymus gland was reported (cf. Goldstein and White, 1971). Since 1966 and continuing until the present time, there have been numerous reports of the isolation of different biologically active thymic extracts. In a symposium held at Rijswijk, The Netherlands (van Bekkum, 1975), many of the aspects of the biological activity of several of the thymic factors were reviewed. Table I summarizes some of the thymic extracts and their biological effects reported so far.

Thymosin, the most extensively studied of the thymic factors, is discussed in detail in the following sections. Three other thymic factors (THF, STF, and thymopoietin) that have been well characterized are now described with reference to their biological activities.

### 9.2.2.1. Thymic Humoral Factor

Nathan Trainin and his colleagues at the Weizmann Institute separated extracts from thymuses of sheep, calves, and rabbits (Trainin *et al.*, 1966; Trainin *et al.*, 1967a,b) that were capable of inducing lymphocytopoiesis and immune reconstitution in normal and thymectomized mice. The active factor was termed thymic humoral factor (THF). The procedures for the extraction of THF are relatively simple (Kook *et al.*, 1975; Trainin and Small, 1970). THF is prepared by homogenization of the thymus gland followed by clarification at 2500 rpm. THF is then passed through gauze and centrifuged again at 105,000 $\times$ $g$ for 5 hr. These

**Table I.**   Some Thymic Extracts and Their Reported Biological Effects

| Year | Authors | Type of thymic extract | Reported biological effects |
|---|---|---|---|
| 1896 | Abelous and Billard | Calf thymus | Restoration of muscle tone and skin color in thymectomized frogs |
| 1905 | Bracci | Rabbit thymus, aqueous | Stimulation of calcium metabolism and reduced calcium excretion in thymectomized rabbits |
| 1930 | Nowinski | Calf thymus, aqueous (thymocresin) | Stimulation of growth and increased size of gonads in rats |
| 1933 | Asher | Calf thymus? | Substitutive in thymectomized guinea pigs. Restored normal growth in rats reared on a poor diet without specific deficiencies |
| 1934 | Rowntree *et al.* | Calf neck thymus, acid aqueous | Increased growth rate and fertility of rats |
| 1940 | Bomskov and Slodovic | Calf thymus, lipid extract (thymus hormone) | Diabetogenic in rats, guinea pigs, and rabbits |
| 1940 | Rehn | Calf thymus | Lymphocytosis in man |
| 1947 | Torda and Wolff | Cat thymus | Depressed acetylcholine synthesis |
| 1949 | Roberts and White | Calf thymus saline extract; ethanol-insoluble fraction | Stimulation of lymphocytopoiesis and increased lymphoid tissue size in adult rats |
| 1949 | Constant *et al.* | Human, dog, and cat thymus. Saline extract | Decreased the neuromuscular contractions (contained curare-like substance) |
| 1953 | Schwartz *et al.* | Calf thymus, lyophilized extract | Increased serum phosphate and calcium levels in man and dog |
| 1953 | Eskelund and Plum | Calf thymus | Accelerated the healing of fractures |
| 1953 | Molnar and Kovacs | Calf thymus | Modified the metastatic trend and localization of transplants of Brown–Pierce carcinomas in rabbits |
| 1955 | Wilson and Wilson | Calf, human, and fetal whale thymus, acetone-soluble saline extract | Inhibiting effects on rat phrenic nerve diaphragm preparation |
| 1955 | Telkkä and Teir | Rat thymus | Stimulation in the mitotic activity of the thymus |
| 1956 | Gregoire and Duchateau | Irradiated pig thymus extract | Production of hyperplastic changes in regional lymph nodes of rats |

**Table I.** (*continued*)

| Year | Authors | Type of thymic extract | Reported biological effects |
|---|---|---|---|
| 1956 | Metcalf | Mouse or human thymus extract; heat labile, non-dialyzable, lymphocyte-stimulating factor (LSF) | Blood lymphocytosis in young mice |
| 1957 | Nakamoto | Cow thymus, lipid rich | Blood lymphocytosis in young rabbits |
| 1957a,b | Comsa | Calf thymus | Lymphopoietic effect on thyroidectomized guinea pigs |
| 1958 | Bezssonoff and Comsa | Veal thymus; ethanol insoluble, protein rich | Prevention of creatinuria in thymectomized, thyroid-ectomized, castrated guinea pigs after exoge-nous thyroxine injection |
| 1962 | Duplan *et al.* | Mouse thymus | Blood lymphocytosis |
| 1962 | Szent-Gyorgyi *et al.* | Thymus and other organs; low-molecular-weight substances (promine, retine, and sterilizing factor) | Stimulation or inhibition of tumor growth; induction of temporary sterility |
| 1963 | DeSomer *et al.* | Cell-free extract from incubated calf thymic slices | Increased blood lympho-cytes; prevention of wast-ing and fatal virus infec-tion in thymectomized mice |
| 1964 | Maisin | Neonatal mouse thymus | Protection of skin of mice against cancer induced by methylcholanthrene |
| 1964 | Camblin and Bridges | Rat and rabbit thymus | Lymphocytosis on X-irradi-ated rats |
| 1965 | Klein *et al.* | Mouse, rat, and calf thy-mus; $105,000 \times g$ supernatant fluid of saline extract | Production of lymphocyto-poiesis and growth of peripheral lymphoid tissue |
| 1965 | Jankovic *et al.* | Rat thymus, lipid-rich extract | Blood lymphocytosis and improved immunological responsiveness of the delayed hypersensitivity type |
| 1965 | Pansky *et al.* | AKR mouse thymus, ace-tone-insoluble fraction | Decreased blood glucose in AKR mice |
| 1965 | Bernardi and Comsa | Calf or sheep thymus; homeostatic thymus hormone (HTH) | Suppressed the conse-quences of thymectomy on lymphatic tissue, ade-nohypophyse, thyroid, and adrenal in guinea pigs and rats |
| 1966 | Goldstein *et al.* | Calf thymus, partially pur-ified protein (thymosin) | Stimulation of lymphocyto-poiesis and lymphoid tis- |

**Table I.** (*continued*)

| Year | Authors | Type of thymic extract | Reported biological effects |
|---|---|---|---|
| | | | sue growth *in vivo* and DNA, RNA, and protein synthesis |
| 1966 | Comsa | Veal thymus; glycopeptide, molecular weight 3000 | Prevention of all consequences of thymectomy in guinea pigs and rats |
| 1966 | Trainin *et al.* | Cell-free extract of sheep, calf, or rabbit thymus (THF) | Stimulation of lymphopoiesis and prevention of wasting in neonatally thymectomized mice |
| 1966 | Potop *et al.* | Calf thymus; aqueous protein and peptide extract | Increased ATP and decreased inorganic phosphate content of muscle and serum of thymectomized rabbits |
| 1967a | Trainin *et al.* | Calf thymus; $105,000 \times g$ supernatant fluid; heat labile, nondialyzable factor | Stimulation of lymphopoiesis in thymectomized mice |
| 1967 | Hand *et al.* | Bovine thymus crystalline basic protein, molecular weight 10,000–30,000 (LSH) | Blood lymphocytosis in mice |
| 1970 | Mizutani *et al.* | Bovine thymus (hypocalcemic factor) | Produced hypocalcemia in rabbits |
| 1971 | Milcu and Potop | Calf thymus (TP, lipid in nature) | Antiblastic activity |
| 1972 | Robey *et al.* | Calf thymus (LSH$_r$) | Accelerated the appearance of hemolysin to sheep erythrocytes in neonatal mice |
| 1972 | Goldstein *et al.* | Calf thymus (thymosin fractions 7 & 8, aggregate of two or more smaller peptides) | Restored the population of azathioprine-sensitive cells in the rosette bioassay |
| 1974 | G. Goldstein | Bovine thymus (thymopoietin I and II, or "thymin") | Caused delayed impairment of neuromuscular transmission *in vivo;* induced bone marrow cells to develop intrathymic lymphocytes |
| 1975 | Bach *et al.* | Normal mouse serum (serum thymic factor) | Induced the appearance of sensitivity to AZ and A$\Theta$S in spleen cells of adult thymectomized mice |
| 1975 | Hooper *et al.* | Calf thymus (thymosin fraction 5) | Induced T cell differentiation and enhanced immunological function |

**Table I.   (_continued_)**

| Year | Authors | Type of thymic extract | Reported biological effects |
|---|---|---|---|
| | | | in animal models and in humans |
| 1977a | Goldstein _et al._ | Calf thymus (thymosin $\alpha_1$, the first purified and sequenced thymosin polypeptide) | Increased mitogenic responsiveness of murine lymphocytes; induced enhancement of MIF production; increased population of Ly 1,2,3 positive cells |
| 1977 | Ernström and Nordlind | Calf thymus | Potent stimulator of DNA synthesis in lymphocytes |
| 1977 | Astaldi _et al._ | Human serum (serum factor, can be induced by thymosin) | Increased cellular levels of cyclic AMP |

supernatants are then dialyzed against water for 60 hr. The dialysate comprising material with molecular weights below 6000 is then lyophilized and constitutes the crude extract. Further purification is achieved by gel filtration on Sephadex G-25 and the active peak is rechromatographed on DEAE–Sephadex A-25. The peak eluted at 0.15 M NaCl contains all the activity. The active polypeptide which is heat stable has a p$I$ of 5.7–5.9 and a molecular weight of approximately 3000. THF survives treatments with ribonucleases and deoxyribonucleases but is destroyed by pronase digestion. This peptide consists of 31 amino acid residues according to the amino acid analysis (Trainin _et al._, 1975). However, the sequence has not yet been reported.

The major assay for THF is based on a model for _in vitro_ graft versus host reaction (GVHR) first introduced by Auerbach and Globerson (1966). Two small (1 mm$^3$) sections of spleen from newborn F1 donors are placed on Millipore filters and immersed in medium. After 24 hr at 37°C, parental spleen cells are placed on one section and syngeneic F1 spleen cells on the other. At the end of 4 days the sections are measured with an ocular micrometer. Ratios of allogeneic to syngeneic splenomegaly of 1.2 or greater are considered positive. While $1 \times 10^6$ normal parental cells give positive GVHR, cells from neonatally thymectomized (NeoTx) mice do not (Trainin _et al._, 1969). THF activity is detected, therefore, by the ability of an extract preparation to restore the GVHR capacity to the cells of NeoTx parental animals. Those extracts producing three out of five positive pairs at a dilution of 1:50 are considered active. This is obviously a qualitative assay, but it has been very effectively applied for purification and characterization of THF preparations.

### 9.2.2.2. Thymopoietin

Thymopoietin was first isolated by G. Goldstein (1974, 1975; Goldstein and Mananaro, 1971) and was initially named thymin. The preparation of this peptide was developed from experimental studies related to the human disease myasthenia gravis. This disease is characterized by a deficit in neuromuscular transmission and thymic malfunction (Lindstrom *et al.*, 1976). Based on the impairment of neuromuscular transmission with thymin (thymopoietin), the neuromuscular blocking substance thymopoietin was isolated from thymus tissue (G. Goldstein, 1975). It can also induce differentiation of bone marrow cells to T cells *in vitro* and hence has been claimed to be a putative thymic hormone. The purification procedures include homogenization, a heat step (70°C, 30 min), and filtration through gauze and cotton. After concentration on Diaflo (XM100A; UM2) and two passages on Sephadex G-50, the eluates (two times the void volume) are lyophilized and fractionated on hydroxyapatite. The active volumes are desalted (G-25) and provide two peaks of activity when eluted from QAE Sephadex. The yield is approximately 1 mg/kg of tissue. The two isopeptides thymopoietin I and II are apparently related by peptide mapping and immunological cross-reactions. Thymopoietin II has a molecular weight of 5562 daltons and a p$I$ of 5.5. The sequence of the molecule has been delineated (Fig. 1) (Schlesinger and Goldstein, 1975). It is composed of 49 amino acids, and a 13 amino acid fragment possessing 3% of the parental activity has been synthesized (Schlesinger *et al.*, 1975).

### 9.2.2.3. Serum Thymic Factor

Following their studies with Goldstein and White showing thymosin induction of theta ($\theta$) antigen and increase in azathioprine sensitivity in rosette-forming cells (FC) from adult thymectomized mice (Bach *et al.*, 1971), Bach and co-workers isolated a serum factor from normal mice which demonstrated the same properties (Bach *et al.*, 1973). They named this activity the circulating thymic factor (TF). Most recently this factor has been purified and the amino acid sequence determined (Bach *et al.*, 1977), and it has been renamed the serum thymic factor (STF) (Fig. 1).

STF is now routinely isolated from pig blood (Bach *et al.*, 1975). The isolation procedure is briefly as follows. Ninety liters of blood from 3- to 4-month-old pigs is defibrinated by mechanical agitation, the serum ultrafiltered by pressure dialysis, and the filtrate concentrated by Amicon diafiltration. At this point the titer as measured by the rosette assay is increased from 1/128 to 1/25,000. Purification is accomplished in five steps: (1) Sephadex chromatography, (2) desalting, (3) carboxymethylcellulose chromatography (eluting in 0.1–0.15 M NaCl with an activity dilution of 1/500,000, (4) desalting, and (5) Sephadex G-25 chromatography in acetic

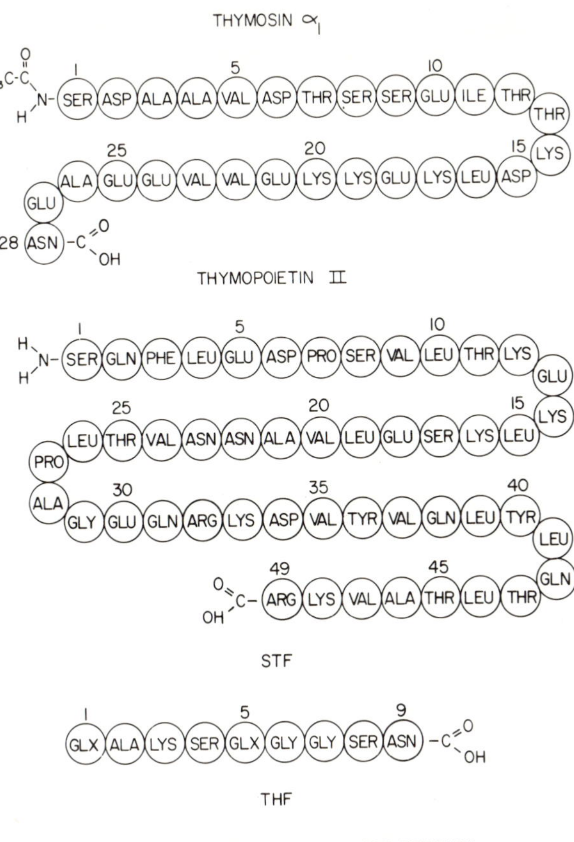



**Fig. 1.** Amino acid sequence of purified thymic factors: thymosin $\alpha_1$ (Goldstein *et al.*, 1977a), thymopoietin II (Schlesinger and Goldstein, 1975), STF (Bach *et al.*, 1977), THF (Trainin *et al.*, 1975). The GLX in positions 1 and 5 of the STF sequence denotes existing uncertainties as to the identity of the amino acids at these positions.

acid. The final titer is $1/10^6$ with a yield of 2 $\mu$g. The molecular weight of STF is 959. It is destroyed by trypsin, chymotrypsin, and pronase, and has a p*I* of 7.5. The amino terminal is blocked.

### 9.2.3. From Postulation to Establishment of the Thymus as an Endocrine Gland

Based on the experimental and clinical data, it is evident that the thymus is an important endocrine gland. It is also clear that at least three regulatory roles are exerted by this organ: (1) the production and export to the peripheral tissues of immunocompetent T cells; (2) the synthesis and secretion of thymic hormones by the epithelial cells; and (3) the provision of a thymic microenvironment suitable for the maturation of T cells which ultimately express functions that deal specifically with parameters of host immunological competence.

## 9.3. Chemical and Biological Characterization of Thymosin

Beginning in 1964, Klein, Goldstein, and White initiated the research which has led to the identification of a lymphopoietic factor in rat and mouse thymus extracts (Klein *et al.*, 1965, 1966). In 1966, an acetone-precipitable stable form of the biologically active fraction was prepared from calf thymus and was termed thymosin fraction 3 (Goldstein *et al.*, 1966). In 1972, after further fractionation of the crude extract, the preparation and characterization of a more purified fraction was achieved including the isolation of one of the active components, a protein with a molecular weight of 12,600 (Goldstein *et al.*, 1972). In 1975 a modified procedure was developed to prepare large quantities of material, termed thymosin fraction 5, for clinical trials (Hooper *et al.*, 1975).

### 9.3.1. Thymosin Fraction 5

Thymosin fraction 5 is prepared from calf thymus as described by Hooper *et al.* (1975). The purification procedures are outlined in Fig. 2. Thymus tissue is thawed and trimmed free of adipose tissue and is processed in batches of 5 kg. The thymus tissue is homogenized in 3 volumes of 0.15 M NaCl and 0.16% octyl alcohol (v/v) in a Waring blender for 3 min at top speed. The homogenate is centrifuged at $14,000 \times g$ to sediment the nuclear materials and 2-liter portions of the supernatant are heated with stirring to 80°C in a boiling water bath. The voluminous precipitate of heat-denatured protein is removed by filtration through Miracloth. The clear yellow filtrate is cooled to 4°C and added slowly, with stirring, to 5 volumes of acetone at $-10°C$. The precipitate is collected on a large Buchner funnel, washed with several volumes of cold $(-10°C)$ acetone, and dried in a desiccator under reduced pressure. The white powder obtained by this procedure is suspended in 10 volumes of 10 mM sodium phosphate, pH 7.0, and stirred at room temperature for 1 hr. A small amount of insoluble residue is removed by centrifugation at 15,000 $\times g$ and the sample is adjusted to a protein concentration of 25 mg/ml as determined by the Lowry procedure (Lowry, 1951). Saturated ammonium sulfate solution adjusted to pH 7.0 with $NH_4OH$ is added (33.3 ml to each 100 ml solution), and the solution is stirred for 1 hr. The

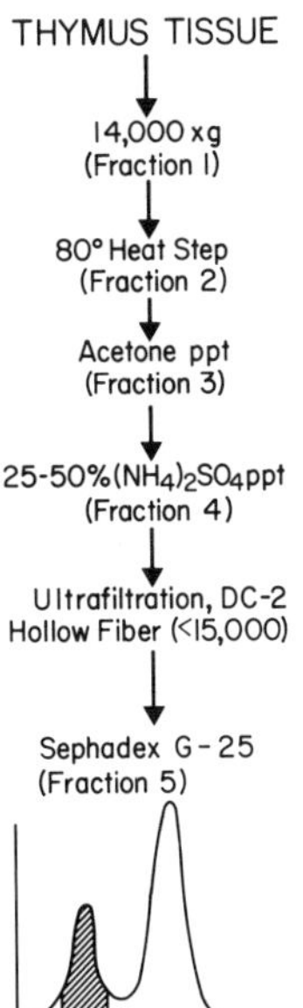


**Fig. 2.** Purification of bovine thymosin fraction 5 (Goldstein *et al.*, 1966; Hooper *et al.*, 1975). One kilogram of thymus tissue homogenized in 3 liters of NaCl provides the sample to initiate the procedure.

precipitate is removed by centrifugation and the supernatant is adjusted to pH 4.0 with acetic acid. Solid ammonium sulfate (14.6 g/100 ml) is added and the suspension is stirred for 1 hr. The precipitate is collected by centrifugation, dissolved in 10 mM tris-HCl (pH 8.0) at a concentration of 10 mg/ml protein, and subjected to ultrafiltration at room temperature in an Amicon DC-2 hollow fiber system (concentration mode, H1DP10 membrane cartridge). The filtrate is collected at 4°C, concentrated by rotary evaporation under reduced pressure, and desalted on a 5 × 80-cm column of Sephadex G-25 (fine) equilibrated with deionized water. The protein peak which elutes in advance of the salt and nucleotide peak is pooled, concentrated by rotary evaporation, and dried by lyophilization.

### 9.3.1.1. Chemical Characterization and Nomenclature of Thymosin Polypeptides

Thymosin fraction 5 is composed of a group of polypeptides with molecular weights ranging from 1000 to 15,000. They are heat stable up to 80°C. The preparation contains a small amount of carbohydrate and is essentially free of lipids and nucleotides.

Our major effort in our continuing biological studies of thymosin is to understand the molecular events by which the thymus gland exerts control over T cell development. In order to understand the detailed mechanism(s) of how each thymosin polypeptide exerts control over the development and senescence of immunological responses, we have been undertaking the isolation and characterization of each polypeptide component in thymosin fraction 5 and a detailed study of their individual biological functions.

To facilitate the identification and comparison of all the thymic peptides from one laboratory to another, we have proposed a nomenclature based on the isoelectric pattern of thymosin fraction 5 in the pH range 3.5–9.5. As shown in Fig. 3, the separated peptides are divided into three regions: the $\alpha$ region consists of peptides with p$I$ below 5.0, the $\beta$

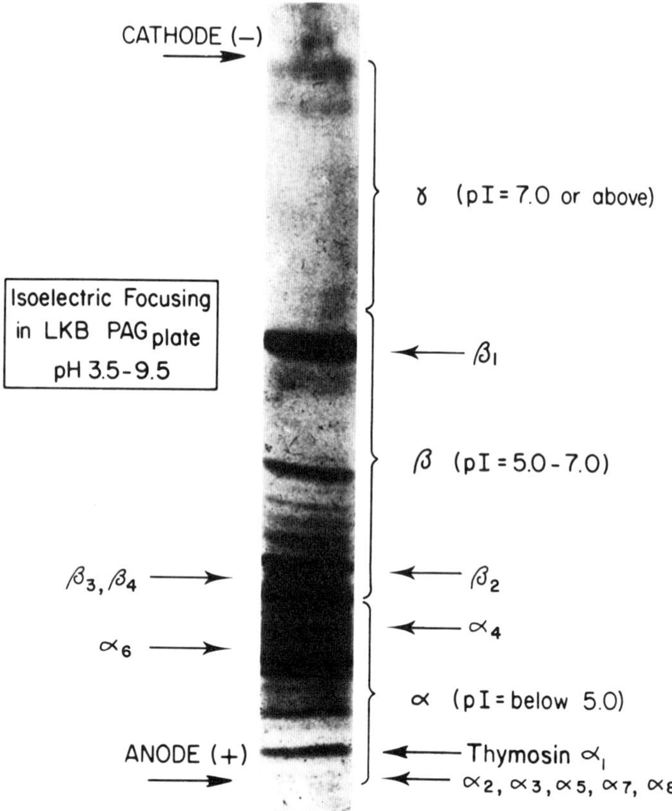


**Fig. 3.** Isoelectrically focused sample of thymosin fraction 5 showing distribution of mostly acidic peptide components. The $\alpha$, $\beta$, and $\gamma$ regions indicate segmentation of the gel based upon isoelectric point (p$I$) ranges suggested for peptide nomenclature to facilitate interlaboratory comparison of purified thymic extracts. (From Goldstein *et al.*, 1977a.)

region 5.0–7.0, and the $\gamma$ region above 7.0. The subscripts (1,2, . . . ) are used to identify the peptides from that region as they are isolated.

With the combination of ion exchange chromatography and gel filtration, we have isolated 12 polypeptide components from fraction 5 for further characterization, eight from the $\alpha$ region ($\alpha_1$–$\alpha_8$) and four from the $\beta$ region ($\beta_1$–$\beta_4$).

Figure 4 shows a schematic drawing of thymosin fraction 5 and the purified peptide components on isoelectric focusing in LKB PAG$_{plate}$ with pH 3.5–9.5. Most of the peptides from the $\alpha$ region have very similar properties. They are all rather acidic with p$I$ around 3.5–4 and with molecular weights around 3000.

## 9.3.1.2. Biological Activities of Thymosin Fraction 5

Thymosin fraction 5 is a potent immunopotentiating preparation and can act in lieu of the thymus gland to reconstitute immune functions in certain thymus-deprived and/or immunodeprived individuals. Thymosin has been found to induce T cell differentiation and enhance immunological functions in genetically athymic mice (Thurman *et al.*, 1975), in adult thymectomized mice (Thurman *et al.*, 1975; Bach *et al.*, 1975), in NZB mice with severe autoimmune reactions (Thurman *et al.*, 1975; Dauphinee *et al.*, 1974), in tumor-bearing mice (Zisblatt *et al.*, 1970; Hardy *et al.*, 1971; Khaw and Rule, 1973), and in mice with casein-induced amyloidosis (Scheinberg *et al.*, 1976).

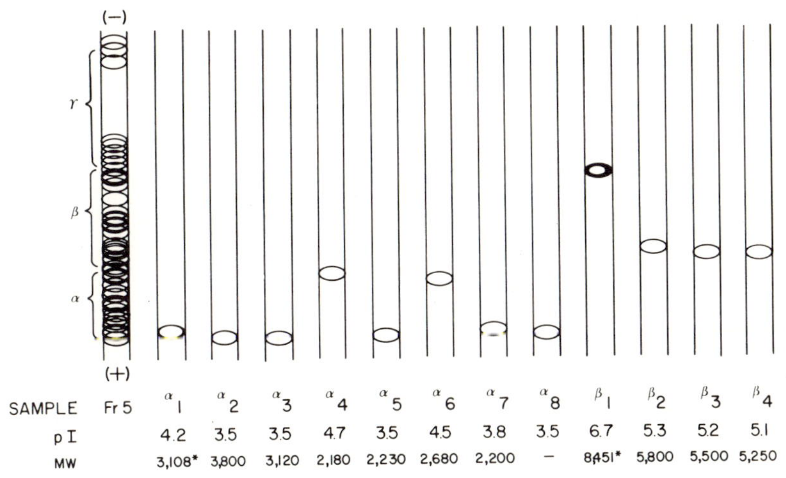


| SAMPLE | Fr 5 | $\alpha_1$ | $\alpha_2$ | $\alpha_3$ | $\alpha_4$ | $\alpha_5$ | $\alpha_6$ | $\alpha_7$ | $\alpha_8$ | $\beta_1$ | $\beta_2$ | $\beta_3$ | $\beta_4$ |
|---|---|---|---|---|---|---|---|---|---|---|---|---|---|
| p$I$ | | 4.2 | 3.5 | 3.5 | 4.7 | 3.5 | 4.5 | 3.8 | 3.5 | 6.7 | 5.3 | 5.2 | 5.1 |
| MW | | 3,108* | 3,800 | 3,120 | 2,180 | 2,230 | 2,680 | 2,200 | − | 8,451* | 5,800 | 5,500 | 5,250 |

**Fig. 4.** Schematic drawing of thymosin fraction 5 and the purified peptide components on isoelectric focusing in LKB PAG$_{plate}$ with pH 3.5–9.5. *Sequence established.

One of the first detectable effects of thymosin fraction 5 on thymocytes is to increase the intracellular cyclic GMP levels (Naylor *et al.*, 1976). Using an acetylation RIA procedure to measure cyclic GMP (Harper and Brooker, 1975), the stimulation is seen as early as 1 min after *in vitro* incubation with thymosin and is maximal between 5 and 10 min. However, by employing various assays, including the RIA kinase binding (Steiner *et al.*, 1972) and prelabeling of intracellular adenine pools, no stimulatory effect of thymosin on cyclic AMP levels has been observed. In contrast to our findings with thymosin, Kook and Trainin (1974), using THF, and Scheid *et al.* (1975), with thymopoietin, have reported that these thymic factors increase cyclic AMP levels.

These studies suggest that both cyclic GMP and cyclic AMP may be important secondary messengers for specific T cell responses. It is anomalous that thymosin does not yet stimulate cyclic AMP directly. Cyclic AMP can mimic thymosin in some *in vitro* systems such as the induction of spontaneous rosette-forming cells in the adult thymectomized spleen (Bach *et al.*, 1975) and the appearance of TL and thy-1 in pre-T-cell-enriched bone marrow (Scheid *et al.*, 1975). In addition, recent studies by Astaldi *et al.* (1977) have shown that thymosin can, in the serum of immunodeficient patients, induce the appearance of a factor that can stimulate cyclic AMP production in mouse thymocytes yet thymosin directly cannot.

Thymosin fraction 5 can also induce certain functional changes in lymphocytes, such as stimulation of macrophage migration inhibitory factor (MIF) and increased production of antibody-forming cells. The thymosin MIF assay (Thurman *et al.*, 1977) was developed based on the observations of Field and Shenton (1975) that the peripheral blood cells (PBL) of thymectomized guinea pigs which had been sensitized 10 days before to tuberculin-purified protein derivative (PPD) rapidly lose their capacity to make MIF. The reactivity could be restored by the addition of serum from thymus-bearing guinea pigs or human serum. We have found that thymosin fraction 5 in concentrations of less than 50 $\mu$g/ml could also restore the capacity of thymectomized guinea pigs to make MIF.

Using a modified Mishell–Dutton (1967) procedure, we have developed an assay to measure the effects of thymosin on antibody production *in vitro* (G. B. Thurman, J. T. Ulrich, and A. L. Goldstein, in preparation). Thymosin fraction 5 at concentrations of less than 100 $\mu$g/ml significantly stimulates spleen cells from normal and thymectomized animals to produce antibody to sheep red blood cells. Furthermore, as previously reported, thymosin fraction 5 was found to be active in an MLR assay (Cohen *et al.*, 1975) measuring the differentiation of murine thymocytes in an allogeneic mixed leukocyte culture, a human E-rosette assay (Wara *et al.*, 1975), and mouse mitogen assays *in vivo* (Thurman and Goldstein, 1975; Thurman *et al.*, 1977).

Thymosin has also been shown to increase phenotypic markers in lymphocyte populations (Bach *et al.*, 1971; Scheid *et al.*, 1973; Komuro and Boyse, 1973). Ahmed *et al.* (1978) incubated C57B1/6 spleen and bone marrow cells with fraction 5 and observed increases in Ly 1 and Ly 2,3 positive cells in A and B layers of bovine serum albumin (BSA) gradients. However, no inductive capacity was observed for the control using spleen fraction 5. Most recently, Pazmiño *et al.* (1978) found that thymosin fraction 5 can induce terminal deoxynucleotidyl transferase [TdT, a DNA polymerase found almost exclusively in cortical thymocytes (Barton *et al.*, 1976)] *in vivo* and *in vitro* in the A and B layers of bone marrow cells of nude mice and adult thymectomized mice.

### 9.3.2. Purified Bovine Thymosin $\alpha_1$

The first thymosin polypeptide isolated from the highly acidic region of fraction 5 has been termed thymosin $\alpha_1$. This peptide is very active in several bioassay systems. The primary structure of thymosin $\alpha_1$ has recently been completely elucidated (Goldstein *et al.*, 1977a).

#### 9.3.2.1. Isolation Procedure for Thymosin $\alpha_1$

The method for the isolation of thymosin $\alpha_1$ is diagrammed in Fig. 5. Lyophilized thymosin fraction 5 is chromatographed on a carboxymethyl-cellulose column at pH 5.0 in 10 mM NaAc, 1.0 mM 2-mercaptoethanol. The void volume is then desalted on a Sephadex G-25 column in water. The second protein peak is further separated on a DEAE-cellulose column in 50 mM Tris, 1.0 mM 2-mercaptoethanol, pH 8.0. A salt gradient of 0–0.8 M NaCl is employed. The first retained peak is desalted and further purified by gel filtration on Sephadex G-75 in guanidine hydrochloride. The first protein peak is then rechromatographed on a column of G-75 and the resulting material is thymosin $\alpha_1$.

#### 9.3.2.2. Chemical Characterization of Thymosin $\alpha_1$

Thymosin $\alpha_1$ prepared as just described migrates as a single band on analytical polyacrylamide gels at pH 8.3 and 2.9 and as a major band with a p*I* of 4.2 on an isoelectric focusing slab gel of pH range 3–5. The yield of thymosin $\alpha_1$ from fraction 5 is about 0.6%. The preparation is free of carbohydrate and nucleotide.

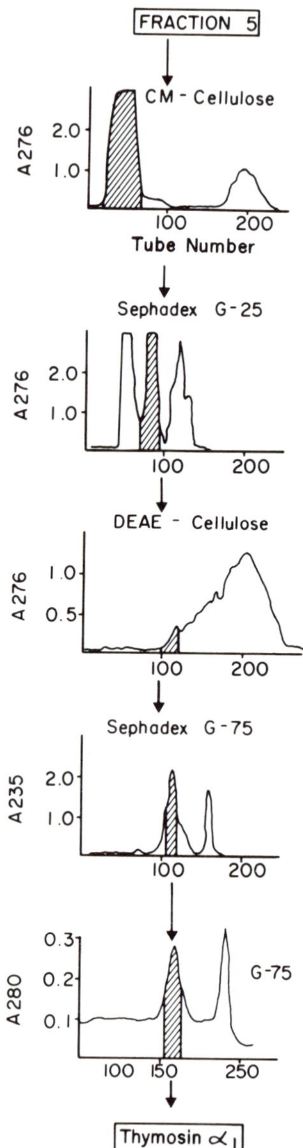



**Fig. 5.** Flow diagram of the fractionation of thymosin $\alpha$ from bovine thymosin fraction 5. Tube numbers are shown on the abscissa, absorbance on the ordinate of each plot. The shaded areas indicate pooled fractions collected for use in the subsequent step. Material from the final step represents a yield of 0.6% and migrates as a single band on analytical PA gels at pH 8.3 or 2.9 and as a major band with p$I$ of 4.2 on isoelectric focusing slab gel, pH 3–5. (From Goldstein *et al.*, 1977a.)

Thymosin $\alpha_1$ is a polypeptide consisting of 28 amino acid residues with a molecular weight of 3108. The complete amino acid sequence of this peptide is shown in Fig. 1. The amino terminus of thymosin $\alpha_1$ is blocked by an acetyl group. Using parameters for the prediction of protein conformation described by Chou and Fasman (1974), it would appear that the carboxy-terminal half of the molecule has a high helical potential.

Comparison of the sequence of thymosin $\alpha_1$ with the published sequence of other thymic factors such as thymopoietin (Schlesinger and Goldstein, 1975) and serum thymic factor (Bach *et al.*, 1977) reveals no homology. Only the amino acid composition but not the sequence has been described for thymic humoral factor, THF (Trainin *et al.*, 1975). It appears that thymosin $\alpha_1$ and THF, although of similar molecular weight, differ greatly in amino acid composition.

Computer analysis of the sequence of $\alpha_1$ has established that $\alpha_1$ bears very little homology to any of the 957 protein sequences that have been published to date (personal communication through National Biomedical Research Foundation). The highest homology was found to be with a segment of tropomyosin $\alpha$ chain from skeletal muscle (score 101 from mutation data matrix) and a segment of 50S ribosomal protein L7 of *Escherichia coli* (score 94). Figure 6 shows these comparisons. Since the comparison is made of short segments out of large proteins with undefined functional relationship, the significance of the homology, if any, is not clear. Nevertheless, it is interesting to note that both tropomyosin and troponin I are shown to be responsible for the calcium-dependent regulation of the actomyosin adenosine triphosphatase in vertebrate striated muscle (Wilkinson *et al.*, 1972).

### 9.3.2.3. Biological Activities of Thymosin $\alpha_1$

As can be seen in Table II, thymosin $\alpha_1$ is from 10 to 1000 times more active than thymosin fraction 5 in a mouse mitogen assay *in vivo* (Thurman and Goldstein, 1975), a lymphokine assay *in vitro* measuring produc-

**Table II.** Thymosin Activity in Various Bioassays[a]

|  | MLR | MIF | E Rosette | Mitogen[b] |
|---|---|---|---|---|
| Thymosin fraction | | | | |
|   5 ($\mu$g) | 1–10 | 1–5 | 1–10 | 1–10 |
| Thymosin $\alpha_1$ ($\mu$g) | NA[c] | 0.01–0.1 | 0.001–0.01 | 0.01–0.1 |

[a]MLR, mixed lymphocyte response; MIF, macrophage inhibiting factor.
[b]Fourteen daily injections *in vivo*.
[c]Not active.

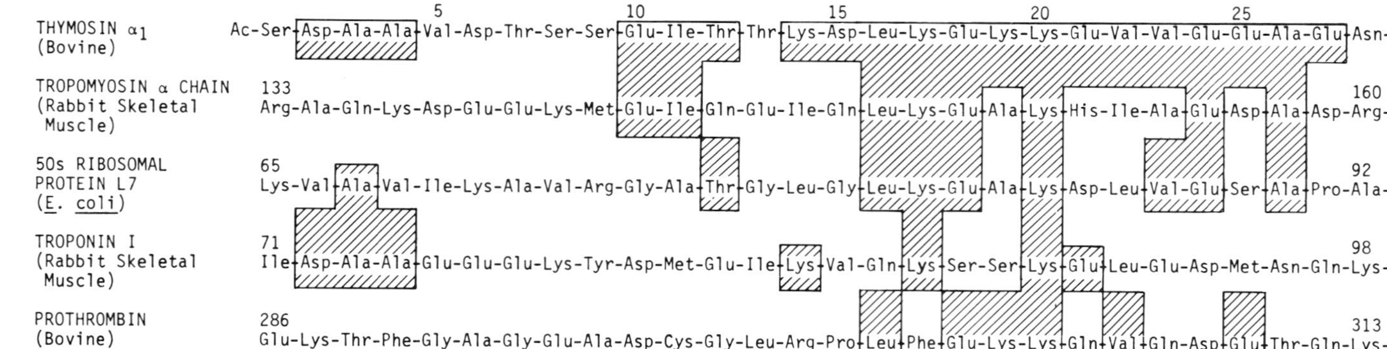



**Fig. 6.** Sequence homology of thymosin $\alpha_1$ to other proteins. Computer search of thymosin $\alpha_1$ against other protein segments of equal length reveals very little homology. The search was made against 957 protein sequences that have been published to date (computer analysis service provided through National Biomedical Research Foundation). The figure shows the sequence of thymosin $\alpha_1$ together with the homologous protein segments with the highest scores from mutation data matrix. The residues that are identical to thymosin $\alpha_1$ are shaded.

tion of macrophage inhibitory factor (Thurman *et al.*, 1977), and a human E-rosette assay *in vitro* (Wara *et al.*, 1975). However, it is not active in the mixed lymphocyte response or Mishell–Dutton assay. Most recently, A. Ahmed (personal communication) has found that thymosin $\alpha_1$ specifically increased the population of Ly 1,2,3 positive cells in the A and B layers of BSA gradient separated spleen cells *in vitro*. Ahmed and co-workers have also found that they could induce the capacity of athymic (nu/nu) mice and adult thymectomized, irradiated bone marrow-restored mice to reconstitute a normal IgM and IgG response to DNP following haptenation to thymosin fraction 5 (Ahmed *et al.*, 1977) and thymosin $\alpha_1$ (personal communication). These studies suggest that the thymosin receptors and the antigen receptors in the cell membrane may be in close proximity. It is postulated that the haptenated hormone, DNP-thymosin, may exert its influence both as a hormone and as a carrier on the development and maturation of precursor T cells to helper cells which influence and induce the formation of anti-DNP antibodies by the DNP-reactive B cells, either by direct presentation of DNP to the antigen-reactive B cells or via the macrophages.

### 9.3.3. Human Thymosin $\alpha_1$

Thymosin fraction 5 preparations have been isolated primarily from calf thymus. In order to evaluate the species variation of thymosin polypeptides we have prepared thymosin fraction 5 from different species including human thymus. It is especially crucial to obtain information from human thymus because of the potential clinical application of thymosin.

#### 9.3.3.1. Preparation

Through the arrangements made with the Departments of Pathology and Surgery here at The University of Texas Medical Branch (UTMB), we receive human thymus tissue obtained from selected autopsies and open heart surgery. Human thymosin fraction 5 has been prepared using extraction and fractionation procedures similar to those used for the isolation of bovine thymosin fraction 5. However, in the ammonium sulfate precipitation step, both 25–50% and 50–95% cuts were collected for biochemical and biological studies.

Owing to the limited amount of human thymosin fraction 5 available, the purification of thymosin $\alpha_1$ was performed by a modified procedure. As shown in Fig. 7, human fraction 5 was chromatographed through a carboxymethylcellulose (CM-22) column equilibrated with 10 mM NaAc, 1 mM 2-mercaptoethanol, pH 3.40. At this low pH, most peptides bind to the column and only the most acidic fractions appeared in the void

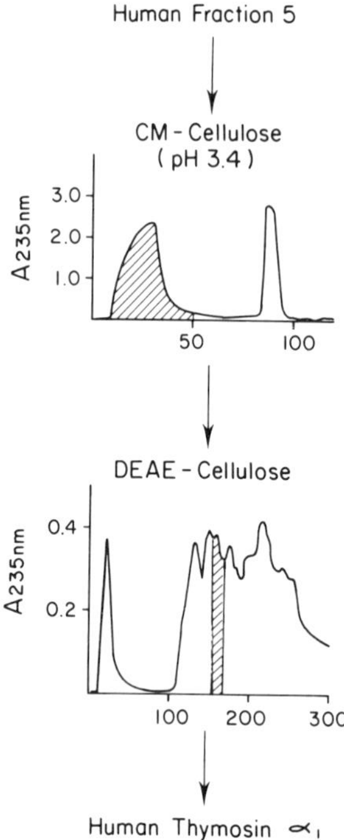



**Fig. 7.** Purification of human thymosin $\alpha_1$ from thymosin fraction 5. This is a modified procedure from the one used for the purification of bovine thymosin presented in Fig. 5. The carboxymethylcellulose column is performed at a much lower pH (pH 3.4 versus pH 5.0) which allows a substantial purification of $\alpha_1$ in one step. The void volume is further purified on a DEAE-cellulose column.

volume. The void volume is then further purified by a DEAE-cellulose column.

### 9.3.3.2. Chemical Characterization

The amount of human thymosin $\alpha_1$ obtained is very low because of the limited supply of human thymosin fraction 5. However, the amount available has permitted the preparation of a tryptic peptide map. The tryptic peptide maps of bovine and human thymosin $\alpha_1$ are shown in Figs. 8 and 9. Although the tryptic map of human $\alpha_1$ contains a few contaminant spots, it has been found that human $\alpha_1$ has all the tryptic peptides present in bovine $\alpha_1$. The tryptic peptides from human $\alpha_1$ have been analyzed and partially sequenced. From the results obtained as summarized in Fig. 10, the human and bovine thymosin $\alpha_1$ appear to have an identical sequence.

### 9.3.4. Other Thymosin Polypeptides

As shown in Fig. 4, we have isolated 12 classes of polypeptides from thymosin fraction 5, eight from the $\alpha$ region and four from the $\beta$ region. Chemical and biological characterizations of these peptides in addition to $\alpha_1$ are in progress. However, a few peptides deserve special attention at this time.

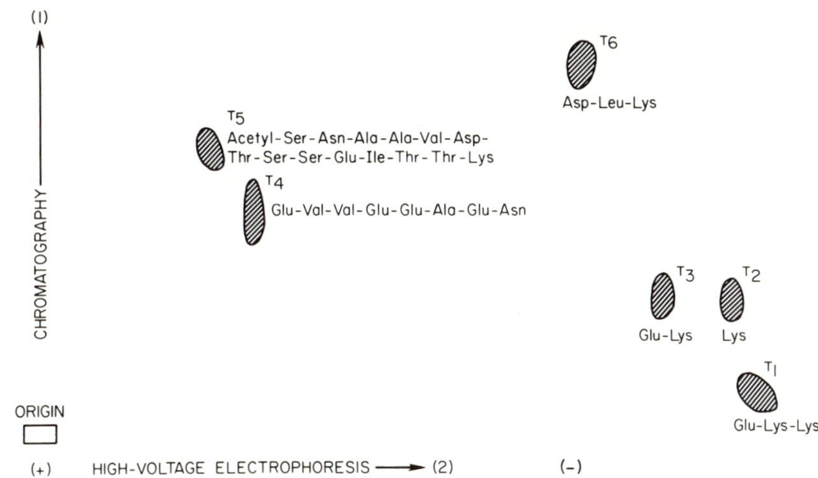



**Fig. 8.** Tryptic peptide map of bovine thymosin $\alpha_1$. The first dimension is conducted by paper chromatography with the solvent system of *n*-butanol–glacial acetic acid–water = 4:1:5 (v/v). This is followed by high-voltage electrophoresis at pH 1.9 for 30–40 min at 60 V/cm. Peptides are detected by staining with either cadmium-ninhydrin reagent or fluorescamine.

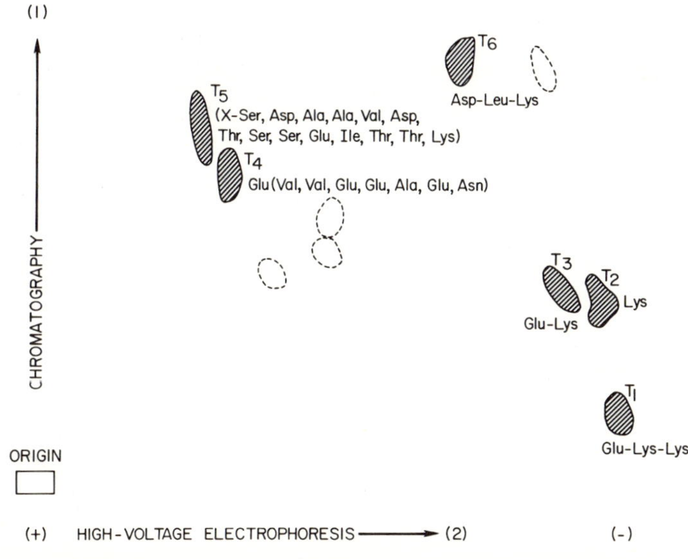



**Fig. 9.** Tryptic peptide map of human thymosin $\alpha_1$. This map shows that human $\alpha_1$ has all the tryptic peptides present in bovine $\alpha_1$ (shown in Fig. 8).

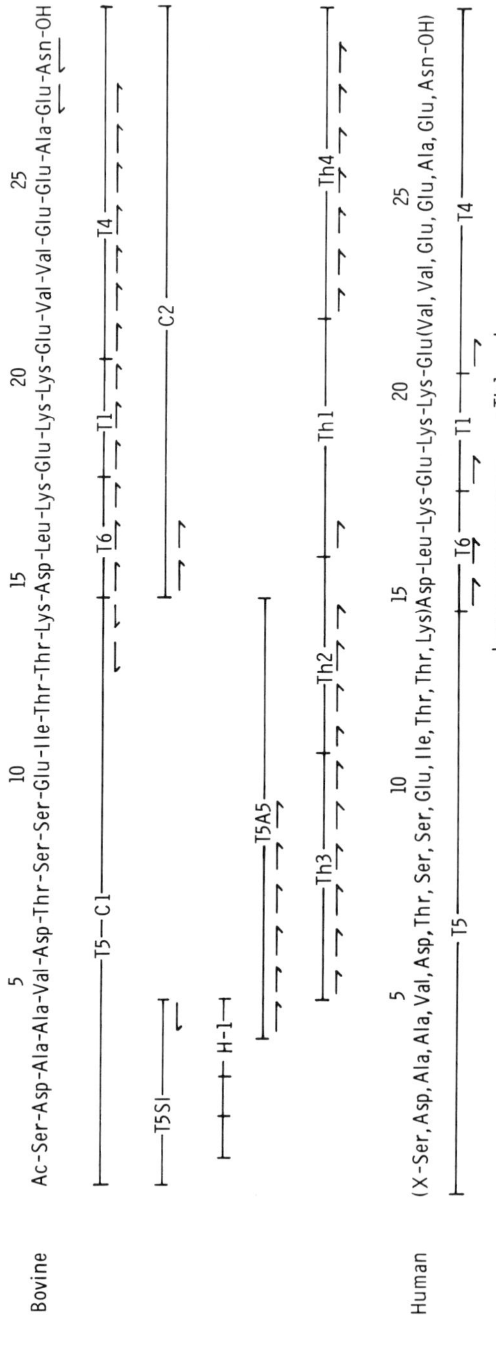



**Fig. 10.** Complete amino acid sequence of bovine thymosin $\alpha_1$ and partial sequence of human thymosin $\alpha_1$. Results show that these two sequences appear to be identical.

### 9.3.4.1. Thymosin $\alpha_5$ and $\alpha_7$

Both partially purified peptides are highly acidic with isoelectric points around 3.5. They are free of carbohydrate and lipid. The thymosin $\alpha_5$ peptides have a molecular weight of 3000 and the $\alpha_7$ peptides of 2200. We have found that some thymosin $\alpha_5$ preparations amplify helper functions and the thymosin $\alpha_7$ preparation has suppressive properties *in vitro* (unpublished observation). These results, if substantiated, would support our hypothesis that there is a family of thymic polypeptides that may act on different T cell subpopulations to influence the maturation sequence. As shown in Fig. 11, thymosin $\alpha_1$ seems to act on immature precursor T cells to form $T_1$ cells. Thymosin $\alpha_5$ converts $T_1$ to $T_2$ helper cells and thymosin $\alpha_7$ changes $T_1$ to $T_2$ cells with suppressor function.

### 9.3.4.2. Peptide $\beta_1$ Isolated from Thymosin Fraction 5

The most predominant band on isoelectric focusing of thymosin fraction 5 is the peptide $\beta_1$ (see Fig. 2). The amino acid sequence of $\beta_1$ has been determined (T. L. K. Low and A. L. Goldstein, in preparation). It is composed of 74 amino acid residues with molecular weight 8451 daltons and isoelectric point 6.7. It is believed that this peptide is a contaminant in thymosin preparations and is not involved in thymic hormone action. The sequence analysis of $\beta_1$ has revealed that this molecule is identical to ubiquitin (Schlesinger *et al.*, 1975) and a portion of protein A24, a nuclear chromosomal protein (Olson *et al.*, 1976). It has been postulated that ubiquitin is a degradative product of A24 (Hunt and Dayhoff, 1977).

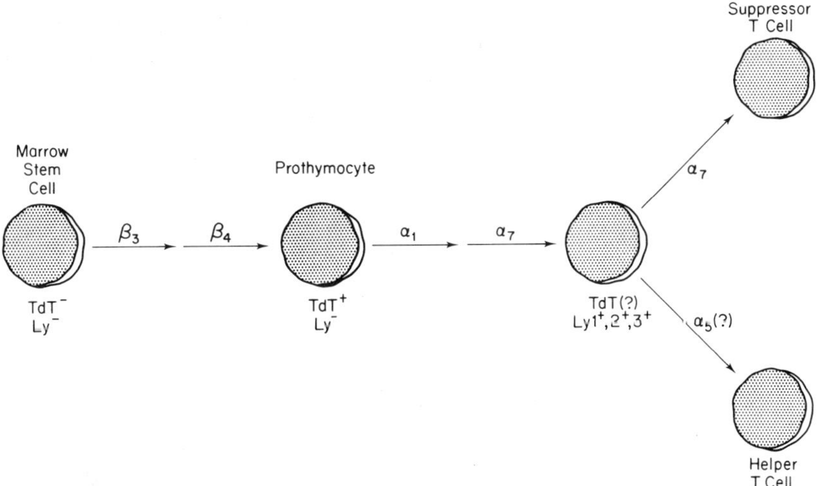


**Fig. 11.** Proposed sites of action of thymosin polypeptides on maturation of T cell subpopulations.

### 9.3.4.3. Thymosin $\beta_3$ and $\beta_4$

The partially purified thymosin $\beta_3$ and $\beta_4$ preparations were found to induce terminal deoxynucleotidyl transferase (TdT)-positive cells in the A and B layers of bovine serum albumin-separated bone marrow cells obtained from genetically athymic mice (N. Pazmino and J. Ihle, personal communication). The thymosin $\beta_3$ peptides have an isoelectric point of 5.2 and a molecular weight of approximately 5500. The thymosin $\beta_4$ peptides have an isoelectric point of 5.1 and a molecular weight of approximately 5250. From the partial sequence obtained for these two classes of polypeptides, they appear to share an identical sequence through most of their amino-terminal part (about 45 amino acid residues) and differ in the carboxyl-terminal ends (about 5 to 10 amino acid residues).

As shown in Fig. 11, thymosin $\beta_3$ and $\beta_4$ may be acting on stem cells to form prothymocytes.

## 9.4. Potential Clinical Application of Thymosin

Short-term incubation of thymosin *in vitro* with the peripheral blood lymphocytes of T cell immunodeficient patients results in a significant increase in the number of T cells (E-rosettes). This observation led to the development of an E-rosette assay for thymosin as well as for the identification of patients with thymosin-dependent immunodeficiency diseases in man (Wara *et al.*, 1975).

The first clinical trial of thymosin was initiated in April 1974 by Dr. Arthur Ammann and Dr. Diane Wara at the University of California Medical Center in San Francisco (Wara *et al.*, 1975). The patient was a 5-year-old female with thymic hypoplasia and hyperimmunoglobulinemia. The patient was treated with transfer factor at age 3½ years without clinical improvement. In view of the substantial increase in the percentage of E-rosettes following *in vitro* incubation with thymosin, it was decided to proceed with thymosin therapy in the patient. The patient has been receiving thymosin for more than 3 years and has improved immunologically and clinically (Wara and Ammann, 1978). It was found that patients with severe combined immunodeficiency do not respond to thymosin *in vitro* (Wara *et al.*, 1975), presumably because of the lack of a lymphoid stem cell population sensitive to thymosin. Patients with active systemic lupus erythematosus (SLE) respond significantly to thymosin *in vitro* in this E-rosette assay whereas individuals with inactive systemic lupus erythematosus are not responsive (Scheinberg *et al.*, 1975). Recently, Horowitz *et al.* (1977) have found that patients with both active and inactive SLE lack suppressor T cells which can be restored *in vitro* with thymosin fraction 5. Other *in vitro* E-rosette studies in patients with other rheumatic diseases such as Sjögren's syndrome and rheumatoid arthritis (Moutsopoulos *et al.*, 1976), acute liver diseases (M. Mutchnick, personal communication), kidney disease (Harris *et al.*, 1975), and burns (Sakai *et al.*, 1975) have similarly shown that thymosin can significantly enhance the number of T cells. Anecdotal reports of the treatment of cancer patients with thymic extracts date back to 1907. In that year Gwyer presented a case of inoperable breast cancer with great relief of symptoms when treated with a water extract of calf thymus. However, these studies were not followed up and until the initiation of clinical trials with thymosin there have been no serious well-controlled clinical trials reported in the literature which documented the efficacy of thymic factors clinically.

Phase I trials of thymosin in cancer patients were initiated in 1974 at The University of Texas Medical Branch in Galveston under the direction of J. J. Costanzi and at the M. D. Anderson Hospital and Tumor Institute in Houston under the direction of E. Hersh. These experimental trials showed that (a) thymosin was not toxic, (b) thymosin treatment significantly increased the percentage of E-rosettes in the peripheral blood of a significant number of patients with initial low T cell numbers, (c) side effects of thymosin administration were mild, and (d) many anergic patients developed positive skin test responses to recall antigens. In 1975–1976, more than 75 patients received thymosin treatment according to phase II protocols (Goldstein *et al.*, 1977b; Schafer *et al.*, 1976a,b, 1977). Preliminary observations have shown that most patients exhibited an increase in circulating T cell numbers when their rosette percentages were initially less than 45%. Some patients exhibited skin test conversion from negative to positive to common recall antigens.

Several trends have emerged from the results of our ongoing clinical trials in pediatric patients. It seems clear that thymosin has no major effect in the amelioration of severe combined immunodeficiency disease (SCID). On the other hand, diseases resulting from aplasia or hypoplasia of the thymus gland have responded well to thymosin therapy (Goldstein *et al.*, 1975a; Rossio and Goldstein, 1977; Wara *et al.*, 1975; Wara and Ammann, 1978). Of particular interest is the efficacy of thymosin in clearing chronic fungal and viral infections in these patients, suggesting a potential major role for thymosin in the treatment of infectious diseases in general.

The first phase II trial of thymosin has been completed in nonresectable small-cell carcinoma of the lungs by Dr. Paul B. Chretien and his associates at the National Cancer Institute (personal communication). In this trial thymosin fraction 5 was found to prolong significantly the survival of cancer patients when given in conjunction with intensive chemotherapy. Mean survival time was increased from 225 days with chemotherapy alone to 450 days with chemotherapy plus 60 mg/M$^2$ thymosin twice per week for the first 6 weeks of the chemotherapy induction period.

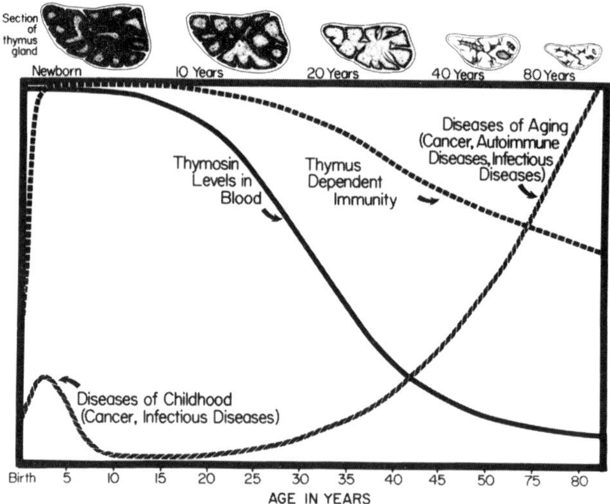


**Fig. 12.** Involution of the thymus with the increasing age of the individual. Thymic factors in the blood and cellular immune mechanisms are shown to decline in similar fashion. The incidence of age-related diseases increases in inverse proportion to the shrinkage of the thymus and to the decrease of thymic-dependent immunity. (From Goldstein *et al.*, 1975b.)

## 9.5. Thymosin and Aging

The involution of the thymus is probably the first noticed indication of aging (Duckworth, 1962). As shown in Fig. 12, numerous immunological studies have demonstrated that there is a concurrent decrease in cellular immunity with increasing age and a corresponding general increase in the incidence of the diseases of aging. Moreover, decrease in thymic function with advancing age causes senescence in T cell immunity directly correlated with an increase in the incidence of cancer. It has been shown that the circulating thymosin and thymosin-like activity (Goldstein *et al.*, 1974; Bach *et al.*, 1971) decreases with age in mouse and in man. These observations suggest that many diseases of the aged may result from an inability of the thymus gland to produce normal amounts of thymic hormones, which in turn results in a decreased resistance to infection. With the advancement in thymic hormone research, the possibility of manipulating the immunological derangements associated with aging may become feasible.

## 9.6. Perspectives

With all the evidence accumulated to date, it is apparent that the thymus gland has come of age as a member of the endocrine family. As illustrated in Fig. 13, the central role of the thymus in the development, growth, and function of lymphoid tissue and in the maintenance of immune balance has also been recognized. Using a partially purified thymic extract termed thymosin fraction 5, we have been able to demonstrate in a number of animal models as well as in humans that these preparations can act in lieu of the thymus gland to reconstitute immune functions. We have now successfully isolated a number of the purified polypeptide components from fraction 5. The observations that these peptides have superior activities in some bioassay systems but not in others (as in the case of thymosin $\alpha_1$) strongly suggest that several chemically distinct peptides in thymosin fraction 5 are necessary for the maintenance of immunological reactivity. As described previously, thymosin fraction 5 induces an increase in the intracellular cyclic GMP level of thymocytes but does not affect cyclic AMP levels. In contrast to these observations with thymosin, it has been reported that THF and thymopoietin stimulate cyclic AMP activity. These findings provide evidence to suggest that the active components in thymosin are not similar to THF or thymopoietin.

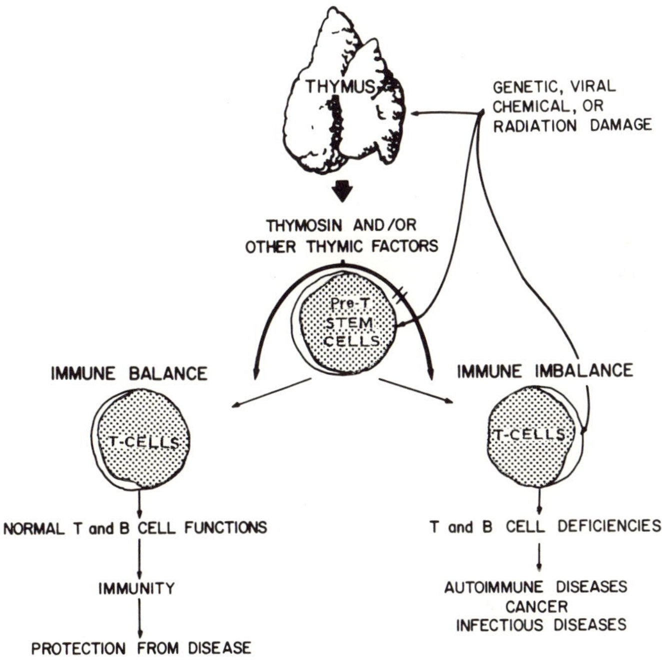


**Fig. 13.** Thymus contribution to immunity. Impairment of lymphoid elements, including the thymus and immunocompetent cells, by various deleterious agents causes deficiencies in immunity which may lead to a variety of disease manifestations. These conditions may in part be the result of a malfunctioning thymus and inadequate levels of thymic secretions.

The isolation and chemical characterization of the individual thymosin polypeptides is vital to our understanding of the mechanism(s) by which the thymus gland exerts control over T cell development. We hope to elucidate the chemical structure of each peptide and correlate their structure to function. The obvious next step will be the chemical synthesis of the biologically active thymic peptides to evaluate the physiological capacity of the synthetic preparations.

The chemical synthesis of the first completely sequenced thymosin peptide, thymosin $\alpha_1$, has been accomplished (S.-S. Wang and J. Meienhofer, personal communication). Preliminary studies have revealed that the synthetic material is as active as the natural peptide.

The long-term goal of our thymosin research program is to dissect the biochemical and molecular processes involved in the development and maintenance of the immune system with the view of developing novel therapeutic approaches to the treatment of diseases. The ongoing basic and clinical studies with thymosin have given us reason to be hopeful that hormonal manipulation of the immune system is possible. Our growing awareness that the thymus produces not one but a family of biologically active peptides (which may interact with each other as well as a multitude of subpopulations of lymphocytes) should provide a stimulus for continued development of this very important new field of endocrinology.

ACKNOWLEDGMENTS

We are greatly indebted to Dr. Gary Thurman for his critical evaluation of the manuscript and for his helpful suggestions. We also wish to acknowledge the excellent secretarial assistance of M. Watson and J. Allen.

This research was supported, in part, by grants from the National Cancer Institute (CA 16964, CA 14108) and Hoffmann–La Roche, Inc., Nutley, New Jersey.

# References

Abelous, J. E., and Billard, A., 1896, Recherches sur les fonctions de thymus, *Arch. Physiol. Norm. Pathol.* **28**:898.

Adler, H., 1937, Thymus und myasthenie, *Arch. Klin. Chir.* **189**:529.

Ahmed, A., Smith, A. H., Sell, K. W., Gershwin, M. E., Steinberg, A. D., Thurman, G. B., and Goldstein, A. L., 1977, Thymic-dependent anti-hapten response in congenitally athymic (nude) mice immunized with DNP-thymosin, *Immunology* **33**:757.

Ahmed, A., Smith, A. H., and Sell, K. W., 1978, Biology of thymosin: Maturation of thymus-derived (T) cells under the influence of thymosin, *in Modulation of*

*Host Resistance in Prevention and Treatment of Neoplasias* (M. A. Chirigos, ed.), Raven Press, New York, in press.

Aisenberg, A. C., and Wilkes, B., 1965, Partial immunological restoration of neonatally thymectomized rats with thymus-containing diffusion chambers, *Nature* **205**:716.

Andreasen, E., 1947, Function of the thymus. I. Critical remarks on the theory and experiments of Bomskov, *Acta Anal.* **2**:275.

Archer, O. K., and Pierce, J. C., 1961, Role of thymus in development of the immune response, *Fed. Proc.* **20**:26.

Asher, D., 1933, Weitere Isolierung des wachstumsfördernden Thymocrescins, *Biochem. Z.* **257**:209.

Astaldi, A., Astaldi, G. C. B., Wijermans, P., Groenewoud, M., Schellekens, P. Th. A., and Eijsvoogel, V. P., 1977, Thymosin-induced serum factor increasing cAMP, *J. Immunol.* **119**:1106.

Auerbach, R., and Globerson, A. G., 1966, *In vitro* induction of the graft-versus-host reaction, *Exp. Cell Res.* **42**:31.

Bach, J. F., Dardenne, M., Goldstein, A., Guha, A., and White, A., 1971, Appearance of T cell markers in bond marrow after incubation with purified thymosin, a thymic hormone, *Proc. Natl. Acad. Sci. U.S.A.* **68**:2734.

Bach, J. F., Dardenne, M., and Bach, M. A., 1973, Demonstration of a circulating thymic hormone in mouse and in man, *Transplant. Proc.* **5**:523.

Bach, J. F., Dardenne, M., Pleau, J. M., and Bach, M. A., 1975, Isolation, biochemical characteristics and biological activity of a circulating thymic hormone in the mouse and in the human, *Ann. N.Y. Acad. Sci.* **249**:186.

Bach, J. F., Dardenne, M., and Pleau, J. M., 1977, Biochemical characterization of a serum thymic factor, *Nature* **266**:55.

Barton, R., Goldschneider, I., and Bollum, F. J., 1976, The distribution of terminal deoxynucleotidyl transferase (TdT) among subsets of thymocytes in the rat, *J. Immunol.* **116**:462.

Beard, J., 1899, The true function of the thymus, *Lancet* **i**:144.

Beard, J., 1900, The source of leucocytes and the true function of the thymus, *Anat. Anz.* **18**:550.

Bernardi, G., and Comsa, J., 1965, Purification chromatographique d'une préparation de thymus douée d'activité hormonale, *Experientia* **21**:416.

Bezssonoff, N. A., and Comsa, J., 1958, Préparation d'un extrait de thymus application á l'urine humaine, *Ann. Endocrinol.* **19**:222.

Bomskov, C., and Sladovic, L., 1940, Der thymus als innersekretorisches organ, *Dtsch. Med. Wochenschr.* **66**:589.

Bracci, C., 1905, Timo e ricambio del calcio, *Riv. Clin. Pediatr.* **3**:572.

Camblin, J. G., and Bridges, J. B., 1964, Effects of cell-free extracts of thymus in leucopenic rats, *Transplantation* **2**:785.

Chou, P. Y., and Fasman, G. D., 1974, Conformational parameters for amino acids in helical, $\beta$-sheet and random coil regions calculated from proteins, *Biochemistry* **13**:211.

Cohen, G. H., Hooper, J. A., and Goldstein, A. L., 1975, Thymosin-induced differentiation of murine thymocytes in allogeneic mixed lymphocyte cultures, *Ann. N.Y. Acad. Sci.* **249**:145.

Comsa, J., 1938, Conséquences de la thymectomie totale chez le cobaye male, *C. R. Soc. Biol.* **127**:903.

Comsa, J., 1940, Action de l'extrait de thymus chez le cobaye thymiprivé, *C.R. Soc. Biol.* **133**:24.

Comsa, J., 1944, Effets de l'extrait de thymectomie totale sur la creatine urinaire du cobaye, *C.R. Soc. Biol.* **138**:773.

Comsa, J., 1955, Action of the purified thymic hormone in thymectomized guinea pigs, *Am. J. Med. Sci.* **250**:79.

Comsa, J., 1956, Influence d'un extrait hautement purifié de thymus sur les conséquences de l'irradiation aux rayons X sur les glandes endocrines du cobaye, *Ann. Endocrinol.* **17**:777.

Comsa, J., 1957a, Wirkung des Thymus Extraktes von Bezssonoff und Comsa beim thyreopriver Meerschweinchen, *Arch. Ges. Physiol.* **264**:383.

Comsa, J., 1957b, Consequences of thymectomy upon the leukopoiesis in guinea pigs, *Acta Endocrinol.* **26**:361.

Comsa, J., 1966, Zur Reindarstellung des Thymushormons, *Arzneim. Forsch.* **16**:18.

Constant, G. A., Porter, E. L., Seybold, H. M., and Andronis, A., 1949, Effect of thymic extracts on neuromuscular response, *Am. J. Physiol.* **159**:565.

Dauphinee, M. J., Talal, N., Goldstein, A. L., and White, A., 1974, Thymosin corrects the abnormal DNA synthetic response of NZB mouse thymocytes, *Proc. Natl. Acad. Sci. U.S.A.* **71**:2637.

DeSomer, P., Denys, P., and Leyten, R., 1963, Activity of a noncellular calf thymus extract in normal and thymectomized mice, *Life Sci.* **II**:810.

DiGeorge, A. M., 1968, Congenital absence of the thymus and its immunologic consequences: Concurrence with congenital hypoparathyroidism, *Birth Defects* **4**:116.

Duckworth, W. L., 1962, *in Galen on Anatomical Procedures, The Later Books* (M. C. Lyons and B. Towers, eds.), p. 160, Cambridge Univ. Press, London and New York.

Duplan, J. F., Foschi, G. V., and Manson, L. A., 1962, The lymphocytosis stimulating factor (LSF), *Proc. Soc. Exp. Biol. Med.* **110**:426.

Ernström, U., and Nordlind, K., 1977, Thymic factors regulating DNA synthesis in lymphocytes cultured *in vitro, Int. Arch. Allergy Appl. Immunol.* **54**:463.

Eskelund, V., and Plum, C. M., 1953, Experimental investigations on the healing of fractures, *Acta Endocrinol.* **12**:171.

Fagraeus, A., 1948a, The plasma cellular reaction and its relation to the formation of antibodies *in vitro, J. Immunol.* **58**:1.

Fagraeus, A., 1948b, Antibody production in relation to the development of plasma cells, *Acta Med. Scand.,* Suppl. 204, p. 3.

Fichtelius, K. E., Laurell, G., and Phillipsson, L., 1961, The influence of thymectomy on antibody formation, *Acta Pathol. Microbiol. Scand.* **51**:81.

Field, E. J., and Shenton, B. K., 1975, Assay of thymosin in blood, *Lancet* **i**:49.

Gershon, R. K., 1975, Immunoregulation by T cells, *in Molecular Approaches to Immunology* (E. E. Smith and D. W. Robbins, eds.), pp. 267–288, Academic Press, New York.

Goldstein, A. L., and White, A., 1970, The thymus as an endocrine gland, *in*

*Biochemical Actions of Hormones* (G. Litwak, ed.), pp. 465–502, Academic Press, New York.

Goldstein, A. L., and White, A., 1971, Role of thymosin and other thymic factors in the development, maturation and functions of lymphoid tissue, *in Current Topics in Experimental Endocrinology* (V. H. T. James and L. Martini, eds.), pp. 121–149, Academic Press, New York.

Goldstein, A. L., Slater, F. D., and White, A., 1966, Preparation, assay and partial purification of a thymic lymphocytopoietic factor (thymosin), *Proc. Natl. Acad. Sci. U.S.A.* **56**:1010.

Goldstein, A. L., Asanuma, Y., and White, A., 1970, The thymus as an endocrine gland: Properties of thymosin, a new thymus hormone, *in Recent Progress in Hormone Research,* Vol. 26 (E. B. Astwood, ed.), pp. 505–538, Academic Press, New York.

Goldstein, A. L., Guha, A., Zatz, M. M., Hardy, A., and White, A., 1972, Purification and biological activity of thymosin, a hormone of the thymus gland, *Proc. Natl. Acad. Sci. U.S.A.* **69**:1800.

Goldstein, A. L., Hooper, J. A., Schulof, R. S., Cohen, G. H., Thurman, G. B., McDaniel, M. C., White, A., and Dardenne, M., 1974, Thymosin and the immunopathology of aging, *Fed. Proc.* **33**:2053.

Goldstein, A. L., Wara, D. W., Ammann, A. J., Sakai, H., Harris, N. S., Thurman, G. B., Hooper, J. A., Cohen, G. H., Goldman, A. S., Costanzi, J. J., and McDaniel, M. C., 1975a, First clinical trial with thymosin: Reconstitution of T cells in patients with cellular immunodeficiency diseases, *Transplant. Proc.* **7**:681.

Goldstein, A. L., Thurman, G. B., Cohen, G. H., and Hooper, J. A., 1975b, Thymosin: Chemistry, biology and clinical applications, *in Biological Activity of Thymic Hormones* (D. W. van Bekkum, ed.), pp. 173–197, Kooyker Scientific Publ., Rotterdam.

Goldstein, A. L., Low, T. L. K., McAdoo, M., McClure, J., Thurman, G. B., Rossio, J. L., Lai, C.-Y., Chang, D., Wang, S.-S., Harvey, C., Ramel, A. H., and Meienhofer, J., 1977a, Thymosin $\alpha_1$: Isolation and sequence analysis of an immunologically active thymic polypeptide. *Proc. Natl. Acad. Sci. U.S.A.* **74**:725.

Goldstein, A. L., Thurman, G. B., Rossio, J. L., and Costanzi, J. J., 1977b, Immunological reconstitution of patients with primary immunodeficiency diseases and cancer after treatment with thymosin, *Transplant Proc.* **9**:1141.

Goldstein, G., 1974, Isolation of bovine thymin: A polypeptide hormone of the thymus, *Nature* **247**:11.

Goldstein, G., 1975, The isolation of thymopoietin (thymin), *Ann. N.Y. Acad. Sci.* **249**:177.

Goldstein, G., and Mananaro, A., 1971, Thymin: A thymic polypeptide causing the neuromuscular block of myasthenia gravis, *Ann. N.Y. Acad. Sci.* **183**:230.

Good, R. A., and Varco, R. L., 1955, A clinical and experimental study of agammaglobulinemia, *J. Lancet* **75**:245.

Good, R. A., Dalmasso, A. P., Martinez, G., Archer, O. K., Pierce, J. C., and Papermaster, B. W., 1962, The role of the thymus in development of immunologic capacity in rabbits and mice, *J. Exp. Med.* **116**:773.

Goslar, H. G., 1958, Über die Wirkung eines standardisierten Thymusextraktes auf die Häutungsvorgänge und auf einige Organe von *Natrix natrix* L., *Arch. Exp. Pathol. Pharmakol.* **233**:201.

Gregoire, C., 1945, Sur le mechanisme de l'atrophie thymique déclenchée par les hormones sexuelles, *Arch. Int. Pharmacodyn. Ther.* **70**:45.

Gregoire, C., and Duchateau, G., 1956, A study on lymphoepithelial symbiosis in thymus. Reaction of the lymphatic tissue to extracts and to implants of epithelial components of thymus, *Arch. Biol., Liege* **68**:269.

Gwyer, F., 1907, Thymus gland treatment of cancer (a preliminary report with a presentation of a case of inoperable cancer with great relief of symptoms), *Ann. Surg.* **56**:86.

Hammar, J. A., 1938, Experimentelle Untersuchung über die Rolle der Thymus bei der Immunisierung, *Z. Mikrosk. Anat. Forsch.* **44**:425.

Hand, T., Caster P., and Luckey, T. D., 1967, Isolation of a thymus hormone, LSH, *Biochem. Biophys. Res. Commun.* **26**:18.

Hardy, M. A., Zisblatt, M., Levine, N., Goldstein, A. L., Lilly, F., and White, A., 1971, Reversal by thymosin of increased susceptibility of immunosuppressed mice to Moloney sarcoma virus, *Transplant. Proc.* **3**:926.

Harper, J. F., and Brooker, G., 1975, Femtomole sensitive radioimmunoassay for cyclic AMP and cyclic GMP after 20 acetylations by acetic anhydride in aqueous solution, *J. Cyclic Nucleotide Res.* **1**:207.

Harris, J., Sengar, D., Hyslop, D., Green, L., and Goldstein, A. L., 1975, Immunodeficiency in chronic uremia: Preliminary evidence for thymosin deficiency, *Transplantation* **20**:176.

Harris, T. N., Rhoads, J., and Stokes, J., 1948, A study of the role of the thymus and spleen in the formation of antibodies in the rabbit, *J. Immunol.* **58**:27.

Hooper, J. A., McDaniel, M. C., Thurman, G. B., Cohen, G. H., Schulof, R. S., and Goldstein, A. L., 1975, The purification and properties of bovine thymosin, *Ann. N.Y. Acad. Sci.* **249**:125.

Horowitz, S., Borcherding, W., Moorthy, A. V., Chesney, R., Schulte-Wissermann, H., Hong, R., and Goldstein, A., 1977, Induction of suppressor T cells in systemic lupus erythematosus by thymosin and cultured thymic epithelium, *Science* **197**:999.

Hunt, L. T., and Dayhoff, M. O., 1977, Amino-terminal sequence identity of ubiquitin and the nonhistone component of nuclear protein A-24, *Biochem. Biophys. Res. Commun.* **74**:650.

Jankovic, B. D., Waksman, B. H., and Arnason, B. G., 1962, Role of the thymus in immune reactions in rats. I. The immunologic response to bovine serum albumin (antibody formation, Arthus reactivity, and delayed hypersensitivity) in rats thymectomized or splenectomized at various times after birth, *J. Exp. Med.* **116**:159.

Jankovic, B. D., Isakovic, K., and Horvat, J., 1965, Effect of a lipid fraction from rat thymus on delayed hypersensitivity reactions of neonatally thymectomized rats, *Nature* **208**:356.

Khaw, B. A., and Rule, A. H., 1973, Immunotherapy of the Dunning leukaemia with thymic extracts, *Br. J. Cancer* **28**:288.

Klein, J. J., Goldstein, A. L., and White, A., 1965, Enhancement of *in vivo* incorporation of labeled precursors into DNA and total protein of mouse lymph nodes after administration of thymic extracts, *Proc. Natl. Acad. Sci. U.S.A.* **53**:812.

Klein, J. J., Goldstein, A. L., and White, A., 1966, Effects of the thymus lymphocytopoietic factor, *Ann. N.Y. Acad. Sci.* **135**:485.

Komuro, K., and Boyse, E. A., 1973, *In vitro* demonstration of thymic hormone in the mouse by conversion of precursor cells into lymphocytes, *Lancet* **1**:740.

Kook, A. I., and Trainin, N., 1974, Hormone-like activity of a thymus humoral factor on the induction of immune competence in lymphoid cells, *J. Exp. Med.* **139**:193.

Kook, A. I., Yakir, Y., and Trainin, N., 1975, Isolation and partial chemical characterization of THF, a thymic hormone involved in immune maturation of lymphoid cells, *Cell. Immunol.* **19**:151.

Levey, R. H., Trainin, N., and Law, L. W., 1963a, Evidence for function of thymic tissue in diffusion chambers implanted in neonatally thymectomized mice. Preliminary report, *J. Natl. Cancer Inst.* **31**:199.

Levey, R. H., Trainin, N., Law, L. W., Black, P. H., and Rowe, W. P., 1963b, Lymphocyte choriomeningitis infection in neonatally thymectomized mice bearing diffusion chambers containing thymus, *Science* **142**:483.

Lindstrom, J. M., Lennon, V. A., Seybold, M. E., and Whittingham, S., 1976, Experimental autoimmune myasthenia gravis: Biochemical and immunological aspects, *Ann. N.Y. Acad. Sci.* **274**:254.

Low, T. L. K., In preparation, The chemistry and biology of thymosin. II. Amino acid sequence analysis of thymosin $\alpha_1$ and peptide $\beta_1$.

Lowry, O. H., Rosenbrough, N. J., Farr, A. L., and Randall, R. J., 1951, Protein measurement with the folin phenol reagent, *J. Biol. Chem.* **193**:265.

MacGillivray, M. H., Jones, V. E., and Leskowitz, S., 1964, Restoration of immunological competence in thymectomized rats by a noncellular thymic factor, *Fed. Proc.* **23**:189.

Maclean, L. D., Zak, S. J., Varco, R. L., and Good, R. A., 1956, Thymic tumor and acquired agammaglobulinemia, a clinical and experimental study of the immune response, *Surgery* **40**:1010.

Maisin, J. H. F., 1964, Role of thymus and thymus factors in the induction of 20-methylcolanthrene: Skin cancer in mice, *Nature* **202**:202.

Metcalf, D., 1956, The thymic origin of the plasma lymphocytosis stimulating factor, *Br. J. Cancer* **10**:442.

Milcu, S. M., and Potop, I., 1971, Isolation of an antiblastic factor from the bovine thymus, *Rev. Roum. Endocrinol.* **8**:1.

Miller, J. F. A. P., 1961, Immunological function of the thymus, *Lancet* **2**:748.

Miller, J. F. A. P., and Osoba, D., 1967, Current concepts of the immunological function of the thymus, *Physiol. Rev.* **47**:437.

Miller, J. F. A. P., Block, M., Rowlands, D. T., Jr., and Kind, P., 1965, Effect of thymectomy on hematopoietic organs of the opossum "embryo," *Proc. Soc. Exp. Biol. Med.* **118**:916.

Mishell, R. I., and Dutton, R. W., 1967, Immunization of dissociated spleen cell cultures from normal mice. *J. Exp. Med.* **126**:423.

Mizutani, A., Saito, Y., Sato, H., and Saito, M., 1970, The search for a hypocalcemic factor in the thymus gland. I. Separation of fractions producing hypocalcemia in rabbits from bovine thymus gland by precipitation with calcium chloride, *J. Pharm. Soc. Jap.* **90**:445.

Molnar, P., and Kovacs, K., 1953, Wirkung eines Thymusextraktes auf das Brown-Pearce-Karzinom des Kaninchens, *Arch. Geschwulstforsh.* **5**:33.

Moutsopoulos, H., Fye, K. H., Sawada, S., Becker, M. J., Goldstein, A., and Talal, N., 1976, *In vitro* effect of thymosin on T-lymphocyte rosette formation in rheumatic diseases, *Clin. Exp. Immunol.* **26**:563.

Nakamoto, O., 1957, Influence of thymus on blood picture especially on lymphocytes, II. Influence of thymic extract on peripheral blood lymphocytes, *Acta Haematol. Jap.* **20**:187.

Naylor, P. H., Sheppard, H., Thurman, G. B., and Goldstein, A. L., 1976, Increase of cyclic GMP induced in murine thymocytes by thymosin fraction 5, *Biochem. Biophys. Res. Commun.* **73**:843.

Nowinski, W. W., 1930, Fortgesezte Beitraege zur Funktion der Thymus. Die Wirkungen des Thymocrescins auf das Wachstum, *Biochem. Z.* **226**:415.

Nowinski, W. W., 1933, Die Bezehungen zwischen Thymocrescin und Thyroxin beim Wachstum der Tiere, *Biochem. Z.* **259**:182.

Olson, M. O. J., Goldknopf, I. L., Guetzow, K. A., James, G. T., Hawkins, T. C., Mays-Rothberg, C. J., and Busch, H., 1976, The $NH_2$- and COOH-terminal amino acid sequence of nuclear protein A24, *J. Biol. Chem.* **251**:5901.

Osoba, D., and Miller, J. F. A. P., 1964, The lymphoid tissues and immune responses of neonatally thymectomized mice bearing thymus tissue in Millipore diffusion chambers, *J. Exp. Med.* **119**:177.

Pansky, B., House, E. L., and Cone, L. A., 1965, An insulin-like thymic factor: A preliminary report, *Diabetes* **14**:325.

Pazmiño, N. H., Ihle, J. N., and Goldstein, A. L., 1978, Induction *in vivo* and *in vitro* of terminal deoxynucleotidyl transferase by thymosin in bone marrow cells from athymic mice, *J. Exp. Med.*, **147**:708.

Potop, I., Boeru, V., and Mreana, G., 1966, The effect of thymus extracts on phosphorus compounds in muscle and serum, and on serum calcium, *Biochem. J.* **101**:454.

Rehn, E., 1940, Die Hyperfunktion der Thymus als Krankheit, *Dtsch. Med. Wochenschr.* **66**:594.

Restelli, D. A., 1845, De thymo observationes anatomico-physiologico-pathologicae, *Ticini Regii Typog. Fusi Soc.* **46**:4.

Roberts, S., and White, A., 1949, Biochemical characterization of lymphoid tissue proteins, *J. Biol. Chem.* **178**:151.

Robey, G., Campbell, B. J., and Luckey, T. D., 1972, Isolation and characterization of a thymic factor, *Infect. Immun.* **6**:682.

Rossio, J. L., and Goldstein, A. L., 1977, Immunotherapy of cancer with thymosin, *World J. Surg.* **1**:605.

Rowntree, L. G., Clark, J. H., and Hanson, A. M., 1934, The biologic effects of thymus extract (Hanson), *JAMA* **103**:1425.

Sakai, H., Costanzi, J. J., Loukas, D. F., Gagliano, R. G., Ritzmann, S. E., and Goldstein, A. L., 1975, Thymosin induced increase in E-rosette forming capacity of lymphocytes in patients with malignant neoplasms, *Cancer* **36**:974.

Schafer, L. A., Goldstein, A. L., Gutterman, J. U., and Hersh, E. M., 1976a, *In vitro* and *in vivo* studies with thymosin in cancer patients, *Ann. N.Y. Acad. Sci.* **277**:609.

Schafer, L. A., Gutterman, J. U., Hersh, E. M., Mavligit, G. M., Dandridge, K., Cohen, G. H., and Goldstein, A. L., 1976b, Partial restoration by *in vivo* thymosin of E-rosettes and delayed-type-hypersensitivity reactions in immunodeficient cancer patients, *Cancer Immunol. Immunother.* **1**:259.

Schafer, L. A., Gutterman, J. U., Hersh, E. M., Mavligit, G. M., and Goldstein, A. L., 1977, *In vitro* and *in vivo* studies of thymosin activity in cancer patients, *in Progress in Cancer Research and Therapy,* Vol. 2 (M. A. Chirigos, ed.), pp. 329–346, Raven Press, New York.

Schaller, R. T., and Stevenson, J. K., 1967, Reversal of post thymectomy wasting syndrome with multiple thymus grafts in diffusion chambers, *Proc. Soc. Exp. Biol. Med.* **124**:199.

Scheid, M. P., Hoffman, M. K., Komuro, K., Hammerling, U., Boyse, E. A., Cohen, G. H., Hooper, J. A., Schulof, R. S., and Goldstein, A. L., 1973, Differentiation of T-lymphocytes induced by preparations from thymus and by non-thymic agents. The determined state of the precursor cell, *J. Exp. Med.* **138**:1027.

Scheid, M. P., Goldstein, G., Hammerling, U., and Boyse, E. A., 1975, Induction of T and B lymphocyte differentiation *in vitro, in Membrane Receptors of Lymphocytes* (M. Seligmann, J. L. Preudhomme, and F. M. Kourilsky, eds.), pp. 353–359, American Elsevier, New York.

Scheinberg, M. A., Cathcart, E. S., and Goldstein, A. L., 1975, Thymosin-induced reduction of "null cells" in peripheral-blood lymphocytes of patients with systemic lupus erythematosus, *Lancet* **1**:424.

Scheinberg, M. A., Goldstein, A. L., and Cathcart, E. S., 1976, Thymosin restores T cell function and reduces the incidence of amyloid disease in casein-treated mice, *J. Immunol.* **116**:156.

Schlesinger, D. H., and Goldstein, G., 1975, The amino acid sequence of thymopoietin II, *Cell* **5**:361.

Schlesinger, D. H., Goldstein, G., Scheid, M. P., and Boyse, E. A., 1975, Chemical synthesis of a peptide fragment of thymopoietin II that induces selective T cell differentiation, *Cell* **5**:367.

Schwartz, H., Price, M., and O'Dell, C. A., 1953, Effect of lyophilized thymic extracts on serum calcium and phosphorus, *Metabolism* **2**:261.

Sherman, J. D., and Dameshek, W., 1963, "Wasting disease" following thymectomy in the hamster, *Nature* **197**:469.

Steiner, A. L., Pagliara, A. S., Chase, L. R., and Kipnis, D. M., 1972, Radioimmunoassay for cyclic nucleotides. II. Adenosine 3′,5′-monophosphate and guanosine 3′,5′-monophosphate in mammalian tissues and body fluids, *J. Biol. Chem.* **274**:1114.

Szent-Gyorgyi, A., Hegyeli, A., and McLaughlin, J. A., 1962, Constituents of the thymus gland and their relation to growth, fertility, muscle, and cancer, *Proc. Natl. Acad. Sci. U.S.A.* **48**:1439.

Telkkä, A., and Teir, H., 1955, Influence of thymus suspension on mitotic rate in the thymus, liver and outer orbital gland of rat, *Acta Pathol. Microbiol. Scand.* **36**:323.

Thurman, G. B., and Goldstein, A. L., 1975, Mitogen bioassay for thymosin: Increased mitogenic responsiveness of murine lymphocytes *in vitro* following *in vivo* treatment with thymosin, in *The Biological Activity of Thymic Hormones* (D. W. van Bekkum, ed.), pp. 261–264, Kooyker Scientific Publ., Rotterdam.

Thurman, G. B., Ahmed, A., Strong, D. M., Gershwin, M. E., Steinberg, A. D., and Goldstein, A. L., 1975, Thymosin-induced increase in mitogenic responsiveness of lymphocytes of C57B1/6J, NZB/W and nude mice, *Transplant. Proc.* **7**:299.

Thurman, G. B., Rossio, J. L., and Goldstein, A. L., 1977, Thymosin-induced enhancement of MIF production by peripheral blood lymphocytes of thymectomized guinea pigs, in *Regulatory Mechanisms in Lymphocyte Activation* (D. O. Lucas, ed.), pp. 629–631, Academic Press, New York.

Thurner, K., 1924, Über den Einfluss des Thymusextrakten auf die Leistungsfähigkeit und Ermuedbarkeit des Säugetiermuskels, *Pfluegers Arch. Gesamte Physiol. Menschen Tiere* **202**:444.

Tilney, N. L., Beattie, E. J., and Econamou, S. G., 1965, The effect of neonatal thymectomy in the dog, *J. Surg. Res.* **5**:23.

Torda, C., and Wolff, H. G., 1947, Effect of organ extracts and their fractions on acetylcholine synthesis, *Am. J. Physiol.* **148**:417.

Trainin, N., 1974, Thymic hormones and the immune response, *Physiol. Rev.* **47**:137.

Trainin, N., and Small, M., 1970, Studies on some physiochemical properties of a thymus humoral factor conferring immunocompetence on lymphoid cells, *J. Exp. Med.* **132**:885.

Trainin, N., Begerano, A., Strahilevitch, M., Goldring, D., and Small, M., 1966, A thymic factor preventing wasting and influencing lymphopoiesis in mice, *Israel J. Med. Sci.* **2**:549.

Trainin, N., Burger, M., and Kaye, A., 1967a, Some characteristics of a thymic humoral factor determined by assay *in vivo* of DNA synthesis in lymph nodes of thymectomized mice, *Biochem. Pharmacol.* **16**:711.

Trainin, N., Burger, M., and Linker-Israeli, M., 1967b, Restoration of homograft response in neonatally thymectomized mice by a thymic humoral factor (THF), in *Proceedings of the International Congress, Transplantation Society, First Advance in Transplantation* (J. Dausset, J. Hamburger, and G. Mathe, eds.), p. 91, Munksgaard, Copenhagen.

Trainin, N., Small, M., and Globerson, A., 1969, Immunocompetence of spleen cells from neonatally thymectomized mice conferred *in vitro* by a syngeneic thymus extract, *J. Exp. Med.* **130**:765.

Trainin, N., Small, M., Zipori, D., Umiel, T., Kook, A. I., and Rotter, V., 1975, Characteristics of THF, a thymic hormone, in *The Biological Activity of Thymic Hormones* (D. K. van Bekkum, ed.), p. 117, Kooyker Scientific Publ., Rotterdam.

Trench, C. A. H., Watson, J. W., Walker, F. C., Gardner, P. S., and Green, C. A., 1966, Evidence for a humoral thymic factor in rabbits, *Immunology* **10**:187.

van Bekkum, D. W., ed., 1975, *The Biological Activity of Thymic Hormones*, Kooyker Scientific Publ., Halsted Press Division, Rotterdam.

Wara, D., and Ammann, A. J., 1978, Thymosin treatment of children with primary immunodeficiency diseases, *Transplant. Proc.*, **10**:203.

Wara, D. W., Goldstein, A. L., Doyle, W., and Ammann, A. J., 1975, Thymosin activity in patients with cellular immunodeficiency, *N. Engl. J. Med.* **292**:70.

White, A., and Goldstein, A. L., 1968, Is the thymus an endocrine gland? Old problem, new data, *Perspect. Biol. Med.* **11**:475.

Wilkinson, J. M., Perry, S. V., Cole, H. A., and Trayer, I. P., 1972, The regulatory proteins of the myofibril, separation and biological activity of the components of inhibitory-factor preparations, *Biochem. J.* **127**:215.

Wilson, A., and Wilson, H., 1955, Thymus and myasthenia gravis, *Am. J. Med.* **19**:697.

Wolf, B., and Erb, S., 1970, *In vitro* stimulation of the secondary antibody response in lymph nodes by normal thymus and thymosin, *in Proceedings Annual Leukocyte Culture Conference, 4th* (O. Ross McIntyre, ed.), pp. 207–216, Appleton-Century-Crofts, New York.

Zisblatt, M., Goldstein, A. L., Lilly, F., and White, A., 1970, Acceleration by thymosin of the development of resistance to murine Sarcoma virus-induced tumor in mice, *Proc. Natl. Acad. Sci. U.S.A.* **66**:1170.

# Chalones and Blood Cells

## Tapio Rytömaa

## 10.1. Introduction

It has become increasingly obvious that cell proliferation is regulated, in part, by means of negative feedback: an inhibitory effect is exerted on cell proliferation within a cell line by the cell line itself. According to the current concept, this communication between the cells is transmitted by an inhibitory signal, now commonly called chalone.

The term chalone, in this particular sense, was proposed by Bullough in 1962, but it has been accepted rather slowly by an increasing number of scientists. Many authors, even if they believed in "specific endogenous mitotic inhibitors," have remained reluctant to use this term, at least partly because of the connotations that the word has continued to invoke. Another factor, and evidently more important in feeding skepticism, is the fact that despite 10–15 years of research nobody seemed to be able to "reasonably" purify and chemically characterize any chalone. Such a lack of success was not reassuring regarding the material reality of chalones. Now, however, the situation has finally changed.

In its broadest sense chalone is only a convenient operational designation for a conceptual factor, or perhaps even for a cascade effect, which

TAPIO RYTÖMAA ● Medical Research Group, Institute of Radiation Protection; Experimental Cell Research, University of Helsinki, Helsinki, Finland.

enables the "mass" of a cell line to be gauged and cell proliferation to be regulated accordingly. Yet chalones are sometimes "defined" as substances even with characteristics such as water solubility, heat lability, and protease sensitivity. These, and many other "characteristics" often associated with chalones, may or not may be properties of some or all chalones; however, these properties should not be included in a meaningful definition of chalones. In my terminology, chalone is defined by four characteristics:

1.  Chalone is generated by the same cell line on which it acts.
2.  Chalone action is cell line specific.
3.  Chalone inhibits cell proliferation *in vivo*.
4.  The inhibitory action of chalone is not based on cytotoxicity.

In the following section I shall elaborate the chalone concept in a little more detail. I hope that the discussion, in spite of some speculation, will help in gaining a more adequate understanding of the general principles of the concept.

## 10.2. The Chalone Concept: General Principles

It is worth noting at once that the definition of chalones does not include any properties related to the chemical nature of the inhibitory signal, its exact mode of action, cell cycle specificity, species nonspecificity, or even reversibility of the action. Thus, for instance, the definition does not require that cell line specificity of chalone action depend on a unique molecular configuration; specificity of action may well be determined by other mechanisms as well, such as anatomical location of another potentially responsive cell line.

It may appear striking that, according to the definition given, chalone action may be irreversible. This is indeed different from the current opinion of most "chalonists" (see, e.g., Bullough, 1973; Houck, 1976), and also from my own earlier definitions (Rytömaa, 1970, 1976). It is now clear, however, that the requirement for reversibility is easily misinterpreted: as far as the whole cell line is considered, the inhibition must be reversible, but this does not mean that chalone-induced inhibition is reversible at the level of individual cells, too. In fact, it has recently been shown (Benestad and Rytömaa, 1977) that granulocytic chalone accelerates maturation of the granulocytic precursor cells. This action, which may be only secondary to the prolongation of the proliferative cell cycle (thus giving the cell a better opportunity to develop the specific cytoplasmic machinery typical of mature cells), means that some cells become nonproliferative end cells during the inhibition and hence they can no longer start a new cell cycle when the inhibition is released. Clearly, chalone has not killed or damaged these cells in a cytotoxic manner, but its inhibitory activity has nevertheless resulted in an irreversible loss of proliferative activity. Interestingly enough, this irreversible effect actually provides direct evidence against any cytotoxic action of granulocytic chalone: the inhibited cells can be traced to the stage of polymorphs, which thus shows that the cells affected by chalone skip divisions but otherwise behave normally (Benestad and Rytömaa, 1977).

In contrast to most earlier definitions of chalones, the present one does not include a lack of species specificity either. Such a property is not inherent in the concept of feedback regulation; hence, in my opinion, it is an unnecessary requirement, even if available evidence shows that chalones actually are species nonspecific.

According to all published definitions, chalones are cell line specific with respect to both source and action. For the time being, there are perhaps good practical reasons for accepting the maxim that the specificity of chalones is even absolute; yet enormous technical difficulties are involved in establishing this property beyond doubt. From the theoretical point of view absolute specificity of chalone action is not at all necessary and some degree of nonspecificity might actually be advantageous, because it would prevent overly strong and biologically useless oscillations in cell proliferation. It should also be noted that a low level of background "noise" does not make the specific signals nondiscriminative or ineffective. Furthermore, if chalone action is tested in artificial conditions *in vitro*, using "unprotected" isolated cells as the target and excessive concentrations of chalone, it would not be too surprising to find that an absolutely specific *in vivo* signal affects nonphysiological targets *in vitro*. A lack of absolute specificity could be remotely similar to the well-known relationship of antibody to homologous antigen and cross-reacting antigen.

At present, a meaningful definition of chalones must leave the chemical nature of these substances completely open. Clearly, there are no obvious reasons which would force the assumption that chalones must have a particular predetermined chemical structure. Although chalones cannot readily be compared with hormones, there is sufficient analogy to warrant the conclusion that chalones affect ongoing processes and, therefore, that the inhibitory activity could be achieved by a variety of molecular configurations. It is highly likely, however, that chalones are chemically not as heterogeneous as hormones, but it is not intuitively obvious why chalones should be proteins or polypeptides. In fact, recent evidence suggests that at least in some chalones the active moiety may be polyamine (Allen *et al.*, 1977; Barfod and Marcker, 1977).

It seems to be a common opinion that chalones act in the $G_1$ phase of the cell cycle by preventing or slowing down the $G_1 \rightarrow S$ transition. However, epidermal chalone, the first to be discovered, was recognized by its effect on the $G_2$ phase of the cell cycle (Bullough and Laurence, 1960, 1964). This is now usually called the $G_2$ inhibitor to distinguish it from the $G_1$ inhibitor, another epidermal chalone. These two chalones appear to be distinct entities with different chemical characteristics (Hondius Boldingh and Laurence, 1968; Marks, 1975), a different source—basal versus keratinizing cells (Elgjo *et al.*, 1972)—and different cell cycle specificity (Thornley and Laurence, 1975, 1976). The role of the $G_1$ chalone seems obvious, whereas that of the $G_2$ chalone is less clear (see Bullough and Mitrani, 1976); consequently, it is the opinion of most workers in this field that the $G_1$ inhibitor is the "real" epidermal chalone and that the existence of the $G_2$ inhibitor is curious and its role has yet to be discovered. However, it is possible, at least in theory, that the $G_1$ and $G_2$ inhibitors are not really two different chalones but rather two different "phenotypes" of the same inhibitor bound to different carrier molecules. Thus the properties distinguishing the two inhibitors (molecular weight, source, and cell cycle specificity) might merely reflect characteristics of the carrier and hence be secondary to the basic concept.

According to the definition given, chalones are physiological, noncytotoxic, cell line specific inhibitors of cell proliferation. As already indicated, all other suggested properties of chalones are generalizations either of some experimental findings or of intuitive ideas. To elaborate the present argument further, we may tentatively assume that chalones act simply by prolonging the cell cycle time (they may, of course, act differently, for instance by diverting cycling cells to postmitosis). Because the cell cycle is an ongoing process, chalones would thus modulate the rate of the expression of an inherent property of the cell. It is of secondary importance whether the traversion of the cell through the cycle is slowed down in $G_1$ or in $G_2$, or in any other phase of the cell cycle; what matters here is that the cycle time is prolonged. We may now consider a hypothetical cell line, or rather an expanding clone somewhat similar to the erythron, characterized by a fixed maturation time and a variable number of successive mitoses during the cells' progression toward full maturity and subsequent permanent loss of the mitotic potential. It is intuitively clear that if the cell cycle time is prolonged enough to result in one skipped mitosis, cell production is halved (see the figure in Section 10.4.4). If the maturation pathway would normally consist of ten successive mitoses, one skipped mitosis is obtained by about 10% prolongation in the cell cycle time. It is, of course, of secondary importance whether the prolongation involves $G_1$ or $G_2$, or any other phase of the cell cycle. It should also be noted that 10% prolongation might be difficult to observe by a direct analysis of the cell cycle, and that some commonly employed indicators of proliferative activity, such as pulse labeling index, would give misleading results if the prolongation is based on changes in the duration of the S phase.

Although this example is fictive and not based on direct experimental evidence, it serves to illustrate some important aspects of the chalone concept. In particular, it is important to realize that the versatility of the concept should not be restricted by unwarranted assumptions regarding the mechanism of the inhibition; these are problems which must be solved experimentally. When it is realized that chalones may merely slow down the rate of an ongoing process (i.e., cell cycle), and that this may be achieved by a number of different mechanisms, it becomes obvious that all chalones are not necessarily similar chemically and that their mode of action can vary from one cell line to another. Furthermore, it is quite possible that more than one chalone exists for each cell line.

In this chapter I shall review what is known of the "blood cell chalones." It may be easier to put some of the findings in more perspective if the reader has in mind at least one possible specific mechanism of chalone action. Although the mechanism proposed herein has not yet been verified for any one of the blood cell chalones, its existence is supported by circumstantial evidence.

In brief, the proposed mechanism of chalone action is inhibition of DNA polymerases. According to a recent report (Nakai, 1976), partially purified Ehrlich ascites tumor (EAT) chalone inhibits nascent DNA synthesis by reversibly inhibiting $\alpha$- and $\beta$-polymerases isolated from the tumor. In contrast to polymerases, DNA ligase is not affected by EAT chalone. Nakai's findings that EAT chalone also inhibits mouse spleen DNA polymerase and, at least partially, mouse kidney polymerase, are neither surprising nor contradictory to the requirement of cell line specificity. As also pointed out by Nakai, the cell line specificity of chalone action is likely to reside at the cell membrane as specific receptors rather than at the level of DNA polymerases. It is interesting, however, that EAT chalone stimulates rather than inhibits *Escherichia coli* DNA polymerase (Nakai, 1976).

I shall not discuss in any detail the different implications of Nakai's findings. However, two general points are worth making: first, the inhibition of DNA polymerases is not inconsistent with the observed inhibition of $G_1 \rightarrow S$ transition, and second, several "odd" findings indicated later would be readily explained by this mechanism of action.


## 10.3. Assay Systems for "Blood Cell Chalones"

### 10.3.1. *In Vitro* Cultures

One of the most commonly used culture methods in the study of blood cell chalones is a short-term coverslip culture of bone marrow (for techniques, see Rytömaa, and Kiviniemi, 1967; Rytömaa, 1969). In brief, in this culture method bone marrow cells attach to a coverslip, hanging from the wall of a horizontally positioned test tube, and form a monolayer onto the upper surface of the coverslip. After predetermined culture times the coverslips are retrieved from the tubes and the cells are fixed *in situ*. The advantages of this assay method include simple preparation of the cultures, a small culture volume (~0.5 ml), and the possibility of analyzing each culture with respect to several endpoints.

The coverslip culture method of bone marrow is a fast and useful screening system in the study of blood cell chalones. However, the method suffers from certain drawbacks which limit the usefulness of this assay system; for instance, the cultures run down in their cellularity with time (at a rate of ~1.5% $hr^{-1}$; see Rytömaa, 1969) and, owing to differences in cell attachment to the glass, the normal balance of bone marrow is slightly upset in favor of granulocytic cells. It has sometimes been claimed that the decreasing cellularity indicates a complete lack of proliferation and, therefore, that this assay system is totally inadequate for demonstrating the action of noncytotoxic inhibitors such as chalones (see, e.g., Maurer *et al.*, 1976). However, decreasing cellularity does not necessarily mean a lack of cell proliferation; it only shows that the rate of cell loss is higher than the rate of cell gain. In the coverslip cultures cell proliferation—and even normal maturation of granulocytic cells—is maintained at a reasonable level for well over 10 hr, i.e., long enough to allow the demonstration of the chalone action. Thus, in continuous labeling with $[^3H]$-TdR, the labeling index increases approximately linearly at a rate of about 2% $hr^{-1}$, the relative number of labeled nonproliferative granulocytes increases at a rate of about 1% $hr^{-1}$ (Rytömaa, 1969), and all mitoses are labeled some 4 hr after the onset of the cultures (T. Rytömaa and K. Kiviniemi, unpublished results).

Although the coverslip cultures, as well as the even simpler suspension cultures (Paukovits, 1973), are useful especially as screening tests for granulocytic chalone, they are far from ideal in elucidating the chalone action in greater detail. In my experience, the best *in vitro* system for analyzing the mode of action of granulocytic chalone is an established culture of chloroma cells (Yunis *et al.*, 1975; P. Foa, W. Paile, and T. Rytömaa, unpublished results). These cells, derived from a transplanted Shay chloroma of the rat, grow exponentially for about 5 days in a suspension culture in Petri dishes ($T \leq 24$ hr, depending on the subline of chloroma cells). A detailed study of the kinetics of the chloroma cell population (P. Foa, W. Paile, and T. Rytömaa, unpublished results) and the use of a nonanalytical mathematical model based on Monte Carlo simulation (Toivonen, 1976; Toivonen and Rytömaa, 1978), seem to make it possible to solve the mode of action of granulocytic chalone in great detail. Figure 1 gives a simple example of the action of granulocytic chalone on chloroma cells in this culture system (P. Foa, W. Paile, H. Toivonen, and T. Rytömaa, unpublished results).

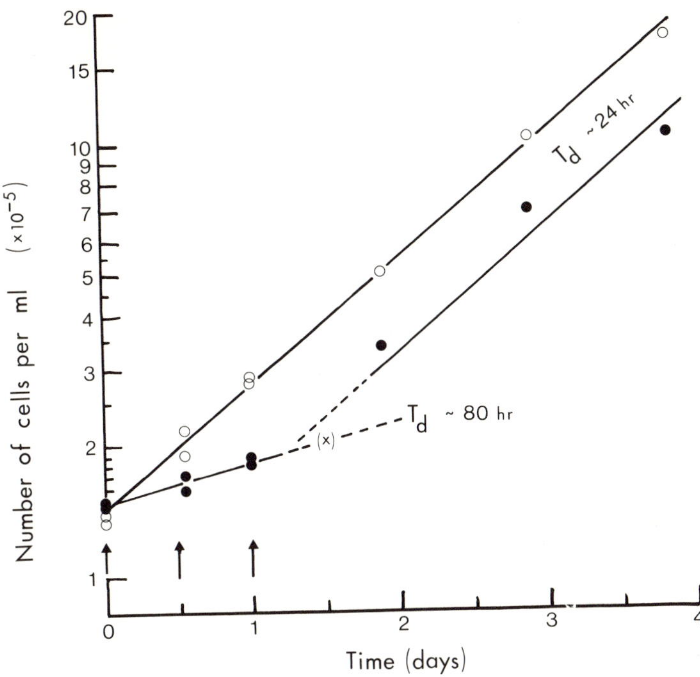



**Fig. 1.** Effect of granulocytic chalone on rat chloroleukemia cells grown in suspension cultures in Petri dishes. The arrows indicate addition of chalone (50 $\mu$g/ml) to the cultures; purity of the preparation was similar to that used in human trials *in vivo* (see text). The least squares regression lines show 70% inhibition in the growth rate, followed by a complete recovery within 12 hr. All points were obtained from independent cultures.

A wide variety of other *in vitro* culture systems have also been used in the study of blood cell chalones. The culture systems in regard to lymphocytes include conventional systems, such as stimulation of blood or spleen cells with phytohemagglutinin (PHA) or other plant lectins. These assays are naturally based on highly standardized culture systems and they also have the additional advantage that only one cell type proliferates. Furthermore, by a suitable choice of the stimulator it is possible to transform preferentially either T cells (PHA being the type example) or B cells (e.g., using $\beta$-lipopolysaccharide from *Salmonella typhosa;* see Peavy *et al.,* 1970). However, these assay systems as well as their extensions, such as the mixed lymphocyte culture, are not always without disadvantages in the study of chalones. Thus, in practice, most investigators have added the test extract at the start of the cultures, i.e., at a time when the cells are not yet proliferating. In these conditions the assay system measures the ability of the test extract to inhibit transformation (i.e., a step that leads to proliferation), rather than cell proliferation itself. Lymphocytic chalone(s) may exert such an effect but, by definition, it is not an inherent property of specific inhibitors of lymphocyte proliferation. It is, however, easy to avoid this complication by adding the test extract to the cultures after allowing the transformation process to be completed.

Another immunologically based *in vitro* technique which has been used in the study of lymphocytic chalone(s) is the inhibition of the macrophage migration inhibitory factor (Houck *et al.*, 1973). From the quantitative point of view this is an excellent assay system, but it is extremely dangerous if applied uncritically to the study of chalones: release of the macrophage migration inhibitory factor is dependent on recognition but not at all on cell proliferation (see Ranney, 1975).

Several established lymphocytic cell lines can be, and have been, used in the study of lymphocytic chalones (see, e.g., Attallah and Houck, 1976). Among these are the NC-37 human lymphoblastic cells, a permanent line with B cell characteristics (see Pattengale *et al.*, 1973); Molt, an established line of human lymphoblastic leukemia with T cell characteristics (see Minowada *et al.*, 1973); EL-4, a mouse leukemic lymphocyte line (see Gorer, 1960); and L-1210, a mouse leukemic line that has been studied extensively.

Permanent cultures of leukemic cells can also be used for a purpose other than targets of different tissue extracts: at least some cell lines appear to be good sources of the chalone of their tissue of origin. For instance, granulocytic chalone has been obtained from rat chloroleukemia cells (see Rytömaa and Kiviniemi, 1968c), and lymphocytic chalone (B cell chalone) has been extracted from human NC-37 leukemia cells (see Attallah *et al.*, 1975).

Several unrelated permanent cell lines have been used as control targets in blood cell chalone testing to reveal specificity and a lack of cytotoxicity. However, it has been claimed that these are of limited value, especially in specificity tests, because many of these cell lines, such as HeLa cells, are far removed even from their own original characteristics (see Lord, 1976). This may be a valid criticism, especially if it is required that cell line specificity of chalone action be absolute. In practice, however, established cultures are still quite useful in chalone testing, because they are likely to reveal at least most of the trivial "inhibitors" of cell proliferation, such as the presence of cold thymidine in the test extracts and crude cytotoxicity. Furthermore, lymphocytic and granulocytic cell lines are not necessarily far removed from each other, at least originally, and they are therefore valuable for cross-checking the inhibitory actions of lymphocytic and granulocytic chalones.

It is well known that normal granulocytic cells can be kept proliferating actively for several days in many different systems *in vitro*. Some of the techniques developed are, however, complicated and their use does not offer dramatic advantages over the simpler techniques commonly adopted in the study of granulocytic chalone. It is self-evident that any *in vitro* system, however advanced it may be, can never fully simulate *in vivo* conditions and the results obtained *in vitro* therefore do not necessarily apply *in vivo*. Every student is, of course, aware of this limitation; yet it seems that there is too strong a tendency in chalone research to "confirm" earlier findings with the aid of new culture systems rather than to develop adequate *in vivo* assays. In my opinion, little important new information has been obtained from the adoption of sophisticated *in vitro* culture methods. Perhaps one notable exception is a long-term liquid suspension culture, based on coculturing of thymocytes and bone marrow cells (Dexter *et al.*, 1973), in which granulocytes proliferate actively for several days and also seem to mature normally. This system has been successfully applied to the study of granulocytic chalone (Lord *et al.*, 1974a,b; Lord, 1975), using the unique technique of measuring changes in the "structuredness" of the cell cytoplasmic matrix (Cercek *et al.*, 1973).

The well-known agar colony technique, in which the colonies develop from primitive cells committed primarily to the granulocytic series, is another advanced culture technique that may appear particularly useful in the study of granulocytic chalone (see MacVittie and McCarthy, 1974; Aardal *et al.*, 1977). It must be noted, however, that colony-stimulating factor (CSF) is needed for the development of agar colonies and the test extracts may thus directly interfere with CSF or, possibly, prevent its production or recognition. Thus the situation is somewhat similar to that seen in PHA-stimulated lymphocyte cultures and the inhibition does not necessarily reflect the defined action of chalones, i.e., direct inhibition of cell proliferation. Furthermore, in contrast to stimulated lymphocyte cultures, in the agar colony technique it is difficult to assay the effect of the test material after the time of plating; i.e., the effect on the colonies which have already begun to grow cannot easily be measured.

Recently a refinement of the conventional agar colony technique has been developed (Maurer and Henry, 1976, 1977) with the particular aim of developing a standardized quantitative assay for granulocytic chalone. In this refinement the cells are grown in agar-containing glass capillaries, and the number and the size of colonies and clusters are determined with the aid of an automated optical scanning system. If indeed it can be shown convincingly that one of the specific actions of granulocytic chalone is to counter CSF, then the new technique may turn out to be a powerful tool in the final purification of granulocytic chalone.

Thus far relatively few *in vitro* methods have been used in testing erythrocytic chalone. Among those already tried are the simple suspension cultures of bone marrow and of proliferating normoblasts from mouse fetal liver. More advanced techniques could be used and, in fact, have already been successfully adopted (D. J. O. Perrins, personal communication). However, compared with appropriate *in vivo* techniques (see Lord *et al.*, 1977), their main value is probably limited to a large-scale screening when it comes to the purification of the erythrocytic chalone.

## 10.3.2. Diffusion Chamber Technique

A closed *in vivo* culture system, utilizing diffusion chambers implanted in the abdominal cavity of mice or rats, was developed by Benestad (1970) for quantitative studies of hematopoietic cells. In brief, the chamber consists of two Millipore membranes sealed on either side of an acrylic ring. The volume of a typical chamber is about 130 $\mu$l and it is usually filled through a hole in the ring by injecting 100 $\mu$l of cell suspension into the chamber. After sealing, the chamber is implanted in the abdominal cavity of the host animal, often pretreated with drugs or irradiation to improve cell growth in the chambers. After a short-lasting initial decrease in cell counts, rapid growth is resumed, which at least in optimal conditions for granulopoiesis continues exponentially for about 1 week. The chambers harvested after predetermined culture times are then usually treated with pronase to dissolve the fibrin clot formed in the chambers.

The diffusion chamber technique is particularly well suited for studying granulocytic chalone. Among the advantages of this technique are the fast proliferation and normal maturation of granulocytic cells, comparable to those found in granulopoietically stimulated bone marrow *in situ* (Bøyum and Breivik, 1973). There are several alternative ways of using the diffusion chamber technique in the study of potential inhibitors of granulopoiesis. Thus, two or more chambers, filled with different cell types, can be implanted into the abdominal cavity of the same host animal to assay the specificity of the inhibitory action. Furthermore, the putative inhibitor can be applied to the target cells in a variety of ways. These include injection of the inhibitor into the host animal; application of the inhibitor directly into the chamber (treatment *in vitro* of the inoculated cells); addition of the potential inhibitor-producing cells to the chamber with the target cells or to another chamber in a double-chamber system; and implantation of the chambers into host animals with an expected high endogenous inhibitor level. As indicated later, all these variations can be further combined with measurements of different endpoints, and hence the diffusion chamber technique can be used to give vital information on many aspects of chalone action. In many ways the diffusion chamber technique is superior to all other assay systems of blood cell chalones. It is natural, however, that it cannot fully substitute for assays performed under nonartificial *in vivo* conditions. In addition, the diffusion chamber technique cannot easily be used as an assay system when large numbers of test fractions are screened for inhibitory activity.

### 10.3.3. *In Vivo* Models

It is self-evident that the true role of chalones in the regulation of cell proliferation cannot be solved with the aid of artificial assay systems, regardless of the precision of the information thus obtained. Clearly, the ultimate reality of chalones can only be proved in an *in vivo* situation.

Because of the complexity of living systems, *in vivo* studies are subjected to experimental pitfalls which make the interpretation of the results difficult. With regard to the blood cell chalones, the effects of the putative erythrocytic chalone are perhaps easiest to establish unequivocally *in vivo*, provided sufficient quantities of reasonably purified material are available for testing. *In vivo* demonstration of the action of erythrocytic chalone is not beset with enormous technical difficulties, owing to the rather detailed knowledge in the kinetics of erythropoiesis and to the relative ease and precision with which various endpoints can be measured. It is thus not surprising that in the study of erythrocytic chalone the progress, although slow, has actually been unique in the "history" of chalones: after only a few *in vitro* experiments, a rather detailed *in vivo* study was successfully conducted (Lord *et al.*, 1977).

In the case of lymphocytic and granulocytic chalones, miscellaneous *in vivo* models have been used. In essence, the models differ from each other merely with respect to the endpoints measured. These include treatment of animals and man with test extracts, followed by measurements of tumor regression and survival times of leukemic individuals, changes in DNA synthesis in different tissues, rate of thymus growth in neonatal animals, changes in blood lymphocyte counts, alterations in the immune response against sheep red blood cells and dinitrophenylated antigens, effects on graft-versus-host reaction, survival times of skin allografts and xenografts, accumulation of granulocytes into an inflammatory focus, and effects on leukemia in man. Many of the *in vivo* studies, however, are open to criticism. In particular, injections of crude tissue extracts at enormous doses (up to ~300 mg/kg) sometimes make the interpretation of the results rather hazardous. Furthermore, the endpoints measured are not always unequivocal indicators of cell proliferation. This is especially true of changes in the immune response of the animal treated, because the material injected may have interfered with activation or recognition phenomena rather than with cell proliferation. Several specific problems involved in the *in vivo* studies are discussed in more detail in the sections on the chalone concerned.

## 10.3.4. Measurement of Chalone Action

Because chalones are, by definition, inhibitors of cell proliferation, their action should in principle be easy to measure. Indeed, the methodological difficulties in chalone research do not depend on a lack of adequate techniques of recording changes in cell proliferation; many simple and advanced techniques are readily available for this purpose.

In addition to obtaining reasonably pure test material, characterized well enough to reassure us as to the material composition of the inhibitor, methodological difficulties in chalone research become formidable when it comes to demonstrating, unequivocally, the cell line specificity of the inhibitory action and the lack of cytotoxicity. For instance, it is obviously impossible, under *in vitro* conditions, to assay the effect of a putative chalone on all cell types under identical conditions. The best practical approach is to test it against closely related cell lines rather than against completely dissimilar cells which just happen to be on hand (see Lord *et al.*, 1974a; Lord, 1976). Under *in vivo* conditions the problem of specificity can, of course, be faced more physiologically, but the complexity of living systems and the need for repeated injections create a number of new problems. Thus far granulocytic and erythrocytic chalones are actually the only chalones which have been studied extensively under *in vivo* conditions (see Sections 10.4.3 and 5).

There is nothing unique in principle in the assay techniques used to reveal the specificity of chalone action. In specificity tests, it would naturally be preferable to measure the same endpoints both in the putative target and in the control cell lines, but this is often simply impossible. Sometimes it is actually advantageous to measure endpoints which are most typical of a particular tissue; the typical example is hemoglobin synthesis in the study of erythropoiesis.

The assay techniques available for measuring cell proliferation *per se* are naturally the same in chalone research as in any field interested in cell proliferation. Most of them are standard methods, such as those measuring incorporation of tritiated thymidine ($[^3H]$-TdR) into the cells synthesizing DNA. It is a little surprising, however, that some of the commonly adopted techniques are occasionally considered totally inadequate when it comes to the demonstration of a chalone effect (see, e.g., Houck, 1973, 1976). This is particularly true of techniques using $[^3H]$TdR uptake as an indicator of cell proliferation. It is clear, of course, that changes in $[^3H]$-TdR uptake cannot always be equated with changes in cell proliferation, but few, if any, of the various pitfalls are unique for chalone tests. Most potential artifacts, such as dilution by cold thymidine and alteration or catabolism of [$^3$H]-TdR by the test extract, do not represent insuperable complications which cannot be readily detected.

Because chalones are, by definition, inhibitors of cell proliferation, the most realistic endpoint in studying chalone action is a direct measurement of cell production. This is easily possible in closed systems where growing cell populations can be studied quantitatively. Many *in vitro* cultures, especially those involving established cell lines, and also *in vivo* cultures utilizing diffusion chambers, are suitable for such measurements and they have also been used extensively in chalone research. In nonartificial *in vivo* conditions direct quantitative studies of cell populations are more complicated; for instance, it is often difficult to control changes in population size caused by cell "migration." In the case of hematopoietic cell lines it is particularly difficult to measure directly the total cell mass in the body. Furthermore, in normal adult animals cell populations do not expand but are in steady state. An injected extract may therefore simply contribute as a similar fictitious "unhappiness" factor, as has been suggested for *in vitro* cultures which run down in their cellularity (see Lord, 1976).

It is a little surprising that chalone effects have only occasionally been tested in neonatal, fast-growing animals. Yet such a model is in many ways nearly ideal, because it provides an opportunity to determine the cell line specificity of the inhibitory action by simple and direct assessment of growth rates simultaneously in a variety of cell populations. In those few instances in which this approach has been used (Rytömaa and Kiviniemi, 1969, 1970; Chung and Hufnagel, 1973), the results have been promising and should encourage further trials of a similar nature. It may already be noted here that in the experiments involving treatment of transplanted chloroleukemia in baby rats (Rytömaa and Kiviniemi, 1969, 1970), the growth of the chalone-injected leukemic animals was as fast as the growth of their untreated nonleukemic littermates. Because there can be no doubt whatsoever that the preparations used in these studies contained at least some inhibitor(s), active both *in vitro* and *in vivo* in a variety of assay conditions (see Section 10.4.3), the apparent total lack of effect on nongranulocytic cell lines in baby rats provides strong evidence for a specific, noncytotoxic action.

As already noted, one of the major difficulties in demonstrating the chalone effect is an unequivocal exclusion of cytotoxicity. Clearly, failure to detect cytotoxic damage to the cells by any direct technique is always open to the criticism that the methods employed were not sensitive enough. The main problem, of course, is the requirement that the results prove a lack of difference, i.e., something which is the opposite of a normal experimental approach. Although several findings are capable of rendering cytotoxicity highly unlikely, such as reversibility of the inhibition, perhaps the best evidence is obtained by showing that inhibition of proliferative activity is not accompanied by concomitant depression of other types of activities in the inhibited cells. In tests with granulocytic chalone, such evidence has been obtained in a rather clear-cut manner. It has been shown that development of the cytoplasmic machinery, characteristic of the maturation of granulocytic cells, is not depressed in chalone-inhibited precursor cells but is actually stimulated (Benestad and Rytömaa, 1977).

It seems unnecessary to discuss in more detail the wide variety of techniques that are available for the direct or indirect measurement of cell proliferation. In addition to the measurements involving direct assessment of population growth, such as cell and colony counting, and the methods involving incorporation of [$^3$H]-TdR or other labeled precursor substances into the cells, these techniques include trapping of the cells in metaphase (stathmokinetic index), measurement of the "structuredness" of the cell cytoplasmic matrix, measurement of the DNA content of single cells with automatic fluorescence cytophotometry, and even measurements involving specific functions of a cell line, such as rejection of a skin graft (see, however, Section 10.6.1).

## 10.4. Granulocytic Chalone

### 10.4.1. Crude Granulocyte Extract

By definition, granulocytic chalone should be obtainable directly from granulocytes. To this end, granulocytes have usually been isolated either from the blood or from an artificially induced inflammatory exudate (Rytömaa and Kiviniemi, 1968a; Bateman, 1974; Lord *et al.*, 1974a; Lord, 1975; MacVittie and McCarthy, 1974; Maiolo *et al.*, 1975; Rytömaa *et al.*, 1976; Løvhaug and Bøyum, 1977; Balázs *et al.*, 1977), but occasionally other sources have also been used, such as bone marrow and even spleen (Rytömaa and Kiviniemi, 1968c; Paukovits, 1971, 1973; Aardal *et al.*, 1977). In these last-mentioned tissues, however, cell populations are unnecessarily heterogeneous and hence crude extracts are rather strongly contaminated by a variety of substances. If granulocytic cells are unequivocally shown to be the specific source of granulocytic chalone, then mixtures of cell populations may naturally be used as starting material, especially if large quantities of granulocytes are then obtained more easily. At present, however, purification techniques for granulocytic chalone are neither easy enough nor sufficiently well standardized to make the use of highly heterogeneous mixtures of cell populations advantageous compared with the use of pure, or almost pure, granulocytic cells. In addition to the direct extraction of cells, granulocytic chalone has also been obtained from natural "granulocyte conditioned media," such as serum and aseptically induced ascitic fluid (Rytömaa and Kiviniemi, 1967, 1968a; Paukovits, 1971; Laerum and Maurer, 1973). However, these sources do not provide obvious advantages for the purification of granulocytic chalone.

Absolutely pure populations of normal granulocytes are difficult to obtain and hence it may be questioned whether these cells are really the specific source of granulocytic chalone. There are several lines of evidence which show that this is the case. Thus, it has been shown that lymphocytes and erythrocytes, i.e., the two cell types most commonly contaminating granulocyte populations isolated from blood, do not release detectable quantities of granulocytic chalone (Kivilaakso and Rytömaa, 1971; Bateman, 1974; MacVittie and McCarthy, 1974; Maiolo et al., 1975; Lord, 1975; Lord et al., 1974a, 1977; Løvhaug and Bøyum, 1977). Monocytes/macrophages (the major contaminant cell type in "ascites cell suspensions") have not yet been directly excluded as a possible additional source of granulocytic chalone, but these cells are definitely not the sole or even the main source of the inhibitor. This is clear from the findings that good inhibitor yields are readily obtained from cell suspensions which are, at least for all practical purposes, totally free of monocytes/macrophages, such as highly purified normal granulocytes isolated from blood (Bøyum et al., 1976; Løvhaug and Bøyum, 1977) and human leukemic granulocytes (Maiolo et al., 1975; Bøyum et al., 1976). Conversely, detectable amounts of granulocytic chalone are not obtainable from blood leukocytes isolated from some leukemic patients (ALL, and CML in blastic crisis; see Maiolo et al., 1975), although the cell suspensions extracted evidently contained some monocytes, but no mature granulocytes. It may also be noted that granulocytic chalone cannot be extracted from tissues such as liver, which contain macrophages but virtually no granulocytes (Rytömaa, 1973a).

In most studies crude granulocyte extracts have been obtained using cell suspensions of which 70–90% are granulocytes; in some cases the purity has been as high as 99% (Bøyum et al., 1976; Løvhaug and Bøyum, 1977). In contrast to the common practice of biochemists of extracting tissue homogenates, granulocytic chalone is usually obtained by incubating intact cells, e.g., in saline. This is naturally more physiological in light of the chalone concept, and it also represents a powerful purification step in the isolation of the substance. The techniques used vary a little among different groups of workers; the "classical" method of obtaining crude granulocyte extracts is to incubate intact cells in saline or in a balanced salt solution for 1–2 hr at 37°C. After collecting the supernatant the same cells can be "reextracted" several times without apparent loss in the inhibitor yield (Rytömaa and Kiviniemi, 1968b).

Extracts made from 1 liter of blood yield approximately 10 mg of (desalted) crude leukocyte extract following a 1-hr incubation period. About one-third of this material comprises proteins/polypeptides and about one-tenth different purine/pyrimidine derivatives (Rytömaa, 1976). It may be noted that crude granulocyte extracts do not contain thymidine detectable with highly sensitive techniques (Rytömaa, 1976; Maurer *et al.*, 1976), and hence the criticism occasionally expressed suggesting thymidine dilution as the cause of the inhibition has no foundation.

Crude (desalted) granulocyte extracts significantly inhibit [$^3$H]-TdR uptake in short-term bone marrow cultures at a concentration of 10$\mu$g/ml or less (see Rytömaa, 1976). Although this figure is of no great interest *per se*, it shows that crude extracts added to the cultures do not significantly upset the composition of an ordinary culture medium. For instance, the total protein/polypeptide content of a medium supplemented with 10% serum is increased by less than 0.1% following the addition of 10 $\mu$g/ml of the crude extract. It is indeed highly unlikely that crude granulocyte extracts would contain any physiological substance in an amount that exerts a pure pharmacological effect on the cells, provided excessive concentrations are not used. It is important to realize, however, that crude extracts nevertheless *do* contain substances which are potentially hazardous. It is possible, although perhaps not likely, that extensive purification of chalone activity leads to marked enrichment of an originally innocent physiological substance which then, at a high test concentration, inhibits cell proliferation in a nonspecific manner. Among such substances are several nucleosides and nucleotides (Rytömaa and Kiviniemi, 1975).

## 10.4.2. Purification of Granulocytic Chalone

Granulocytic chalone has not yet been isolated in a pure form and its chemical nature remains to be determined. It is a matter of opinion, however, whether or not the purity reached thus far is reasonable to warrant a conclusion of the chemical "reality" of this substance. If it is required that the substance at least be characterized as to its composition, granulocytic chalone is perhaps not yet chemically "real." On the other hand, if it is sufficient that a factor, at extremely low test concentrations, produces detectable effects *in vitro* and *in vivo*, granulocytic chalone is definitely real chemically as well. In this latter sense, the material existence of granulocytic chalone is indicated by the finding that a partially purified preparation causes measurable effects *in vitro* at a concentration of 50 pg/ml which, if the average molecular weight of the cocktail is 1000 daltons, represents a $5 \times 10^{-11}$ M solution (Lord, 1975). In regard to the *in vivo* effects, more highly purified preparations have been shown to inhibit leukemia in man after intravenous injections of doses as low as 80 $\mu$g/kg

(Rytömaa *et al.*, 1976). Because even these preparations still are cocktails of many different substances, the biologically active factor may well be effective at dose levels of 1 $\mu$g/kg. Clearly, therefore, granulocytic chalone is active both *in vitro* and *in vivo* at concentrations that are very much smaller than those commonly needed for unphysiological substances with a pharmacological action. Furthermore, in sharp contrast to most unphysiological substances, the biologically active dose of granulocytic chalone can be increased 1000-fold without detectable side effects *in vivo* (Rytömaa *et al.*, 1976, 1977). Compared, for example, with cytotoxic substances used in the treatment of human malignancies, a very much smaller increase in dose would be immediately fatal to the patient. It may also be noted in passing that a 1000-fold increase in the therapeutic dose of such an "innocent" drug as aspirin would kill the patient rather quickly. Under *in vitro* conditions an effective concentration of granulocytic chalone can be increased at least $10^6$-fold without signs of cell damage (Lord, 1975). All these findings indicate that inhibition of cell proliferation by granulocytic chalone is clearly unique and definitely not explicable in terms of trivial pharmacological effects.

In spite of high purification, the evidence for the chemical nature of granulocytic chalone now available is not yet conclusive. According to Paukovits (1973; Paukovits and Paukovits, 1975a, 1976), granulocytic chalone is a strongly acidic peptide or possibly a glycopeptide. Paukovits has even reported a preliminary amino acid composition for an inhibitor, believed to be the granulocytic chalone (Paukovits and Paukovits, 1976). This substance, capable of inhibiting $[^3H]$-TdR uptake in short-term bone marrow cultures, was extracted by incubating nonhomogenized rabbit marrow cells in Hanks' solution, and then extensively purified using ultrafiltrations (500–20,000 daltons fraction) and successive steps of gel filtration chromatography (Sephadex G-25 and G-15), followed by electrophoresis and thin-layer chromatography. The total yield from 1.3 $\times$ $10^{10}$ bone marrow cells was 9–10 $\mu$g, i.e., rather small for an accurate analysis of amino acid composition. However, a preliminary analysis revealed 22 amino acid residues and the presence of glucosamine or galactosamine, or both, and probably glucose. The molecular weight of the purified material, as estimated from the amino acid composition, was about 3000 daltons.

Unfortunately, the total yield of the purified inhibitor was too small for adequate biological testing and hence the evidence is not yet sufficient to warrant the conclusion that the amino acid composition detected represents granulocytic chalone. In fact it is quite likely that it does not, e.g., because granulocytic chalone seems to be considerably smaller than 3000 daltons; approximately 1000 daltons is probably much closer to the true value (unpublished observations).

It follows from these uncertainties that the preliminary amino acid composition may not only misrepresent the true composition, but that it does not even prove the peptide nature of granulocytic chalone. Although it is likely that this inhibitor really is a small peptide, hard facts are still lacking. Perhaps the only direct evidence indicating the peptide nature of the inhibitor is its apparent susceptibility to the action of trypsin (Paukovits and Paukovits, 1975a). However, even this evidence may not be fully convincing, because an unusually long period of treatment with trypsin (0.05%, 8 hr at 37°C) was necessary in order to destroy the inhibitory activity.

Thus, despite energetic attempts to purify and chemically characterize granulocytic chalone, surprisingly little is known with certainty. Critical evaluation of the evidence available shows that almost the only characteristic which has been demonstrated beyond a reasonable doubt is a low molecular weight. The behavior of the inhibitor even in basically simple systems, such as gel filtration chromatography, displays certain peculiarities which warrant caution, e.g., regarding the reported exact elution volumes. It is not possible to discuss these problems in detail here, but it is worth noting that almost all chemical characteristics associated with granulocytic chalone are uncertain. This does not mean that all, or even most, of the observations reported are wrong; however, some of them seem to be misleading. The reasons for this peculiar situation are not clear, but they may be remotely similar to the difficulties encountered in the application of various purification procedures to lymphocytic and fibroblastic chalones (Houck *et al.*, 1977).

In view of the foregoing, it is clearly risky to suggest anything about the chemistry of granulocytic chalone. However, it would be unwise not to mention that Burzynski *et al.* (1976), who have isolated 119 medium-sized peptides from human urine, point out that the action of some of their peptides is similar to that of chalones. In particular, one of the peptides inhibited DNA synthesis in human myeloid leukemia *in vitro* in an apparently cell line specific manner. Whether or not this strongly acidic peptide (probably a sulfated glycopeptide containing as much as 40% carbohydrate moiety) has anything to do with granulocytic chalone remains to be shown.

## 10.4.3. Specificity of Action

The first reports showing specific inhibition of granulocytic precursor cells by extracts obtainable directly from granulocytes were published in the late 1960s (Rytömaa and Kiviniemi, 1967, 1968a,b,c,d). Measuring [³H]-TdR uptake in short-term bone marrow cultures, together with autoradiographic analysis of the cells, we demonstrated that crude and partially purified granulocyte extracts depressed specifically the proliferation of granulocytic precursor cells. These findings were later confirmed and extended by different groups of workers utilizing a variety of techniques. In addition to those based on essentially similar nonideal *in vitro* models and assay techniques used by us (e.g., Paukovits, 1971, 1973; Shadduck, 1971; Cross 1972, 1974; Balázs *et al.*, 1972, 1977; Bateman, 1974; Maiolo *et al.*, 1975), the specific inhibitory effect of granulocyte extracts on granulocytic precursor cells was also demonstrated by more advanced assay techniques. Regarding *in vitro* models, Lord *et al.* (1974a,b) used the unique technique of measuring "structuredness" of the cell cytoplasmic matrix (SCM) to investigate the specificity and reversibility of the inhibition of hematopoietic cell proliferation by blood cell extracts. They showed that granulocyte extracts did indeed affect granulocytic precursor cells in a highly specific manner. These extracts, purified partially by ultrafiltrations, had no effect on erythroid and lymphoid cells and, conversely, extracts of erythrocytes and lymphocytes had no effect on proliferating granulocytes but affected their own types of precursor cells. Furthermore, the actions of the different extracts were not based on cytotoxicity because the effects were fully reversible simply by washing the cells.

The effect of granulocyte extracts on granulocyte growth has also been studied using the agar colony technique. The results showed that in the presence of granulocyte extracts the action of colony-stimulating factor (CSF) was blocked (MacVittie and McCarthy, 1974). Colony formation was also inhibited by incubating bone marrow cells together with partially purified extracts for a short time prior to plating (Aardal *et al.*, 1977). This effect could be reversed by washing the bone marrow cells after incubation for 1 hr, but not after incubation for 5 hr. Aardal *et al.* (1977) also demonstrated that by increasing the dose of CSF the inhibitory effect of granulocyte extracts was prevented; however, at high concentrations the effect of granulocyte extracts could not be released by excess CSF. Judging from the trypan blue exclusion test, granulocyte extracts were not toxic to bone marrow cells (incubation for 24 hr) nor did they inhibit Sc-1 lymphoblastic leukemia cells growing exponentially (Aardal *et al.*, 1977), lymphocyte response to PHA, rat marrow response to erythropoietin, and proliferation of mouse L-929 fibroblasts (MacVittie and McCarthy, 1974).

It is thus clear that granulocyte extracts inhibit agar colony formation in an apparently nontoxic manner, but it is not yet certain that this is a chalone effect. Because colony growth is dependent on CSF, the inhibitory effect represents competition with the colony-stimulating factor rather than direct inhibition of cell proliferation. It is possible, however, that granulocytic chalone and CSF compete for the same receptor sites on the cell membrane (see Paukovits, 1976). If this is the case, then the blocking of CSF action would be a most useful, although indirect, assay of granulocytic chalone. It may be noted in this context that there is indeed some evidence for cell-surface receptors of granulocytic chalone (Paukovits and Paukovits, 1975b), but it remains to be shown whether or not CSF acts via the same receptor sites.

The complicated situation found in granulopoiesis in living systems does not easily allow convincing direct demonstration of the direct effects of granulocytic chalone *in vivo*. However, the closed *in vivo* culture system, utilizing diffusion chambers implanted in the abdominal cavity of mice or rats, provides an excellent assay system for the granulocytic chalone. In the first experiments utilizing this technique, granulocyte extracts were shown to inhibit DNA synthesis in proliferating granulocytes (Benestad *et al.*, 1973). The extracts had no effect on proliferating immunoblasts and macrophages cultured in another chamber in the same mice (twin chamber system) and hence the inhibitory effect was cell line specific.

The lack of effect of granulocyte extracts on macrophage proliferation in diffusion chamber cultures was later confirmed by other workers (Laerum and Maurer, 1973; Løvhaug and Bøyum, 1977). This finding provides very strong evidence in favor of absolute specificity of granulocytic chalone action, because macrophages are probably more closely related to granulocytes than any other cell line in the body. In view of this it may not seem particularly impressive that granulocytic chalone has also been shown to be without effect on a number of other cell lines cultured in diffusion chambers. These include the pluripotent stem cell or CFU-S (MacVittie and McCarthy, 1975; Løvhaug and Bøyum, 1977)—which have also been shown to be insensitive to granulocytic chalone in other assay systems (Lord, 1975)—HeLa cells and mouse mastocytoma cells (Vilpo *et al.*, 1973), Ehrlich ascites carcinoma cells (Ferris *et al.*, 1973), and human psoriatic skin (Kariniemi, 1976).

Owing to the timing of chalone administration in the first experiments utilizing diffusion chambers (Benestad *et al.*, 1973), no reduction could even be expected in the granulocyte yields. However, using more appropriate treatment schedules such an effect was readily demonstrated (Laerum and Maurer, 1973; Vilpo *et al.*, 1973; MacVittie and McCarthy, 1974; Løvhaug and Bøyum, 1977). This is important because direct demonstration of reduced cell production is naturally the best endpoint in chalone studies.

In addition to showing cell line specificity and a lack of cytotoxicity (regarding the latter, see Section 10.4.4), the diffusion chamber technique has given much new information on the effects of granulocytic chalone. Perhaps the most interesting of these is the finding that chalone-inhibited proliferative granulocytes mature at an accelerated rate (Benestad and Rytömaa, 1977). It is possible, or even probable, that the faster maturation is not directly caused by chalone, but that it merely reflects improved development of the functional machinery in the presence of reduced "proliferative metabolism" and reduced "dilution" associated with each mitotic division. Another finding of considerable interest is the demonstration that granulocytic chalone inhibits the growth of proliferating committed granulocytic progenitor cells or CFU-C (MacVittie and McCarthy, 1975; Bøyum *et al.*, 1976). It remains to be shown whether this effect is based on direct inhibition of proliferative activity of CFU-C or on competition with CSF for the same receptor sites on the cell membrane (cf. Section 10.4.4).

In spite of the superiority of the diffusion chamber technique over *in vitro* cultures, it is still an artificial assay system and not fully comparable to genuine living systems. Consequently, the ultimate reality of granulocytic chalone requires direct demonstration of the inhibitory activity *in vivo*. Early attempts to show this by injecting chalone into mice indicated that DNA synthesis was inhibited in granulocytic precursor cells, but not in the other types of bone marrow cells (Rytömaa and Kiviniemi, 1968d). Schütt and Langen (1972) confirmed a little later that crude granulocyte extracts do indeed inhibit granulopoiesis *in vivo*. These authors showed that injection of the test material depressed [$^3$H]-TdR uptake by granulocytic precursor cells in the bone marrow and reduced labeling of granulocytes recovered later from an induced inflammatory focus.

These early studies of the effects of granulocytic chalone in living systems were not fully convincing and they are rarely noted even by those who support the chalone theory. However, later studies have established that granulocyte extracts are certainly effective *in vivo* and that the inhibition is both cell line specific and noncytotoxic. Thus, it was demonstrated by Lord (1975) that partially purified granulocytic chalone (500–2000 mol. wt. range fraction) reduced the labeling index ([$^3$H]-TdR) in the granulocytic cell population of regenerating mouse spleen within 0.5–1 hr, followed by a slow return to normal within 12 hr. Lymphocyte and erythrocyte extracts were without effect and, conversely, granulocyte extract had no effect on lymphoid cell labeling in regenerating spleen. Repeated labeling experiments showed that proliferating granulocytes in regenerating spleen had a cell cycle time of 15 hr with an S-phase duration of about 4.5 hr; treatment with granulocytic chalone prolonged the cycle time to 30 hr and the S-phase duration to 6 hr. Cell production in developing granulocytic spleen colonies in polycythemic mice was reduced by repeated injections of granulocytic chalone over a period of 4 days; approximately two cell doublings were lost during this treatment period. CFU-S was not affected by granulocytic chalone; the inhibited colony growth was based on reduced colony cellularity. It may also be noted that Lord *et al.* (1977) later demonstrated that granulocytic chalone does not affect labeling of erythroid cells in regenerating spleen colonies, spleen colony growth, and radioiron incorporation into erythroid cells.

Further studies of the *in vivo* effects of granulocytic chalone, in both animals and man, are discussed in Section 10.10 in detail. It may be noted here that repeated injections of partially purified granulocytic chalone have been shown to lead to a selective inhibition of proliferating normal and leukemic granulocytes without any inhibition of lymphopoiesis, erythropoiesis, megakaryopoiesis, and, in fact, any nongranulocytic cell line in the body (Rytömaa and Kiviniemi, 1969, 1970; Rytömaa *et al.*, 1976, 1977).

### 10.4.4. Mechanism of Action

An essential part of the granulocyte system consists of a series of transit populations in which cell proliferation takes place. In such a system one skipped mitosis means that the output (i.e., the production of postmitotic end cells) is halved. The average number of successive mitoses thus determines the degree of amplification when the cells proceed through the transit populations. It is intuitively obvious that the number of successive mitoses is subject to regulation and is not a biologically unique invariate (see Rytömaa, 1973b, 1976).

One of the simplest ways to alter the degree of amplification is to modulate the duration of the cell cycle:

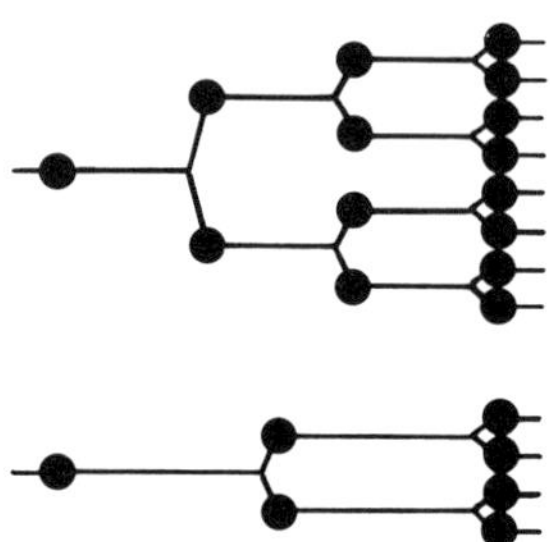

The role of granulocytic chalone in granulopoiesis is thus easily recognized: chalone prolongs cell cycle time. Consequently, an understanding of the mechanism of chalone action, even at the molecular level, does not require fundamental new discoveries. Clearly, any reaction in the chain of events leading to cell division can be made rate limiting, and thus the number of theoretically possible molecular targets for chalone action is huge. One candidate, supported by some experimental evidence

(Nakai, 1976), is DNA polymerase. It may be noted that the simplistic model for granulocytic chalone action shows that there is no obvious need to make the rate of the limiting reaction zero: depending on the average number of successive mitoses, even a minor (a few percent) decrease in the rate of the reaction can easily halve cell production.

The evidence available suggests that granulocytic chalone does indeed act by prolonging the cell cycle. For instance, repeated labeling of granulocytic colonies in regenerating mouse spleen showed that granulocytic chalone doubled the cell cycle time, mainly by prolonging the duration of the $G_1$ phase (Lord, 1975). Similarly, granulocytic chalone also seems to lengthen the cell cycle in rat chloroleukemia cells without blocking cell proliferation completely (Fig.1) (P. Foa, W. Paile, H. Toivonen, and T. Rytömaa, unpublished results).

According to the *in vivo* results reported by Lord (1975), the main effect of granulocytic chalone was on the $G_1$ phase of the cycle; the S phase was moderately affected. It has often been reported that chalone-induced inhibition also leads to a decreased mean grain count of [3H]-TdR-labeled cells (Rytömaa and Kiviniemi, 1968a; Laerum and Maurer, 1973; Vilpo *et al.*, 1973; Bateman, 1974). This is not an unequivocal demonstration of prolonged S-phase duration, but such an explanation is an apparent possibility. The findings of Ferris *et al.* (1973) also support this conclusion. These authors determined the fraction of labeled mitosis (FLM) curve for chloroleukemia cells grown in diffusion chambers in leukemic hosts and observed prolongation of the S phase. In the assay conditions used by Ferris *et al.* (1973), chloroleukemic cells are strongly inhibited by granulocytic chalone, owing to the high endogenous level of chalone produced by the tumor cells of the host animal (Rytömaa and Kiviniemi, 1967, 1968c; Vilpo *et al.*, 1973). It may be noted that nongranulocytic cell lines are not affected when grown in diffusion chambers in these hosts and, conversely, that chloroleukemia cells are not inhibited in animals bearing nongranulocytic tumors (Vilpo *et al.*, 1973; Ferris *et al.*, 1973).

Thus a reduction in the mean grain count, the FLM curves, and the continuous labeling indicates prolongation of the S phase by granulocytic chalone. This effect was less marked than the effect on the $G_1$ phase, especially in granulocytic colonies in regenerating mouse spleen (Lord, 1975). Judging from the FLM curves, the $G_1$ phase of chloroleukemia cells was not prolonged at all (Ferris *et al.*, 1973), but this finding is not necessarily at variance with Lord's (1975) results. It is possible that strongly inhibited chloroleukemia cells become quiescent in the $G_1$ phase. These noncycling or resting cells cannot then enter mitosis and hence they are not detected from the FLM curves. The response of chloroleukemia cells would thus be similar to that seen in JB-1 ascites plasmacytoma cells (see Bichel, 1976).

Prolongation of the S phase by granulocytic chalone could be explained in terms of inhibition of DNA polymerases (cf. Nakai, 1976). Such an explanation would also be consistent with the finding that granulocytic chalone does not directly inhibit the progress of cells through the $G_2$ phase (Laerum and Maurer, 1973; Lord, 1975). Ferris *et al.* (1973), however, observed prolongation of the $G_2$ phase in chloroleukemia cells, and hence the results obtained from the FLM curves are again different from those obtained by other techniques. However, it is possible that cells which are inhibited in the $G_1$ or S phase proceed more slowly through $G_2$. The possibility that granulocytic chalone would affect cells in the $G_2$ phase during the next rounds of the cell cycle may well be an indication that the durations of the different cell cycle phases are not independent.

One more point is worth noting with regard to the mechanism of granulocytic chalone action: the granulocytic chalone content in the bone marrow is evidently of more physiological importance than that in the blood. There are several reasons for suggesting this (cf. Cross, 1974) such as the great excess of granulocytic cells in the bone marrow compared with the total number of granulocytes in the peripheral blood. In addition, the local concentration of granulocytic chalone would evidently be higher in the bone marrow than in the blood even if both compartments contained the same number of cells, e.g., because in the blood the chalone would be subject to more dilution. Furthermore, a possible endogenous lability of the chalone molecule, as well as its probable loss by excretion and enzymatic degradation, would mean that each marrow-produced chalone molecule has a greater chance of acting on the target cells than a chalone molecule present in the blood.

## 10.4.5. Granulocytic Chalone and Immune Reactions

Preparations of granulocytic chalone, or leukocyte extracts with a small molecular weight in general, are nonimmunogenic in animals and man. Thus attempts to produce antibodies by injecting partially purified granulocytic chalone in Freund's complete adjuvant into rabbits were unsuccessful (Rytömaa *et al.*, 1977). Furthermore, antibodies to the chalone preparations were not detectable in a leukemic patient's serum after three courses of chalone injections over a period of more than 1 year (Rytömaa *et al.*, 1976, 1977). Finally, the chalone preparations did not cause blastic transformation of normal human lymphocytes *in vitro* (Rytömaa *et al.*, 1977).

It is of interest to note that in studies concerned with transfer factor, dialysates of leukocyte extracts failed to elicit antibody production in man by repeated injections in high weekly doses, over a period of about 1 year

(Lawrence, 1969). These extracts, which were clearly purified less than those containing granulocytic chalone, also failed to produce antibodies when injected in Freund's adjuvant into rabbits (Lawrence, 1969); furthermore, they did not cause blastic transformation of human lymphocytes *in vitro* (Fireman *et al.*, 1967) and were incapable of actively immunizing recipients to reject a skin homograft from the leukocyte donor (Rapaport *et al.*, 1965). Clearly, therefore, leukocyte extracts from which substances with a large molecular weight ($>$10,000 daltons) have been removed are nonimmunogenic in both animals and man. Because the preparations of granulocytic chalone used in the recent *in vivo* studies (Rytömaa *et al.*, 1976, 1977) were purified much more highly than merely by dialysis, the apparent total lack of immunogenicity of these preparations is not surprising.

However, the major criticism of *in vivo* studies of granulocytic chalone has been related to possible immunological complications caused by the injection of a variety of foreign materials into an animal or man (Houck and Attallah, 1976; Houck and Hunt, 1976). It was suggested that this greatly stimulates immunological rejection mechanisms and, therefore, that the inhibition of tumor growth is not via inhibition of cell proliferation by chalones but rather via rejection phenomena. Yet it is not immediately obvious how injections of a nonimmunogenic material could lead to marked immunological stimulation. Houck suggests that this may be accomplished by a transfer factor which, according to this author, is very similar to granulocytic chalone and presumably a contaminant in the chalone preparations.

It is indeed true that the methods of isolating transfer factor (for a review, see Lawrence, 1969) appear somewhat similar to those used for isolating granulocytic chalone. However, it is highly unlikely that transfer factor is a common contaminant in chalone preparations—and even if it were, it certainly does not cause the effects obtained in the *in vivo* studies of granulocytic chalone. For instance, transfer factor is isolated from lymphocytes rather than from granulocytes, and at least in some cases the cell populations used for isolating granulocytic chalone have been free of lymphocytes. However, more important than this is the well-established fact that transfer factor is not present at all in leukocyte extracts obtained from nonsensitive donors. It is absurd to assume that, e.g., ox might be a "sensitive donor" which could provide transfer factor capable of effecting passive transfer of homograft sensitivity to reject leukemic cells in man. In fact, it has been shown that in the transfer of homograft rejection in humans it is obligatory for another individual to be actively sensitized via a homograft before the appearance of a new transfer factor for that graft (see, e.g., Lawrence *et al.*, 1960; Nadler and Moore, 1965; Lawrence, 1969). Furthermore, the transfer factor produced in this fashion is highly

individual specific, with specificity directed only against the transplantation antigens of the individual providing the homograft for sensitization.
It is thus virtually impossible that oxen in England possess a transfer
factor specific for the antigenic configuration of leukemic cells of a
Finnish patient. Transfer factor does not even cross the species barrier *in
vivo* (see Lawrence, 1969).

Interestingly enough, transfer factor is not yet chemically more "real"
than granulocytic chalone (see Rainer and Moser, 1977).

## 10.5. Erythrocytic Chalone

As already noted several times, one of the essential properties of a
chalone is the specificity of the source, i.e., the inhibitor must be obtainable from the same cell line on which it acts. Because it is usually difficult to
isolate pure cell populations for chalone extraction, red cells provide a
welcome exception. Furthermore, incubation of intact nonnucleated red
cells for 1–2 hr in saline and then collecting the supernatant—which is the
common procedure in obtaining erythrocytic chalone (Kivilaakso and
Rytömaa, 1971; Bateman, 1974; Bateman and Goodwin, 1976; Lord *et al.*,
1974a, 1977)—results in a crude extract which is clearly contaminated
much less than most "normal" chalone-containing cocktails prepared by
extracting homogenized tissues rich in several different cell types.

A little surprisingly, essentially nothing is known of the chemical
properties of erythrocytic chalone. The only property that is known with
any certainty is its low molecular weight; judging from gel filtration
chromatography and ultrafiltrations (see Kivilaakso and Rytömaa, 1971;
Bateman, 1974; Bateman and Goodwin, 1976; Lord *et al.*, 1974a. 1977),
erythrocytic chalone has a molecular weight somewhere between 500 and
10,000 daltons, most likely near 1000. An almost complete lack of information of this type is surprising, because erythrocytic chalone is presumably the easiest of all chalones to purify and characterize. In addition to
the practically unlimited supply of red cells and their easy isolation, and
the apparent relative purity of crude red cell extracts, the availability of
several unambiguous assay techniques for erythropoiesis should make the
chemical characterization of erythrocytic chalone rather easy. It is possible
that such work has been delayed, because evidence for the material reality
of erythrocytic chalone may not have been convincing until now.

The existence of erythrocytic chalone was first suggested by circumstantial evidence showing that serum of polycythemic rats inhibits [3H]-
TdR uptake by bone marrow cells *in vitro* (Rytömaa and Kiviniemi, 1967;
Kivilaakso and Rytömaa, 1970). Further studies demonstrated that a
similar inhibitor of erythrocytic precursor cells is also obtainable directly

from mature red cells. Results obtained from measuring incorporation of [$^3$H]-TdR into cultured bone marrow combined with autoradiographic analysis of the cells, indicated that partially purified red cell extracts depressed proliferation of the erythroid cells and that this effect was cell line specific (Kivilaakso and Rytömaa, 1971). These results were later confirmed by Bateman (1974) who used basically similar assay techniques, and at the same time also by Lord *et al.* (1974a) who used the technique of measuring "structuredness" of the cell cytoplasmic matrix (SCM). Lord *et al.* (1974a) demonstrated that partially purified red cell extracts do indeed have a highly specific effect on erythroid population, and that this effect is not based on cytotoxicity, because the inhibition was fully reversible simply by washing the cells. As judged from the changes in SCM, red cell extracts had no effect on proliferative granulocytic or on lymphocytic cells; conversely, granulocyte and lymphocyte extracts did not affect erythroid cells (proliferating normoblasts from mouse fetal liver).

As already stated several times, the ultimate reality of a chalone can only be proved by its biological activity under *in vivo* conditions. From this viewpoint erythrocytic chalone, together with granulocytic chalone, is clearly much better established than any other chalone studied thus far. The *in vivo* evidence for erythrocytic chalone action comes from the recent work of Lord *et al.* (1977) who assayed partially purified erythrocytic chalone *in vivo* by a variety of techniques. (It may be noted in passing that the Manchester group rarely uses the term chalone, although it is clear that they are studying inhibitors which fulfill the present definition exactly.) Using granulocyte and lymphocyte extracts as controls, the specific effect of erythrocytic chalone on the proliferation of erythrocytic precursor cells was confirmed by measuring autoradiographic labeling indices of erythroid and lymphoid cells in regenerating spleens of mice, spleen colony growth, and $^{59}$Fe incorporation. The results showed that partially purified erythrocytic chalone reduced the labeling index of the erythroid cells significantly within 1.5 hr, followed by a slow return to normal within 5–6 hr. The labeling index of the lymphoid cells was not affected by erythrocytic chalone; conversely, granulocyte and lymphocyte extracts did not affect erythroid cells. As judged from repeated labeling with [$^3$H]-TdR, erythroid cells in regenerating spleens of mice had a cell cycle time of about 11–12 hr with 4–4.5 hr spent in the S phase; treatment with erythrocytic chalone prolonged the cell cycle time to about 30 hr and the duration of the S phase to about 5–6 hr. Measurement of the stathmokinetic index using vinblastine indicated that erythrocytic chalone had no effect on the cells in the $G_2$ phase; however, the flow of cells to mitosis was strongly reduced by the time late $G_1$ and early S cells were expected to reach mitosis. Treatment of irradiated mice for a period of 4 days with erythrocytic chalone, which had earlier been shown to have no direct effect on CFU-S, the spleen colony-forming stem cell (Lord, 1975), reduced the mean cellularity of erythroid spleen colonies by about 50%. Erythrocytic chalone also caused a dramatic reduction in erythrocyte release into the circulation, as revealed by [59]Fe incorporation over a 24-hr period; the effect was maximal (60–70% depression) 2 days after erythrocytic chalone. A fivefold increase in dose did not cause stronger depression in radioiron incorporation, but retarded the recovery to normal an extra day. It was also reported that erythrocytic chalone had no effect on erythropoietin-responsive cells as revealed by [59]Fe incorporation in polycythemic mice given erythropoietin. This may warrant some caution regarding the effect of granulocytic chalone on committed granulocytic precursor cells (see Section 10.4.3), although the unresponsiveness of the committed erythroid cells is not yet clear. This reservation seems necessary because administering erythrocytic chalone to polycythemic mice with a high endogenous chalone content and no active erythropoiesis is likely to have no effect. Thus the finding that injecting erythropoietin 3 hr later normally stimulated erythropoiesis (Lord *et al.*, 1977) does not yet prove the unresponsiveness of committed erythroid progenitor cells to erythrocytic chalone.

The preparations used by Lord *et al.* (1977) were partially purified by ultrafiltrations (fraction of rat and pig erythrocyte extracts with a nominal molecular weight range of 500–10,000 daltons), but clearly they were far from being pure erythrocytic chalone. Nevertheless, intravenous injection of as little as 10 $\mu$g per mouse produced a maximum effect on iron incorporation. This dose, about 400 $\mu$g/kg, is comparable to the dose of partially purified granulocytic chalone effective against myeloid leukemia in man (lowest dose used 80 $\mu$g/kg; see Rytömaa *et al.*, 1976), and nearly 1000 times smaller than the doses commonly used in the *in vivo* studies of lymphocytic chalone. Because 1 liter of rat blood yields about 25 mg of red cell extract of this purity per hour (Lord *et al.*, 1977), it does not seem enormously difficult to obtain enough material for full chemical characterization of erythrocytic chalone.

## 10.6. Lymphocytic Chalone(s)

### 10.6.1. Specificity of Source and Action

The existence of two distinct types of lymphocytes, T and B cells, has now been firmly established. Because T- and B-lymphocytes respond to different functional stimuli, it may be expected that the proliferation of T and B cells is also regulated by different chalones. As indicated in the following, some evidence has been obtained to support this idea. However, in most studies distinct separation between the responses of T and B cells has not been possible and in the discussion that ensues the term lymphocytic chalone is used to refer to either one or both of the two putative types of chalones.

The first evidence for a lymphocytic chalone was reported by Moorhead *et al.* (1969), who showed that extracts of pig lymph nodes were capable of inhibiting the morphologically demonstrable transformation and [$^3$H]-TdR uptake by PHA-stimulated human lymphocytes *in vitro*. At the same time Bullough and Laurence (1970) observed that lymphocyte extracts inhibited mitotic activity of mouse lymphoma cells, as revealed by trapping the cells in metaphase. In this study lymphocyte extracts affected cells in the $G_2$ phase of the cell cycle. Olsson and Claësson (1975) have also shown that lymphocyte extracts inhibit the progression of normal thymocytes through the $G_2$ phase under *in vivo* conditions, hence confirming the findings of Bullough and Laurence (1970) with leukemic cells *in vitro*. Although not yet confirmed more extensively, these results suggest that lymphocyte proliferation may be controlled by two different chalones, one acting in $G_1$ and the other in $G_2$. A similar situation seems to exist in some other cell lines as well, such as epidermis (Elgjo *et al.*, 1971, 1972; Thornley and Laurence, 1976) and transplanted JB-1 ascites plasmacytoma (Bichel, 1973).

The existence of specific and endogenous inhibitors of lymphocyte transformation and proliferation was soon confirmed in different laboratories (e.g., Jones *et al.*, 1970; Lasalvia *et al.*, 1970; Garcia-Giralt *et al.*, 1970; Houck *et al.*, 1971; Kiger *et al.*, 1972a; Lord *et al.*, 1974a; Maiolo *et al.*, 1975; Olsson and Claësson, 1975; Heideman *et al.*, 1976; Blazsek *et al.*, 1976). The evidence published thus far on lymphocytic chalone is more extensive than that dealing with other blood cell chalones but the overall picture is, if anything, less clear.

In regard to the source of lymphocytic chalone, it is apparent that a cell line specific inhibitor is obtainable from thymus, spleen, lymph nodes, and from at least some established lymphoblastic cell lines; no similar inhibitor can be extracted, e.g., from brain, muscle, lung, kidney, skin, erythrocytes, and granulocytes (see, e.g., Attallah and Houck, 1976; Lord *et al.*, 1974a). Conversely, lymphoid cell extracts have no inhibitory effect on a variety of nonlymphoid cell lines, such as diploid human fibroblasts, HeLa cells, choriocarcinoma cells, and erythrocytic and granulocytic precursor cells (e.g., Attallah and Houck, 1976; Lord, 1975; Lord *et al.*, 1974a, 1977). Some authors have reported that lymphocyte extracts inhibit [$^3$H]-TdR uptake by nonlymphoid cells (Jones *et al.*, 1970; Garcia-Giralt and Macieira-Coelho, 1974; Aoyama *et al.*, 1975), but such results do not indicate the nonexistence of specific and endogenous inhibitors of lymphocyte proliferation. It is self-evident that a failure to demonstrate cell line specific actions only applies to the particular extract tested and that this does not give any basis at all for concluding that other lymphocyte extracts are similarly nonspecific. Clearly, if 10–15 independent groups of workers have been able to obtain lymphocyte extracts that display essentially absolute cell line specificity in a variety of assay systems, it is highly unlikely that the inhibition is real but the specificity somehow artifactual. Isolation of any authentic chalone is associated with considerable difficulties, and certain nonspecific inhibitors, such as free spermine and spermidine (see Section 10.6.3), might have survived some extraction procedures used for obtaining lymphocytic chalone. It is thus possible, if not probable, that the amount of inhibitory polyamines in different extracts varies and that the lack of specificity occasionally observed is merely an indication of high concentrations of free spermine/spermidine in such extracts (see Allen *et al.*, 1977).

Another type of "failure" reported in the study of lymphocytic chalone is the observation that some lymphocyte extracts act as immunosuppressive agents both *in vitro* and *in vivo* but that the same extracts do not decrease lymphocyte proliferation (Garcia-Giralt *et al.* 1973, 1975; Kiger *et al.*, 1975). Although this dichotomy of action has not been commonly observed in the study of lymphocytic chalone, its existence is by no means unlikely. In my opinion, the dichotomy may actually be expected because the prevention of lymphocyte response to different physiological and nonphysiological stimuli of transformation is not necessarily associated with direct inhibition of cell proliferation. Kiger *et al.* (1975) have actually reported evidence which suggests that the immunosuppressive activity and the direct inhibition of lymphocyte proliferation are indeed based on two different factors. According to the results published, the two molecules seem to form a complex which then breaks down by further purification. Judging from the variable nominal molecular weights of different preparations with apparent lymphocytic chalone activity (cf. Section 10.6.3), it is tempting to speculate that both an "antiactivator" and an "antiproliferative agent" can also rebind to other unrelated substances. This behavior would explain the enormous difficulties encountered in the purification of lymphocytic chalone (Houck *et al.*, 1977), as well as the seemingly discrepant results regarding immunosuppression and inhibition of cell proliferation.

It has sometimes been stated that the "classic" lymphocytic chalone does not inhibit the rate of cell division at all (Ranney, 1975). This is, of course, absurd in view of the definition of chalones; yet it may well be asked whether or not the demonstration of a direct decrease in cell proliferation by lymphocyte extracts is unequivocal. Ranney (1975) supports his claim by the findings of Garcia-Giralt and Macieira-Coelho (1974), who showed that spleen extracts profoundly suppressed $[^3H]$-TdR uptake by malignant lymphoid cell lines without actually decreasing their growth rate. It is not possible to offer any definite explanation for these findings, although it now seems probable that Garcia-Giralt and Macieira-Coelho may have measured the effects of free spermine or spermidine rather than genuine lymphocytic chalone. Nevertheless, there can be no doubt whatsoever that lymphocyte extracts do not simply interfere with [$^3$H]-TdR uptake by lymphoid cells. For instance, lymphocyte extracts cause absolutely cell line specific and reversible changes in the "structuredness" of the cell cytoplasmic matrix, similar to those caused by granulocyte and erythrocyte extracts in proliferating granulocytes and erythrocytes, respectively (Lord *et al.*, 1974a,b; Lord, 1975). Furthermore, intraperitoneal injections of partially purified thymus and lymph node extracts significantly inhibited thymus growth in neonatal rabbits (Chung and Hufnagel, 1973; Chung, 1976). Lymph node extracts have also been observed to cause a decrease, although small, in the labeling index of lymphoid cells in regenerating mouse spleen without any effect on the labeling index of granulocytic and erythrocytic cells in the same spleen (Lord, 1975; Lord *et al.*, 1977). Finally, cell proliferation in the murine thymus has been shown to be inhibited *in vivo* after a single injection of crude thymus extracts as revealed by autoradiography and microspectrophotometry, and by trapping the cells in metaphase (Olsson and Claësson, 1975). Crude spleen extracts were found to have a weaker inhibitory effect, and skin extracts had no such effect; conversely, thymus and spleen extracts had no inhibitory effect on the skin.

Despite the well-demonstrated lack of cytotoxicity of lymphocyte extracts against normal lymphocytes, similar extracts were found to kill several mouse and human lymphoblastic cell lines under crowded conditions *in vitro* (Attallah and Houck, 1975, 1976). In sparse cultures lymphocyte extracts no longer demonstrated cytotoxicity nor did they inhibit proliferation of leukemic lymphocytes. Attallah and Houck (1975, 1976) concluded that the lymphocytotoxicity for leukemic cells is specific for the $G_1$–$G_0$ phase of the cell cycle. In my opinion, these findings of Attallah and Houck are curious and it is difficult to believe that lymphocytic chalone would be selectively cytotoxic for different types of leukemic cells in the $G_1$–$G_0$ phase but not for normal lymphoid cells in the same phase (note that normal lymphocytes are definitely in the $G_1$–$G_0$ phase at the onset of conventional leukocyte cultures). I cannot offer a more plausible alternative to the explanation suggested by Attallah and Houck (1975, 1976), but without further confirmation their interpretation must be considered highly uncertain. This is true because their conclusion is totally at variance with the definition of chalones and, in particular, because all other chalones studied have been observed to inhibit malignant cell proliferation without killing the cells (see Bullough and Laurence, 1970; Rytömaa and Kiviniemi, 1970; Laurence and Elgjo, 1971; Bichel, 1973, 1976; Cooper and Smith, 1973; Rytömaa *et al.*, 1976).

It has been reported by several authors that lymphocyte extracts exert immunosuppressive properties *in vivo*. Thus, thymus extracts inhibit thymus-dependent antibody formation, such as IgM production against dinitrophenylated human IgG, and IgG production against dinitrophenylated human γ-globulin or against sheep red blood cells (Florentin *et al.*, 1973; Kiger *et al.*, 1975). The same extracts do not affect IgM-antibody production against dinitrophenylated polymerized flagellin which does not require T-lymphocyte interaction, hence suggesting specificity between T and B chalones (Florentin *et al.*, 1973). Both spleen and thymus extracts have been shown to suppress a graft-versus-host reaction with treatment of the lymphocyte donor (Garcia-Giralt *et al.*, 1970, 1972, 1973; Kiger *et al.*, 1972a,b, 1973a,b), of the recipient (Garcia-Giralt *et al.*, 1972), or of the donor lymphocytes themselves before cell transfer (Garcia-Giralt *et al.*, 1973; Kiger *et al.*, 1973a,b). Furthermore, lymphocyte extracts also prolong skin-graft rejection (Kiger *et al.*, 1972a,b; Houck *et al.*, 1973; Chung and Hufragel, 1973; Allen *et al.*, 1977). All these results show that the effects of lymphocyte extracts are readily demonstrable *in vivo* by measuring specific endpoints of immune reactions. However, suppression *in vivo* of immune responses does not prove that the extracts function by directly inhibiting lymphocyte proliferation; it is possible, if not even likely, that they prevent activation or recognition phenomena. Such an effect would be similar to the inhibitory action of lymphocyte extracts on different mitogenic stimuli *in vitro*. These phenomena may be caused by lymphocytic chalone proper but they do not represent a defined property of direct inhibitors of cell proliferation.

## 10.6.2. Mechanism of Action

Attallah and Houck (1977) have shown that the incorporation of $[^3H]$-TdR into acid-soluble precursor pool and into acid-insoluble DNA of PHA-stimulated human lymphocytes is inhibited both by cyclic AMP (cAMP) and by lymphocytic chalone (splenic ultrafiltrate, 30,000–50,000 dalton fraction). When a mixture of both substances was added to the culture medium, DNA synthesis was dependent solely on the concentration of chalone and the cells did not respond further to exogenous cAMP. However, theophylline significantly increased the inhibition caused by lymphocytic chalone, and it was therefore speculated that chalone changes either the cell membrane or the phosphodiesterase system in such a way that the cells become insensitive to cAMP added. In conclusion the authors suggest that lymphocytic chalone maintains a high level of activity of adenyl cyclase and, consequently, a high intracellular concentration of cAMP. This, in turn, would inhibit nucleoside kinases and hence the synthesis of DNA.

It is clear, of course, that the findings of Attallah and Houck (1977) are not yet sufficient to prove the mechanism of lymphocytic chalone action, and this is also clearly stated by the authors themselves. In my opinion, the mechanism tentatively proposed appears somewhat questionable for two main reasons. First, theophylline was used at a very high concentration ($\geqslant 10^{-3}$ M) and hence a direct pharmacological effect is probable and was certainly not excluded (see Rytömaa and Kiviniemi, 1975). Second, an increase in the intracellular concentration of cAMP has been reported to stimulate rather than inhibit DNA synthesis in many cell lines including thymocytes (MacManus and Whitfield, 1969; Whitfield *et al.*, 1973). On the other hand, however, some experimental evidence has been obtained which seems to suggest that cAMP may play a role in the epidermal chalone mechanism (Brønstad *et al.*, 1971; Vorhees *et al.*, 1973).

### 10.6.3. Purification and Biochemical Nature

During the past several years various groups of workers have attempted to purify lymphocytic chalones but, until recently, they have met with little success. In a typical case, crude extracts have been obtained from thymus, spleen, or lymph node cells by extracting homogenized or acetone powdered tissues with distilled water. After centrifugation at 15,000–20,000 $\times$ *g* for 0.5–1 hr, the supernatant is collected and the crude extract thus obtained is either lyophilized for direct testing or else subjected to further purification using a variety of techniques.

It seems useful at this stage to give a few quantitative values which may help in evaluating the "meaning" of the different dose levels used in tests *in vitro* and *in vivo*. According to Olsson and Claësson (1975), crude aqueous extract of one mouse thymus yields 1 mg of lyophilized powder, one mouse spleen yields 1.5 mg, and the whole skin of one mouse 5 mg. Judging from these values, in the *in vivo* tests the doses injected into mice have been equivalent to up to 20 "thymuses" per injection, and in the *in vitro* tests up to "one mouse thymus per milliliter." In principle these amounts are reasonable and likely to upset the appropriate chalone status enough to result in easily measurable changes. It may be estimated from the data available that 50% inhibition in PHA-stimulated lymphocytes is obtained at a concentration of about "one-third mouse thymus per milliliter." This seems to correspond to approximately 50 $\mu$g/ml of chalone concentrate prepared by membrane ultrafiltrations of crude aqueous extracts (30,000–50,000 dalton fraction; see, e.g., Houck *et al.*, 1977).

Two main approaches have been adopted in the attempts to purify lymphocytic chalone, both with some success. In the first of these, the essential steps are based on molecular sieving using ultrafilters with different cutoff limits. Houck (see, e.g., Houck *et al.*, 1971, 1977; Attallah and Houck, 1976) has shown that lymphocytic chalone activity passes rapidly through a 50,000-dalton filter, very slowly through a 30,000-dalton filter, and not at all through a 10,000-dalton filter. The activity recovered in the range 30,000–50,000 daltons is destroyed by trypsin and chymotrypsin, but not by ribonuclease and desoxyribonuclease, hence indicating that the biological activity requires peptide bonds involving both basic and aromatic amino acids (Attallah and Houck, 1976). After ribonuclease treatment (10 $\mu$g/ml for 4 hr at 37°C), however, the lymphocytic chalone activity was found exclusively in the molecular range of 1000–10,000 daltons (Houck *et al.*, 1977). This finding thus suggests that the chalone polypeptide was tightly bound to relatively small molecules of RNA, possibly transfer RNA with a molecular weight of about 25,000 daltons. Consequently, Houck *et al.* (1977) concluded that lymphocytic chalone has a molecular weight of about 5000 daltons and, owing to its binding to the anionic polyelectrolyte RNA, must be strongly cationically charged. The behavior of lymphocytic chalone in concanavalin A–Sepharose column (affinity chromatography) further suggested that the chalone activity involves covalently bound mannose (Houck *et al.*, 1977).

The other main approach adopted in the purification of lymphocytic chalone is based on ethanol fractionation, followed by ion exchange chromatography on DEAE–Sephadex A-50 columns (Kiger *et al.*, 1973 a,b). Using this technique, Allen *et al.* (1977) were able to isolate from pig thymus a nondialyzable inhibitor which, according to *in vitro* and *in vivo* tests, appeared to be lymphocytic chalone (see also Kiger *et al.*, 1973 a,b, 1975; Garcia-Giralt *et al.*, 1973). The active moiety of the inhibitor was identified biologically and chemically as spermine; the carrier responsible for the tissue specificity of the spermine complex was not identified (Allen *et al.*, 1977). It has also been demonstrated by others (Byrd *et al.*, 1977) that spermine and spermidine reversibly inhibit *in vitro* parameters of immunity, such as the lymphocyte response to PHA and other stimulators commonly used. As expected, however, the inhibitory effect of unbound spermine and spermidine on [³H]-TdR uptake was not cell line specific (Allen *et al.*, 1977).

The thymic extracts with tightly bound spermine (Allen *et al.*, 1977) and free spermine and spermidine (Byrd *et al.*, 1977; Allen *et al.*, 1977) were inhibitory *in vitro* only if the cultures were supplemented with calf or fetal calf serum. For instance, in mouse and human sera no inhibition could be demonstrated *in vitro;* nevertheless, the injection of 1.0-mg doses of spermidine into mice prolonged skin-graft survival in a way similar to the spermine-containing complex isolated from thymus (Allen *et al.*, 1977). It may be worth noting that in the *in vivo* tests Allen *et al.* (1977) used spermidine rather than spermine, although the latter was the active moiety in the complex. Although not mentioned by the authors, the apparent reason is that spermine is toxic when injected into mice.

Because free spermine and spermidine, as well as the complex, were not inhibitory *in vitro* in nonruminant sera, they were probably converted into some other active moieties by the bovine serum. Allen *et al.* (1977) suggested that the active moieties are the corresponding aldehydes produced enzymatically by amine oxidase, although it has been previously shown that the aminoaldehydes are toxic to cultured cells (Alarcon, 1964; Bachrach, 1973). Nevertheless, the inhibition of lymphoid cells *in vitro* by converted spermine and spermidine or, alternatively, by an unrelated molecule released from bovine serum, was not based on toxicity (Byrd *et al.*, 1977).

In many ways the inhibitory effect of spermine and spermidine, and that of the spermine-containing complex isolated from thymus, is perplexing at present, especially because polyamines are commonly associated with stimulatory actions (Bachrach, 1973; Raina and Jänne, 1975). Yet Dewey (1977) has also recently reported that "melanocytic chalone" (see Dewey, 1973), capable of inhibiting Harding–Passey melanoma cells in culture and even of inducing complete regression of the tumor in mice (Dewey, *et al.*, 1977), is nothing but free spermidine. Because Allen *et al.* (1977) showed that spermine (spermidine was not tested) also inhibited [$^3$H]-TdR uptake by rat bone marrow cells in suspension cultures supplemented with fetal calf serum (assayed by the method of Paukovits, 1971), it may seem that even granulocytic chalone is or contains spermine or spermidine. It has been shown, however, that the inhibitory effect of granulocytic chalone is definitely not based on contaminating polyamines and, furthermore, that granulocytic chalone does not seem to contain tightly bound polyamine either (P. Foa, W. Paile, T. L. S. Tse Hing Yuen, W. A. Jones, J. Jänne, and T. Rytömaa, unpublished results). A trace amount of spermine is present in semipurified preparations of granulocytic chalone (0.1 nmol/mg or less) which is several orders of magnitude less than an effective concentration of authentic spermine capable of causing detectable inhibition of granulocytic cells cultured in presence of fetal calf serum. It is also worth noting that partially purified granulocytic chalone is active in all types of sera used by us and even in serum-free culture media (Rytömaa and Kiviniemi, 1968a, 1970, unpublished results).

In many ways the results obtained by Allen *et al.* (1977) are most interesting, but nevertheless it is not yet certain that lymphocytic chalone contains spermine as the true active moiety. It should be remembered that, according to Houck (Houck *et al.*, 1971, 1977; Attallah and Houck, 1976), lymphocytic chalone is readily inactivated by trypsin and chymotrypsin and hence its biological activity is dependent on peptide bonds. Allen *et al.* (1977) prepared their complex containing spermine by the method of Kiger *et al.* (1973a), which is different from that used by Houck; this, however, does not seem to explain the discrepancy. Kiger herself has reported (Kiger *et al.*, 1975) that her material, too, capable of inhibiting DNA synthesis in thymocytes *in vitro,* is sensitive to trypsin (and to pronase). This particular fraction, with a nominal molecular weight of 10,000–15,000 daltons, was completely devoid of immunosuppressive activity *in vivo*, but Kiger has suggested that the inhibitor of DNA synthesis is part of a larger molecule (>300,000 daltons) that possesses both immunosuppressive activity on T-lymphocytes *in vivo* and an inhibitory action on DNA synthesis in thymocytes *in vitro* (Kiger *et al.*, 1975).

The wide variety of molecular weights and the apparently different chemical nature of substances isolated from lymphoid cells, capable of inhibiting lymphocyte proliferation in a cell line specific manner, make one wonder whether there really are several lymphocytic chalones. As discussed earlier (Section 10.2), there are no obvious reasons why this could not be the case. However, it is perhaps more likely that the inconsistencies observed regarding the biochemical properties of lymphocytic chalone(s) are more apparent than real, i.e., that they only reflect a peculiar property of chalones to form strong complexes with other substances (see Houck *et al.*, 1977). Owing to this, the exact amino acid composition reported for B- and T-lymphocytic chalones (Grundboeck-Juśko, 1976) must be viewed with skepticism. The possibility that the two glycoproteins isolated from supernatants of smooth microsomes of bovine spleen do not represent true compositions for T and B cell chalones receives further support from the observation that as much as 16 mg/kg of pure protein was needed for distinct inhibition in mitotic activity in lymphoid organs of mice (Grundboeck-Juśko, 1976). Such a dose appears enormous for a pure lymphocytic chalone because even impure preparations of granulocytic chalone were strongly active in doses 100–1000 times smaller (see Rytömaa *et al.*, 1976, 1977). Similarly, a cocktail containing erythrocytic chalone was maximally effective at a dose level which was 40 times smaller than that used in testing "pure" lymphocytic chalones (see Lord *et al.*, 1977).

## 10.7. Stem Cell Chalone

As expected from the chalone concept, pluripotent stem cells, or hematopoietic spleen colony-forming units (CFU-S), are not inhibited by granulocytic and erythrocytic chalones (Lord, 1975; Lord *et al.*, 1977; MacVittie and McCarthy, 1975; Bøyum *et al.*, 1976; Løvhaug and Bøyum, 1977). It has recently been reported, however, that extracts from normal bone marrow, but not from regenerating bone marrow, specifically inhibit stem cell proliferation (Lord *et al.*, 1976). The stem cell chalone, obtained by incubating normal bone marrow cells in saline for 2 hr at 37°C, was partially purified by ultrafiltrations (50,000–100,000 dalton fraction). It protected rapidly proliferating CFU-S from the lethal effects of large doses of [$^3$H]-TdR ("thymidine suicide technique"), but had no effect on committed granulocytic progenitor cells (CFU-C) or on the whole bone marrow cell population (note that the proportion of CFU-S in the bone marrow is <0.5% and hence too low to have a detectable effect on the overall response). According to preliminary data, stem cell chalone seems to be protein because its activity is destroyed by trypsin (Lord *et al.*, 1976).

## 10.8. Other Blood Cell Chalones

Experimental evidence for the existence of chalones regulating hematopoietic cells other than those already mentioned is scanty at present. However, a few findings may be worth noting here.

Laerum and Maurer (1973) have reported that when extracts made from suspensions of granulocytes contaminated with macrophages (ascites inflammatory exudate) were injected into mice, the proliferation of granulocytic precursor cells as well as macrophages was inhibited in diffusion chamber cultures. When the extracts were made from suspensions of granulocytes containing no macrophages (cells separated from blood), the proliferation of granulocytic cells was again inhibited without detectable effects on macrophages. Essentially similar results were also obtained by Benestad *et al.* (1973) using the diffusion chamber technique.

One of the cell lines studied in great detail regarding growth regulation in general is the JB-1 ascites tumor in AKR mice (see Bichel, 1976). This ascites tumor is a transplanted plasmacytoma and hence JB-1 ascites tumor chalone(s) may actually represent plasma cell chalone(s). Two chalone-type inhibitors, one acting primarily in the $G_1$ phase and the other in the $G_2$ phase of the cell cycle, have been isolated from the ascites fluid of JB-1 tumor-bearing mice. Both substances have also been partially purified and are probably of a protein nature with different molecular weights, 10,000–50,000 daltons ($G_1$ chalone) and 1000–10,000 daltons ($G_2$ chalone) (see Bichel, 1976). Interestingly enough, recent attempts to purify more extensively the $G_1$ inhibitor have led to the isolation of a polyamine-containing complex (cf. Section 10.6.3) with a low molecular weight of 600–1000 daltons (Barfod and Marcker, 1977).

Bichel (1976) has suggested that tumor cells, when maintained for long periods of time by serial passages, develop a new tumor-specific feedback control. In my opinion, however, it is highly unlikely that clonal evolution of tumor cells leads to the development of a new specific feedback-regulation mechanism, i.e., to the appearance of a new tumor-specific chalone. Such a development is at least not supported by experimental evidence; in contrast, several observations indicate that tumor cells both produce and respond to the chalone of their tissue of origin (e.g., Bullough and Laurence, 1968; Rytömaa and Kiviniemi, 1968c; Laurence and Elgjo, 1971; Bullough and Deol, 1971; Vilpo *et al.*, 1973; Ferris *et al.*, 1973; Maiolo *et al.*, 1975; Kariniemi and Rytömaa, 1976; Rytömaa *et al.*, 1977). Furthermore, advanced clonal evolution of chloroleukemia in rat (K. Stenstrand, P. Foa, W. Paile, and T. Rytömaa, unpublished results) has not been associated with the development of a new tumor-specific chalone mechanism (see Fig. 1). Although it may not be fully justified to generalize from these findings, they nevertheless strongly support the possibility that JB-1 ascites tumor chalone is, in fact, plasma cell chalone.

## 10.9. Chalones and Other Inhibitors of Hematopoiesis

In addition to granulocytic chalone, other inhibitors of granulopoiesis have also been reported. Among these are nondialyzable lipoprotein inhibitors, present in serum, which inactivate CSF (Chan, 1971; Chan *et al.*, 1971; Beran, 1975). Lipoprotein inhibitors are evidently different from granulocytic chalone and also from another inhibitor with a small molecular weight, CIA (colony-inhibiting activity), which is released from polymorphonuclear neutrophils (Baker *et al.*, 1975; Broxmeyer *et al.*, 1976a). CIA acts directly on colony-stimulating cells and inhibits either CSF production or release, or both (Broxmeyer *et al.*, 1976b). It remains to be shown directly whether or not CIA and granulocytic chalone are related; the indirect evidence available suggests that they are not. For instance, Aardal *et al.* (1977) have reported that partially purified granulocytic chalone inhibited CSF action in assay conditions where an indirect action on CSF-producing cells was excluded. Furthermore, in diffusion chamber cultures *in vivo* granulocytic chalone accelerates the maturation of proliferating granulocytes (Benestad and Rytömaa, 1977), an effect not exerted by CIA in agar cultures *in vitro* (Broxmeyer *et al.*, 1976b). Granulocytes isolated from leukemic patients (e.g., CML) often do not condition media with CIA (Broxmeyer *et al.*, 1976a,b); granulocytic chalone, however, has been present in all cases studied thus far. Finally, in view of the mode of action of CIA (inhibition of CSF production or release), it seems virtually impossible that intravenous injections of CIA into leukemic patients could inhibit proliferation of leukemic cells (probably requiring no CSF at all for proliferation) and even induce regression of the leukemia in 24 hr; yet granulocytic chalone, a direct inhibitor of cell proliferation, is active in this test (Rytömaa *et al.*, 1976, 1977). Thus CIA and granulocytic chalone are evidently two different factors which inhibit granulopoiesis by different mechanisms. Nevertheless, owing to the source of CIA and its low molecular weight, it is quite possible, or even likely, that CIA is a common contaminant in many preparations of granulocytic chalone. Consequently, some effects believed to be caused by granulocytic chalone may have actually been caused by CIA.

Interferon, which also can inhibit colony formation *in vitro* (Fleming *et al.*, 1972), is definitely different from granulocytic chalone. This is clear from several findings, such as those related to the source, action, and species specificity of interferon and granulocytic chalone, respectively, and even to the chemical properties of the two substances (regarding the properties of interferon, see, e.g., Ng and Vilcek, 1972; Valle *et al.*, 1975; Knight, 1976).

Lindeman (1971, 1975) has reported the existence of an inhibitor of erythropoiesis with a low molecular weight extracted from normal human urine. This substance is active *in vivo*, and its action is cell line specific and noncytotoxic. However, this factor does not affect erythropoiesis by directly inhibiting cell proliferation; it interferes with erythropoietin action. Other inhibitors of purified erythropoietin have also been isolated from a number of tissues, such as kidney. The inhibitor isolated from kidney seems to be a complex lipid which binds to erythropoietin, causing a loss of erythropoietic activity (Erslev *et al.*, 1972). It should also be noted that injecting physiological doses of estradiol into male rats reduces erythropoietin plasma titers; this suggests that the lower erythropoietin response to hypoxia in female rodents as compared with males is based on an inhibitory effect of estrogens on erythropoietin-producing organs (Peschle *et al.*, 1972).

Ranney (1975) has recently published a review on biological inhibitors of lymphoid cell division, other than chalones. One of these factors is a compound with a low molecular weight released by lymphoid tissues. It inhibits [³H]-TdR uptake by lymphoid cells in a reversible and apparently noncytotoxic manner; the inhibitor does not seem to affect nonlymphoid cells and it is species nonspecific (see Ranney, 1975). The possible identity of this inhibitor (molecular weight $\leq 1000$ daltons) with lymphocytic chalone remains to be shown. It may be noted, however, that the inhibitor seems to be produced either by "null cells" (lymphocytes lacking B or T surface markers) or macrophage-like cells. According to Ranney (1975), the inhibitor is different from lymphocytic chalone because it is insensitive to heat and trypsin. These characteristics are naturally unable to differentiate this inhibitor from chalones, but it is true, of course, that lymphocytic chalone has been reported to be sensitive to heat and to tryptic digestion. The inhibitor differs from the lymphocytic chalone isolated by Houck *et al.* (1977) in some other respects as well, such as molecular weight and charge, but the only property which directly suggests its nonchalone nature is the possibly nonspecific source. The true role of this inhibitor under *in vivo* conditions has not yet been demonstrated.

## 10.10. Leukemia and Chalones

The main characteristic of a growing tumor is an excess of cell production over cell loss. Clearly, if in a tumor the rate of cell production is so suppressed that it becomes less than the rate of cell loss, the tumor will regress. One approach to achieve such a reversion is to inhibit cell production by the chalone of the parent tissue.

It is intuitively obvious that the reversion should be obtainable merely by prolonging the cell cycle time (reducing the rate of cell production), provided cell loss is not correspondingly decreased. It is perhaps more difficult to reach the conclusion that even a moderate lengthening of the cell cycle can result in an exceedingly fast regression of a tumor. Yet, a Monte Carlo simulation of tumor growth, based on realistic parameter values and—owing to the nonanalytical nature of the simulation—free of simplifying assumptions, has shown that at least rat chloroleukemia can disappear completely in 4–5 days if the cell cycle time is about doubled (Toivonen, 1976; Toivonen and Rytömaa, 1978). It is understandable that a sudden extensive necrosis in a tumor following injections of relatively crude cell extracts may not seem to be due to a noncytotoxic inhibition of cell production (chalone effect) but is instead believed to be caused by the direct or indirect killing of cells (see Iversen, 1970, 1976). However, although the Monte Carlo simulation cannot prove that a sudden necrosis is not caused by artificially accelerated cell death, it does show that in biological reality this result can nevertheless be an automatic outcome after such a simple change as the prolongation of the cell cycle time.

It should be apparent from the foregoing that the theoretical basis for using chalones in the treatment of leukemia is by no means unique. The main principle is extremely simple and, in fact, analogous to that involved in the use of bacterio*static* antibiotics in the treatment of infections. Owing to this basic simplicity, it is a little surprising that several authors have considered the working hypothesis as being highly speculative and have tried to prove, with the aid of various theoretical arguments, that the model cannot work in biological reality (see, e.g., Iversen, 1970, 1976; Houck, 1976). There is no longer any need to answer this criticism with theoretical counterarguments: experimental evidence has shown that the model does work.

In the first attempts to treat leukemia with chalone, extracts containing granulocytic chalone were injected into young rats with transplanted Shay chloroma (Rytömaa and Kiviniemi, 1969). It was observed that following intraperitoncal chalone injections, subcutaneous chloroma tumors became necrotic, ulcerated, and regressed. Sometimes the rate of tumor regression was fast, although never as fast as might have been achieved by higher doses of chalone, as judged from the kinetic parameters of chloroma cell populations (see later in this chapter, and Toivonen and Rytömaa, 1978). Interestingly enough, in all cases in which the tumor regression was complete, it was also permanent. It was apparent even to the naked eye that the chalone treatment did not influence several nongranulocytic cell lines: for instance, fur renewal was activated, anemia disappeared (readily detectable, e.g., from the ear color), and body growth was accelerated compared with control animals.

The experiments with Shay chloroleukemia were later continued by treating rats suffering from generalized leukemia (induced by intraperitoneal transplantation of leukemic cells) with granulocytic chalone (Rytömaa and Kiviniemi, 1970). The first results were less dramatic than in the treatment of solid tumors; the injections produced only a small, though significant prolongation of the mean survival time. However, when larger amounts of more purified chalone material were obtained, the doses could be increased and the effect of the treatment became more marked. Thus, in 9 rats out of 40 the leukemia regressed completely and this led to a permanent cure of the animals; in the remaining rats the survival time was prolonged compared with controls, all 42 of which died after a mean survival time of 12.2 days. It was again observed that chalone treatment did not inhibit nongranulocytic cell lines; in particular, body growth of these baby rats was much faster in the chalone- treated than in the control group, and actually as fast as in the untreated nonleukemic litters. Furthermore, rats that were cured of leukemia by chalone injections bred normally and eventually died of "old age."

These experiments with transplanted leukemia gave promising results regarding the possibilities of inhibiting spontaneous human tumors by chalone. However, transplanted animal tumors are not necessarily adequate models from which one can deduce the response of spontaneous human tumors. In particular, it is an absolute requirement for the successful treatment of tumors with chalones that the spontaneous rate of cell loss be higher than zero. Clearly, if the rate of cell loss is just a few percent of the rate of cell production, only a profound inhibition can result in a negative imbalance (cell production smaller than cell loss). It has been established that the rate of cell loss from our chloroleukemia population was 12–64% of the rate of cell production even in a relatively well-protected environment in diffusion chambers (Vilpo and Rytömaa, 1973). Hence it could be expected that a moderate inhibition of cell production was likely to result in a negative imbalance at least in some animals; on the other hand, in animals in which chloroleukemia cells were lost at a rate of 12% of the rate of cell production, a moderate inhibition was not able to stop tumor growth and hence only a marginal prolongation of survival time was to be expected. The results obtained in the actual experiments (Rytömaa and Kiviniemi, 1969, 1970) were exactly those suggested by theoretical reasoning.

It seems important in this context to elaborate in a little more detail the crucial role of spontaneous cell death for an expected outcome of chalone treatment. Malignant tumors, expecially those maintained by serial passages in animals, undergo clonal evolution which is associated with a progressive increase in "clinical" malignancy; this has also been observed in the Shay chloroleukemia maintained by us (Rytömaa and Kiviniemi, 1968c; K. Stenstrand, P. Foa, W. Paile, and T. Rytömaa, unpublished results). At present, the leukemia is extremely fatal, killing a young rat in about 7 days (transplanted with $10^6$ cells); the leukemia cell population now grows with a doubling time of about 24 hr almost without any cell loss both *in vitro* and *in vivo* (P. Foa, W. Paile, and T. Rytömaa, unpublished results). Although the cells have retained good responsiveness to granulocytic chalone (see Fig.1), it would nevertheless be useless to attempt chalone treatment now, hoping for more than just a marginal prolongation of the mean survival time. This is because, owing to zero cell loss, even a 100% inhibition of cell production could not result in a regression of leukemia. This example may also be taken as a warning: there is absolutely no sense in trying to treat transplanted animal tumors by the appropriate chalone, regardless of an established responsiveness of the cells, unless it has been confirmed that spontaneous cell loss from the tumor is sufficiently high in relation to the expected inhibition obtainable by chalone injections.

This situation was fully realized by us when the first attempts were made to treat leukemia in man by granulocytic chalone (Rytömaa *et al.*, 1976, 1977). It was not, of course, possible to make a direct measurement of the rate of cell loss in the patients, but it was hoped that the earlier findings indicating a high rate of cell loss from spontaneous human tumors (Steel, 1967; Refsum and Berdal, 1967; Iversen, 1967; Cooper, 1973) would also hold true in our patients. In retrospect, this was evidently the case in at least five of the seven patients; in two of these five patients, however, the rate of cell loss became smaller with time, as judged from the decreased cellular serum enzyme and urate values in spite of an increased leukemic mass. Consequently, in the first of these patients retreatment with chalone failed to induce another regression of the leukemia (the cells had also become less responsive *in vitro* to the chalone added; see Rytömaa *et al.*, 1976), and in the second patient, retreatment with chalone produced results that were somewhat less dramatic than those obtained with the original chalone therapy (Rytömaa *et al.*, 1977).

Granulocytic chalone used in these trials with human leukemia (five patients with AML and two with CML in blastic crisis) had been prepared by Weddel Pharmaceuticals Ltd., London. The chalone was extracted from nonhomogenized leukocytes (the majority being granulocytes) isolated from ox blood; after separation of the conditioned medium, the fraction with a nominal molecular weight of 500–10,000 daltons was isolated by ultrafiltrations, lyophilized, further purified by gel filtration chromatography, and the appropriate fractions desalted and lyophilized. The first three batches of granulocytic chalone (see Rytömaa *et al.*, 1976) were pyrogenic in tests with rabbits, and they also elicited a febrile reaction in most of the patients. After further purification it was possible to eliminate the pyrogenicity completely (see Rytömaa *et al.*, 1977) and these preparations caused no side effects at all.

The patients were not selected for treatment using any particular criteria; they were simply seven consecutive cases of myeloid leukemia seen in the hospital when chalone was available. The chalone doses and the injection schedules varied widely among the patients, for different clinical reasons. Most commonly, two daily intravenous injections were given with an average dose of about 200 $\mu$/kg (largest dose 1.5 mg/kg and smallest 80 $\mu$g/kg).

It was observed that granulocytic chalone strongly inhibited proliferation of normal and leukemic granulocytes, leaving all other cell types unaffected. The inhibition of leukemic growth was distinct in six of the seven patients; in five cases the inhibition was followed by actual regression of the leukemia, lasting up to several months in the absence of any maintenance therapy, and in one case the treatment, quite unexpectedly, led to complete remission of the disease (Rytömaa *et al.*, 1976, 1977). In three of the patients the regression of leukemia was followed by a dramatic improvement in the patients' general condition; in the case of complete remission, the patient lived normally for 10 months without any maintenance therapy. It must be emphasized that the short-term treatments of leukemic patients with granulocytic chalone were not conducted as true therapeutic trials, and hence the real therapeutic value of granulocytic chalone cannot be deduced either from the remarkable improvement of the patients' general condition or from their significantly prolonged survival times (see Rytömaa *et al.*, 1977).

In addition to the profound inhibition of normal and leukemic granulocytes, chalone treatment did not inhibit any other cell types. Erythropoiesis and megakaryopoiesis were often strongly stimulated, but these effects were naturally secondary to the regression of the leukemia. In some cases immunostimulation was also observed, as judged from an increase in serum innumoglobulin values, within 2 weeks after the onset of chalone injections. The reason for this phenomenon is not clear, but it was definitely not directly caused by chalone injections (see Rytömaa *et al.*, 1976, 1977; see also Section 10.4.5) and it had nothing to do with the inhibition of the proliferation of leukemic cells (sometimes detectable within 24 hr after the onset of injections; furthermore, regression of leukemia occurred even in cases in which signs of subsequent immunostimulation were not seen). Another totally unexpected finding was that the patients were remarkably resistant to bacterial infections even in the presence of extreme chalone-induced granulocytopenia ($\leq 100$ cells/$\mu$l). It is possible that this resistance was associated with the total lack of chalone-induced damage to different cell lines in the body. Apart from the pyrogenic reaction seen in most of the patients treated with the first three batches of chalone, the injections did not cause any side effects.

The results obtained in these first clinical trials (Rytömaa *et al.*, 1976, 1977) showed unequivocally that granulocytic chalone inhibits human myeloid leukemia. A more extensive clinical study is therefore warranted to elucidate the true therapeutic role of granulocytic chalone.

## 10.11. Conclusions

One of the main purposes of this chapter has been to present an overview of the experimental evidence bearing on blood cell chalones. Let the following three comments summarize the message of the article:

1. Modifying "Humpty Dumpty" and Iversen (1976): When I use the word chalone, it means just what I choose it to mean. For my choice, see Section 10.1.
2. The time has come to purify and chemically fully characterize at least one chalone. I suggest that the easiest is erythrocytic chalone.
3. It has been demonstrated that granulocytic chalone inhibits myeloid leukemia in man without side effects. A more extensive clinical study is thus certainly warranted.

## References

Aardal, N. P., Laerum, O. D., Paukovits, W. R., and Maurer, H. R., 1977, Inhibition of agar colony formation by partially purified granulocyte extracts (chalone), *Virchows Arch. B. Zellpathol.* **24**:27.

Alarcon, R. A., 1964, Isolation of acrolein from incubated mixtures of spermine with calf serum and its effects on mammalian cells, *Arch. Biochem. Biophys.* **137**:365.

Allen, J. C., Smith, C. J., Curry, M. C., and Gaugas, J. M., 1977, Identification of a thymic inhibitor ("chalone") of lymphocyte transformation as a spermine complex, *Nature* **267**:623.

Attallah, A. M., and Houck, J. C., 1975, Lymphocyte chalone concentrates and their effects upon leukemic cells in vitro, *Boll. Ist. Sieroter. Milan.* **54**:227.

Attallah, A. M., and Houck, J. C., 1976, Lymphocyte chalone, in *Chalones* (J. C. Houck, ed.), pp. 353–383, North-Holland/ American Elsevier, New York.

Attallah, A. M., and Houck, J. C., 1977, Tentative mechanism of lymphocyte chalone action, *Exp. Cell Res.* **105**:137.

Attallah, A. M., Sunshine, G. H., Hunt, C. V., and Houck, J. C., 1975, The specific and endogenous mitotic inhibitor of lymphocytes (chalone), *Exp. Cell Res.* **93**:283.

Aoyama, T., Kihara, K., and Nishiguchi, K., 1975, Dual effects of thymic substance(s) on growth of cultured mammalian cells, *Exp. Cell Res.* **93**:427.

Bachrach, U., 1973, *Function of Naturally Occurring Polyamines*, Academic Press, New York.

Baker, F. L., Broxmeyer, H. E., and Gailbraith, P. R., 1975, Control of granulopoiesis in man. III. Inhibition of colony formation by dense leukocytes, *J. Cell. Physiol.* **86**:337.

Balázs, A., Fazekas, I., Bukulya, B., Blazsek, I., and Rappay, G., 1972, An intracellular factor (DCI) controlling differentiation and cell division, *Mech. Ageing Dev.* **1**:175.

Balázs, A., Klupp, T., Zsila, G., Blazsek, I., Holczinger, L., and Gaál, D., 1977, Modulative effect of endogenous granuloid inhibitors on cell proliferation, *Mech. Ageing Dev.* **6**:207.

Barfod, N. M., and Marcker, K., 1977, Partial purification and characterization of $G_1$ chalone from JB-1 plasmacytoma cells, in Abstracts of Papers, International Symposium on Molecular Control of Proliferation in Eukaryotic Cells, April 17–20, Dobogókö, Hungary.

Bateman, A., 1974, Cell specificity of chalone-type inhibitors of DNA synthesis released by blood leucocytes and erythrocytes, *Cell Tissue Kinet.* **7**:451.

Bateman, A. E., and Goodwin, B. C., 1976, An inhibitor of DNA synthesis in erythrocyte-conditioned medium and its separation from haemoglobin, *Biomedicine* **25**:77.

Benestad, H. B. 1970, Formation of granulocytes and macrophages in diffusion chamber cultures of mouse blood leukocytes, *Scand. J. Haematol.* **7**:279.

Benestad, H. B. and Rytömaa, T., 1977, Regulation of maturation rate of mouse granulocytes, *Cell Tissue Kinet.* **10**:461.

Benestad, H. B., Rytömaa, T., and Kiviniemi, K., 1973, The cell specific effect of the granulocyte chalone demonstrated with the diffusion chamber technique, *Cell Tissue Kinet.* **6**:147.

Beran, M., 1975, The influence of mouse sera on colony formation and on the production of colony stimulating factor *in vitro*, *Exp. Hematol.* **3**:309.

Bichel, P., 1973, Further studies on the self-limiting of growth of JB-1 ascites tumours, *Eur. J. Cancer* **8**:167.

Bichel, P., 1976, Ascites tumours and chalones, *in Chalones* (J. C. Houck, ed.), pp. 429–449, North-Holland/American Elsevier, New York.

Blazsek, I., Balázs, A., Gaál, D., and Holczinger, L., 1976, A multifactorial system controlling myeloid cell differentiation and division, *Mech. Ageing Dev.* **5**:57.

Bøyum, A., and Breivik, H., 1973, Kinetics of murine haemopoietic cell proliferation in diffusion chambers, *Cell Tissue Kinet.* **6**:101.

Bøyum, A., Løvhaug, D., and Boecker, W. R., 1976, Regulation of bone marrow cell growth in diffusion chambers: The effect of adding normal and leukemic (CML) polymorphonuclear granulocytes, *Blood* **48**:373.

Broxmeyer, H. E., Moore, M. A. S., and Ralph, P., 1976a, Cell-free granulocyte colony inhibiting activity derived from human polymorphonuclear neutrophils, *Exp. Hematol.* **5**:87.

Broxmeyer, H. E., Baker, F. L., and Galbraith, P. R., 1976b, *In vitro* regulation of granulopoiesis in human leukemia: Application of an assay for colony inhibiting cells, *Blood* **47**:389.

Brønstad, G. O., Elgjo, K., and Øye, I., 1971, Adrenalin increases cyclic 3′,5′-AMP formation in hamster epidermis, *Nature New Biol.* **233**:78.

Bullough, W. S., 1962, The control of mitotic activity in adult mammalian tissues, *Biol. Rev.* **37**:307.

Bullough, W. S., 1973, Epidermal chalone mechanism, *Natl. Cancer Inst. Monogr.* **38**:99.

Bullough, W. S., and Deol, J. U. R., 1971, Chalone-induced mitotic inhibition in the Hewitt keratinising epidermal carcinoma of the mouse, *Eur. J. Cancer* **7**:425.

Bullough, W. S., and Laurence, E. B., 1960, The control of epidermal mitotic activity in the mouse, *Proc. Roy. Soc. B* **151**:517.

Bullough, W. S., and Laurence, E. B., 1964, Mitotic control by internal secretion: The role of the chalone-adrenalin complex, *Exp. Cell Res.* **33**:176.

Bullough, W. S., and Laurence, E. B., 1968, Control of mitosis in rabbit Vx2 epidermal tumours by means of epidermal chalone, *Eur. J. Cancer* **4**:587.

Bullough, W. S., and Laurence, E. B., 1970, The lymphocytic chalone and its antimitotic action on a mouse lymphoma *in vitro, Eur. J. Cancer* **6**:525.

Bullough, W. S., and Mitrani, E., 1976, An analysis of the epidermal chalone control mechanism, *in Chalones* (J. C. Houck, ed.), pp. 7–36, North-Holland/American Elsevier, New York.

Burzynski, S. R., Loo, T. L., Ho, D. H., Rao, P. N., Georgiades, G., and Kratzenstein, H., 1976, Biologically active peptides in human urine: III. Inhibitors of the growth of human leukemia, osteosarcoma, and HeLa cells, *Physiol. Chem. Phys.* **8**:13.

Byrd, W. J., Jacobs, D. M., and Amoss, M. S., 1977, Synthetic polyamines added to cultures containing bovine sera reversibly inhibit *in vitro* parameters of immunity, *Nature* **267**: 621.

Cercek, L., Cercek, B., and Ockey, C. H., 1973, Structuredness of the cytoplasmic matrix and Michaelis-Menten constants for the hydrolysis of FDA during the cell cycle in Chinese hamster ovary cells, *Biophysik* **10**:187.

Chan, S. H., 1971, Influence of serum inhibitors on colony development *in vitro* by bone marrow cells, *Aust. J. Exp. Biol. Med. Sci.* **49**:553.

Chan, S. H., Metcalf, D., and Stanley, E. R., 1971, Stimulation and inhibition by normal human serum of colony formation *in vitro* by bone marrow cells, *Br. J. Haematol* **20**:329.

Chung, A. C., 1976, The *in vivo* effects of lymphoid chalone(s) and its immuno-suppressive properties, in *Chalones* (J. C. Houck, ed.), pp. 385–393, North-Holland/American Elsevier, New York.

Chung, A. C., and Hufnagel, C. A., 1973, Some *in vivo* effects of chalone (mitotic inhibitor) obtained from lymphoid tissues, *Natl. Cancer Inst. Monogr.* **38**:131.

Cooper, E. H., 1973, The biology of cell death in tumours, *Cell Tissue Kinet.* **6**:87.

Cooper, P. R., and Smith, H., 1973, Influence of cell-free ascites fluid and adenosine 3'5'-cyclic monophosphate upon the cell kinetics of Ehrlich's ascites carcinoma, *Nature* **241**:457.

Cross, J. P., 1972, A technique for the assay of granulocytic chalone and antichalone, *J. Anat.* **111**:336.

Cross, J. P., 1974, The physiological control of neutrophil production with special reference to granulocytic chalone, in *Proceedings of the Advanced Haematology Seminar*, pp. 16–28, Regional Technical College, Galway, England.

Dewey, D. L., 1973, The melanocyte chalone, *Natl. Cancer Inst. Monogr.* **38**:213.

Dewey, D. L., 1977, The nature of an inhibitor extracted from melanoma tumours, in Abstracts of Papers, International Symposium on Molecular Control of Proliferation in Eukaryotic Cells, April 17–20, Dobogókö, Hungary.

Dewey, D. L., Butcher, F. W., and Galpine, A. R., 1977, Control of melanoma cells, in Annual Report, Gray Laboratories, Mount Vernon Hospital, pp. 95–100, Northwood, Middlesex, England.

Dexter, T. M., Allen, T. D., Lajtha, L. G., Schofield, R., and Lord, B. I., 1973, Stimulation of proliferation and differentiation of haemopoietic cells *in vitro*, *J. Cell. Physiol.* **82**:461.

Elgjo, K., Laerum, O. D., and Edgehill, W., 1971, Growth regulation in mouse epidermis. I. $G_2$ inhibitor present in the basal cell layer. *Virchows Arch. B Zellpathol.* **8**:277.

Elgjo, K., Laerum, O. D., and Edgehill, W., 1972, Growth regulation in mouse epidermis. II. $G_1$ inhibitor present in the differentiating cell layer, *Virchows Arch. B Zellpathol.* **10**:229.

Erslev, A. J., Kazal, L. A., Miller, O. P., and Abaidoo, K.-J. R., 1972, The renal erythropoietin inhibitor, in *Regulation of Erythropoiesis* (A. S. Gordon, M. Condorelli, and C. Peschle, eds.), pp. 217–222, The Publishing House "Il Ponte," Milano.

Ferris, P., LoBue, J., and Gordon, A. S., 1973, Possible feedback inhibition of leukemic cell growth: Kinetics of Shay chloroleukemia grown in diffusion chambers and intraperitoneally in rodents, in *Humoral Control of Growth and Differentiation*, Vol. I (J. LoBue and A. S. Gordon, eds.), pp. 213–225, Academic Press, New York.

Fireman, P., Boesman, M., Haddad, Z. H., and Gitlin, D., 1967, Passive transfer of tuberculin reactivity *in vitro*, *Science* **155**:337.

Fleming, W. A., McNeill, T. A., and Killen, M., 1972, The effects of an inhibitory factor (interferon) on the *in vitro* growth of granulocyte-macrophage colonies, *Immunology* **23**:429.

Florentin, I., Kiger, N., and Mathe, G., 1973, T lymphocyte specificity of a lymphocyte-inhibiting factor (chalone) extracted from the thymus, *Eur. J. Immunol.* **3**:624.

Garcia-Giralt, E., and Macieira-Coelho, A., 1974, Differential effect of a lymphoid chalone on the target and nontarget cells *in vitro*, in *Proceedings of the Eighth Leucocyte Culture Conference: Lymphocyte Recognition and Effector Mechanisms* (K. Lindahl-Kiessling and D. Osobu, eds.), pp. 457–474, Academic Press, New York.

Garcia-Giralt, E., Lasalvia, E., Florentin, I., and Mathe, G., 1970, Evidence for a lymphocyte chalone, *Eur. J. Clin. Biol. Res.* **15** :1012.

Garcia-Giralt, E., Morales, V. H., Lasalvia, E., and Mathe, G., 1972, Suppression of graft-vs.-host reaction by spleen extract, *J. Immunol.* **109**:878.

Garcia-Giralt, E., Rella, W., Morales, V. H., Diaz-Rubio, E., and Richard, F., 1973, Extraction from bovine spleen of immunosuppressant with no activity on hematopoietic spleen colony formation, *Natl. Cancer Inst. Monogr.* **38**: 125.

Garcia-Giralt, E., Diza-Rubio, E., and Rappaport, H., 1975, Evaluation of the specificity of a lymphoid chalone, *Cell Tissue Kinet.* **8**:589.

Gorer, P. A., 1960, The isoantigens of malignant cells, *in Biological Approaches to Cancer Chemotherapy* (R. J. C. Harris, ed.), pp. 219–230, Academic Press, New York.

Grundboeck-Juśko, J., 1976, Chemical characteristics of chalones isolated from bovine spleen, *Acta Biochim. Pol.* **23**:165.

Heideman, E., Jung, A., and Wilms, K., 1976, Gewebsspezifische Hemmung der Lymphocytenproliferation durch Milzextrakt (Lymphocytenchalon), *Klin. Wochenschr.* **54**:221.

Hondius Boldingh, W., and Laurence, E. B., 1968, Extraction, purification and preliminary characterization of the epidermal chalone. A tissue-specific mitotic inhibitor obtained from vertebrate skin. *Eur. J. Biochem.* **5**:191.

Houck, J. C., 1973, General introduction to the true chalone concept, *Natl. Cancer Inst. Monogr.* **38**:1.

Houck, J. C., 1976, Introduction, *in Chalones* (J. C. Houck, ed.), pp. 1–5, North-Holland/American Elsevier, New York.

Houck, J. C., and Attallah, A. M., 1976, Chalones (specific and endogenous mitotic inhibitors) and cancer, *in Cancer, A Comprehensive Treatise*, Vol. 3 (F. F. Becker, ed.), pp. 287–326, Plenum Press, New York.

Houck, J. C., and Hunt, C. V., 1976, Critique, *in Chalones* (J. C. Houck, ed.), pp. 483–491, North-Holland/American Elsevier, New York.

Houck, J. C., Irasquin, H., and Leikin, S., 1971, Lymphocyte DNA synthesis inhibition, *Science* **173**:1139.

Houck, J. C., Attallah, A. M., and Lilly, J. R., 1973, Immunosuppressive properties of the lymphocyte chalone, *Nature* **245**:148.

Houck, J. C., Kanagalingam, K., Hunt, C. V., Attallah, A. M., and Chung, A., 1977, Lymphocyte and fibroblast chalones: Some chemical properties, *Science* **196**:896.

Iversen, O. H., 1967, Kinetics of cellular proliferation and cell loss in human carcinomas: A discussion of methods available for *in vivo* studies, *Eur. J. Cancer* **3**:389.

Iversen, O. H., 1970, Some theoretical considerations on chalones and the treatment of cancer: A review, *Cancer Res.* **30**:1481.

Iversen, O. H., 1976, The history of chalones, in *Chalones* (J. C. Houck, ed.), pp. 37–69, North-Holland/American Elsevier, New York.

Jones, J., Paraskova-Tchernozenska, E., and Moorhead, J. F., 1970, In vitro inhibition of DNA synthesis in human leukaemic cells by a lymphoid cell extract, *Lancet* **ii**:654.

Kariniemi, A.-L., 1976, Chalone-induced inhibition in DNA synthesis of human psoriatic epidermal cells cultured in diffusion chambers in mice, *Ann. Clin. Res.* **8**:340.

Kariniemi, A.-L., and Rytömaa, T., 1976, Effect of the Hewitt keratinizing epidermal carcinoma on cell proliferation in different organs of the host mouse and in human psoriatic skin cultured in diffusion chambers, *Br. J. Dermatol.* **94**:515.

Kiger, N., Florentin, I., and Mathe, G., 1972a, Some effects of a partially purified lymphocyte-inhibiting factor from calf thymus, *Transplantation* **14**:448.

Kiger, N., Florentin, I., Garcia-Giralt, E., and Mathe, G., 1972b, Lymphocyte inhibitory factors (chalones) extracted from lymphoid organs. Extraction, partial purification and immunosuppressive properties. *Transplant. Proc.* **4**:531.

Kiger, N., Florentin, I., Garcia-Giralt, E., and Mathe, G., 1973a, Inhibition of graft-versus-host reaction (GVHR) by *in vitro* incubation of donor lymphoctyes with thymic or splenic chalone(s), *Exp. Hematol.* **1**:22.

Kiger, N., Florentin, I., and Mathe, G., 1973b, Inhibition of graft-versus-host reaction by preincubation of the graft with a thymic extract (lymphocyte chalone), *Transplantation* **16**:393.

Kiger, N., Florentin, I., and Mathe, G., 1975, Further purification of the lymphocyte inhibiting extract from the thymus, *Boll. Ist. Sieroter, Milan.* **54**:244.

Kivilaakso, E., and Rytömaa, T., 1970, The effect of polycythaemic serum on the proliferation of rat bone marrow cells *in vitro, Cell Tissue Kinet.* **3**:385.

Kivilaakso, E., and Rytömaa, T., 1971, Erythrocytic chalone, a tissue-specific inhibitor of cell proliferation in the erythron, *Cell Tissue Kinet.* **4**:1.

Knight, E., Jr., 1976, Antiviral and cell growth inhibitory activities reside in the same glycoprotein of human fibroblast interferon, *Nature* **262**:302.

Laerum, O. D., and Maurer, H. R., 1973, Proliferation kinetics of myelopoietic cells and macrophages in diffusion chambers after treatment with granulocyte extracts (chalone), *Virchows Arch. B Zellpath.* **14**:293.

Lasalvia, E., Garcia-Giralt, E., and Macieira-Coelho, A., 1970, Extraction of an inhibitor of DNA synthesis from human peripheral blood lymphocytes and bovine spleen, *Eur. J. Clin. Biol. Res.* **15**:789.

Laurence, E. B., and Elgjo, K., 1971, Epidermal chalone and cell proliferation in a transplantable squamous cell carcinoma in hamsters. II. *In vitro* results, *Virchows Arch. B Zellpathol.* **7**:8.

Lawrence, H. S., 1969, Transfer factor, *Adv. Immunol.* **11**:195.

Lawrence, H. S., Rapaport, F. T., Converse, J. M., and Tillett, W. S., 1960, Transfer of delayed hypersensivity to skin homografts with leukocyte extracts in man, *J. Clin. Invest.* **39**:185.

Lindeman, R., 1971, Erythropoiesis inhibiting factor (EIF). I. Fractionation and demonstration of urinary EIF, *Br. J. Haematol.* **21**:623.

Lindeman, R., 1975, Erythropoiesis-inhibiting factor(s) (EIF): Methodologic studies, *Blood* **47**:155.

Lord, B. I., 1975, Modification of granulopoietic cell proliferation by granulocyte extracts, *Boll. Ist. Sieroter. Milan.* **54**:187.

Lord, B. I., 1976, The assay of cell proliferation inhibitors, *in Chalones* (J. C. Houck, ed.), pp. 97–139, North-Holland/American Elsevier, New York.

Lord, B. I., Cercek, L., Cercek, B., Shah, G. P., Dexter, T. P., and Lajtha, L. G., 1974a, Inhibitors of haemopoietic cell proliferation: Specificity of action within the haemopoietic system, *Br. J. Cancer* **29**:168.

Lord, B. I., Cercek, L., Cercek, B., Shah, G. P., and Lajtha, L. G., 1974b, Inhibitors of haemopoietic cell proliferation. Reversibility of action, *Br. J. Cancer* **29**:407.

Lord, B. I., Mori, K. J., Wright, E. G., and Lajtha, L. G., 1976, An inhibitor of stem cell proliferation in normal bone marrow, *Br. J. Haematol.* **34**:441.

Lord, B. I., Shah, G. P., and Lajtha, L. G., 1977, The effects of red blood cell extracts on the proliferation of erythrocyte precursor cells, *in vivo, Cell Tissue Kinet.* **10**:215.

Løvhaug, D., and Bøyum, A., 1977, Regulation of bone marrow cell growth in diffusion chambers: The effect of granulocyte extracts, *Cell Tissue Kinet.* **10**:137.

MacManus, J. P., and Whitfield, J. F., 1969, Stimulation of DNA synthesis and mitotic activity of thymic lymphocytes by cyclic adenosine $3',5'$ monophosphate, *Exp. Cell Res.* **58**:188.

MacVittie, T. J., and McCarthy, K. F., 1974, Inhibition of granulopoiesis in diffusion chambers by a granulocyte chalone, *Exp. Hematol.* **2**:182.

MacVittie, T. J., and McCarthy, K. F., 1975, The influence of a granulocytic inhibitor(s) on hematopoiesis in an *in vivo* culture system, *Cell Tissue Kinet.* **8**:553.

Maiolo, A. T., Cazzaniga, E., Cortelezzi, A., DePangher, V., Foa, P., Lombardi, L., Mozzana, R., and Polli, E. E., 1975, *In vitro* production of lymphocyte and granulocyte proliferation inhibitors (chalones?) from living cells, *Boll. Ist. Sieroter. Milan.* **54**: 235.

Marks, F., 1975, Isolation of an endogeneous inhibitor of epidermal DNA synthesis ($G_1$ chalone) from pig skin, *Hoppe Seylers Z. Physiol. Chem.* **356**:1989.

Maurer, H. R., and Henry, R., 1976, Automated scanning of bone marrow cell colonies growing in agar-containing glass capillaries, *Exp. Cell Res.* **103**:271.

Maurer, H. R., and Henry, R., 1977, Growth kinetics by scanning of granulocytic cell colonies in glass capillaries, *Blut* **34**:89.

Maurer, H. R., Weiss, G., and Laerum, O. D., 1976, Evaluation of a short term *in vitro* test for granulocytic chalone activity, *Virchows Arch. B Zellpathol.* **20**: 229.

Minowada, J., Ohnuma, T., and Moore, G. E., 1973, Rosette-forming human lymphoid cell lines. I. Establishment and evidence for origin of thymus-derived lymphocytes, *J. Natl. Cancer Inst.* **49**:891.

Moorhead, J. J., Paraskova-Tchernozenska, E., Pirrie, A. J., and Hayes, C., 1969, Lymphoid inhibitor of human lymphocyte DNA synthesis and mitosis *in vitro*, *Nature* **224**:1207.

Nadler, S. H., and Moore, G. E., 1965, Autotransplantation of human cancer, *JAMA* **191**:105.

Nakai, G., 1976, Ehrlich ascites tumor (EAT) chalone effects on nascent DNA synthesis and DNA polymerases alpha and beta, *Cell Tissue Kinet.* **9**:553.

Ng, M. H., and Vilcek, J., 1972, Interferons, *Adv. Protein Chem.* **26**:173.

Olsson, L., and Claësson, M. H., 1975, Studies on the regulation of lymphocyte production in the murine thymus and some effects of a crude thymus extract, *Cell Tissue Kinet.* **8**:491.

Pattengale, P. K., Smith, R. W., and Gerber, P., 1973, Selective transformation of B lymphocytes by EB virus, *Lancet* **ii**:93.

Paukovits, W. R., 1971, Control of granulocyte production: Separation and chemical identification of a specific inhibitor (chalone), *Cell Tissue Kinet.* **4**:539.

Paukovits, W. R., 1973, Granulopoiesis-inhibiting factor: Demonstration and preliminary chemical characterization of a specific polypeptide (chalone), *Natl. Cancer Inst. Monogr.* **38**:147.

Paukovits, W. R., 1976, *In vitro* biological and chemical properties of the granulocytic chalone, in *Chalones* (J. C. Houck, ed.), pp. 311–330, North-Holland/American Elsevier, New York.

Paukovits, W. R., and Paukovits, J. B., 1975a, Separation, identification and mechanism of action of the granulocytic chalone, *Boll. Ist. Sieroter. Milan.* **54**:177.

Paukovits, W. R., and Paukovits, J. B., 1975b, Mechanism of action of granulopoiesis inhibiting factor (chalone). I. Evidence for a receptor protein on bone marrow cells. *Exp. Pathol.* **10**:348.

Paukovits, W. R., and Paukovits, J. B., 1976, The granulocytic chalone, *IRCS Med. Sci.* **4**:44.

Peavy, D. L., Adler, W. H., and Smith, R. T., 1970, The mitogenic effect of endotoxin and staphylococcal endotoxin B on mouse spleen cells and human peripheral lymphocytes, *J. Immunol.* **105**:1453.

Peschle, C., Sasso, G. F., Rappaport, I. A., Rossanigo, F., Gordon, A. S., and Condorelli, M., 1972, Hormonal influences on erythropoiesis and erythropoietin production, in *Regulation of Erythropoiesis* (A. S. Gordon, M. Condorelli, and C. Peschle, eds.), pp. 269–299, The Publishing House "Il Ponte," Milano.

Raina, A., and Jänne, J., 1975, Physiology of the natural polyamines putrescine, spermidine and spermine, *Med. Biol.* **53**:121.

Rainer, H., and Moser, K., 1977, *In vitro*—Untersuchungen mit menschlichem Transferfactor, *Blut* **34**:471.

Ranney, D. F., 1975, Biological inhibitors of lymphoid cell division, in *Advances in Pharmacology and Chemotherapy*, Vol. 13 (S. Garattini, A. Goldin, F. Hawking, and I. J. Kopin, eds.), pp. 359–408, Academic Press, New York.

Rapaport, F. T., Dausset, J., Converse, J. M., and Lawrence, H. S., 1965, Biological and ultrastructural studies of leucocyte fractions as transplantation antigens in man, *Transplantation* **3**:490.

Refsum, S. B., and Berdal, P., 1967, Cell loss in malignant tumours in man, *Eur. J. Cancer* **3**:235.

Rytömaa, T., 1969, Granulocytic chalone and antichalone, *In Vitro* **4**:47.

Rytömaa, T., 1970, Regulation of cell production by chalones, *Ann. Clin. Res.* **2**:94.

Rytömaa, T., 1973a, Chalone of the granulocyte system, *Natl. Cancer Inst. Monogr.* **38**:143.

Rytömaa, T., 1973b, Role of chalone in granulopoiesis, *Br. J. Haematol.* **24**:141.

Rytömaa, T., 1976, The chalone concept, *in International Review of Experimental Pathology*, Vol. 16 (G. W. Richter and M. A. Epstein, eds.), pp. 155–206, Academic Press, New York.

Rytömaa, T., and Kiviniemi, K., 1967, Regulation system of blood cell production, *in Control of Cellular Growth in Adult Organisms* (H. Teir and T. Rytömaa, eds.), pp. 106–138, Academic Press, New York.

Rytömaa, T., and Kiviniemi, K., 1968a, Control of granulocyte production I. Chalone and antichalone, two specific humoral regulators, *Cell Tissue Kinet.* **1**:329.

Rytömaa, T., and Kiviniemi, K., 1968b, Control of granulocyte production. II. Mode of action of chalone and antichalone, *Cell Tissue Kinet.* **1**:341.

Rytömaa, T., and Kiviniemi, K., 1968c, Control of DNA duplication in rat chloroleukemia by means of the granulocytic chalone, *Eur. J. Cancer* **4**:595.

Rytömaa, T., and Kiviniemi, K., 1968d, Control of cell production in rat chloroleukemia by means of the granulocytic chalone, *Nature* **220**:136.

Rytömaa, T., and Kiviniemi, K., 1969, Chloroma regression induced by the granulocytic chalone, *Nature* **222**:995.

Rytömaa, T., and Kiviniemi, K., 1970, Regression of generalized leukaemia in rat induced by the granulocytic chalone, *Eur. J. Cancer* **6**:401.

Rytömaa, T., and Kiviniemi, K., 1975, Cyclic adenosine 3':5'-monophosphate and inhibition of deoxyribonucleic acid synthesis *in vitro, In Vitro* **11**:1.

Rytömaa, T., Vilpo, J. A., Levanto, A., and Jones, W. A., 1976, Effect of granulocyte chalone on acute and chronic granulocytic leukaemia in man. Report of seven cases, *Scand. J. Haematol.*, Suppl.27, pp. 5–28.

Rytömaa, T., Vilpo, J. A., Levanto. A., and Jones, W. A., 1977, Effect of granulocytic chalone on acute myeloid leukaemia in man. A follow-up study, *Lancet* **i**:771.

Schütt, M., and Langen, P., 1972, Comments on granulocytic chalone action, *Stud. Biophys.* **31/32**:311.

Shadduck, R. K., 1971, Granulocyte stimulating and inhibiting activity from neutrophils (PMS's): Possibly dual feedback control of granulopoiesis, *Blood* **38**:820.

Steel, G. G., 1967, Cell loss as a factor in the growth rate of human tumours, *Eur. J. Cancer* **3**:381.

Thornley, A. L., and Laurence, E. B., 1975, Chalone regulation of the epidermal cell cycle, *Experientia* **31**:1024.

Thornley, A. L., and Laurence, E. B., 1976, The specificity of epidermal chalone action: The results of *in vivo* experimentation with two purified skin extracts, *Dev. Biol.* **51**:10.

Toivonen, H., 1976, Leukemian kasvun matemaattinen malli ja merkkiaine-mittauksia, Diploma Thesis, pp. 1–56, Department of Technical Physics, Helsinki University of Technology.

Toivonen, H., and Rytömaa, T., 1978, Monte Carlo simulation of malignant growth, *J. Theor. Biol.* **71**, in press.

Valle, M. J., Jordan, G. W., Haahr, S., and Merigan, T. C., 1975, Characteristics of immune interferon produced by human lymphocyte cultures compared to other human interferons, *J. Immunol.* **115**: 230.

Vilpo, J. A., and Rytömaa, T., 1973, Proliferation kinetics of Shay chloroleukaemia cells grown in diffusion chambers *in vivo, Cell Tissue Kinet.* **6**:489.

Vilpo, J. A., Kiviniemi, K., and Rytömaa, T., 1973, Inhibition of granulopoiesis by endogenous granulocyte chalone studied with the diffusion chamber technique, *Eur. J. Cancer* **9**:515.

Vorhees, J. J., Duell, E. A., Bass, L. J., and Harrell, E. R., 1973, Role of cyclic AMP in the control of epidermal growth and differentiation, *Natl. Cancer Inst. Monogr.* **38**:47.

Whitfield, J. F., MacManus, J. P., and Gillan, D. J., 1973, The ability of calcium to change cyclic AMP from a stimulator to an inhibitor of thymic lymphoblast proliferation, *J. Cell. Physiol.* **81**:241.

Yunis, A. A., Arimura, G. K., Haines, H. G., Ratzen, R. J., and Cross, M. A., 1975, Characteristics of rat chloroma in culture, *Cancer Res.* **35**:337.

11

# Cytogenetic Studies in Leukemia

## Jacqueline Whang-Peng and Robert C. Young

## 11.1. Introduction

In 1902, Boveri published a paper on the dispermic sea urchin egg and proposed the theory that malignant tumors could be due to an abnormal chromosome constitution. This theory received considerable credence in 1960 when Nowell and Hungerford discovered a minute chromosome, later designated the Philadelphia (Ph$^1$) chromosome, in cultured blood cells from two patients with chronic myelogenous leukemia. Encouraged by the possibility of identifying a specific chromosome abnormality for each malignancy and determining the relationship of the characteristic abnormality to a particular disease, numerous investigators have conducted cytogenetic studies in many types of leukemia but, unfortunately, no other unique chromosome abnormalities have been found. However, the association of a variety of chromosome abnormalities with human leukemia is now well established.

Significant technical advances in the past decade, led by the introduction of the quinacrine fluorescence stain for the chemical differentiation of the metaphase chromosome by Caspersson *et al.* in 1968 and followed by the Giemsa banding technique in 1971 (Seabright, 1971; Dutrillaux

JACQUELINE WHANG-PENG and ROBERT C. YOUNG • Medicine Branch, National Cancer Institute, National Institutes of Health, Bethesda, Maryland.

375

and Lejeune, 1971), have added a new dimension to the field of cytogenetics. These techniques made it possible, for the first time, to identify precisely each pair of chromosomes, and some chromosome changes previously thought to be of a random nature have not been found to be nonrandom (Rowley, 1975). Certain chromosomes of the C group, #7, #8, and #9, appear to be associated with abnormalities of the erythroid and myeloid systems. Monosomy of the #7 chromosome has been reported in several closely related myeloproliferative diseases: in erythroleukemia (Petit *et al.*, 1973), in a case of preleukemia which progressed to AML (Kaufman *et al.*, 1974), in AMMoL (Macdougall *et al.*, 1974), and in a case of pancytopenia without leukemia (Rowley, 1973a). Trisomy 8 has been seen in AML, AMMoL, and erythroleukemia (Rowley and Potter, 1976), as well as in the blastic phase of CML (Rowley, 1975) and in polycythemia vera (Hsu *et al.*, 1974). Trisomy 9 has been identified in patients with myelosclerosis (Davidson and Knight, 1973), AMMoL (Rutten *et al.*, 1974), thrombocytosis (Rowley, 1973b), and polycythemia vera (Knight *et al.*, 1974). Several investigators have also noted specific chromosome deletions: a partial deletion of the long arm of chromosome #5 has been found in several cases of refractory anemia exhibiting thrombocytopenia, peripheral leukocytosis, and normal or low alkaline phosphatase (Verhest *et al.*, 1976); and deleted long arms of the #20 chromosome have been reported in polycythemia and one case of AML (Reeves *et al.*, 1972; Whang-Peng *et al.*, 1977). Finally, an isochromosome, formed from the long (q) arms of chromosome #17, has been observed in AML, Hodgkin's disease, and CML (Engel *et al.*, 1975). While these abnormalities are not exclusively confined to a specific disease, they appear to have a greater than expected association with certain types of hematologic disorders.

## 11.2. Materials and Methods

### 11.2.1. Materials

#### 11.2.1.1. Introduction

Cytogenetics is the field of investigation which studies the chromosomes during mitosis and meiosis. The cytogenetics of malignant disorders is generally confined to mitotic division, preferably in the late prophase and early metaphase when the chromosomes are not overly contracted. Tissues containing a sufficient quantity of actively dividing cells can be processed directly without prior *in vitro* culture, whereas short- or long-term cultures, with or without mitogenic stimulation, are usually required for those tissues with low mitotic rates.

### 11.2.1.2. Bone Marrow

Because of its great cellularity and high mitotic activity, the bone marrow can be processed directly and it has proven to be a very useful tool in the study of hematologic disorders such as leukemia. A much more accurate picture of the abnormalities present and their relative numbers can be obtained from such specimens than from those which require *in vitro* culture. The procedure is a simple one which requires only a small amount of aspirated tissue and basic laboratory equipment. Also of importance is the fact that results can be available within a matter of hours.

### 11.2.1.3. Other Tissues

There are several other tissues which, if diseased, quite often yield considerable numbers of dividing cells and can also be processed directly; these include tumors, infiltrated lymph nodes, pleural effusions, ascites fluid, and peripheral blood. Good results can also be obtained from peripheral blood cultured for 1–2 days without a mitotic inducer if there are sufficient quantities of circulating immature cells.

### 11.2.2. Methods

The preparation of slides for chromosome analysis is a unique process, one in which only minimal variations are encountered from one laboratory to another. The purpose of each procedural step can be summarized as follows:

1. The initial step is treatment with a mitotic arresting agent which disrupts the spindle formation, allowing the chromosomes to become unattached from one another. The most commonly used agent is colchicine, in concentrations varying from 0.1 to 1.0 $\mu$g/ml; vincristine, proresid, and maytansine are also used. These agents are made up in medium or buffered saline solutions and the tissue is exposed to this treatment for 1–2 hr or longer if necessary.
2. The cells are next transferred to a hypotonic solution, the purpose of which is to swell the cells. The most popular hypotonic solutions are 1% sodium citrate (for 30 min) and 0.075 M KCl (for 10–15 min). Various concentrations of a mixture of distilled water and medium or serum are also occasionally employed.
3. Fixation is the final step prior to making the slides; it fixes the cells and, in bone marrow specimens, denatures and hemolyzes the erythrocytes which can then be discarded with the supernatant. Most fixatives are a 3:1 absolute alcohol–glacial acetic acid mixture, although some investigators prefer to use 45–60% glacial acetic acid only. The fixation step is generally repeated two to three times.

4. The final step, preparing the slides, is the one in which the most individual variation is seen. The purpose of all the methods is to break the cytoplasmic membrane, allowing the chromosomes to spread out in one plane. Air-dried preparations can be made by placing a few drops on an alcohol-cleaned slide and then blowing directly on the slide or by dropping the cells onto a prechilled slide from various heights; some prefer merely to swing the slides in the air. Flaming the slide over a Bunsen burner, a once popular method, is no longer widely used because it hardens the chromosomes, which interferes with chromosome banding.

### 11.2.2.1. Specific Methods

*11.2.2.1a. Bone Marrow.* The method outlined briefly herein is a slight modification of the one reported by Tjio and Whang in 1962, and is the one used in our laboratory:

1. Using no anticoagulants, collect 0.25–0.50 ml of bone marrow aspirate and transfer to a 0.2 $\mu$g/ml colchicine solution for 45–60 min; reduce time if the patient is receiving intensive chemotherapy.
2. Centrifuge the specimen, remove the supernatant, and resuspend the cells in 1% sodium citrate for 30 min.
3. Centrifuge, remove the supernatant, and resuspend the cells in freshly prepared 3:1 absolute ethanol–glacial acetic acid fixative. Repeat this step once, or twice if the specimen contained a lot of blood.
4. Centrifuge, remove all the supernatant, and resuspend the cells in a small amount of fixative.
5. Place a few drops of the cell suspension on each slide and blow on the slides. Make slides at varying cell concentrations.

*11.2.2.1b. In Vitro Peripheral Blood Culture.* The most widely used method for *in vitro* short-term culture is that of Moorhead *et al.* (1960). The modification described here is the one used in our laboratory. Heparinized blood (20 units/ml blood) is dispensed into sterile tubes which are then placed in an incubator to facilitate the sedimentation of the erythrocytes. The leukocyte-rich plasma remaining in the upper portion of the tube is collected (10 ml of blood will ordinarily yield 2–3 ml of cells). Leukocyte-free plasma is obtained by centrifuging the remaining blood at high speeds. To each 4 ml of medium (McCoy's 5A), add 1 ml of leukocyte-rich plasma and 1 ml of cell-free plasma. If the patient's WBC is higher or lower than normal (5000–10,000 mm$^{-3}$) the amount of leukocyte-rich plasma must be adjusted so that the final concentration of leukocytes is 1000–2000 mm$^{-3}$ of culture. If mitogenic stimulation is desired, add 4 drops of phytohemagglutinin M (PHA) to each 6 ml culture. Incubate at 37°C for 24–72 hr. Longer culture times are not generally used for leukemia patients except for conditions, such as CLL or Sezary syndrome, in which spontaneous division and response to mitogenic stimulation are poor and are often delayed. In those cases, the cells should be cultured for 6–7 days, with one change of medium after 3 or 4 days.

## 11.2.3. Staining

The orcein and Giemsa stains were both widely used for cytogenetic preparations for many years. Orcein stains were used mainly for chromosome squash preparations, a technique rarely used today.

### 11.2.3.1. Standard Giemsa Stain

Most nonbanding preparations are stained with Giemsa stains, of which there are numerous types. The one employed in our laboratory is Giemsa stain, azure B type; it is supplied in liquid form. The working stain is made from 6 ml stock Giemsa, 6 ml of pH 6.2 buffer, and 138 ml of distilled water. The slides are stained for 10 min, rinsed under running tap water, allowed to dry, and then coverslipped with Permount.

### 11.2.3.2. Quinacrine Fluorescence Banding Stain

Introduced by Caspersson *et al.* in 1968, this method made possible the precise identification of each chromosome pair for the first time. The detailed structure of each chromosome was characterized by the differential affinity of various segments of a chromosome for a fluorescent stain, and each chromosome shows a different pattern of fluorescent (or Q) bands when exposed to ultraviolet light. The original method has undergone many variations and is used by many laboratories only to demonstrate the Y body, which fluoresces brightly. Its primary disadvantage is that it is an expensive, time-consuming technique that requires considerable photographic experience. In our laboratory we use the following method: A few drops of 50 $\mu$g/ml quinacrine mustard (dissolved in McIlvaine's disodium phosphate–citric acid buffer, pH 7.0) are placed on the slide, which is then coverslipped and allowed to stand for 20 or 30 min. The coverslip is removed and the slide is placed in distilled water for 3 min, then rinsed in running water two to three times, and finally allowed to air-dry. Immediately prior to examination under the fluorescent microscope, a few drops of buffer solution or distilled water are placed on the slide which is then coverslipped; the excess fluid is removed by blotting the slide with filter paper.

### 11.2.3.3. Giemsa Banding Techniques

Of much broader application are the Giemsa banding techniques which were introduced by Dutrillaux and Lejeune (1971) and Seabright (1971). In all these techniques the preparations are subjected to various chemical and/or physical treatments in order to disrupt nucleoprotein associations which produce characteristic banding patterns when the slides are stained with Giemsa stain. There are currently four different procedures, each producing a different banding pattern referred to as G-, R-, C-, and T-bands.

*11.2.3.3a. G-Banding (Giemsa Trypsin).* This is the most widely used banding method and was the one initially described by Seabright (1971). It is based on the preferential binding of stain to chromosome regions containing DNA rich in dA-dT residues. Most techniques use proteolytic enzymes, such as trypsin, but a variety of other agents, such as urea and various salt solutions have also been employed. The method used in our laboratory is a modification of the one described by Seabright. Air-dried slides which have been aged for 1–2 weeks are placed in a 37°C incubator for 4–5 hr. While still warm, they are immersed in a 0.025% trypsin solution for a specific time (10–30 sec for bone marrow and 10–20 sec for peripheral blood preparations), immediately immersed and rinsed in cold saline, and then stained in a 2% Gurr's Giemsa stain (R66) for 30–45 min; they are then lightly rinsed in tap water and allowed to dry.

*11.2.3.3b. R-Banding (Reverse Banding).* In the R-banding technique, the bands produced correspond to the nonfluorescent regions seen in Q banding and the nonbanded regions of G-banding. It is based on thermal denaturation of DNA and the preparations are observed under phase contrast. It is most useful for determining the exact location of terminal translocation sites. The most popular method is that of Dutrillaux and Lejeune (1971). The slides are immersed in a 20mM phosphate buffer, pH 6.5, at 87°C for 10–12 min and are then stained with dilute Giemsa at room temperature for 10 min. Van De Sande *et al.* (1977) recently described a method for R-banding using Olivomycin, a guanosine-cytosine specific DNA binding antibiotic, which is very encouraging. The slides are simply treated with a 1-mg/ml solution of Olivomycin in a phosphate buffer, pH 6.8, for 20 min at room temperature, washed in two changes of buffer solution for a total of 2 min, mounted with the same buffer, and then examined under the fluorescent microscope.

*11.2.3.3c. C-Banding (Constitutive Heterochromatin Banding).* The bands produced in this technique correspond to the centromeric regions which are composed of highly repetitive DNA sequences called constitutive heterochromatin. Originally described by Arrighi and Hsu (1971), the procedure involves DNA denaturation with HCl, RNase, and NaOH, and the renaturation of the DNA in a saline citrate solution at 65°C. This stain is best used to demonstrate polymorphism at the heterochromatic region.

*11.2.3.3d. T-Banding (Terminal Banding).* In 1973, Dutrillaux introduced two methods of T-banding, both of which are similar to the R-banding method. The origin of the terminal bands produced by this technique are unknown but are thought to represent the parts of the R-bands most resistant to the denaturation process. One of Dutrillaux's methods requires a longer incubation time (up to 30 min) than the R-banding technique; the other uses a more acidic buffer solution (pH 5.1 rather than the pH 6.5 buffer used in R-banding). T-banding is chiefly used to precisely identify juxtatelomeric break points.

## 11.2.4. Nomenclature

The normal human karyotype was established by the Denver convention in 1960 and has since become universally accepted. The participants proposed that the 46 human chromosomes be divided into eight broad categories, designated groups A to G including the sex chromosomes, on a morphological basis dependent on chromosome size and centromeric location. The three largest pairs (#1–3) comprise group A; the two large submedium pairs (#4 and 5), group B; the medium-sized chromosomes (pairs #6–12 and the X), group C; the three large acrocentric pairs (#13–15), group D; the metacentric to submetacentric pairs (#16–18), group E; the small metacentric (#19 and 20), group F; and the smaller acrocentric chromosomes (pairs #21 and 22, and the Y), group G. Only pairs 1, 2, 3, and 16 could be identified with certainty. The introduction of chromosome autoradiography (German, 1962), in which [$^3$H]thymidine is used to label newly replicated DNA, expanded precise identification to pairs 4, 5, 13, 14, and 15, and to the late-labeling (hot) X (in cells with more than one X chromosome). The introduction of the quinacrine fluorescence banding stain by Caspersson *et al.* in 1968, followed by the Giemsa banding techniques, made possible the precise identification of each chromosome pair.

### 11.2.4.1. Paris Conference

In 1971, the Paris Conference established a standardized system of nomenclature for human cytogenetics; it described the various chromosome regions revealed by the new banding techniques. Only the most frequently used symbols are described here.

All the symbols for rearrangement are placed before the chromosome involved and this chromosome is then placed in parentheses (many authors, for the purpose of simplification, eliminate the parenthesis). The + or − sign placed before the chromosome number indicates additional or missing whole chromosomes; when placed after the chromosome number, the + or − means an increase or decrease (deletion) in length. The symbol $p$ represents the short arm of the chromosome and $q$ represents the long arm. The secondary constriction region is represented by $h$ and it can be increased (h+) or decreased (h−) in length; when a secondary constriction alters the length of the short arm it is abbreviated $ph+$ or $ph−$ and alteration of the long arm is $qh+$ or $qh−$.

*11.2.4.1a. Translocation.* The $t$ stands for translocation; the lowest number chromosome in a translocation should be listed first, the only exception being a rearrangement involving the X chromosome, in which case the X is listed first; for example, a translocation from a #6 to an X and a translocation from an X to a #6 are both designated t(X;6), whereas a translocation from a #9 to a #22 or a translocation from a #22 to a #9 are both designated t(9;22). There are several types of translocation, including *rob* (Robertsonian, which results from centric fusion of two acrocentrics), *rcp* (reciprocal or balanced translocation), and *tan* (tandem translocation); where these are specified, the abbreviation replaces the $t$.

*11.2.4.1b. Other Symbols.* Three-break rearrangements involving one or two chromosomes are referred to as insertions (*ins*) and result from the excision of a segment after two breaks in one chromosome and its insertion at a point of breakage in the same or another chromosome; the receptor chromosome is listed first. An inverted insertion is *inv ins*.

A dicentric chromosome has two centromeres, formed by breakage and reunion involving two chromatids; it is designated *dic*, and a dicentric chromosome formed after a translocation would be *tdic*. A ring chromosome is represented by $r$ and, for example, a ring chromosome formed from a #8 chromosome would be $r(8)$. An isochromosome (*iso* or *i*) is a symmetrical chromosome composed of the duplicated long or short arms formed after misdivision of the centromere in a transverse plane; for example, an isochromosome formed from the long arms of chromosome #17 would be *iso*(17q) or *i*(17q). Other abbreviations include *del* (deletion), *der* (derivative chromosome, a structurally rearranged chromosome generated by a single rearrangement involving two or more chromosomes), *dup* (duplication), and *rec* (recombinant chromosome, a structurally rearranged chromosome with a new segmental composition); *ter* represents the terminal portion of a chromosome, so *pter* means the ends of the short arms and *qter* the ends of the long arms. A single ":" means a break and a double one "::" break and join; → means from–to and ";" is used to separate designations.

## 11.3. Myeloproliferative Diseases

### 11.3.1. Acute Myelogenous Leukemia

#### 11.3.1.1. Introduction

Compared to the technical difficulties encountered in acute lymphocytic leukemia (ALL), it is relatively easy to produce good chromosome preparations from the bone marrow of patients with acute myelogenous leukemia (AML). By applying the banding technique, it is possible to identify each chromosome pair precisely and to determine which chromosomes are involved in aneuploidy. In 1975, Rowley, on the basis of published data on chromosomal banding, suggested that there exists a nonrandom relationship between certain chromosomal abnormalities and hematologic disorders.

#### 11.3.1.2. Congenital AML

Cengenital leukemia, though rare, is a well-described phenomenon, and it has been reported in normal infants as well as in those with congenital defects such as Down's syndrome. There is a high incidence of aneuploidy in the reported cases of congenital AML. In a case described in 1967 by Zussman *et al.*, myeloblastic-promyelocytic leukemia was diagnosed in a male newborn who had cutaneous lesions and blood dyscrasia; 50% of the metaphases in the direct bone marrow preparation were pseudodiploid with a deleted $A_3$. The infant survived only 30 days. In a study of 52 cases of leukemia, Reisman *et al.* (1964a) included four patients with congenital AML. In two of the cases, aged 2 weeks and 1 year, no congenital anomalies were present; both cases exhibited aneuploidy with modal numbers of 45 and 53 chromosomes, respectively. The remaining two cases had trisomy 21 Down's syndrome; one of them had no additional chromosomal abnormalities whereas the other had a cell line with 48 chromosomes including an extra C group chromosome. In all four of these cases, the aneuploid lines were seen only during the active phase of the disease and no abnormalities (other than the trisomy 21) were observed during remission.

#### 11.3.1.3. Evidence for Stem Cell Origin of AML

Cytogenetic studies have been employed to demonstrate that erythroid as well as myeloid precursors are involved in the leukemia process, indicating a common stem cell abnormality in AML. The first indirect evidence was provided by Krogh Jensen and Killmann in 1971: they reported that in five patients with numerous erythroblasts, the proportion of erythroblastic mitoses exceeded the proportion of normal metaphases. Direct evidence for the involvement of the red cell series was provided by Blackstock and Garson in 1974 when they were able to show that aneuploid metaphases in three cases of AML incorporated radioactive iron ($^{55}$Fe), thus proving that they were erythroid precursors.

### 11.3.1.4. Cytogenetic Studies with Nonbanding Stains

Between 1962 and 1976 a combined total of 328 cases of AML were reported by Hungerford and Nowell (1962), Kiossoglou *et al.* (1965a), Sandberg *et al.* (1968), Whang-Peng *et al.* (1970), and Fitzgerald and Hamer (1976). Of the 328 cases, 141 (43%) were aneuploid and 19 of the 31 cases in whom a detailed analysis was reported had both normal and abnormal karyotypes. In two of the studies, aneuploidy was shown to have little effect on survival: Fitzgerald and Hamer reported a mean survival of 6.8 ($\pm1.7$) months in the aneuploid group versus a survival of 7.4 ($\pm1.9$) months in those patients with normal karyotypes; our results (Whang-Peng *et al.*, 1970) showed median survivals of 9 and 10 months in the two groups, respectively. Age appears to be more of a determining factor in survival. In Fitzgerald and Hamer's study, patients over the age of 50 had survivals of 8–9 months in contrast to median survivals of only 4 months in the younger group, regardless of the karyotype. Evidence for an association between chromosomal abnormalities and malignant transformation were presented by Reisman *et al.* (1964b). These authors performed serial cytogenetic studies on 13 aneuploid patients with acute stem cell or granulocytic leukemia and found that aneuploid lines which were consistently seen during active stages of the leukemia disappeared or were suppressed during remission; on subsequent relapse, the same or a closely related line frequently reappeared.

### 11.3.1.5. Chromosome Banding Studies in AML

In 1976, two large series of chromosome studies with banding results were published, one by Rowley and Potter, the other by Mitelman *et al.*; a summary of their combined data is shown in Table I. Of the 52 cases, 58.2% were aneuploid. This is higher than the percentage of aneuploidy seen in studies done with conventional stains and demonstrates the improved sensitivity afforded by the banding techniques in detecting minor abnormalities. Both normal and abnormal metaphases were seen in 14 (48.3%) of the 29 aneuploid cases and hyperdiploidy was the most

**Table I.**   Results from Banding Studies in AML

| Reference | Total | N[a] | A + N | A | Hypo | Pseudo | Hyper | ? |
|---|---|---|---|---|---|---|---|---|
| | | | A[a] | | | A | | |
| Rowley and Potter, 1976 | 22 | 10 | 7 | 5 | 5 | 3 | 3 | 1 |
| Mitelman *et al.*, 1976 | 30 | 13 | 7 | 10 | 3 | 3 | 11 | 0 |
| Total | 53 | 23 | 14 | 15 | 8 | 6 | 14 | 1 |
| | | 41.8% | 58.2% | | | | | |

[a]N, normal karyotype; A, aneuploidy.

common form of aneuploidy. In another paper, Rowley (1976b) correlated her banding studies with survival in AML: 87% of the patients with a
normal karyotype achieved a complete remission and had a median
survival of 18 months; this was in comparison to a remission rate of only
20% and a median survival of 2 months in those patients with abnormal
karyotypes.

The selected data in Table II are drawn from banding studies in 69
patients from 17 different papers (Rowley and Potter, 1976; Kaufman *et
al.*, 1974; Yamada and Furnsawa, 1976; Engel *et al.*, 1975; Rutten *et al.*,
1974; Mitelman *et al.*, 1976; Kohn *et al.*, 1975; Littefield, 1976; Lampert

**Table II.**   Detailed Banding Data in 69 Patients with AML

| Chromosome involved | Specific findings | Number of cases | Total |
|---|---|---|---|
| 8 | +8 | 18 | 28 |
| | + 8 and others | 2 | |
| | t(8;21)(q22;q22) | 8 | |
| 7 | −7 | 10 | 11 |
| | del(7)(q22) | 1 | |
| 9 | +9 | 5 | 12 |
| | −9 | 3 | |
| | t(6;9)(q23;q34) | 2 | |
| | t(4;9)(p16;q22) | 1 | |
| | t(9;10)(q34;q22) or (q22; q11) | 1 | |
| 21 | +21 | 5 | 11 |
| | −21 | 6 | |
| 17 | Iso 17q | 2 | 4 |
| | −17 | 2 | |
| X | −X | 4 | 4 |
| Y | −Y | 5 | 5 |

*et al.*, 1972; Sakurai *et al.*, 1974; Jonasson *et al.*, 1974; de la Chapelle *et al.*, 1971; van den Berghe, 1976; Philip, 1975b; Pan, 1976; Berger *et al.*, 1973; Oshimura *et al.*, 1976); the table summarizes the specific chromosomal abnormalities most frequently observed in AML. Chromosome #8 was by far the most commonly involved in aneuploidy: 20 cases demonstrated trisomy 8, and in eight additional cases there was a translocation of the #8 chromosome, t(8;21)(q22;q22). Monosomy 7 was the next most common abnormality, followed by abnormalities of chromosomes #9, #21, X, Y, and #17.

A missing Y chromosome has been frequently noted in both Ph[1] positive and negative CML but rarely in ALL (only one of our 332 ALL patients had a missing Y chromosome; Whang-Peng *et al.*, 1976a). It has been suggested that abnormalities of the myeloid series may contribute to premature aging of the bone marrow cells. In order to determine the frequency of a missing Y in AML, Sakurai and Sandberg (1976c) studied the marrows of 73 male AML patients. A missing Y chromosome was found in eight patients: in six patients the cells with a missing Y had additional chromosomal abnormalities but in the remaining two patients, both of whom were over 70 years of age, the cells had a 45,X karyotype. It was felt that these cells were not involved in the leukemic process. The increased involvement of a missing Y in myeloid leukemias may be due to the difference in age distribution between ALL and the myeloid leukemias, but three of the patients in Sakurai and Sandberg's study were under 60 years of age and a missing Y is not commonly found in control groups of similar ages.

## 11.3.1.6. The 45 Chromosome Syndrome

The term "45 chromosome syndrome" was first proposed by Freireich *et al.* (1964) and is characterized by a missing C group chromosome in patients with anemia or preleukemia whose disease terminates in AML or AMMoL. Freireich's three patients had refractory anemia of 1, 2, and 6 years duration, granulocytic hyperplasia of the bone marrow, low or absent leukocyte alkaline phosphatase, and a missing C group chromosome; the disease was at various times classified as preleukemia. Immature leukocytes resembling those found in CML were eventually seen in the peripheral blood and all three patients developed acute myelomonocytic leukemia. Teasdale *et al.* (1970) reported three similar cases, all children (aged 7 months, 1 year, and 13 years, respectively) with anemia, thrombocytopenia, increased myeloid elements in the bone marrow, and a missing C; all three patients died from acute myeloblastic leukemia. A seventh case, and the only one in whom banding studies were available, was described in 1974 by Macdougall *et al.;* the missing C in this case was identified as a #7 chromosome.

### 11.3.1.7. The Ph[1] in AML

The Ph[1] chromosome has been observed in nine patients with illnesses classified clinically as AML (Kiossoglou *et al.*, 1965b; Mastrangelo *et al.*, 1967; Hossfeld *et al.*, 1971; Whang-Peng *et al.*, 1970; Khan, 1972a) and their cytogenetic findings and clinical data are summarized in Table III; banding studies were not performed in any of these cases. The Ph[1] was the sole chromosomal abnormality in three patients, one of whom had two Ph[1] chromosomes. Only two of the nine patients were 100% Ph[1] positive; in the remaining seven patients the percentage of Ph[1] positive cells varied from 20 to 100%. Although there were two rather distinct age groups (three patients under the age of 10, and six patients over 40), there was no apparent relationship between age and chromosomal or clinical findings. There are several distinctive features in these patients which appear to set their disease apart from classical CML. The varying percentage of Ph[1] positive cells during the course of the disease, reflecting perhaps remission and relapse phases, and the high proportion of patients (7/9) with both Ph[1] positive and negative cells, are quite different from the findings in classical CML; in our 179 cases of CML (Whang-Peng *et al.*, 1968), only 5.6% were not 100% Ph[1] positive. A diagnosis of AML is also favored by the fact that the majority of these patients had a low to normal WBC, a normal to high LAP, and a short survival (the median survival was 5 months compared to a median of approximately 40 months in CML). The presence of hepatosplenomegaly and lymphadenopathy, which was observed in five of these patients, however, suggests a diagnosis of CML. Because it is currently impossible to separate completely this small group of patients from atypical CML presenting with blastic transformation, we (Whang-Peng *et al.*, 1970) have proposed that Ph[1] positive AML be reclassified as a rare manifestation of blastic crisis in CML.

### 11.3.1.8. Conclusion

Combining the cytogenetic results from studies with both conventional and banding techniques reveals that about 50% of all AML cases demonstrate some degree of aneuploidy, hypo- and hyperdiploidy being the most common forms. Approximately half of those patients exhibiting aneuploidy have both normal and abnormal cell lines, and the abnormal cells tend to disappear or be reduced in number during remission and to reappear on relapse. A normal karyotype is more conducive to achieving a complete remission than an abnormal one and chromosomes #8, #7, #9, #21, X, Y, and iso-17, listed in order of frequency, are the ones most commonly involved in aneuploidy. Although the myeloblast is the typical leukemic cell in this disease, there is cytogenetic evidence that the erythroid cells are also directly involved in the leukemic process.

**Table III.** Survival and Clinical Data in Nine AML Patients with the Ph[1] Chromosome

| Reference | Age/sex | Modal number chromosome | Number of Ph[1] chromosomes | % Ph[1] cells | Hgb (g/ 100 ml) | WBC X 10³ | LAP[a] | Initial size | | | Survival (months) |
|---|---|---|---|---|---|---|---|---|---|---|---|
| | | | | | | | | Liver | Spleen | LN[a] | |
| Kiossoglou *et al.*, 1965b | 65/F | 39–46 | 2 | 100 | 7.5 | 9.7 | — | 0 | 0 | 0 | 1 |
| Mastrangelo *et al.*, 1967 | 5/M | 46, 48 | 1 | 57–20, 88–22, 100 | 8.3 | 3.4 | — | +[a] | 2 cm | + | 21 |
| Hossfeld *et al.*, 1971 | 42/M | 46 | 1 | 80 | — | 100.0 | — | 0 | 0 | 0 | 6 |
| | 43/M | 46 | 1 | 100–80 | 9.5 | 430.0 | — | 4 cm | 12 cm | min. | 6 |
| Whang-Peng *et al.*, 1970 | 9/M | 46, 65–70 | 1 | 50–26, 100 | 7.5 | 10.3 | N | 3 cm | 3 cm | 0 | 24 |
| | 68/F | 46–49 | 1 | 100 | 13.1 | 17.0 | N | 0 | <1 cm | 0 | 3 |
| | 3/M | 46 | 1 | 83 | 10.1 | 5.1 | H[a] | 2 cm | 3 cm | ++[a] | 4+ |
| | 46/F | 46 (2 large D group) | 1 | 74–100 | 9.5 | 13.0 | H+[a] | 1 cm | 1 cm | 0 | 4+ |
| Khan, 1972a | 61/M | 44–53 (2 markers) | 1 | 21 | 8.1 | 3.7 | — | 0 | 0 | 0 | 5 |

[a]LAP, leukocyte alkaline phosphatase; LN, lymph node; N, normal; H, high; H+, very high; +, <2-cm enlargement in normal and lymph node areas; ++, 2–4-cm enlargement in normal lymph node-bearing sites.

## 11.3.2. Acute Myelomonocytic Leukemia

The primary difference between acute myelocytic leukemia and acute myelomonocytic leukemia (AMMoL) is the presence of atypical and/or increased numbers of abnormal monocytes. The demarcation between the two diseases is not clear and they are frequently treated as one disease, with AMMoL considered as an atypical variant of AML. There are, therefore, few reports of cytogenetic studies of patients identified strictly as AMMoL.

### 11.3.2.1. Cytogenetic Studies

A total of 24 cases have been reported in which banding studies were not performed (Atkins and Goulian, 1965; Kiossoglou *et al.*, 1965a; Sakurai, 1970a; Pierre *et al.*, 1971). Of the eight cases reported by Kiossoglou, five had a normal karyotype, two cases had pseudodiploid lines, and one case was hyperdiploid. Extensive chromosomal abnormalities were seen in the one case reported by Atkins and Goulian and the seven cases of Pierre *et al.*: four to six chromosomes were either lost or gained and all chromosomal groups including the Y chromosome were involved in aneuploidy; 1–11 microchromosomes were seen in Pierre's cases, some of whom also had ring chromosomes (three cases) and/or one to two submetacentric markers (two cases). Sakurai observed aneuploidy in five of his eight cases of AMMoL: two had hypodiploidy, two had hyperdiploidy, and one had both hypo- and hyperdiploid cell lines; four, and possibly five, of these cases had abnormalities involving the G group chromosomes.

The 13 cases (Rowley and Potter, 1976; Whang-Peng *et al.*, 1977; Bourgeois and Hill, 1977; Brandt *et al.*, 1974) in whom banding studies were done are listed in Table IV. Five cases had abnormalities involving more than three chromosomes and one case had very complex abnormalities. A missing Y chromosome was noted in two males, aged 61 and 58. The limited data available indicate that no specific chromosome abnormality is associated with this disease with the possible exception of the microchromosomes reported by Pierre *et al.* (1971). Of the nine cases in whom they observed microchromosomes, which they defined as very small chromatin structures with no clear centromeric site (sometimes referred to as minute chromosomes), seven had myelomonocytic leukemia, one had a preleukemic syndrome which subsequently evolved into acute leukemia, and one case was believed to be in a preleukemic phase of myelomonocytic leukemia. Microchromosomes have been occasionally observed in tumors, such as neuroblastoma, medulloblastoma, bronchogenic carcinoma, and metastatic carcinoma (Cox *et al.*, 1965; Levan *et al.*, 1968; Lubs *et al.*, 1966; Martineau, 1966; Spriggs *et al.*, 1962), in ALL

**Table IV.**  Banding Studies in Acute Myelomonocytic Leukemia

| Reference | Case number | Age/sex | Specific findings |
| --- | --- | --- | --- |
| Rowley and Potter, 1976 | 1 | 26/M | 46XY,t(1;9)(p34?;q34),inv(8)(p11q12) |
| | 2 | 40/F | 46,XX,ins(3;3)(q21;q21q26) |
| | 3 | 32/M | 46,XY,t(3;5)(q25;q33?) |
| | 4 | 32/F | 46,XX,t(?;11)(?;q23) |
| | 5 | 25/F | 45,X,t(8;17)(q22;q25) |
| | 6 | 61/M | 45,X |
| | 7 | 58/M | 45,X |
| | 8 | 21/M | 45,X,r(21) |
| | 9 | 68/F | 45,XXdel(2)(q31?)del(7)(p13),−13 |
| | 10 | 42/M | 42,XY,−7,i(8q),−16,−17,−18, t(21;21)(q12;q11),+mar,+1 to 2 frag/43,same karyotype + second i(8q) |
| Brandt *et al.*, 1974 | 11 | 57/M | 47,XY,+21 |
| Bourgeois and Hill, 1977 | 12 | 6/M | 46,XY,t(5;18) |
| Whang-Peng *et al.*, 1977 | 13 | 76/M | 46,XY,19p−q− 47,XY,+G or 47,XY,+C |

(Whang-Peng *et al.*, 1976a) and other leukemias (Crossen *et al.*, 1969; Todd *et al.*, 1969), and in the Sezary syndrome (Whang-Peng *et al.*, 1976b). Pierre considers them to be definite marker chromosomes which identify leukemic clones.

The incidence of polyploidy in the bone marrow was recently investigated by Borgstrom *et al.* (1976) who examined a consecutive series of 841 patients with various hematologic disorders; 11 of the patients were found to have at least 10% polyploidy. Of the 11 patients, three had acute myelomonocytic leukemia, with frequencies of 34, 63, and 95% of the metaphases, respectively. Increased polyploidy is apparently a rare phenomenon, even in leukemia, and was associated in these cases with a poor prognosis and short survival.

There is some evidence to suggest a relatively higher incidence of AMMoL, as opposed to other types of leukemia, in Fanconi's anemia. Bourgeois and Hill (1977) have reported such an association in a 6-year-old boy with a pseudodiploid cell line in the bone marrow. Of the six other reported cases (Bloom *et al.*, 1966; Dosik *et al.*, 1970; Gmyrek *et al.*, 1968; Silver *et al.*, 1952; Cowdell *et al.*, 1955) of leukemia in Fanconi's anemia, three were of the AMMoL type.

In a study of survival in 50 cases of acute nonlymphocytic leukemia in adults, Golomb *et al.* (1976) noted some differences between the AML (22 cases) and AMMoL (24 cases) groups. Although similar median survival times were obtained for the two diseases, the effect of aneuploidy was markedly different: no differences in median survivals were observed when the AMMoL patients were subgrouped according to the presence or absence of chromosomal abnormalities, whereas the AML patients, when so subgrouped, showed median survival times of 2 months in the aneuploid group versus 18 months in the normal group.

### 11.3.2.2. Conclusions

There is great variety in the cytogenetic findings in AMMoL, the high incidence of microchromosomes being found in one group contrasting sharply with the increased involvement of G group chromosomes reported in another group. This variety may be a reflection of the differences in cytologic interpretation of the bone marrow in this type of leukemia.

### 11.3.3. Acute Promyelocytic Leukemia

Acute promyelocytic leukemia (APL) is an unusual form of acute myeloid leukemia; cytogenetic studies have been published in only ten cases. Three of these cases (Sakurai, 1970a; Kiossoglou et al., 1965a; Obara et al., 1969) were karyotypically normal. Of the seven cases with aneuploidy, five or possibly six cases had abnormalities involving chromosome #17. Three patients were reported by Rowley: two of them (a 22-year-old female and a 25-year-old male) had a deletion of the long arm of #17, del(17)(q11q21) (Rowley and Potter, 1976) and the third had a 46,XY,ins(15;17) (q22?;q21),del(7)(q22),del(9)(q22) karyotype (Rowley et al., 1977). In letters to the editor, Okada et al. (1977) and Kaneko and Sakurai (1977) each reported a case of APL with two abnormal chromosomes in a majority of the bone marrow or peripheral blood cells which they interpreted as resulting from a reciprocal translocation, t(15;17)(q22;q21). In a case of APL in a 6-year-old girl, Engel et al. (1967) observed a partial deletion of the long arm of chromosome 17 or 18. The seventh aneuploid case was that of a 35-year-old male reported by Krogh Jensen (1967): 80% of the cells contained 44 chromosomes (none of which was analyzable) and 80% of the metaphases contained a small acro- or metacentric marker which was half the size of a G group chromosome. With such a small number of cases it is difficult to reach any conclusions as to the cytogenetic findings in this disease, but the involvement of chromosome 17 in aneuploidy in five, and possibly six, out of ten cases is certainly of interest. Translocations between chromosomes 15 and 17 have not been reported in any other types of leukemia, and despite the discrepancies among the cases the mechanism producing this abnormality may well be the same in all three cases. The relationship between these translocations and APL merits further exploration.

### 11.3.4. Chronic Myelocytic Leukemia

Chronic myelocytic leukemia (CML) is the only known malignancy with a specific chromosomal abnormality, the Philadelphia (Ph[1]) chromosome. Originally described in the peripheral blood of two patients by Nowell and Hungerford in 1960 as a G group chromosome with partially deleted long arms, it has since been shown to be present in the bone marrow of 85–90% of all CML patients (Nowell and Hungerford, 1961; Fitzgerald *et al.*, 1963a; Tough *et al.*, 1961; Sandberg *et al.*, 1962; Whang-Peng *et al.*, 1968).

#### 11.3.4.1. Characterization of the Ph[1]

The recently developed banding techniques have further characterized the Ph[1] chromosome, which was found to be a #22 chromosome. It was thought for many years that the genetic material deleted from this chromosome was lost to the cell. However, in 1973, Rowley (1973c), employing fluorescence and Giemsa banding techniques, proved that the deleted material had been translocated onto one of the #9 chromosomes, and was seen as additional dull fluorescing material at the end of the long arm of the #9; the amount of additional material was approximately equal to the amount deleted from the long arms of the Ph[1] chromosome (Fig. 1). More details became available shortly thereafter when we (Whang-Peng *et al.*, 1974a) demonstrated that the distal portion of the #22 is broken at the 12 band location (between bands 11 and 12); the resulting translocation can be abbreviated as t(9;22)(q34;q12) (Fig. 2). Additional Ph[1] chromosomes in the same cell do not result in further lengthening of the #9 chromosome. Pravtcheva and Manolov (1975) suggested that the long arm of the Ph[1] chromosome was longer than the band 22q11, and made two alternative proposals for the location of the break point and recombination position: (1) there is a reciprocal translocation between #9 and #22, with break points in the light band 9q34 and at the boundary between 22q11 and the terminal light segment of 9q34; or (2) an insertion of the 22q12 into the 9q34 results in a Ph[1] chromosome which includes 22q11 and q13. Neither of these two proposals has been widely accepted. On gross appearance, this translocation seems to be a balanced one but there are currently no known methods available which could detect mutation or deletion of only a few gene sequences.

#### 11.3.4.2. Nature of Ph[1] Translocations

All the initial studies on the translocation of the Ph[1] reported exclusive involvement of chromosomes 9 and 22. In the past few years, how-

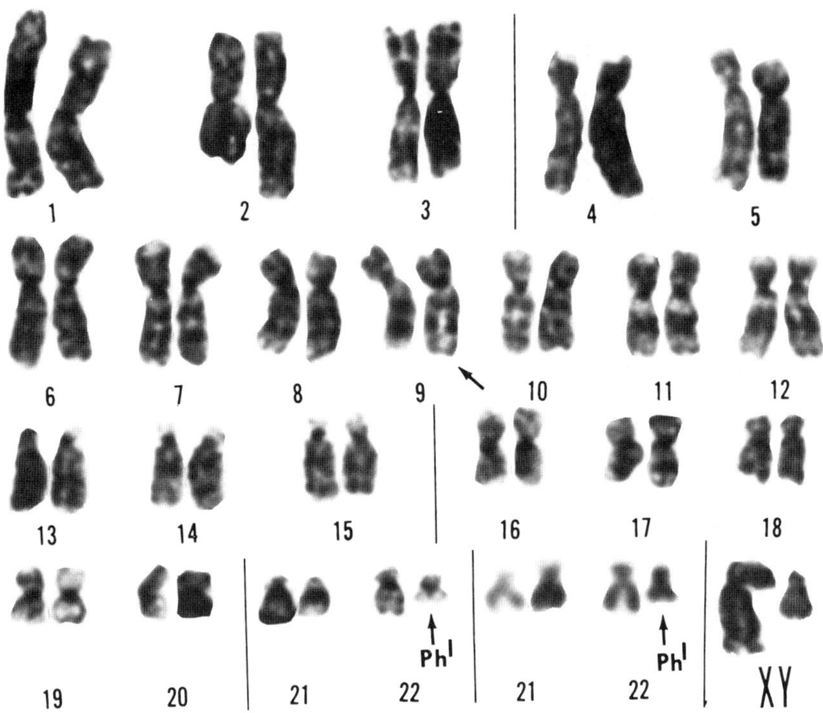

**Fig. 1.** Giemsa banding karyotype of a Ph[1] positive male cell with translocation t(9;22), including regular Giemsa-stained G group chromosomes.

ever, there have been an increasing number of examples in which the deleted portion of #22 was translocated to other chromosomes. Although it is now apparent that the mechanism producing the Ph[1] chromosome is not necessarily universal, Rowley (1976a) reported that 94% of her 440 cases of CML exhibited the now typical 9;22 translocation. In a very recent communication, Sonta and Sandberg (1977) summarized both the simple and complex translocations of the Ph[1] chromosome which have been reported in the literature. The simple translocations, including those reported in two other papers (Matsunaga *et al.*, 1976; Engel *et al.*, 1977), involve the chromosome arms: 2q, 6p, 9p, 9q, 11p, 12p, 13p, 14q, 16p, 17p, 17q, 19q, 21q, 22p, and 22q (Fig. 3); the translocation to the short arm of a #22 in one case and to the short arm of a #7 in another case resulted in the formation of a dicentric chromosome (Whang-Peng *et al.*, 1973,1976d) (Figs. 4 and 5). The complex translocations in CML (i.e., translocations in addition to those involving the deleted portion of the Ph[1]) involved the following chromosomes in each particular case: #3,9;

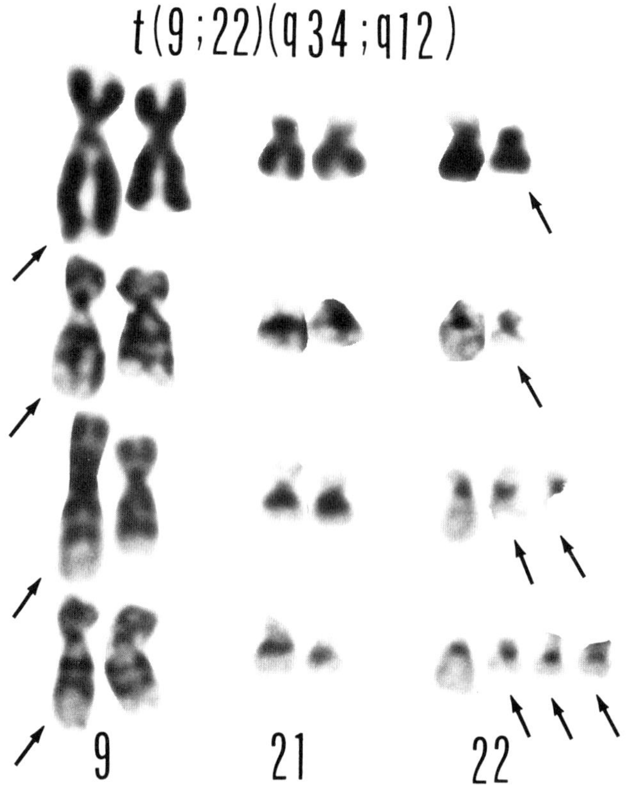



**Fig. 2.**  Partial karyotypes from regular Giemsa and trypsin banding with one, two, and three Ph[1] chromosomes from four cells showing the translocation t(9;22)(q34;q12).

#4; #5,9; #9; #6,9; #10,9; #10,15,19,9; #13,9; #13,15,9; #14,9; #17,9; #21,22; and their own case, #9,22,17 (Nowell *et al.*, 1975; Horland *et al.*, 1976; Hayata *et al.*, 1975; Potter *et al.*, 1975; Hayata and Sasaki, 1976; Ishihara *et al.*, 1974). In Ph[1] negative CML, no additional material is noted on the #9 chromosome (Rowley, 1974) but other abnormalities can occur: both a translocation involving a #17 chromosome (Engel *et al.*, 1974) and a reciprocal translocation between chromosomes 3 and 22 (Pravtcheva *et al.*, 1976) have been reported.

### 11.3.4.3. Location of the Gene Regulating Myeloid Proliferation

In 1976, Fitzgerald observed an abnormally short #22 chromosome, which closely resembled the Ph[1], in a family free of any hematologic

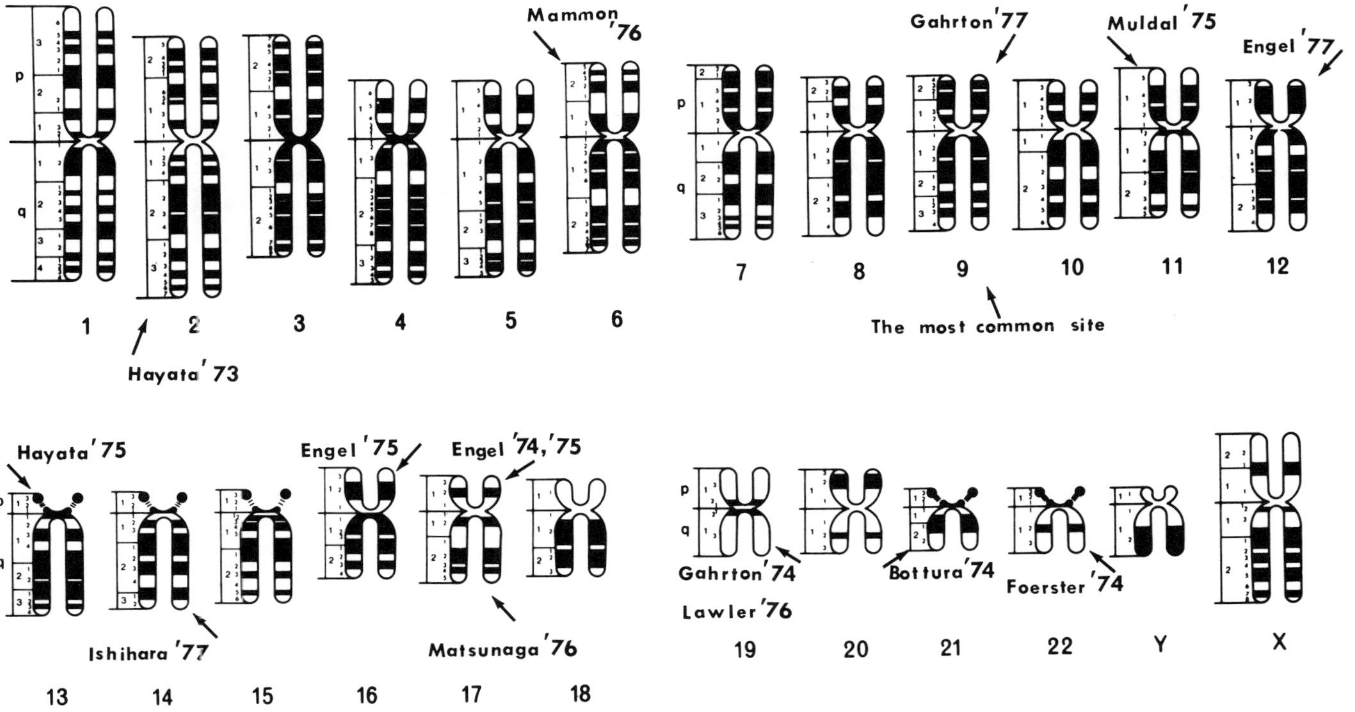


**Fig. 3.** Reported translocation sites for the deleted portion of the $Ph^1$ chromosome.

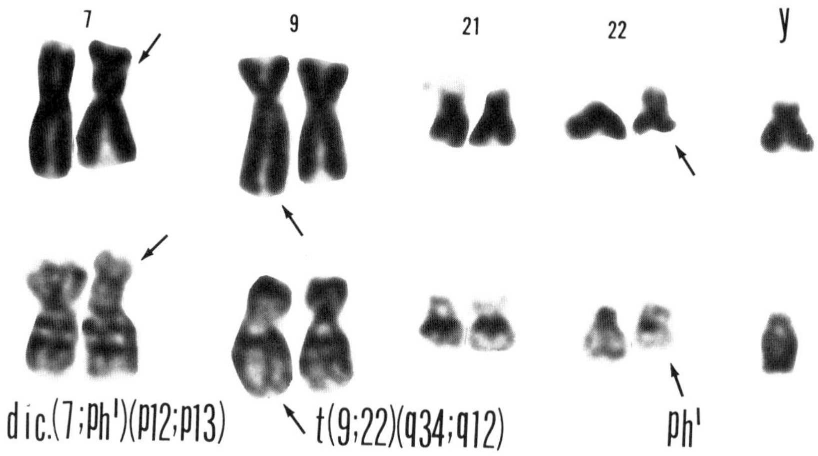


**Fig. 4.** Partial karyotype from regular Giemsa and trypsin banding showing dic(7;Ph¹)(p12;p13) and t(9;22)(q34;q12).

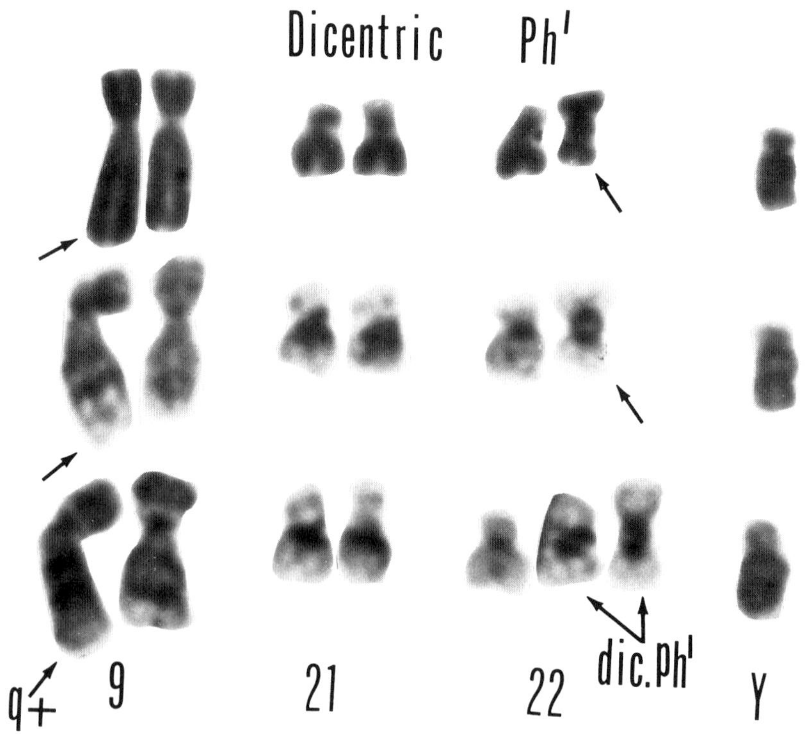


**Fig. 5.** Partial karyotype from regular Giemsa and trypsin banding showing dicentric Ph¹ chromosomes.

disorders. Giemsa banding demonstrated that this abnormal chromosome resulted from the translocation t(11;22)(q25;q13). The break point on the #22 was at the q12/q13 band interface compared with the Ph[1] chromosome break point at the q11/q12 band interface. He postulated that since this family showed no evidence of hematologic abnormalities, this case is an indication that the genes regulating myeloid proliferation are located in the 22q12 band.

### 11.3.4.4. Cellular Distribution of the Ph[1] Chromosome

The presence of the Ph[1] chromosome in the myeloid series has been well established; however, it has been demonstrated in other types of hematologic cells as well. Ultraviolet spectrophotometry (Whang *et al.*, 1963) and direct labeling of bone marrow cells *in vitro* with iron (Rastrick *et al.*, 1968) have shown that precursor cells possessing hemoglobulin contain the Ph[1] chromosome and its presence in polyploid cells strongly suggests occurrence in the megakaryocytic series. Golde *et al.* (1977) concluded that macrophages also contain the Ph[1] chromosome. These authors studied bone marrow cells from three patients cultured under conditions favoring macrophage proliferation and found Ph[1] positive metaphases at a time when 80% of the metaphases were identifiable macrophages.

In peripheral blood, the frequency of Ph[1] positive metaphases roughly corresponds to the percentage of circulating immature granulocytes. In 1-day unstimulated cultures of leukocytes from CML patients, when the dividing cells are immature granulocytes, there is a much higher percentage of Ph[1] positive metaphases compared to the number found in 3-day cultures stimulated with phytohemagglutinin, whose mitogenic properties activate division of the lymphocytic series. The lymphocyte does not appear to possess this chromosomal defect nor do tissues other than hematopoietic elements. Studies have failed to demonstrate the Ph[1] chromosome in skin cultures from CML patients. The existence of a precursor cell, common to the erythrocytic, myelocytic, megakaryocytic, and macrophage series, is supported by the observed distribution of the Ph[1] chromosome; it is also likely that this precursor cell is generally unrelated to the lymphoid series or to other tissues of the body.

### 11.3.4.5. Origin of the Ph[1]

Although, to date, it has not been possible to determine when the Ph[1] positive cell makes its first appearance, several factors point to a unicellular origin of CML. In those cases in which it has been possible to distinguish one #22 chromosome from the other, the Ph[1] chromosome has consistently been confined to only one or the other. This was demonstrated by Gahrton *et al.* (1974a) who used the satellite on the #22 to demonstrate that the Ph[1] chromosome was the maternal #22 in one case and the paternal #22 in a second case. In CML patients with cytogenetic mosaicism due to congenital abnormalities (Fitzgerald *et al.*, 1971; Moore *et al.*, 1974), the Ph[1] chromosome has been found in only one of the cell lines, and in a female CML patient the 9q+;22q− translocation was consistently seen only in the #9 which had an unusually long secondary constriction (Hossfeld, 1975). Studies of CML in identical twins (Dougan *et al.*, 1966; Goh and Swisher, 1965), in which only the affected twins are found to be Ph[1] positive, also prove that the Ph[1] chromosome is an acquired abnormality.

It is assumed that the Ph[1] chromosome arises in bone marrow cells and that the karyotypic evolution which heralds blastic transformation also occurs in this organ. There is some evidence, however, which implicates a primary role for the spleen. Armenta *et al.* (1976) reported a case of polycythemia vera of 10 years duration which evolved into CML. Cytogenetic studies of the bone marrow 4 years prior to and after the development of CML showed a normal karyotype; the Ph[1] chromosome was, however, seen in the splenic tissue when the CML was diagnosed. It later appeared in cervical lymph nodes as well. Several studies (Hossfeld and Schmidt, 1973; Gomez *et al.*, 1975; Mitelman *et al.*, 1974) employing serial chromosomal analysis of both bone marrow and spleen have established other instances in which the karyotypic evolution first appeared in the spleen.

### 11.3.4.6. The Significance of the Ph[1] Chromosome

In patients with obvious hematologic disorders, the presence of the Ph[1] chromosome is virtually diagnostic of CML. Its presence in asymptomatic individuals who show no evidence of CML, however, can be indicative of the preleukemic state. A representative case was reported by us in 1972 (Canellos and Whang-Peng, 1972): for 5 years prior to the development of a leukemic phase, the patient had harbored the Ph[1] chromosome in marrow cells but had no significant hematologic changes. A similar case with 100% Ph[1] positive cells in the bone marrow was reported by Baccarani *et al.* (1973).

### 11.3.4.7. The Ph[1] and Age

CML in infants or in young children differs in some clinical and hematologic aspects from the disease seen in older children and adults, and is termed the juvenile type of CML. The high percentage of Ph[1] positive cases seen in CML patients overall drops considerably when patients over the age of 60 or below the age of 10 are examined; in these groups, Ph[1] negative CML predominates. The youngest patients reported to be Ph[1] positive were 1, 5½, 7, and 9 years old at the time of diagnosis (Saffhill *et al.*, 1976; Reisman and Trujillo, 1963; Hardisty *et al.*, 1964; Whang-Peng *et al.*, 1968).

### 11.3.4.8. Presence of the Ph[1] Chromosome in Diseases Other than CML

In a recent report, Forman *et al.* (1977) presented two children with Ph[1] positive leukemia, confirmed by Giemsa banding as 22q−. These children had blast cells possessing both lymphoid and myeloid characteristics as demonstrated by determinations for histochemical, biochemical, or cell surface receptors. These authors suggested that Ph[1] positive childhood leukemia may represent a complex biological stem cell relationship, and that further investigations of such patients should include comprehensive studies of their cytogenetic, histochemical, and enzymatic properties, surface receptor sites, and *in vitro* maturation. Tests for the presence of terminal deoxynucleotidyl transferase have already yielded interesting findings. This enzyme is thought to be specific for thymic or prethymic lymphocytes and the elevated levels found in ALL are to be expected. Surprisingly, however, McCaffrey *et al.* (1975) found comparably elevated levels in one of four CML cases undergoing blastic transformation, and Saffhill *et al.* (1976) reported similar results in a case of Ph[1] positive CML in the chronic stage in an infant. Either the leukemic cells in these cases represent primitive cell lines, a phenomenon not unknown in malignant cells, possessing elevated levels of this enzyme, or the enzyme is not specific for pre-T cells and thymocytes but is elevated in the undifferentiated cells of certain disease states.

Despite the fact that the Ph[1] chromosome is almost pathognomonic for CML, it has been reported in other diseases as well. In cases like the two reports (Ricci *et al.*, 1970; Weiner, 1965) involving the familial transmission of a Ph[1]-like chromosome (Gq−), banding studies are required to differentiate the true Ph[1] from other deletions of the G group (Fitzgerald, 1976).

Ph[1] chromosomes have also been reported in acute leukemias and are discussed in greater detail in those sections. Radiation or drug exposure may play a role in the development of the Ph[1]: one case discussed earlier had a history of radiation exposure, and a radiologist who developed ALL (Propp and Lizzi, 1970) had some Ph[1] positive cells in his marrow; Ph[1] chromosomes have also been found in a patient with acute leukemia who had previously been an LSD user (Irwin and Egozcue, 1967). Unfortunately, banding studies were unavailable in all these cases.

### 11.3.4.9. Clinical Aspects of the Ph[1] Chromosome

There appears to be a definite relationship between chromosomal abnormalities and the course of the disease in CML. In one of our reports on CML (Whang-Peng *et al.*, 1968) the patients were divided into two major chromosomal groups: (1) Ph[1] negative and (2) Ph[1] positive; both groups contained patients with or without additional aneuploidy. The Ph[1] negative patients, including even those with normal karyotypes, had the poorest prognosis, with a median survival of 12 months compared to a median survival of 40 months in the Ph[1] positive groups.

A high incidence of chromosomal abnormalities has been observed prior to, or during, blastic crisis in CML by many investigators (Kemp *et al.*, 1964; Sandberg *et al.*, 1971). The development of these abnormalities, which are in addition to the Ph[1], can precede the identification of definite hematologic change (Krompotic *et al.*, 1968) and can therefore be useful in predicting the blastic phase. Specifically, duplication of the Ph[1] chromosome seems to be associated with a higher incidence of leukemic infiltration of the lymph nodes (Duvall *et al.*, 1967). Hyperdiploidy and a high degree of G group involvement, usually a duplication of the Ph[1] chromosome, were the most common forms of abnormalities observed in a series of CML patients studied prior to or during blast crisis (J. Whang-Peng, unpublished data). Duplication of the Ph[1] has also been reported by several other investigators (Engel and McKee, 1966; Kiossoglou *et al.*, 1966a; Kamada and Uchino, 1967) and even three Ph[1] chromosomes have been observed on rare occasions (Fig. 2) (Whang-Peng *et al.*, 1971). Abnormalities of the C group are second only to the G group in frequency and the new staining techniques have made possible the identification of the specific pairs involved, such as #8 (Hsu *et al.*, 1974; Rowley, 1973c), #9 (Davidson and Knight, 1973; Rutten *et al.*, 1974; Rowley, 1973b), #10 (Beck and Chesney , 1973), #11 (Philip, 1975a), and #7,12 (Kaffe *et al.*, 1974). In hematologic diseases, especially CML and polycythemia vera, trisomy #8 and trisomy #9 are the most common acquired abnormalities of the C group. A missing Y chromosome, reported in at least 30 cases of CML (Hossfeld and Wendehorst, 1974; Shiffman *et al.*, 1974), about one-third of whom were close to or over 60 years of age, appears to have no effect on prognosis. It has also been reported in the bone marrow and peripheral blood of normal males by several groups (Pierre and Hoagland, 1971; Jacobs *et al.*, 1964) and it has been suggested that it is associated with premature aging of the bone marrow.

### 11.3.4.10. Conclusion

Once observed, the Ph[1] chromosome rarely disappears from the bone marrow, even during remission; it is not seen in the blood, however, when there are no immature cells in the peripheral circulation. Other chromosomal abnormalities occasionally disappear when remission is achieved following intensive chemotherapy (Canellos *et al.*, 1971). This behavior of the Ph[1] chromosome contrasts sharply with the findings in acute leukemia where aneuploidy, present in 40–50% of the cases, can occasionally revert to a completely normal karyology during remission. The disappearance of the Ph[1] has been reported in only three cases, two of which were studied by Clarkson *et al.* (1974); it was achieved only after intensive chemo- and radiotherapy and was only of a transitory nature.

The presence or absence of a demonstrable translocation of the deleted portion of the Ph[1] chromosome has no observable bearing on the clinical course or hematologic pattern in CML (Gahrton *et al.*, 1974b) but the late appearance of other chromosomal abnormalities indicates the emergence of blastic transformation, a highly malignant and aggressive terminal phase of the disease.

## 11.3.5. Hypereosinophilic Syndrome (Eosinophilic Leukemia)

### 11.3.5.1. Disease Definition and Criteria

The criteria used to define the hypereosinophilic syndrome are variable. Several authors (Hardy and Anderson, 1968; Benvenisti and Ultmann, 1969; Chusid *et al.*, 1975) have written extensive reviews on the subject. Some authors prefer to include only those cases which can definitely be described as eosinophilic leukemia, whereas others include a wide spectrum of disorders which have been variously diagnosed as eosinophilic leukemia (Benvenisti and Ultmann, 1969), disseminated eosinophilic collagen disease (Odeberg, 1965), and Loeffler's fibroplastic endocarditis with eosinophilia (Brink and Weber, 1963). Eosinophilia is frequently seen in CML, and some authors (Kauer and Engle, 1964; Gruenwald *et al.*, 1965; Chusid *et al.*, 1975) have suggested that the hypereosinophilic syndrome is actually a variant of CML; others (Goh *et al.*, 1965), however, disagree and believe it to be a separate disease entity. It can also sometimes be difficult to distinguish from some nonhematologic disorders which can cause secondary eosinophilia such as parasitic infestations, and collagen and hypersensitivity diseases (Benvenisti and Ultmann, 1969).

Basically, the disease is characterized by persistent hypereosinophilia of the peripheral blood, associated with diffuse organ infiltration by eosinophils, progressive heart failure, respiratory distress, central nervous system abnormalities, and fever. It is frequently refractory to treatment and the prognosis is generally poor.

### 11.3.5.2. Cytogenetic Findings in Nonbanding Studies

In the few cytogenetic reports published, three cases have been Ph[1] positive (Kauer and Engle, 1964; Gruenwald *et al.*, 1965; Chusid *et al.*, 1975). In the case reported by Gruenwald, the Ph[1] was present in 88–91% of the bone marrow cells, and 51% of the cells had a 47,+C karyotype. Cytogenetic studies in 13 of the 14 cases studied by Chusid *et al.* (1975) showed one patient with a Ph[1] chromosome in 100% of his bone marrow cells, two patients with missing C group chromosomes, and three patients with unspecified aneuploidy. In none of these cases were banding studies performed.

Goh *et al.* (1965) reported a very large acrocentric chromosome in 10 and 20%, respectively, of the analyzed metaphases in two patients, one with a definite and one with a probable diagnosis of eosinophilic leukemia.

A case of probable chronic eosinophilic leukemia of 12 years duration was reported by Lisker *et al.* (1973). Serial cytogenetic studies performed over a 4-year period demonstrated a normal bone marrow (BM) karyotype at first presentation; 2 years later she had a 46,XX,Dq+ karyotype in three of the eight cells analyzed, and 2 years after that, at which time Myleran treatment was instituted, the same abnormality was present in all five BM cells analyzed. The patient was still alive 1 year after the last chromosome study.

### 11.3.5.3. Banding Studies

In a case report by Mitelman *et al.* (1975) banding studies revealed a chromosomal abnormality, an isochromosome 17, i(17q), in all bone marrow cells. The authors felt that this was not an atypical case of CML but rather a true eosinophilic leukemia. The cytogenetic findings offer evidence that this type of leukemia also has a clonal origin. The isochromosome was found to be present in all metaphases on two separate occasions: in the first BM 94% of the cells were neutrophilic and 2% were eosinophils, and in the second sample, 75% of the cells were eosinophils and only 25% were neutrophilic cells. Obviously, both cell types were of leukemic origin.

In a study of the morphologic composition of the eosinophilic series in the bone marrow in 10 cases of reactive eosinophilia (RE) and two cases of eosinophilic leukemia (EL), Brandt *et al.* (1977) found a distinct difference between the two types of patients: a more pronounced maturation of the eosinophilic series was observed in the RE patients compared to defective differentiation of the eosinophilic bone marrow cells in EL patients. Cytogenetic studies were performed only in the EL patients, one of whom had been reported previously by Mitelman *et al.*, 1975 (see preceding paragraph); the other had an extra C group chromosome in his peripheral blood metaphases.

The high incidence of chromosomal aneuploidy and evidence of a selective process favoring the replacement of normal cells with abnormal ones indicate that the hypereosinophilic syndrome is truly a neoplastic disease. The presence of the Ph[1] chromosome in some cases suggests that it is a variant of CML but this viewpoint is far from being generally accepted.

## 11.3.6. Erythroleukemia

### 11.3.6.1. Introduction

Cytogenetic studies of acute erythroleukemia (DiGuglielmo's disease, erythremic myelosis) have been combined in this section. These terms are frequently applied interchangeably, owing in part to the variable morphologic picture presented. Generally, DiGuglielmo's disease and erythremic myelosis are used when the erythroid series predominates in the leukemic process; the term erythroleukemia (EL), on the other hand, indicates involvement of both myeloid and erythroid precursors. Occasionally, these diseases are considered to be variants of AML. Chromosome studies in these diseases have been few in number and the quantity of banding results is especially limited. There appears to be a high incidence of aneuploidy and no specific abnormal patterns with the possible exception of increased occurrences of isochromosome 17 (see Table V), a long acrocentric marker (Castoldi *et al.*, 1968; Heath *et al.*, 1969; Kroll and Schlesinger, 1970), and a small F chromosome. The small F chromosome

**Table V.**    Detailed Chromosome Banding in Nine Cases of Erythroleukemia

| Reference | Age/sex | Specific findings |
|---|---|---|
| Petit *et al.*, 1973 | 4½/M | 45,XY,−7 |
| Macdougall *et al.*, 1974 | 8 mo/F | 45,XX,−7   (preleukemia to EL) |
| Yamada and Furnsawa, 1976 | 38/M | 44,XY,−3,−18 |
| | 41/F | 45,XX,−18 |
| | 40/M | 49,XY,+8,+12,+17,t(17;21)(p11;q22) |
| | 36/M | 47,XY,+8 |
| | 72/M | 45,XY,del(4)(q23?),del(5)(q13?),−6,del(6)(q21), del7(p14),del(8)(p21),del(9)(q31),16q+  (55%) |
| | | Same karyotype except −4+mar          (35%) |
| Najfeld, 1976 | 57/F | Major clone: 47,XX,−5,i(17q),−19,+3mar |
| Whang-Peng *et al.*, 1977 | 50/F | 46,XX,19p−q−,11q+ |
| | | 47,XX,19p−q−,+21 |

has been reported in several types of abnormal erythropoiesis, such as idiopathic sideroblastic anemia (DeGrouchy *et al.*, 1966), DiGuglielmo's syndrome (Hossfeld *et al.*, 1972; Whang-Peng *et al.*, 1977), polycythemia vera (Hossfeld *et al.*, 1972; Reeves *et al.*, 1972; Visfeldt, 1971; Wurster-Hill *et al.*, 1976), erythroleukemia (Whang-Peng *et al.*, 1977) (Fig. 6), and in a case of AML which had been preceded for 1 year by erythroid hyperplasia (Whang-Peng *et al.*, 1977) (Fig. 7).

### 11.3.6.2. Cytogenetic Studies

Eighty-four cases were reported from 1961 to 1976 and were analyzed only by use of the conventional Giemsa stain: results from these 84 cases up to 1967 were reviewed in three of the larger studies (Kiossoglou *et al.*, 1965a; Castoldi *et al.*, 1968; Heath *et al.*, 1969); the remainder, except for nine cases by Sakurai and Sandberg (1976a), were case reports of one to two individuals (Krogh Jensen, 1967; Dyment *et al.*, 1968; Crossen *et al.*, 1969; Khan and Martin, 1970; Kroll and Schlesinger, 1970; Hossfeld *et al.*, 1972; Krogh Jensen and Killmann, 1971; Inoue *et al.*, 1975; Lawler *et al.*, 1975; Golomb *et al.*, 1976). Aneuploidy was seen in 75% of the cases, hypodiploidy (37%) being the most common form, followed by hyperdiploidy (17%) and pseudodiploidy (7%); 20% had a high incidence of polyploidy and 28% had increased minor and/or major chromosomal aberrations such as breaks, fragments, minutes, and ring or dicentric chromosomes. Marker chromosomes included several instances

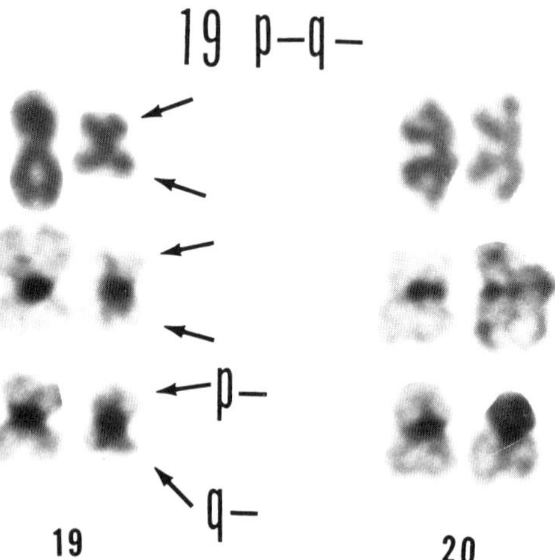


**Fig. 6.** Partial karyotype from regular Giemsa and trypsin banding from two patients, one with erythroleukemia and one with AMMoL, showing 19p-q-.

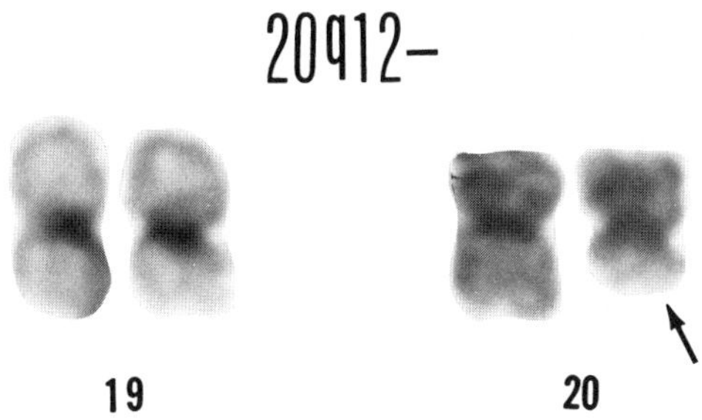


**Fig. 7.** Partial karyotype from trypsin Giemsa banding from a patient with AML showing 20q12−.

of large acrocentrics and two reports of Ph¹-like chromosomes. Table V includes the 10 cases studied from 1974 to 1976 on whom banding analyses were performed; the chromosomes most often involved in aneuploidy appear to be those of the C, D, E, and F groups, especially chromosomes #7, #8, #17, #18, and #19.

### 11.3.6.3. Discussion

Sakurai and Sandberg (1976b) reported the relationship between major karyotypic abnormalities (MAKA) and erythroleukemia (EL). They noted that 15 of the 30 patients with MAKA in their study had a diagnosis of EL or probable EL. The remaining cases had refractory anemia, AML, monocytic leukemia, stem cell leukemia, acute leukemia, or myeloproliferative disease. The MAKA in the 15 EL patients were characterized by hypodiploidy, karyotypic instability, and polyploidy in leukemic cells; "the extent of the polyploidy appeared to be correlated with the proportion of erythroid precursors in the marrow and with karyotypic instability." They also noted a decreased survival in their patients with MAKA: they died within 1 month of study compared to survivals of 4.8 and 9.1 months in the groups without MAKA.

In their study of two children with EL, Inoue *et al.* (1975) suggested that the increased erythropoiesis represents a response to unknown stimuli rather than an involvement in the malignant process. This idea was based on their observation that aneuploidy was minimal or absent during the erythroid phase whereas a high percentage of aneuploidy was found during the myeloblastic stage of the disease.

Erythroleukemia is currently thought to be one of the myeloproliferative diseases and is characterized by varying degrees of ineffective erythropoiesis, megaloblastic erythroid hyperplasia, and the presence in the bone marrow of multinucleated red cell precursors and bizarre mitotic figures; the clinical features range from those of AGL to erythroleukemia. Cytogenetically, this disease shows a high degree of aneuploidy, and increased polyploidy and chromosomal breakage; chromosomes #7, #8, #17, #18, and #19 appear to be especially involved in abnormalities.

### 11.3.7. Polycythemia Vera

Polycythemia vera (PV) is a chronic myeloproliferative disorder with an insidious onset. It is characterized by excessive proliferation of the erythrocytic elements and, usually, by abnormal myeloid and megakaryocytic elements as well. A number of PV patients eventually develop leukemia, regardless of treatment. Some consider leukemia to be part of the natural course of the disease while others consider leukemia in PV to be primarily the results of treatment. The interrelationship of PV, myeloid metaplasia, and leukemia is complex and has been under discussion for many years (Modan, 1975). It is hoped that cytogenetic studies may help to differentiate and more clearly define each of these disease entities.

### 11.3.7.1. Cytogenetic Studies

A combined total of 239 untreated cases of PV were reported in five recently published papers (Lawler *et al.*, 1970; Shiraishi *et al.*, 1975; Wurster-Hill *et al.*, 1976; Westin *et al.*, 1976; Zech *et al.*, 1976). Aneuploidy was observed in 53 (22.2%) of the 239 cases. In contrast, aneuploidy was seen in 42 (67.7%) of the 62 treated ($^{32}$P and/or chemotherapy) patients. This increase appears to be the result of treatment but it could be due to a more severe form of the disease in the treated group.

A small F group chromosome has frequently been reported in PV and also in idiopathic sideroblastic anemia. Reeves *et al.* (1972) reported abnormal F group chromosomes in four cases of PV; banding studies showed it to be a 20q− chromosome in each case (possibly a 20q12− chromosome). All four of these patients had been irradiated and two of them also had other structural chromosomal rearrangements. A study of 66 patients by Millard *et al.* (1968) revealed a deleted F chromosome in seven cases (10.6%); the deleted F was seen in 22–100% of the bone marrow metaphases. Six of the seven patients had received $^{32}$P treatment, and one patient had received only busulfan. Two cases with the abnormal F developed leukemia and both of them had additional chromosomal abnormalities of the C group (a C deletion in one patient and an extra C in the other). Although radiation-induced abnormalities were seen in the blood cultures from most of these patients, almost all of the peripheral blood metaphases had normal F group chromosomes. A follow-up study was done by Lawler *et al.* (1970), in which 13 new cases were added, making a total of 79 cases. These authors found a deleted F group chromosome in three patients who had had normal karyotypes when they were first included in the series. This brings the number of patients with the deleted F to 10 out of a total of 79 patients studied, or 12.6%. Nine of the 10 patients with the deleted F chromosome had received $^{32}$P treatment; the one exception was treated only with busulfan. In the three patients with normal karyotypes initially, the interval between the first dose of $^{32}$P or irradiation and the appearance of the deleted F ranged from 28 to 35 months; no cytogenetic studies were done in the intervening periods, however. The frequency of cells with a small F tended to increase with time except in the case that had been treated with busulfan only, where the percentage dropped from 100 to 50%. None of the three new cases in this report had developed leukemia.

Visfeldt (1971) studied 50 patients with primary polycythemia; abnormal clone formation was found in 21 patients, all of whom had been treated ($^{32}$P treatment in 20 cases, and Myleran with splenic irradiation in one case). Eight of the 21 patients (16%) had a small F. Of the eight patients who died of leukemia, five had abnormal clones showing the following karyotypes: 46,XY,−B,+16; 46,XY,F?−; 46,XX,1?+,−B, −C,−C,+16,+16,+16; 46,XX,−2,+3,Bq+; 45,XY,−3,ring C.

### 11.3.7.2. Chromosome Banding Studies

The results of chromosome banding in 35 patients were compiled from nine different papers (Shiraishi *et al.*, 1975; Wurster-Hill *et al.*, 1976; Westin *et al.*, 1976; Westin, 1976; Zech *et al.*, 1976; Tsuchimoto *et al.*, 1974; Hsu *et al.*, 1974; Rowley, 1973a,b). The involvement of each specific chromosome in aneuploidy, with the number of times it has been observed in parentheses, is as follows: #1 (5), #7q− (2), #8 (7), #9 (14), #10 (1), #11 (2), #12 (3), #13 (2), #15 (1), #16 (3), #17 (3), #18 (1), #20q− (7), #20 (1), #21 (1), #22 (2), and Y (4). As can be seen, the chromosomes most commonly involved in abnormalities are the #9, #8, #20q−, #1, and the Y, listed in descending order of frequency.

### 11.3.7.3. Nonspecific Aberrations and Effect of Treatment

Frequent aneuploidy associated with a multitude of nonspecific chromosomal aberrations, such as breaks, fragments, and abnormal chromosomes, has been reported in untreated PV patients (Lawler *et al.*, 1970; Wurster-Hill *et al.*, 1976; Visfeldt, 1971; Zech *et al.*, 1976; Modan *et al.*, 1970). In a study of 50 (unselected) untreated PV patients, Westin *et al.* (1976) found abnormal clones in seven patients (all but one being hyperdiploid) ranging from 18 to 100% of the total cells studied; one patient had a deleted #20, del(20)(q11). Six other patients had one hyperdiploid cell each.

The chromosomal effect of $^{32}$P was reported in a study of 14 PV cases by MacDiarmid (1965) who analyzed metaphases from cultured peripheral blood before and after $^{32}$P administration. All patients demonstrated chromosomal aberrations after treatment, such as acentric fragments, discentric and ring chromosomes, and numerical abnormalities ranging from 2 to 22.5%. The level of aberrations was highest shortly after treatment and gradually diminished with time, probably due to death of the damaged cells.

The preexisting chromosomal instability in PV may greatly enhance the development of abnormalities after radiation. In a previous report we (Whang-Peng *et al.*, 1977) noted a small F chromosome in cases with abnormal erythropoiesis. It is possible that erythroid disease may have a predisposition to formation of the small F which is enhanced by irradiation (three of our five cases had had radiation therapy) and $^{32}$P. The small F chromosome (20q−) appears to be quite stable and sometimes can replace karyotypically normal cells without affecting the clinical course of the disease. In this aspect, the small F resembles the Ph[1] chromosome in CML.

Ph[1] positive CML has been reported in several cases of PV. Radiation has been known to induce CML (Gavosto *et al.*, 1965) and most of these PV patients had been treated with $^{32}$P (Hoppin and Lewis, 1975; Kemp *et al.*, 1964; Koulischer *et al.*, 1967; Brill *et al.*, 1962). However, CML has been known to occur in untreated PV (Nicoara *et al.*, 1967) and Nicoara proposed that Ph[1] positive PV is a transitory form between primary PV and CML.

## 11.3.8. Myelofibrosis with Myeloid Metaplasia

Myelofibrosis with myeloid metaplasia, a myeloproliferative disorder, is characterized by anemia, abnormal proliferation of hematopoietic precursors, varying degrees of fibrosis of the bone marrow, and extramedullary hematopoiesis in the liver, spleen, and other organs. The number of cytogenetic reports has been limited because of the difficulty in obtaining adequate quantities of dividing marrow cells due to the fibrotic nature of the bone marrow in this condition. However, these patients frequently have circulating immature cells in the peripheral blood which are capable of division without mitogenic stimulation and most results have come from chromosome studies of a 1- and 2-day peripheral blood cultures.

### 11.3.8.1. Cytogenetic Studies

A review of cytogenetic studies in 87 patients drawn from 18 different reports (Nowell and Hungerford, 1962; Sandberg *et al.*, 1962,1964;

Goh and Swisher, 1963; Better *et al.*, 1965; Kiossoglou *et al.*, 1966b; Forrester and Louro, 1966; Jackson and Higgins, 1967; Engel *et al.*, 1968; Mitus *et al.*, 1969; Van Slyck *et al.*, 1970; Sakurai, 1970b; Holden *et al.*, 1971; Woodliff *et al.*, 1975; Davidson and Knight, 1973; Moake *et al.*, 1974; Rowley, 1976c; Nowell *et al.*, 1976; Whang-Peng *et al.*, 1977) from 1962 to 1977 demonstrated that aneuploidy was present in 46 patients (53%). There was considerable individual diversity in the observed aneuploidy which involved every chromosome pair, including the sex chromosomes; no consistent findings could be discerned. When only the reports with banding data (see the last six references just cited) are considered, chromosomes #7 and #8 were most frequently involved in abnormalities, followed by chromosomes #1, #5, #11, #12, iso17q, #18, and a minute marker.

The chromosome results in myelofibrosis are very similar to those observed in leukemia in regard to both the particular chromosomes involved and their relative frequencies in abnormalities. This undoubtedly is a reflection of the relationship that exists between the leukemias and the various myeloproliferative disorders. An extra C group chromosome is one of the most common cytogenetic abnormalities in leukemia. Abnormality of the #7 chromosome has been reported in the 45 chromosome syndrome (Macdougall *et al.*, 1974), in erythroleukemia (Petit *et al.*, 1973), in a case which progressed from preleukemia to AML (Kaufman *et al.*, 1974), and in pancytopenia without leukemia (Rowley, 1973a). Trisomy 8 has been found in AML, AMMoL, CML, and PV (Rowley and Potter, 1976; Rowley, 1975; Hsu *et al.*, 1974).

Chromosome #1 abnormalities have been reported in several cases of myeloproliferative disorders and leukemia (Nowell *et al.*, 1976; Wurster-Hill *et al.*, 1976; Spriggs *et al.*, 1976). There have been very few reports of abnormalities of the B group (chromosomes #4 and #5) but a 5q− chromosome has been noted in aregenerative anemia (Sokal *et al.*, 1975) and in preleukemia terminating in AML (Rowley, 1976c). An isochromosome, iso-17q, has been reported in both myeloproliferative and lymphoproliferative diseases (Engel *et al.*, 1975; Lobb *et al.*, 1972; Mitelman *et al.*, 1975). Minute chromosomes have been described in AMMoL, Sezary syndrome, and ALL (Pierre *et al.*, 1971; Whang-Peng *et al.*, 1976a,b).


### 11.3.8.2. Leukemia in Myelofibrosis with Myeloid Metaplasia

The nine cases of leukemia observed in the 87 patients discussed at the beginning of the preceding section can be categorized into three cases of terminal leukemia (one of which was identified as myeloblastic), and two cases of CML. Six of the leukemic cases were reported by Whang-

Peng *et al.* (in press). Two of these six cases, one with unclassified leukemia terminally and another with AML, had normal karyotypes. Of the two cases with CML, one had a normal karyotype initially and then was found to have developed aneuploidy 32 months later, when the clinical and hematologic pictures were those of CML; the other CML patient had 49 chromosomes, including three extra chromosomes in the C group. One of the cases with unclassified leukemia terminally had an abnormal karyotype, 47,XX,+21. Initially the case with AMMoL had a major clone with a minute marker chromosome and a minor clone with an isochromosome, iso-17q; 12 months later, when a diagnosis of AMMoL was made, the clone with the iso-17q had replaced the clone with the minute marker. Of the total of 20 cases listed in this report, 14 showed no definite evidence of leukemia and 11 of these 14 were aneuploid.

None of the 18 cases of myelofibrosis reported by Nowell *et al.* (1976) had progressed to leukemia; 16 of these cases had been followed for more than 1 year or until death from other causes. Eight individuals had abnormal clones in their peripheral blood. The authors concluded, therefore, that although chromosome abnormalitites are common in myelofibrosis, they do not necessarily indicate that a leukemic phase is imminent.

### 11.3.8.3. Conclusion

The cytogenetic data in myelofibrosis with myeloid metaplasia indicate that this disorder is very heterogeneous. It should perhaps be considered only a symptom of another underlying myeloproliferative disorder rather than a separate disease. This may explain the curious observation that those cases which progress to leukemia do not all develop the same type of leukemia.

### 11.3.9. Thrombocythemia

Primary or essentail thrombocythemia is a chronic disease whose chief symptoms are either thrombotic or hemorrhagic. Whether it is a separate disease entity or a manifestation of another myeloproliferative disorder is still controversial. It can, however, be simply characterized as a condition in which there is a high platelet count (over 1 million/mm$^3$) with no clinical or hematological evidence of any other disease.

### 11.3.9.1. Cytogenetic Studies

Thirteen cases of primary thrombocythemia were studied by Frick (1969). Chromosome analysis was performed in eight of the patients; none had a Ph$^1$ chromosome but six patients had a G-21 chromosome with elongated short arms in a majority of the metaphases (in one patient it was present in 100% of the cells). No chromosome banding was done in this study. Ten patients were treated with $^{32}$P or chemotherapy and three patients were untreated, including the one patient who died of a pulmonary embolism before she could be treated. The more indolent nature of the disease is reflected in the low mortality (death in only one case) in this study where the average follow-up was 6 years.

Rowley and Blaisdell (1966) reported thrombocythemia in a 57-year-old female whose first marrow (prior to treatment) showed cells with 47, 48, and 49 chromosomes with a model number of 48, including two extra C group chromosomes. After successful treatment with $^{32}$P, the abnormal cells completely disappeared and a second posttreatment sample showed only one cell (out of a total of 10) with 47,+C. Banding studies in this same patient (Rowley, 1973c) revealed that one of the extra C group chromosomes was a #9 and the other either a #8 or a #10.

Three cases studied by Kiossoglou *et al.* (1966b) were karyotypically normal.

The Ph$^1$ chromosome has been observed in thrombocythemia only rarely. Two cases were reported by Nicoara *et al.* (1967), one of whom eventually developed CML. It has also been reported by Hossfeld *et al.* (1975) in megakaryoblastic leukemia. Hyperdiploidy with chromosome counts of 47, 48, and 50 in one cell each, a metacentric marker, and extra chromosomes in groups C, E, and G, were seen in the first marrow specimen. On two subsequent marrows after chemotherapy, the hyperdiploidy had disappeared but all metaphases were still Ph$^1$ positive; 4% of the cells were tetraploid and 5% were octoploid.

Aneuploidy of a nonextensive nature is obviously common in thrombocythemia, but it apparently does not indicate a poor prognosis. Clones of cells with abnormal chromosomes behave in a manner similar to those seen in acute leukemia in that they can sometimes be eradicated by treatment.

## 11.3.10. Atypical Myeloproliferative Syndrome

In some hematologic disorders, no diagnosis other than myeloproliferative syndrome can be made. Patients with this syndrome exhibit hepatosplenomegaly, anemia, and thrombocytopenia of variable degrees, a tendency to develop infections, and a hypercellular bone marrow which cannot be diagnosed as leukemia.

### 11.3.10.1. Cytogenetic Studies

Cytogenetic studies have been carried out in nine patients, six of whom had abnormal karyotypes. Berger *et al.* (1975) described a case of atypical myeloproliferative syndrome with polymorphonuclear hyperplasia in the blood and a 46,XY,t(4;12),i(17q),(20q−) karyotype. This patient died 2 years later in what was probably an acute phase of CML. Atypical myeloproliferative disorder was reported in two sisters (aged 12 and 14 years) by Kamiyama *et al.* (1973); they both had marked leukocytosis and proliferation of the granulocytic series. A diagnosis of tentative CML was made on autopsy when infiltration with cells of the granulocytic series was found in both spleen and lymph nodes. Both sisters, however, had normal leukocyte alkaline phosphatase levels and were Ph[1] negative. They also had the same abnormal karyotype, 45XX,−C or 45,X; in one sister this abnormality was found in both bone marrow and peripheral blood specimens and in the other sister only the bone marrow was studied.

Six cases of atypical myeloproliferative syndrome were reported by Lisker *et al.* (1973). These patients were followed from 4 months to 2 years and none showed any evidence of leukemia. Three patients had chromosomal abnormalities. One patient had one cell (out of a total of seven analyzed) with 47,XY,+E in the bone marrow; he died 2 years later of bronchopneumonia. The second patient had karyotypes with a missing C group chromosome, and some cells had a marker chromosome; he died of hemorrhage 7 months after the chromosomal study. The third patient had two abnormal clones, 47,XX,+marker and 46,XX?,−C,+marker; this patient was alive 15 months after study with no evidence of leukemia. The three patients with normal diploid cells were lost to follow-up 4 months to 1½ years after study.

As was also seen in the patients with myelofibrosis with myeloid metaplasia, chromosomal abnormalities in the atypical myeloproliferative syndrome do not necessarily signify that a leukemic transformation is imminent.

## 11.4. Lymphoproliferative Diseases

### 11.4.1. Acute Lymphocytic Leukemia

#### 11.4.1.1. Introduction

The study of cytogenetic alterations associated with acute lymphocytic leukemia (ALL) has been limited by difficulties encountered in producing good chromosome preparations. While the cells with normal karyotypes are generally of good quality, the aneuploid cells often display stickiness and an ill-defined blurred appearance, frequently making it impossible even to enumerate the chromosomes; good banding studies are usually unobtainable in such cases. In spite of these difficulties, the studies performed indicate that approximately half of all ALL patients exhibit chromosomal abnormalities in their bone marrow metaphases.

## 11.4.1.2. Chromosome Findings Prior to the Banding Technique

One of the earliest reports on cytogenetic studies in ALL was that of Kiossoglou *et al.* (1965a), who included three ALL cases in a series on acute leukemia. All three had some degree of aneuploidy. The first case had two cell lines, a pseudodiploid one $(46,-C,+G)$ and one with 47 chromosomes $(47,+G)$, with a $Ph^1$-like chromosome in 64% of the cells. The remaining two cases had normal diploid cells and cells with 45 chromosomes $(45,-\#9)$ as well; in each case, the abnormal karyotype developed after induction of treatment. The authors were unable to discern any correlation between the chromosomal abnormalities and the clinical or hematologic features of the disease, and they felt that the presence of normal as well as abnormal chromosomal patterns suggested that ALL is not a single disease entity but comprises a variety of morphologic responses to various etiologic agents.

Krogh Jensen (1967) included six cases of ALL in his comprehensive study of 30 cases of acute leukemia. Four of them had hyperdiploid lines, mainly cells with 47 chromosomes, ranging from 2 to 62% of the total metaphases. In his first case, serial studies revealed a progression toward aneuploidy: during partial remission, all cells were normal diploid; 2 months later, 1% of the cells were aneuploid; and 9 months later, on relapse, 62% were aneuploid. On the basis of these studies, the author concluded that there was no correlation between the percentage of aneuploid metaphases and the percentage of blast cells seen in direct marrow smears. He felt, however, that cytogenetic studies could provide valuable information concerning the nature and pathogeneis of acute leukemia.

In 1968, Sandberg *et al.* reported the results of chromosome studies in 219 acute leukemia patients, 106 of whom had ALL. Aneuploidy was observed in 50% of the ALL patients and was characterized by hyperdiploidy. The karyotypes showed remarkable variability from one case to another, and except for a small number of cases with trisomy C, no consistent or characteristic chromosomal changes were found which were of statistical significance.

In a report of five cases of ALL, Sakurai (1970a) suggested that there may be a tendency for greater loss or gain in the C and G groups than would be expected if such involvement were purely random. Three of the cases had a minute chromosome; in two cases it was difficult to differentiate the minute from a $Ph^1$ chromosome but in the third case it appeared to be a #18 with deleted short arms. Both the other cases had cell lines with $45,XY,-C$ karyotypes.

In a study of adult acute leukemia, Hart *et al.* (1971) found that chromosomal abnormalities were not influenced by the histologic type of leukemia. However, they did note certain characteristic features that were statistically significant: increased numbers of chromosomes in groups D and E and decreased numbers in group G, and longer survivals in patients with extra D or E compared to patients with deleted chromosomes in the same groups.

Cytogenetic studies in two cases of ALL with eosinophilia were reported by Spitzer and Garson (1973). Both cases exhibited aneuploidy: in case 1, 86% of the cells had a normal karyotype and 12% had a 45,XX,−C,+D,+E,−F,−G karyotype; in case 2, the initial examination showed that all cells were hyperdiploid with chromosome numbers ranging from 47 to 51 and a major cell line of 47,XX,−A,−B,+C,+D,+G.

### 11.4.1.3. Banding Studies in ALL

Lawler *et al.* (1975) examined 49 cases of ALL, 39 (79.6%) of whom were observed to be aneuploid. Nine patients had no normal cells while 30 patients exhibited both normal and abnormal cells. Of the 39 aneuploid patients, 19 had definite clones. Banding studies in three of the cytogenetically abnormal patients (Table VI) revealed: one case with del(7)(q22), one case with del(6)(q13), and one case with 19p+. These authors concluded that a large proportion of ALL patients are hyperdiploid, that this hyperdiploidy often accounts for as many as 30% of the cells, and that the higher the frequency of hyperdiploidy, the greater the chromosome number is per cell.

**Table VI.**  Detail Banding Analysis in 18 Aneuploid Cases of ALL

| Reference | Age/sex | Specific findings |
|---|---|---|
| Mandel *et al.*, 1977 | 56/F | Monosomy 7,Ph$^1$+,t(9;22)(q34;q11) |
| | | del 7(q11),Ph$^1$+,t(9;22)(q34;q11) |
| Whang-Peng *et al.*, 1976a | 3/M | −8 |
| | 4/M | 21q−(Ph$^1$-like), 13q+ |
| | 8/M | 4q−, +17q+ |
| | 5/F | 2q−,4q−,4q−,12p+,13q+,14q+,−20,+21 |
| | 31/F | 21q−(Ph$^1$-like) |
| Yamada and Furnsawa, 1976 | 44/F | 47,XX,+21,i(17q) |
| | 8/F | 45,XX,−21 (52 unknown) |
| | 32/F | 47,XX,+16 |
| | 34/M | 46,XY,1q+ |
| | 23/F | 45,X,−X |
| Oshimura and Sandberg, 1976 | 2 cases | 6q− (missing q21−q25) |
| | 2 cases | 6q−, and others |
| Lawler *et al.*, 1975 | 3 cases | del(6)(q13) |
| | | del(7)(q22) |
| | | 19p+ |

Four cases of ALL reported by Oshimura and Sandberg (1976) had a common abnormality, a partial deletion of the long arm of chromosome 6 (6q−) with break points varying from q21 to q25. In two cases (one an atypical T cell leukemia, and the other the null cell variety) the 6q− was the sole karyotypic abnormality; the other two patients had additional chromosomal abnormalities. These authors also examined the chromosomes from cell lines which were established from the T cells of seven patients with ALL: four of these lines had the 6q− abnormality. They postulated that "the frequency of the 6q− abnormality in ALL is at least as common as that of the so-called nonrandom changes described for AML."

Of 50 ALL patients studied by Fitzgerald and Hamer (1976), 26 were karyotypically normal, 12 had both normal and abnormal karyotypes, and 12 had abnormal karyotypes only. The mean survival for patients with aneuploidy was almost 7 months shorter than that for patients with only normal cells, and patients over 20 years of age had a shorter mean survival than patients below 20 regardless of the cytogenetic findings.

Our recent paper on 331 cases of ALL (Whang-Peng *et al.*, 1976a) included four patients with congenital abnormalities, three of whom had Down's syndrome and one a D/G translocation. Aneuploidy was present in 42.6% of the bone marrows examined prior to treatment, and the G group, followed by the B group, chromosomes were most commonly involved in abnormalities. A $Ph^1$-like chromosome (Gq−) was noted in four patients; banding studies were possible in two of these patients and demonstrated that the Gq− was actually a 21q− (Table VI) (Fig. 8) in contrast to the true $Ph^1$ chromosome which is 22q−. Aneuploidy was observed to be higher in patients under 1 year or more than 20 years of age and in patients with low or elevated WBCs at diagnosis. One patient had a missing Y chromosome and one had an extra Y. Although a missing Y has been reported in leukemia (Vass and Sellyei, 1973; Sandberg and Sakurai, 1973), involvement of this chromosome is not common in ALL.

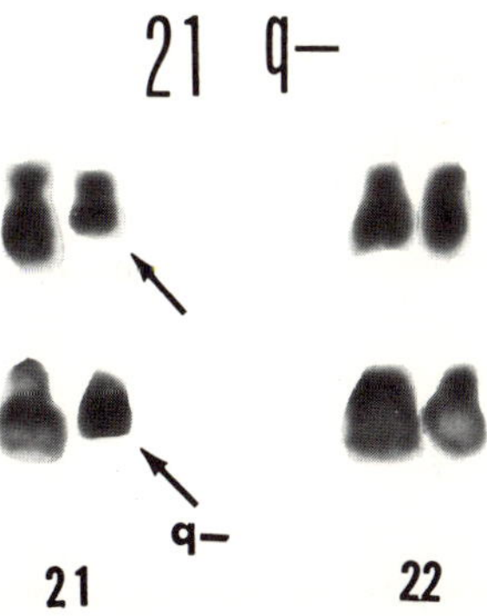


**Fig. 8.**   Partial karyotype from trypsin Giemsa banding showing 21q− in a patient with ALL.

The very limited amount of results from banding studies in ALL (Oshimura and Sandberg, 1976; Whang-Peng et al., 1976a; Lawler *et al.*, 1975; Yamada and Furnsawa, 1976; Mandel *et al.*, 1977) are shown in Table VI. Of the 18 cases, five had abnormalities in chromosomes #6 and #21; two had abnormalities in chromosomes #4, #13, and #17; and chromosomes #1, #2, #8, #9, #12, #19, #20, and X were involved in aneuploidy in only one case each. With so few cases, it is not possible to draw any definite statistical conclusions as to which chromosome is most frequently involved in abnormalities although chromosomes #6 and #21 appear to be frequently involved.

### 11.4.1.4. Polyploidy and Nonspecific Aberrations

Polyploidy occurs occasionally in ALL (Kiossoglou *et al.*, 1965a; Krogh Jensen, 1967; Whang-Peng *et al.*, 1976a). In our series of ALLs, seven patients had a high percentage of tetraploidy, ranging from 12 to 87% of the metaphases, and six had cells in the near-tetraploid range. In these patients, the tetraploidy was found to have no noticeable effect on survival. In comparison, Trujillo *et al.* (1971) described a patient with tetraploid leukemia who died within a month of diagnosis despite intensive chemotherapy.

Chromosomal breakage and fragmentation have also been repeatedly seen in this disease. Krogh Jensen (1967) observed a frequency involving up to 20% of the cells in individual patients, 29 of the 49 patients in Lawler *et al.*'s (1975) series had such findings, and three of our cases (Whang-Peng *et al.*, 1976a) had a high percentage of such aberrations in their bone marrow cells. This phenomenon could be due to the disturbance of DNA synthesis, which is a feature of leukemia, or could be brought about by exposure to chemotherapeutic agents which disrupt DNA synthesis and are known to cause chromosomal breakage and fragmentation.

### 11.4.1.5. The Ph¹ in ALL

The Ph¹ chromosome has been observed in ALL occasionally but its significance is still unclear. Some cases were reported prior to the development of the banding technique and differentiation from CML in blastic transformation is in doubt. Examples include the case of the 53-year-old roentgenologist with Ph¹ and ALL who died 4 months after onset of symptoms without a terminal diagnosis of CML (Propp and Lizzi, 1970), and two of our Ph¹ positive ALLs (Whang-Peng *et al.*, 1976a). Certain of these patients may actually have had a 21q− abnormality, as proved to be the case in our two other ALL patients. Recently, however, banding studies have shown a true $Ph^1$ chromosome (22q−) in several cases of ALL; all except one involved the now classical 9;22 translocation (Mandel *et al.*, 1977; Schmidt *et al.*, 1975; Secker-Walker *et al.*, 1976; Rausen *et al.*, 1977; Secker-Walker and Hardy, 1976; van Biervliet *et al.*, 1975). The one exception showed a 14;22 translocation (Aubert *et al.*, 1975). In 1976, Secker-Walker and co-workers reported four cases of childhood leukemia who were originally diagnosed as ALL but who were subsequently found to be $Ph^1$ positive. One of the cases was indistinguishable from classic ALL; in the remaining three cases the diagnosis was changed to CML in blast crisis, either because the diagnostic features, which consisted predominantly of poorly differentiated blasts in the bone marrow, and/or the clinical course (i.e., failure to respond to standard ALL therapy within 3 months) were uncharacteristic of childhood ALL. Another case of classic ALL with a $Ph^1$ chromosome was reported by Mandel *et al.* (1977): this 56-year-old woman also had abnormalities of the #7 chromosome (monosomy 7 or 7q11−) (Table VI); she responded well to ALL treatment consisting of vincristine and prednisone, with a resulting decrease of the $Ph^1$ positive cells in her bone marrow. $Ph^1$ positive ALL may represent an atypical or occult form of CML, especially in the adult cases, or it may be the result of the coexistence of two types of leukemia. A third, and increasingly popular theory, proposes that the $Ph^1$ clone originates in a lymphoid or prelymphoid stem cell.

### 11.4.1.6. Congenital Lymphoblastic Leukemia

Congenital leukemia, especially the lymphoid type, is rare and is usually found in female infants. Although it is most commonly seen in individuals with congenitally abnormal genotypes (Garson and Milligan, 1974; Hinkes *et al.*, 1973; van den Berghe, *et al.*, 1972) such as Down's syndrome (Conen and Erkman, 1966; Schunk and Lehman, 1954) and trisomy D (Schade *et al.*, 1962), it has been reported without accompanying congenital errors (Whang-Peng *et al.*, 1976a). ALL in a 6-week-old male infant, who survived for only 8 months after diagnosis, was reported by Sharp *et al.* (1973); direct chromosome analysis of the bone marrow obtained prior to treatment revealed a complement of 46,XY,+C, +Mar,−E,−2G. Wagner and Greyerz-Gloor (1968) reported ALL in a 1-day-old female; successful chromosome studies on two separate occasions showed 21 and 18% aneuploidy involving chromosome groups A, B, E, F, and G in the first culture, and the same abnormalities, with the addition of a C group aneuploidy, in the second culture. A case of congenital leukemia described by Bouton *et al.* (1961) was cytogenetically normal. Of the five patients in our ALL series (Whang-Peng *et al.*, 1976a) who were less than a year old, four demonstrated aneuploidy; the survival in these five patients ranged from 2 to 15 months, with a median of 14 months, considerably shorter than the median survival of 21 months (range 1 to 204+ months) seen in the ALL group as a whole.

### 11.4.1.7. Conclusion

Despite the wide variability in the published chromosome date on ALL (Kiossoglou *et al.*, 1965a; Krogh Jensen, 1967; Sandberg *et al.*, 1968; Sakurai, 1970a; Hart *et al.*, 1971; Spitzer and Garson, 1973; Oshimura and Sandberg, 1976; Fitzgerald and Hamer, 1976; Whang-Peng *et al.*, 1976a; Lawler *et al.*, 1975), several general characteristics are apparent. Aneuploidy is present in approximately 50% of all cases, is usually hyperdiploid in nature, and shows no consistent specific pattern. The aneuploid cells, which usually coexist with normal diploid cells, have a tendency to disappear during remission with subsequent reappearance on relapse. The limited banding results available indicate that chromosomes #6 and #21 may be more involved in aneuploidy but more cases will have to be examined before the significance of these findings can be known. The significance of increased numbers of chromosome aberrations, such as breaks and fragments, is also unknown. Whether or not there is any relationship between aneuploidy and the clinical course and prognosis of ALL is at present debatable: some investigators feel that the presence or absence of aneuploid cells has no apparent bearing on the disease (Fitzgerald *et al.*, 1963b; Krogh Jensen, 1967, Kiossoglou *et al.*, 1965a; Reisman *et al.*, 1964a) while others (Hart *et al.*, 1971) state that aneuploidy indicates a poor prognosis. We (Whang-Peng *et al.*, 1976a) believe that the presence of aneuploid cells in the bone marrow at the onset or the appearance later in the disease is of no prognostic significance. However, persistence of these lines and the development of total aneuploidy signal a poor prognosis. The occurrence of new clones during relapse and the development of leukemia in donor cells following bone marrow transplantation (Fialkow *et al.*, 1971; Goh, 1975; Thomas *et al.*, 1972) indicate a continuing effect of a causative agent or agents on the bone marrow cell.

### 11.4.2. Lymphosarcoma Cell Leukemia

Lymphosarcoma cell leukemia (LSA leukemia) is a rare disease. It is sometimes very difficult to differentiate from ALL purely on morphologic grounds. However, the LSA cells contain more cytoplasm than the lymphoblasts of ALL, the nuclear chromatin structure is less delicate, and nucleoli are more clearly demarcated.

All three of the reported cases with chromosome studies were adults (aged 19, 69, and 78 years). They were also all aneuploid and showed the following abnormalities: a large acrocentric chromosome (Goh,

1968c); 46,XX,−D,+long acrocentric marker (Sakurai, 1970a); and 46,XX,−14,−18,?i(14q),?i(18q) (Siegal *et al.*, 1976). An abnormality of the D group chromosomes, manifesting itself either as a long acrocentric or metacentric marker, was observed in all three patients, and banding studies in one case showed the involved D to be a #14 chromosome. More cases with banding studies are needed to evaluate further the possible relationship between the D group chromosomes and this type of leukemia.

## 11.4.3. Stem Cell Leukemia

There is some controversy over the use of the term "stem cell leukemia" and an acute leukemia classified as such in one institution could possibly be categorized as acute lymphocytic, myelocytic, myelomonocytic, or erythroleukemia in another (Hayhoe, 1968).

Cytogenetic studies have been reported in 12 cases of stem cell leukemia, none of which contained banding results (Kiossoglou *et al.*, 1965a; Obara *et al.*, 1969; Fitzgerald and Hamer, 1976). Seven of the 12 (58%) had normal karyotypes. Aneuploidy consisted of hypodiploidy (one case), pseudodiploidy (minute chromosomes in one case), and hyperdiploidy (one case); in the two aneuploid cases of Fitzgerald and Hamer, the type of aneuploidy was not specified but one had both normal and abnormal cells while the other had total aneuploidy. Survival and response to treatment in this type of leukemia are generally very poor as was demonstrated by Fitzgerald and Hamer's study: six of their seven patients were dead within 2 weeks after diagnosis and the remaining patient, who had a normal karyotype, survived for 3 months.

## 11.4.4. Plasma Cell Leukemia

Plasma cell leukemia is usually diagnosed in patients who present with a leukocyte count in excess of 15,000 in which more than 50% of the cells are plasma cells. Hepatosplenomegaly is common. Morphologically the leukemic cell ranges from a typical plasmacyte to immature and atypical forms (Pruzanski *et al.*, 1969). Clinical symptoms differ little from those of other leukemias, weakness, anemia, and bleeding being the most common manifestations.

### 11.4.4.1. Cytogenetic Studies

Cytogenetic studies have been reported in only two cases of plasma cell leukemia. The first case was one reported by Fitzgerald *et al.* (1973). Plasma cell leukemia was diagnosed shortly before death in a 68-year-old woman, a Gp− (Ch[1]) chromosome carrier, who had had chronic lymphocytic leukemia (CLL) for 8½ years and had received treatment with chlorambucil. Chromosome studies were normal (except for the Gp− which was present in all cells) at the time of diagnosis of CLL and again 4 years later. The number of lymphocytes had begun to increase steadily in the final 3 years of life and they had become more immature. Seven years postdiagnosis of CLL, 14% of the cells had an abnormal karyotype, 47,XX,+2C,−E. A year later, 1 week prior to death, a long submetacentric marker chromosome was also found in the abnormal cells.

The second patient (Wurster-Hill *et al.*, 1973) also had marker chromosomes and banding studies revealed one of them to be a #14 chromosome with two extra bands terminally. The model number was 46 and the abnormal #14 replaced a normal #14 in 6 out of 35 cells. The origin of the extra bands could not be determined. This is in contrast to the #14q+ marker seen in Burkitt's lymphoma which is formed by a 8;14 translocation.

## 11.4.5. Chronic Lymphocytic Leukemia

There have not been a great many cytogenetic studies conducted in chronic lymphocytic leukemia (CLL) due primarily to the difficulties encountered in obtaining good cytogenetic preparations from both bone marrow and peripheral blood (PB); even stimulated cultures of PB yield few mitoses because of the poor response of the CLL lymphocyte to mitogenic stimulation.

### 11.4.5.1. Ch¹ Chromosome

In 1962, Gunz *et al.* reported the observation of an abnormal chromosome, the Christchurch or Ch¹ chromosome (a G group chromosome with a total deletion of the short arms), in several members of a family, two of whom had CLL. The authors suggested an association of this Ch¹ chromosome with CLL analogous to that of the Ph¹ and CML. This, however, was not confirmed (Court Brown, 1964) and in two other reports of familial CLL (Heni and Siebner, 1964; Fraumeni *et al.*, 1969), only normal karyotypes were observed. Of interest is the report of a virtually identical G group abnormality in a family with Down's syndrome in three siblings but with no history of CLL (Shaw, 1962). After studying 12 families with multiple occurrences of leukemia and related disorders and finding no other Ch¹ positive cases with CLL, Fitzgerald and Gunz concluded that this abnormal chromosome was of no particular significance as a predisposing factor in CLL. However, individuals with congenital chromosome abnormalities (e.g., Down's syndrome) do have a higher incidence of leukemia so the relationship between the Ch¹ and CLL may not be entirely fortuitous.

### 11.4.5.2. Cytogenetic Studies

In a study of 30 cases of CLL, Fitzgerald and Adams (1965) found definite chromosomal abnormalities in only one case, who had 6 out of a total of 10 cells with 46 chromosomes and a deletion of the long arms of a G or Y chromosome; a second case, with a history of radiation therapy, had a minute fragment in three cells. All the cytogenetic preparations in this study, with the exception of one case, were obtained from peripheral blood cultures; few or no dividing cells were seen in 1- or 2-day cultures, and the most satisfactory metaphases were obtained from 3-day cultures. Direct bone marrow preparations had failed to yield mitotic figures, due to the heavy infiltration of the marrow by mature nondividing lymphocytes. By lengthening the culture period of the PB to 6 days, with one change of media at 72 hr, Ducos and Colombies (1968) were able to get successful cytogenetic preparations in three cases of CLL, and were able to show chromosomal abnormalities in two of the cases. Goh (1968a) confirmed their observation that CLL lymphocytes have a slower response to phytohemagglutinin than normal lymphocytes and he found that 40% of the metaphases from six patients with CLL had a pseudodiploid karyotype.

Six-day PB cultures were also used in a study of seven CLL patients by Rozynkowa and Marczak (1970). Although no specific abnormalities characteristic for CLL were found, all but one patient exhibited hyperdiploidy (47–48 chromosomes) and five had a low frequency of hypodiploidy (one to two cells); two patients had pseudodiploidy and one patient had a marker chromosome (16q+) which was identified on two separate occasions. Lymph node (LN) cultures (stimulated with PHA) were successful in two patients and in one of them the LN showed the same abnormalities as seen in the PB culture (pseudo- and hyperdiploidy) but with differing proportions. In a study of 10 cases of CLL, Berger and Parmentier (1971) cultured the PB for 2, 3, and 6 days. Most of the metaphases were normal and in the few abnormal karyotypes, the aneuploidy was more frequent in the C and D group chromosomes (particularily Dq+ and Dq−) when compared to their normal controls.

### 11.4.5.3. Secondary Leukemia

Secondary acute leukemia has been reported in a total of 20 patients (Lawrence *et al.*, 1949; Diamond *et al.*, 1950; Osgood and Seaman, 1952; Osgood, 1964; Lortholary *et al.*, 1966; Catovsky and Galtor, 1971) with CLL, all of whom had been treated: 17 patients had received radiophosphorus, one patient was treated with total body irradiation and chlorambucil, and two patients had received only chlorambucil. Two other cases of CLL have developed Ph[1] positive CML (Whang-Peng *et al.*, 1974b); only one of these patients had received treatment for CLL, in that instance with total body irradiation. Therapy is obviously, therefore, not a prerequisite for the development of CGL or (probably other) second malignancies in CLL.

In conclusion, because of technical problems cytogenetic studies in CLL have been confined to analysis of peripheral blood cells, and a considerable degree of aneuploidy is observed if the cells are cultured for 5–7 days. Hypodiploidy, pseudodiploidy, hyperdiploidy, and marker chromosomes (e.g., 16p−, Dq+ and Dq−, and minutes) have all been reported in several cases.

## 11.4.6. Sezary Syndrome

The Sezary syndrome was first described by Sezary and Bouvrain in 1938; leonine facies, intensive erythroderma, lymphadenopathy, and the presence of abnormal cells in the peripheral blood are the characteristic clinical features of this syndrome. The typical Sezary cell shows a cerebriform and serpentine nucleus, and recent studies have indicated it to be an abnormal lymphocyte. Cell surface marker studies in 14 cases (Whang-Peng *et al.*, 1976b; Brouet *et al.*, 1973) have identified the Sezary cell as a T-lymphocyte in all but one case, which was found to have both B and T membrane markers. This serves to distinguish the disease from CLL, which is thought to have a B-lymphocyte origin.

### 11.4.6.1. Cytogenetic Studies

There are only a small number of reports of cytogenetic studies in the Sezary syndrome, due primarily to the rarity of the disease and the difficulties encountered in obtaining satisfactory specimens. In some cases the leukocytes from these patients grow very poorly, whereas in other cases there is abundant spontaneous division from unstimulated as well as stimulated cultures. The latter cases provide many metaphases for analysis, but these cells, which are usually aneuploid, often produce indistinct banding patterns. A total of 24 cases of successful cytogenetic studies in the Sezary syndrome were published between 1971 and 1976 (Whang-Peng *et al.*, 1976b; Brouet *et al.*, 1973; Crossen *et al.*, 1971; Dewald *et al.*, 1974; Bosman and van Vloten, 1976; Lutzner *et al.*, 1973). The patients' ages ranged from 28 to 80 years, with a median age of 61. The characteristic chromosome finding was heteroploidy with a broad range of chromosome numbers from the hypodiploid to the tetraploid range. Approximately half of the aneuploid cases (12 out of 22 cases) showed clonal formation. Hypodiploidy was seen in three cases (with cell lines of 39, 40,

44, 45, and 45 chromosomes), three cases had pseudodiploid lines, four cases had hyperdiploidy (with cell lines of 47 and 48 chromosomes), and four cases had chromosome numbers in the near-tetraploid range (72, 75, 76, near-80, and 88). All but one case exhibited marker chromosomes which varied from one to eight markers per patient. Of the 11 cases reported by Whang-Peng *et al.* (1976b), three had rings and four had minute chromosomes in addition to other markers.

The eight patients in whom banding studies were successful are listed in Table VII. The definitions of the various markers are as follows: Marker A is slightly larger than a number $A_2$ chromosome; marker B is somewhat larger than a group B chromosome and the centromere has a more subtelocentric position; $M_1$–$M_5$ are various kinds of submetacentric and metacentric chromosomes including an iso-17q,i(17q) marker. Three of Lutzner and co-workers' (1973) four cases had A and B markers, and the iso-17q was also present in three cases. In the single case of Dewald *et al.* (1974), there were three markers: in the A type, most of the short arm resembled a 6p and the long arm resembled a 2q chromosome arm; the B type was formed from 1q and 13q; and the C type was a 2q− chromosome. Two of the three cases from Bosman and van Vloten (1976) had extensive chromosomal rearrangements.

The observation of a large marker chromosome is apparently very common in the Sezary syndrome but the banding studies have not precisely identified its origin. The i(17q) marker has been seen in four of the eight cases, a frequency which suggests a nonrandom relationship in this lymphoproliferative disease.

Dewald *et al.* (1974) have proposed that hyperdiploid cells are associated with an active malignant phase and, conversely, that hypodiploid cells indicate a remission in the malignant process. From our studies (Whang-Peng *et al.*, 1976b), we feel that the presence of heteroploidy and marker chromosomes is cytogenetically characteristic of the disease but is of no prognostic value; clonal formation, however, is a sign of a fulminating process which rapidly leads to the terminal phase of the disease.

**Table VII.**  Chromosome Banding Studies in Sezary Syndrome

| Reference | Specific findings |
| --- | --- |
| Lutzner *et al.*, 1973 | Markers A, B, $M_1$, $M_2$, $M_3$, $M_4$, $M_5$ |
| Dewald *et al.*, 1974 | Type A, type B, type C markers |
| Bosman and van Vloten, 1976 | #1. t(4q; 3p)(6q;3q)(9q;13q)i17q<br>t(9q;13q)(9q;14q)(9q;12q)i17q?<br>#2. 7+, t(9q;14q)(9q;15q)(11q;2q)i17q<br>#3. t(Xq;10q)i? |

## 11.4.7. Leukemic Transformation of Lymphoma

### 11.4.7.1. Introduction

The occurrence of leukemia in patients with lymphoma is quite rare, but the incidence is considerably higher than would be expected by coincidence alone and several factors indicate that such leukemia is radiation-induced. The higher incidence seen in recent years can be explained by the higher doses of irradiation now being used, and the increased percentage of long survivors. The average latent period between irradiation and the development of leukemia in lymphoma is very similar to that seen in the atomic bomb survivors in Japan (Ezdinli *et al.*, 1969). Secondary leukemia in lymphoma can be either of the myeloid or lymphoid variety.

### 11.4.7.2. Cytogenetic Studies in Lymphoma

In a cytogenetic study of the bone marrow in 28 patients with Hodgkin's disease, Ezdinli *et al.* (1969) observed no chromosomal abnormalities. Aneuploidy has, however, been observed in the lymphoid tissue of lymphoma patients: Seif and Spriggs (1967) reported hypotetraploid and tetraploid clones in the lymph node cells of a patient with Hodgkin's disease, and Spiers and Baikie (1968) reported deletion of the short arms of the 17–18 group in patients with lymphoma and related neoplasms.

### 11.4.7.3. Cytogenetic Studies in Leukemic Transformation of Lymphoma

Canellos *et al.* (1975) investigated the incidence of second tumors in 452 patients with Hodgkin's disease who had been treated with chemotherapy or radiotherapy, alone, in combination, or in sequence. The data were calculated on the basis of age, sex, and man-years of observations. A total of 16 tumors were observed, and the highest incidences, 14.5 and 18.5 times the expected, were seen in the groups which had received both radio- and chemotherapy. Of the 16 secondary malignancies, there were two cases of leukemia, both AML. Cytogenetic studies revealed similar abnormalities in both patients, each of whom had clones missing a C group chromosome; unfortunately, banding studies were unavailable. The authors postulated that secondary neoplasms in such patients may represent a combination of the immunosuppressive and cellular effects of such treatment.

In 1969, Ezdinli *et al.* reported chromosome studies in three cases of myeloid leukemia complicating Hodgkin's disease. All three cases had been treated with irradiation and all showed chromosomal abnormalities. Case 1 had AML and almost all the cells had a pseudodiploid karyotype, 46,XX,−C,+D,+E,−G. Case 2 developed erythroleukemia and had a small metacentric marker chromosome in most of the cells and considerable hyperdiploidy. Case 3 had Ph¹ positive CML. The median latent period between the first course of irradiation and the onset of leukemia was 7 years (7, 2, and 9 years, respectively), a time lag which supports the concept that the leukemia in these cases was radiation-induced. The authors reviewed five additional cases of coexistent Hodgkin's disease and myeloid leukemia reported in the literature and noted that all but one of them also had had previous irradiation.

The only report of chromosome banding studies in a patient with leukemia associated with Hodgkin's disease was that reported by Lundh *et al.* (1975). A case of AML had an abnormal karyotype in all bone marrow metaphases. The major cell line had a 47,XY,+14,−17,+18 karyotype: cells with 46, 48, and 49 chromosomes also showed +14,−17,+18 plus other abnormalities. A pathogenetic relationship between the two disorders was suggested by the karyotypic similarities in this case and those observed in other malignant lymphomas, an example of which is the abnormalities of the #14 chromosome reported in Burkitt's lymphoma. Of interest in this case was the fact that the patient had had infectious mononucleosis 12 years prior to his lymphoma.

Careful cytogenetic investigations in this area of leukemia can perhaps determine whether in fact these leukemias are radiation-induced or are the result of inherent predisposition of patients with lymphoma to the development of leukemia.


## 11.5. Preleukemia

### 11.5.1. Introduction

Preleukemia is a diagnosis which can best be made in retrospect. One of the earliest reports describing this condition was that of Mallarme in 1949; he reported a case of acute leukemia following marrow aplasia. Although some investigators use the term "preleukemia" to describe myeloproliferative disorders (such as polycythemia vera and myeloid metaplasia) and cases of anemia and pancytopenia with abnormal marrows which cannot be definitely classified as leukemia on clinical grounds, others use the term more restrictively. A more definitive description was proposed by Block *et al.* in 1953. The predominant hematologic features they described included anemia, leukopenia with neutropenia, and thrombocytopenia extending for variable periods of time. The bone marrow morphology was characterized by granulocytic hypoplasia and maturation arrest accompanied by erythrocytic changes varying from extreme aplasia to extreme hyperplasia. The terms smoldering acute leukemia, subacute leukemia, and atypical leukemia are also used to describe this condition. When preleukemia proceeds to leukemia, the leukemia is usually of the granulocytic type.

## 11.5.2. Cytogenetic Studies

Nowell (1965) proposed that, since it is extremely difficult to predict from the clinical or hematologic observations which of these patients will develop leukemia or when this will occur, cytogenetic studies might possibly be of prognostic value. He published the first large study in preleukemia, which he divided into two major groups, myeloproliferative and pancytopenic. Other cases have been reported by Rowley *et al.* (1966), Sakurai (1970b), Freireich *et al.* (1964), McClure *et al.* (1965), Jackson and Higgins (1967), Teasdale *et al.* (1970), Humbert *et al.* (1971), Khan (1972b), Kaufman *et al.* (1974), and Pierre (1975). The C and D group chromosomes are those most frequently involved in chromosomal abnormalities in preleukemia.

## 11.5.3. Banding Studies

Chromosome banding results from five patients with preleukemia disorders were reported by Yamada and Furnsawa (1976). Trisomy 8 was the sole chromosomal abnormality in three patients: one with aplastic anemia, one with pancytopenia which later converted to possible AML, and one with aplastic anemia which converted to possible erythroleukemia. The fourth patient, who had sideroblastic anemia, showed chromosomal mosaicism $(44,X,-Y,-21/45,XY,-21/46,XY,1q+)$. The fifth patient had myelodysplasia with a $44,XY,-8,-21$ karyotype; he later developed AML. These five cases demonstrated preferential involvement of chromosomes #8 (four cases) and #21 (two cases).

A deletion of the long arm of chromosome #5 (5q−) was first described by van den Berghe *et al.* (1974) in three cases of refractory anemia. A more detailed study of these three cases plus two additional cases was reported by Sokal *et al.* (1975). Detailed banding studies in a case with refractory anemia reported by Verhest *et al.* (1976) revealed that the deletion was interstitial: del(5) (pter→q12::q31→qter). Although refractory anemia can be considered a preleukemic condition, none of the six reported cases had developed leukemia. Rowley (1976c), however, described a 5q− chromosome in five patients with AML; in three of these patients, the 5q− was observed in a preleukemic state.

## 11.5.4. The 45 Chromosome Syndrome

In 1971, Humbert *et al.* reported the development of probable AML in a child who had had a 3-year history of a myeloproliferative disorder characterized by hepatosplenomegaly with myeloid metaplasia, refractory anemia, leukocytosis, and thrombocytopenia. This child also had a $45, -C$ karyotype in 9–100% of her bone marrow metaphases. These authors also reviewed the other eight cases of this "45 chromosome syndrome" which had been reported by: Freireich *et al.* (1964), three cases; McClure *et al.* (1965), one case; Teasdale *et al.* (1970), two cases; Jackson and Higgins (1967), one case; and Rowley *et al.* (1966), one case. This syndrome was first described by Freireich and co-workers and all nine reported cases exhibited refractory anemia, thrombocytopenia, immaturity of the granulocytic, erythrocytic, and monocytic elements in the peripheral blood, and all but one case had leukocytosis at one point in their disease. Four of the cases died from AML, one from erythroleukemia, and one from sepsis. Of the three patients who were still alive, two had no evidence of leukemia after 18 months and 6 years, respectively, and one had a diagnosis of questionable AML after 44 months. In a similar case described by Macdougall *et al.* (1974) the missing C group chromosome was identified as a #7.

## 11.5.5. Preleukemia in Atomic Bomb Survivors

A survey of preleukemia in atomic bomb survivors in Japan was reported by Kamada and Uchino (1976). Eighty-five patients were in apparent good health; 14 of these patients had stable chromosome aberrations and 11 of the 14 had transient clone formation. Of the 12 patients with prolonged periods of blood disorders, six developed acute leukemia. Chromosome studies had been performed in all of the leukemia patients when they had still been in a preleukemic state and all but one of them had had abnormal clones. Six patients with hematologic disorders who did not develop leukemia also had chromosome aberrations; they were similar to those seen in the leukemia group but the frequencies were a little less. The authors stated that the persistence of high percentages of cytogenetic abnormalities in patients with prolonged periods of blood disorders suggests a preleukemic state, regardless of radiation exposure.

## 11.5.6. Preleukemia and the Ph[1] Chromosome

Paroxysmal nocturnal hemoglobinuria (PNH) terminating in AML has been reported on several occasions. Cytogenetic studies revealing a

$Ph^1$-like chromosome and other chromosomal abnormalities in a case of PNH led Tsuchimoto *et al.* (1970) to suggest that this disorder may also be considered a preleukemic condition.

The $Ph^1$ has been reported in several patients with no apparent evidence of leukemia. Canellos and Whang-Peng (1972) and Baccarini *et al.* (1973) have described a $Ph^1$ chromosome in two patients who had little or no hematologic disease; in the former case, this condition lasted for over 5 years before the development of the blastic phase of CML. A $Ph^1$ chromosome was observed in 10% of the marrow metaphases in a case of PV at diagnosis (Verhest and van Schoubroeck, 1973). Repeat cytogenetic studies failed to reveal any $Ph^1$ positive cells in samples obtained 5 and 6 years later; 7 years postdiagnosis, the patient's condition remained quiescent with no evidence of leukemia. The authors suggested that the $Ph^1$ chromosome is a specific marker of the preleukemic state, regardless of its percentage in marrow cells, and that the chronic phase of CML could itself be considered a preleukemic condition.

### 11.5.7. Conclusion

Two large cytogenetic studies of preleukemia were conducted by Nowell (1971) and Pierre (1975). In the study by Nowell (1971) there were 51 patients, including 26 patients with myeloproliferative disorders, 16 with idiopathic thrombocytopenia, and nine patients with unexplained anemia, neutropenia, leukocytosis, or thrombocytopenia; no chromosomal changes were seen in the last group and no leukemia developed in these patients. In his 205 cases Pierre (1975) included patients with unexplained hematologic abnormalities and excluded those with agnogenic myeloid metaplasia, PV, or CML. Of the combined total of 256 patients from both studies, 90 (35%) had chromosomal abnormalities. Leukemia developed in 30 (33%) of the 90 aneuploid patients and in 13 (8%) of the 166 patients with normal karyotypes. This indicates a much higher incidence of leukemia in those patients exhibiting chromosomal abnormalities. Nowell concluded that these aneuploid preleukemia patients have a high risk of developing clinical leukemia within a few months of study; if however, leukemia does not appear within 3 months, such patients are thereafter at no greater risk than comparable patients with no chromosomal abnormalities. Pierre's study showed that, of the patients whose preleukemia had progressed to frank leukemia, those with initial cytogenetic abnormalities had a poorer prognosis than those who were karyotypically normal.

## 11.6. Predisposition to Leukemia

### 11.6.1. Genetic Inborn Errors

There is considerable evidence that certain congenital disorders are associated with an increased risk of leukemia or lymphoma. While lymphoma is seen more frequently in individuals with immune deficiency syndromes (Miller, 1966), most congenital disorders linked to leukemia have chromosomal abnormalities (Fraumeni and Miller, 1967). Studies of twins also demonstrate the influence of inheritance: the fraternal twin of an affected child has no increased leukemia risk, whereas the risk for an identical twin is 20–25% (MacMahon and Levy, 1964). Fraumeni (1968) coined the term "leukemogenic genes" to explain the remarkable family aggregation which is occasionally seen in leukemia; this phenomenon can also occur in families without congenital chromosome disorders (Gunz *et al.*, 1966; Lundmark *et al.*, 1967).

### 11.6.1.1. Sex Chromosome Anomalies

That there is an increased risk of leukemia in patients with abnormalities of the sex chromosomes is uncertain. There have been only a few reports of hematologic abnormalities in Turner's syndrome. Newman and Gross (1967) reported the observation of congenital erythroid hypoplasia in one such individual, and AML in a Turner's patient who was also a dizygous twin has been described (Wertelecki and Shapiro, 1970). There appears to be a greater possibility for increased risk in Klinefelter's syndrome. At least five cases of leukemia have been reported (Mamunes *et al.*, 1961; Bousser and Tanzer, 1963; Tough *et al.*, 1961; Borges *et al.*, 1967) and a study by Borges *et al.* (1967), in which Klinefelter's syndrome and three cases of other congenital chromosome abnormalities (a probable XYY, an elongated Y, and an F trisomy) were observed in a cytogenetic survey of 25 children with leukemia, suggests that many cases of Klinefelter's syndrome with leukemia may go undetected; this would result in an observed incidence well below the true one. Two cases of AML have been observed in sex chromosome mosaics, one with 45,XO/46,XY (Cardini *et al.*, 1968) and the other with an 45,XO/47,XXX karyotype (Lewis *et al.*, 1963).

Sex chromosome abnormalities and familial leukemia have also been described. Baikie *et al.* (1961) reported a sibship with two cases of acute leukemia (both males) and a male with XY/XXY mosaicism, and Miller *et al.* (1961) reported a family with an XXXXY male, two Down's syndrome females, and a male CLL. A familial tendency of meiotic nondisjunction may be a predisposing factor to the development of leukemia in such cases.

## 11.6.1.2. Autosomal Anomalies

*11.6.1.2a. Down's Syndrome.* In 1954, Bernard *et al.*, in a description of three cases, suggested an etiological relationship between Down's syndrome and leukemia. Subsequently, the risk of leukemia in Down's syndrome was found to be at least 20 times greater than the rate for the general population (Wald *et al.*, 1961). Occasionally a hematologic abnormality resembling acute leukemia is present at birth in Down's syndrome. This disorder of the newborn is usually self-limiting and it is thought to be the result of ineffective regulation of the production and maturation of myeloid cells in the bone marrow (Ross *et al.*, 1963). Although it was previously believed that leukemia in Down's syndrome was more often of the myelogenous type, two studies, one British (Lashof and Stewart, 1965) and one in the United States (Miller, 1970), have shown that the proportion of myeloid to lymphocytic leukemia in this syndrome is similar to that found in the general population. Lashof and Stewart (1965) also reported that the peak of leukemia mortality occurs at 1 year as compared to a peak at 3 to 4 years in the general population (Ederer *et al.*, 1965). An increased risk of leukemia in the siblings of Down's individuals is uncertain (Miller, 1964).

*11.6.1.2b. G Group Abnormalities.* A high incidence of leukemia may also exist in individuals with mosaicism and translocation involving the G group chromosomes. Behrman *et al.* (1966) have described a self-limiting leukemoid reaction and congenital CML (death occurred at 10 days of age) in two siblings with a G/G translocation. ALL has been observed in a D/G translocation carrier (Whang-Peng *et al.*, 1976a) and in a child with three Down's syndrome siblings whose mother was a D/G translocation carrier (Buckton *et al.*, 1961). ALL was also diagnosed in a male with a balanced C/G translocation, t(Cp−;Gp+) (Hinkes *et al.*, 1973); one of his daughters was also a carrier and the other, who was mentally retarded with a peculiar physical appearance, had partial trisomy of the #17 chromosome. The proband's father had a normal karyotype and his mother had died at the age of 47 of ALL. No chromosomal studies had been performed on the mother so it is not possible to ascertain whether or not the proband's chromosomal abnormalities represented a *de novo* appearance of the translocation.

The Gp− or "Christchurch" chromosome (Gunz *et al.*, 1962), originally thought to be an acquired abnormality related to CLL, was found to be an inherited anomaly. Fitzgerald *et al.* (1966) suggested it may represent another instance of increased risk of leukemia in congenital chromosome disorders. A Gp− chromosome with a Gp−;Dp+ translocation has been reported by Goh (1968b) in three members of a family, one of whom had CLL; autoradiographic studies indicated the involved G and D chromosomes were a #21 and a #15, respectively. Juberg and Jones (1970) described a Gp− chromosome in four generations of a family in which 5 out of 37 progeny from 18 carriers of the Gp− had Down's syndrome. One of these five Down's individuals developed erythremic myelosis at 18 months and died of AML at 21 months of age; he had two aneuploid cell lines in his bone marrow and peripheral blood: one with 47 chromosomes and two Gp− chromosomes, the other with 51 chromosomes and three Gp− chromosomes.

*11.6.1.2c. Trisomy C.* Four cases of leukemia with congenital C group trisomy have been described in the literature; all four cases had very short survival times. The first two cases were reported in 1970 by Hilton *et al.*, and involved identical twin boys. One twin was anemic at birth, subsequently developed AML, and died 4 days after admission at less than 1 month of age; the second twin died from AML at the age of 6 months. Studies for sex chromatin bodies and neutrophil drumsticks were negative in each twin, making a 47,XXY karyotype unlikely. The other two cases included banding studies. Trisomy 8 mosaicism (Riccardi, 1976) was found in the bone marrow and skin fibroblasts of a 42-year-old male with AGL and a heritable, balanced translocation, t(7p;20). The translocation was present in at least three generations, and although the trisomy 8 was discovered after diagnosis, its presence in the skin fibroblasts indicates that it was not a consequence of the leukemia. Trisomy 9 mosaicism (Djernes *et al.*, 1976) was observed in the skin fibroblasts (no other tissues could be studied) of a phenotypically normal male infant with congenital leukemia; diagnosis was made at 13 days of age and he died 1 day later. There were aneuploid lines totaling 25% of the metaphases: 47,XY,+9 and 47,XY,+9p−; both parents and a brother had normal PB karyotypes.

*11.6.1.2d. Trisomy D.* Trisomy of the D group chromosomes results in severe congenital abnormalities and most infants are stillborn or die shortly after birth. Two cases of AML in infancy were reported to have trisomy D (Schade *et al.*, 1962; Zuelzer *et al.*, 1968).

*11.6.1.2e. D/D Translocation.* In a chromosome population study of 1020 adult males, Court Brown *et al.* (1966) found an incidence of congenital chromosomal rearrangements of 0.5%, the most common rearrangement being the D/D translocation, t(DqDq) (0.1% or more). Leukemia has been reported in several carriers of D/D translocations. In a review of 100 cases of acute leukemia, Prigogina *et al.* (1970) found one individual with a D translocation, t(DqDq), and another with enlarged short arms of one of the D group chromosomes. One case each of CML (Engel *et al.*, 1965) and DiGuglielmo's syndrome (Dallapiccola and Malacarne, 1971) in individuals with a D/D translocation have also been reported. Since this most common structural abnormality has as incidence of 1/1000 in the human population and it has been seen only rarely in leukemia, the relationship could well be fortuitous.

*11.6.1.2f. Other Autosomal Anomalies.* A reciprocal translocation between chromosomes B4 and D14, t(4;14), was found in a phenotypically normal female with ALL and her father and twin sisters, all of whom were disease-free (Garson and Milligan, 1974). Additional chromosomal abnormalities present in the leukemic cells of the propositus disappeared with therapy and reappeared upon relapse.

### 11.6.1.3. Structural Aberrations

Spontaneous chromosomal aberrations have been observed in several inherited diseases, all of which predispose to cancer, especially leukemia. Most of them, such as xeroderma pigmentosum, ataxia-telangiectasia, Bloom's syndrome, Fanconi's anemia, and Kostmann's agranulocytosis, are autosomal recessive. Glutathione reductase deficiency is autosomal dominant, and in pernicious anemia, the linkage is unknown but the disease is heritable. The chromosomal breakage in these diseases has been studied primarily *in vitro*. Recently, four new chromosome instability syndromes were reviewed by Hecht and McCaw (1977): porokeratosis of Mibelli, nevoid basal cell carcinoma syndrome, incontinentia pigmenti, and scleroderma; these diseases are not discussed in this section.

*11.6.1.3a. Xeroderma Pigmentosum (XP).* XP is characterized by hypersensitivity to sunlight early in life, dry and scaly skin, and a high incidence of sunlight-induced skin cancers; the incidence of XP is approximately 1 per 250,000 in the general population (Heston, 1976). Although there is no spontaneous increase in chromosomal aberrations, XP cells are more sensitive to ultraviolet light due to a defect in DNA repair mechanisms (Cleaver, 1968). The disease has several clinical forms which are associated with different types of repair mechanisms. When exposed to ultraviolet light, the XP cell has higher rates for mortality, production of chromosome aberrations, and mutation than normal cells (Parrington *et al.* 1971).

*11.6.1.3b. Ataxia-telangiectasia.* Ataxia-telangiectasia is an autosomal recessive disease with a variety of clinical manifestations, chief among them being progressive cerebellar ataxia, oculocutaneous telangiectases, and recurrent sinopulmonary infections. There is an increased risk of lymphoreticular neoplasms such as ALL, CLL, and Hodgkin's disease (Hecht and McCaw, 1977). There is increased random chromosome breakage in the peripheral blood lymphocytes and, in 1975, McCaw *et al.* reported the chromosome findings in eight selected cases, as well as reviewing the published data in 14 other cases. All 22 patients had abnormal clones, and in all but two patients, the abnormality involved rearrangements of the D group chromosomes; the two exceptions had a 47,+C karyotype and since no banding studies were available, the possibility exists that the "+C" could have been an abnormal D. Banding studies in nine patients showed a ring 14 chromosome in one patient, a 14q+ in a second, and a translocation involving the 14q− in the remaining seven patients. Detailed analysis of the translocation in six cases showed break points clustered in the 14q12 band: in three cases the 14q− translocated to the other #14 (14q+); in the other cases chromosomes #6, #7, and the X were involved. The proportion of lymphocytes containing the rearrangements varied from case to case, and generally increased in percentage with time in those cases studied serially. One of the cases who developed CLL had the abnormality before and after the onset of CLL, and a case reported by Bochkov *et al.* (1974) with a translocation, t(Dq−;Cq+), had A–T and "lymphoreticular neoplasia." The relationship between this abnormal chromosome and malignancy is currently unknown, but it may be a step toward malignant development.

*11.6.1.3c. Bloom's Syndrome.* This rare autosomal recessive disease is characterized by growth retardation and sensitivity to sunlight causing a reddish rash (telangiectatic erythema) and formation of blisters. Of the 50 reported cases, eight have developed neoplasms, four of which were acute leukemia (German, 1974). In 1971, Schroeder and Kurth reviewed the chromosome breakage syndromes. Of the 35 reported cases of Bloom's syndrome, 26 had cytogenetic studies, and all of them showed increased spontaneous breakage in *in vitro* blood and fibroblast cultures; direct bone marrow studies had been done in only one patient, who showed chromosomal breakage in that tissue also. The most characteristic aberration is the quadriradial figure, which is symmetrical with centromeres in opposite arms of the figure; it results from exchange of chromatid segments of two homologous chromosomes. Certain chromosomes are most commonly involved and this abnormality is rarely seen, even in the other chromosome breakage syndromes.

*11.6.1.3d. Fanconi's Anemia.* This syndrome was first described by Fanconi in 1927 in three brothers with pancytopenia and multiple congenital abnormalities. It is an autosomal recessive condition and is the only one of the breakage syndromes associated with progressive marrow failure. Other characteristic clinical findings include distinctive skeletal malformations (e.g., hypoplasia or plasia of the radius and thumb), congenital heart and kidney defects, and faults in skin pigmentation. There is an increased risk of acute leukemia, especially myelomonocytic. In a study of a Scottish family by Hill (1976), a high incidence of cancer, including leukemia, was observed in the relations of a child with Fanconi's anemia.

In Schroeder and Kurth's review (1971), 44 of the 170 reported cases had been studied cytogenetically; 39 of the 44 had chromosomal breakage *in vitro* (blood and fibroblast cultures) and five were normal; of the seven cases in whom direct bone marrow studies had been performed, four showed breakage. Four of these patients showed chromosome breakage *in vitro* prior to the development of anemia. Almost all the structural changes are chromatid lesions resulting almost exclusively from non-homologous exchanges.

*11.6.1.3e. Glutathione Reductase Deficiency.* This is an autosomal dominant defect resulting in anemia in some cases. The extent of chromosomal breakage *in vitro* is dependent on the stage of disease. The deficiency is found in blood cells, and when confined to the erythropoietic system, mitotic abnormalities are found in immature red blood cells in the bone marrow but not in cultured leukocytes. *In vitro* chromosomal abnormalities are observed when pancytopenia is present and Hampel *et al.* (1969) showed that choramphenicol, an anemia-inducing drug in this disease, increases the frequency of chromosomal breakage *in vitro*. Of 100 reported cases, Schroeder and Kurth (1971) found cytogenetic studies of *in vitro* blood and fibroblast cultures in eight patients, five of whom exhibited chromosomal breakage; all eight patients showed mitotic disorders in bone marrow smears. The structural changes are similar to those seen in Fanconi's anemia, i.e., chromatid lesions.

Elevated levels of glutathione reductase have also been reported. In a study of 841 patients with hematologic disorders, de la Chapelle *et al.* (1976) found that ten cases with leukemia, cytopenias, or preleukemia had an extra C group chromosome which was found to be trisomy 8 in eight patients. Four of the eight patients had elevated levels of the enzyme and the authors proposed that the gene for the enzyme is located on the #8 chromosome.

*11.6.1.3f. Kostmann's Infantile Genetic Agranulocytosis.* This is a very rare autosomal recessive disorder. Only 15 cases were reviewed by Schroeder and Kurth (1971). Of the seven cases known to have survived to more than 3 years of age, one developed acute monocytic leukemia (Gilman *et al.*, 1970). Increased cancer rates are also known for other forms of familial agranulocytosis. Of the 15 cases, only one had cytogenetic studies, a baby who had 20% aberrant cells in a direct bone marrow preparation (Matsaniotis *et al.*, 1966).

*11.6.1.3g. Pernicious Anemia.* This chromosomal breakage syndrome is hereditary but the pattern of inheritance is undefined. It is not a rare disorder and is especially prevalent in northern Europe where the incidence is greater than 2% of the population. There is an increased incidence of leukemia, other cancers, and cancer in family members. Of the 19 cases with cytogenetic studies reviewed by Schroeder and Kurth (1971), 17 showed chromosomal breakage in direct bone marrow preparations and two were cytogenetically normal.

*11.6.1.3h. Conclusion.* The etiology of the chromosome breakage seen in these diseases and their relationship to neoplasia are still unknown. In pernicious anemia the biochemical defect is known and treatment with vitamin $B_{12}$ and/or folic acid can correct this defect which in turn leads to a disappearance of *in vivo* chromosomal breakage (Heath, 1966). On the other hand, in glutathione reductase deficiency, the drug chloramphenicol increases the frequency of chromosomal breakage *in vitro*. In the other hereditary diseases discussed here, the biochemical investigations remain in a preliminary stage.

Although normal diploid karyotypes are still found in neoplastic cells, despite the greater precision afforded by the new banding techniques, the higher incidence of chromosome rearrangements and cancer seen in this group of patients indicates a link between genetic defects and neoplasia.

### 11.6.1.4. Other Genetic Inborn Errors

*11.6.1.4a. Familial Myeloproliferative Disease.* Randall *et al.* (1965) reported the clinical and laboratory findings in a severe myeloproliferative disorder, suggestive of chronic or subacute myelogenous leukemia, observed in nine children who were related as first or second cousins. Early death was seen in three of the children and six had chronic symptoms; two of the latter children recovered completely during adolescence following illnesses of 10-12 years. The main features of the disease included early onset, marked splenomegaly, hepatomegaly, anemia, thrombocytopenia, and leukocytosis. Antileukemic therapy was essentially ineffective.

*11.6.1.4b. Paroxysmal Nocturnal Hemoglobinuria (PNH).* PNH is characterized by an abnormality of the membrane of the erythrocyte but the nature of this defect is unknown. It causes a remarkable susceptibility to the lytic activity of complement. There appears to be an increased incidence of leukemia in this syndrome, either acute (Jenkins and Hartmann, 1969; Holden and Lichtman, 1969) or chronic (Tso and Chan, 1973). The relationship of the two diseases is not clear; only one of the four cases of PNH with leukemia had chromosome studies. In a report of a case of PNH with 46XY/45XO mosaicism, we (Whang-Peng *et al.*, 1976c) reviewed the chromosomal findings in 19 reported cases (including our own) of PNH. Of the ten cases with bone marrow studies, three were karyotypically normal and seven had both abnormal and normal cells; of the 18 cases with peripheral blood studies, three had normal and abnormal karyotypes and the remaining were normal diploid.

## 11.6.2. Chemical or Therapeutic Agents

Any agent that is capable of producing chromosome damage or bone marrow depression should be evaluated for a possible leukemogenic effect. In 1970, Shaw introduced, in a comprehensive review of chemical agents that produced human chromosome damage, the term "clastogens" to describe agents which break chromosomes; this term is distinguished from the term mutagen because not all clastogens have mutagenic activity. Many, if not all, of these drugs are used in the treatment of leukemia and their effects should be borne in mind when analyzing cytogenetic preparations from patients undergoing chemo- or radiotherapy. A more extensive review of the various effects of antineoplastic agents was given by Sieber and Adamson in 1975.

### 11.6.2.1. Antitumor Antibiotics

These antibiotics are derived from streptomyces organisms and can be divided into three groups on the basis of their action, inhibition of DNA, RNA, or protein synthesis.

*11.6.2.1a. Mitomycin C.* This antibiotic is a DNA inhibitor that induces extensive morphologic abnormalities in mammalian cells, such as nuclear fragmentation and partial DNA depolymerization (Shatkin *et al.*, 1962). Cohen and Shaw (1964) reported that the breaks induced by mitomycin C were nonrandom and that the areas most susceptible to breakage were the regions of the secondary constriction in chromosomes #1, #9, and #16.

*11.6.2.1b. Phleomycin.* This is also a DNA inhibitor. *In vitro* human leukocyte studies (Jacobs *et al.*, 1969) have shown a dose-related depression of the mitotic index and an increase in the incidence of chromosomal aberrations, primarily of the chromatid type.

*11.6.2.1c. Daunomycin.* This RNA inhibitor causes morphologic and cytogenetic abnormalities in bone marrow and peripheral blood *in vivo*. The chromosomal effects (Whang-Peng *et al.*, 1969) include chromatid breaks, fragments, chromatid exchanges, ring and dicentric chromosomes, and extensive fragmentation.

*11.6.2.1d. Actinomycin D.* Another RNA inhibitor, actinomycin D is also a potent clastogen (Ostertag and Kersten, 1965).

*11.6.2.1e. Adriamycin.* This compound is closely related to daunomycin and has even greater clastogenic activity. *In vitro* human leukocyte studies showed that the aberrations produced were nonrandom and that chromosome #3 and the Y were more resistant than other chromosomes to the drug's action (Vig, 1971).

*11.6.2.1f. Bleomycin.* Although this drug does not inhibit DNA synthesis, it does induce chromosome aberrations. Chromatid and chromosome gaps, breaks, and dicentric and ring chromosomes were observed in cultured human leukocytes; chromosome #2 demonstrated the most sensitivity to these effects (Ohama and Kadotani, 1970).

*11.6.2.1g. Chloramphenicol.* No clastogenic effect has been observed for this drug (Shaw, 1970) but it is well known for producing bone marrow depression in humans. Of 124 patients with marrow depression due to chloramphenicol reviewed by Fraumeni (1969), three developed leukemia. In one of these patients there was a definite indication of causal relationship between the drug exposure and leukemia, and in a second patient in this series (reported by Cohen and Creger, 1967), AML developed after a 7-year course of aplastic anemia which had been induced by chloramphenicol. Other cases in which this drug has been linked to leukemia with accompanying chromosomal aberrations have been reported by Brauer and Dameshek (1967) and Rowley *et al.* (1966).

### 11.6.2.2. Chemical Agents

*11.6.2.2a. Benzene.* Benzene is a well-known bone marrow depressant, and over 100 cases of leukemia have been attributed to chronic benzene exposure (Vigliani and Forni, 1976); acute leukemia is more common than the chronic varieties. Chromosome changes (breaks and rearrangements) observed both in *in vivo* and *in vitro* studies are similar to those produced by ionizing radiation. Two of our cases (Whang-Peng *et al.*, in press) of myelofibrosis with myeloid metaplasia had occupational exposures to benzene. One patient had a minute chromosome and a i(17q) marker and developed AMMoL; the other had hypodiploid and pseudodiploid cells in both bone marrow and peripheral blood preparations.

*11.6.2.2b. Antineoplastic Agents.* Many of these agents are known to damage human chromosomes. The observed chromosomal abnormalities include both minor (gaps, breaks, and fragments) and major (ring and dicentric chromosomes, and chromatid exchanges or rearrangements) aberrations. These drugs can be divided into two groups on the basis of their mode of action. The potential for producing secondary neoplasia is inherent in all of these agents.

The following alkylating agents have been shown to produce chromosome damage, *in vivo* and/or *in vitro*: nitrogen mustard (Nasjleti and Spencer, 1966), Cytoxan (Nasjleti and Spencer, 1967), melphalan (Stevenson *et al.*, 1973), triethylene-thiophosphoramide or thio-TEPA (Hampel *et al.*, 1966), busulfan (Richmond and Kaufmann, 1969), and chlorambucil or CMBL (Stevenson and Patel, 1973).

Several antimetabolites also cause chromosomal aberrations, including methotrexate or MTX (Voorhees *et al.*, 1969), cytosine arabinoside or ara-C (Kihlman *et al.*, 1963), and 6-mercaptopurine or 6-MP (Nasjleti and Spencer, 1966). *In vivo* clastogenic effects have been reported in azathioprine or Imuran, a drug widely used for immunosuppression in renal transplantation, by vanZyl and Wissmüller (1974), but other *in vivo* studies (Eberle *et al.*, 1968) have had negative findings.

### 11.6.2.3. Radiation

Radiation, in various forms, is a well-recognized leukemogen.

*11.6.2.3a. Thorotrast.* Thorotrast is a radioactive contrast agent used in radioarteriography. A Danish series of 1005 Thorotrast patients was reviewed by Faber (1973); out of 756 patients who survived the primary disease, 312 had died, 11 of leukemia. The time interval between Thorotrast administration and the development of leukemia is variable, ranging from 6 years (Grebe, 1954) to 36 years (Trübestein and Citoler, 1973).

Myeloid, lymphatic, and erythroid leukemia have all been reported (Bastrup-Madsen *et al.*, 1971). Chromosome studies have been done in a few of the Thorotrast induced leukemia cases. Visfeldt *et al.* (1975) reported myeloid leukemia in a 62-year-old woman who had received 40 ml of Thorotrast 34 years earlier; 97% of the marrow cells had a dicentric chromosome probably resulting from a pericentric inversion in a #1 chromosome, a marker characteristic of radiation damage. Trübestein and Citoler (1973) reported a case of $Ph^1$ positive CML following Thorotrast exposure; no other chromosomal abnormalities were observed. Serial bone marrow and peripheral blood cytogenetic studies showed no chromosomal abnormalities in a patient who had developed AML 15 years after injection of Thorotrast: the course of leukemia in this patient was unusual in that the patient has never relapsed and is alive and well 17 years after her leukemia was diagnosed (Mabry *et al.*, 1976). In a study of four Thorotrast patients by Hennekeuser *et al.* (1970), no chromosomal abnormalities were found in bone marrow preparations.

*11.6.2.3b.* $^{32}P$. $^{32}P$ is used extensively to treat polycythemia vera (PV), and a discussion of its leukemogenic effect has been covered in that section. In a review of 1222 cases, Modan and Lilienfeld (1965) noted a marked predisposition to leukemia in patients with PV, an incidence of approximately 1 in 6 after an interval of 10–15 years. Abnormal clones are found in a great many $^{32}P$-treated patients. These clones are presumed to be radiation-induced and sometimes are seen in 100% of the metaphases in the terminal stages of disease; the leukemia is usually of the acute or subacute myeloid form.

*11.6.2.3c. Radiation.* Ionizing radiation, the first recognized human leukemogen, is known to cause acute leukemia and CML. In a review of high-risk factors in leukemia, Miller (1967) listed the probability of developing leukemia in various congenital disorders and in several types of human radiation exposure. In patients treated with radiation for ankylosing spondylitis, the approximate risk is 1 in 270 with a time interval of 15 years (Court Brown and Doll, 1965), and in Hiroshima survivors who were within 1000 m of the hypocenter, the risk was 1 in 60 with a time interval of 12 years (Brill *et al.*, 1962). That diagnostic X-rays during pregnancy may double the risk of childhood leukemia has been indicated by several retrospective and prospective studies (Borges *et al.*, 1967; MacMahon, 1962) and a high incidence of leukemia has also been seen in survivors of Wilm's tumor after radiation treatment (Miller, 1975).

There is some indication that abnormalities of the G group chromosomes can be induced by radiation. Several cases of $Ph^1$ positive CML may have been radiation-induced (Gavosto *et al.*, 1965; Engel, 1965; Whang-Peng *et al.*, 1974b). In other studies, however, no $Ph^1$ chromosomes were found in radiation-induced CML (Court Brown and Tough, 1963; Krauss *et al.,* 1964). In a report by Goh (1966) a smaller G group chromosome was observed in three of eight workers accidently exposed to doses ranging from 68.5 to 339 rads of total body irradiation.

### 11.6.2.4. Both Chemical and Radiation

Arseneau *et al.* (1972) noted that there was a significant increase in the incidence of secondary tumors in patients who received intensive combination treatment. Of 48 cases of Hodgkin's disease who received both intensive chemotherapy (MOPP—nitrogen mustard, vincristine, prednisone, and procarbazine) and radiotherapy (>3500 rads), five developed secondary neoplasia 5–42 months after the diagnosis of Hodgkin's disease (Canellos *et al.,* 1974). These five cases included two cases of skin cancer and one case of lung cancer, 5, 9, and 26 months, respectively, after diagnosis, and two cases of acute myeloid leukemia. In one of the leukemia cases (AMMoL), radiation treatment had been administered first, in the other (AML), chemotherapy had been the initial treatment. Cytogenetic studies revealed a missing C group chromosome in both leukemia patients (no banding studies were available). Monosomy C is a common occurrence in myeloproliferative disorders but a causal relationship between the two remains unclear. Serial cytogenetic studies may reveal the significance of these chromosomal abnormalities to leukemia development in these patients.

**Table VIII.**   Summary of Specific Chromosomes Frequently Involved in Aneuploidy

| Disorder | 1 | 2 | 3 | 5 | 5q− | 6 | 7 | 8 | 8;21 | 9 | 10 | 11 | 12 |
|---|---|---|---|---|---|---|---|---|---|---|---|---|---|
| AML | | | | | | | ++ | +++ | + | + | | | |
| AMMoL | | | | | | | | + | | | | | |
| APL | | | | | | | | | | | | | |
| CML | | | | | | | + | ++ | | ++ | + | + | + |
| Eos. L. | | | | | | | | | | | | | |
| EL | | | | | | | + | + | | | | | |
| PV | + | | | | | | | + | | ++ | | | |
| MF | + | | | + | | | ++ | ++ | | | | + | + |
| Throm. | | | | | | | | +(?) | | +(?) | +(?) | | |
| ALL | | | | | | + | | | | | | | |
| LSA | | | | | | | | | | | | | |
| PL | | | | | | | | | | | | | |
| CLL | | | | | | | | | | | | | |
| Sezary | +(?) | +(?) | +(?) | | | +(?) | | | | +(?) | | | |
| Preleuk. | | | | | + | | | + | | | | | |

[a]+, Involved; ++, frequently involved; +++, most frequently involved.

## 11.7. Significance of Cytogenetic Studies

The development of chromosome banding techniques in the early 1970s added a new dimension to the field of cytogenetics. Analysis was no longer confined to the morphology alone but was extended to include the structure and configuration of each individual chromosome pair.

Aneuploidy is the most common chromosomal abnormality found in leukemia, but its relationship to the disease process remains at present obscure. One of the more important questions still to be resolved is whether or not chromosomal abnormalities precede neoplastic transformation. Approximately half of all leukemia cases demonstrate normal karyotypes; this phenomenon could be due to one of two factors: either the abnormalities in these cases are too small to be detected by techniques currently available or such abnormalities are not essential for malignant transformation. The presence of the Ph[1] chromosome in preleukemia, and the high incidence of leukemia and neoplasia in conditions with congenital chromosome abnormalities and in those cases with a history of genetic injury by irradiation or chemical and physical agents, strongly support the former explanation.

The only consistent chromosomal abnormality correlated with a specific disease is the well-known Ph[1] chromosome which is present in CML. Until the advent of the banding techniques, chromosomal abnormalities were thought to be of a random nature in acute leukemia. Now, however, there is some evidence that the involvement of certain chromosomes is

n Various Hematologic Disorders[a]

| 13 | 14 | 14q+ | 15 | 17 | i(17q) | 18 | 19 | 20q− | 21 | Ph[1]<br>22q− | Y<br>(X) | min<br>(ring) |
|---|---|---|---|---|---|---|---|---|---|---|---|---|
|  |  |  |  |  |  |  |  |  |  |  | + |  |
|  |  |  |  |  | + |  |  |  | + |  | (+?) |  |
|  |  |  |  |  |  |  |  |  |  |  |  | + |
|  |  |  |  |  |  |  |  |  | + |  |  | (+?) |
|  |  |  |  | + |  |  |  |  |  |  |  |  |
|  |  |  |  |  |  |  |  |  |  | +++ | + |  |
|  | Dq+(?) |  |  |  | +(?) |  |  |  |  |  |  |  |
|  |  |  |  | + |  | + | + |  |  |  |  |  |
|  |  |  |  |  |  |  |  | + |  |  | + |  |
|  |  |  |  |  | + | + |  |  |  |  |  | + |
|  |  |  |  |  |  |  |  |  | + |  | + |  |
|  | +(?) |  |  |  |  |  |  |  |  |  |  |  |
|  |  | +(?) |  |  |  |  |  |  |  |  |  |  |
| Dq+,Dq− |  |  |  |  |  |  |  |  |  |  |  |  |
|  |  |  |  |  |  |  |  |  |  |  |  | + |
| +(?) |  |  |  |  | + |  |  |  |  |  |  | (+) |
|  |  |  |  |  |  |  |  |  | + |  |  |  |

greater than would be expected by chance alone. Table VIII summarizes the available banding data in each type of leukemia with respect to each chromosome pair and a few specific abnormalities which have been repeatedly implicated in certain leukemias.

Generally, the description of cytogenetic abnormalities on a single occasion is of little prognostic value. Much more relevant to the disease process is the observation of karyotypic change, either replacement of a normal line by an abnormal one or the emergence of a new clone in addition to existing abnormalities; such changes often but not invariably indicate a poor prognosis. The effectiveness of treatment can frequently be assessed by a decrease or even total eradication of aneuploid cells in the bone marrow. Reappearance of the same or new clones usually portends a failure of treatment resulting in subsequent leukemic relapse.

ACKNOWLEDGMENTS

The authors are most grateful to Mrs. Turid Knutsen for search of the literature and for editing the manuscript, to Mrs. Elaine Lee for assistance with the references, and to Mrs. Le Esta Moran for typing the manuscript.

# References

Armenta, D., Cadotte, M., Beaulieu, R., Neemeh, J., Long, L., Pretty, H., and Gosselin, G., 1976, Cytogenetic evidence for the splenic origin of chronic myeloid leukemia, *Union Med. Can.* **105**:922–927.

Arrighi, F. W., and Hsu, T. C., 1971, Localization of heterochromatin in human chromosomes, *Cytogenetics* **10**:81–86.

Arseneau, J. C., Sponzo, R. W., Levin, D. L., Schnipper, L. E., Bonner, H., Young, R. C., Canellos, G. P., Johnson, R. E., and DeVita, V. T., 1972, Nonlymphomatous malignant tumors complicating Hodgkin's disease, *N. Engl. J. Med.* **287**:1119–1122.

Atkins, L., and Goulian, M., 1965, Multiple clones with increase in number of chromosomes in the G group in a case of myelomonocytic leukemia, *Cytogenetics* **4**:321–328.

Aubert, L., Arroyo, H., and Gharbi, G., 1975, Leucémie aigüe lymphoblastique avec chromosome Philadelphie. Rôle probable d'une translocation 14–22, *Nouv. Presse Med.* **4**:3013.

Baccarani, M., Zaccaria, A., and Tura, S., 1973, Philadelphia-chromosome-positive preleukaemic state, *Lancet* **2**:1094.

Baikie, A. G., Buckton, K. E., Court Brown, W. M., and Harnden, D. G., 1961, Two cases of leukemia and a case of sex-chromosome abnormality in the same sibship, *Lancet* **2**:1003.

Bastrup-Madsen, P., Nielsen, K., and Mose, C. B., 1971, Acute erythraemia (Di

Guglielmo's syndrome) after thorotrast injection, *Acta Med. Scand.* **189**:349–353.

Beck, W. S., and Chesney, T. M., 1973, Myelocytic leukemia with an unusual chromosomal pattern, *N. Engl. J. Med.* **288**:957–963.

Behrman, R. E., Sigler, A. T., and Patchefsky, A. S., 1966, Abnormal hematopoiesis in 2 of 3 siblings with mongolism, *J. Pediatr.* **68**:569–577.

Benvenisti, D. S., and Ultmann, J. E., 1969, Eosinophilic leukemia, report of 5 cases and review of the literature, *Ann. Intern. Med.* **71**:731–745.

Berger, R., and Parmentier, C., 1971, Chromosomes and chronic lymphatic leukemia, *Nouv. Rev. Fr. Hematol.* **11**:261–278.

Berger, R., Weisgerber, C., and Bernard, J., 1973, Clonal evolution during acute leukemia in a mongol child, *Nouv. Rev. Fr. Hematol.* **13**:229–236.

Berger, P. R., Briere, J., and Clauvel, J. P., 1975, Homozygotie et syndrome myéloprolifératif, *Nouv. Rev. Fr. Hematol.* **15**:667–676.

Bernardé J., Mathé, G., and Delorme, J. D., 1954, Les leucoses des trés jeunes enfants, *Arch. Fr. Pediatr.* **12**:470–502.

Better, O., Brandstaetter, S., Padeh, B., and Bianu, G., 1965, Myeloid metaplasia: Clinical, laboratory and cytogenetic observations, *Isr. J. Med. Sci.* **1**:810–817.

Blackstock, A. M., and Garson, O. M., 1974, Direct evidence for involvement of erythroid cells in acute myeloblastic leukaemia, *Lancet* **2**:1178.

Block, M., Jacobson, L. O., and Bethard, W. F., 1953, Preleukemic acute human leukemia, *JAMA* **152**:1018–1028.

Bloom, G. E., Warner, S., Gerald, P. S., and Diamond, L. K., 1966, Chromosome abnormalities in constitutional aplastic anemia, *N. Engl. J. Med.* **274**:8–14.

Bochkov, N. P., Lopukhin, Y. M., Kuleshov, N. P., and Kovalchuk, L. V., 1974, Cytogenetic study of patients with ataxia-telangiectasia, *Humangenetik* **24**:115–128.

Borges, W. H., Nichlas, J. W., and Hamm, C. W., 1967, Prezygotic determinants in acute leukemia, *J. Pediatr.* **70**:180–184.

Borgstrom, G. H., Vuopio, P., and de la Chapelle, A., 1976, Polyploidy of the bone marrow, *Scand. J. Haematol.* **17**:123–131.

Bosman, F. T., and van Vloten, W. A., 1976, Sezary's syndrome: A cytogenetic cytophotometric and autoradiographic study, *J. Pathol.* **118**:49–57.

Bourgeois, C. A., and Hill, F. G. H., 1977, Fanconi anemia leading to acute myelomonocytic leukemia. Cytogenetic studies, *Cancer* **39**:1163–1167.

Bousser, J., and Tanzer, J., 1963, Syndrome de klinefelter et leucémie aiguë, à propos d'un cas, *Nouv. Rev. Fr. Hematol.* **3**:194–197.

Bouton, M. J., Phillips, H. J., Smithells, R. W., and Walker, S., 1961, Congenital leukaemia with parental consanguinity. Case report with chromosome studies, *Br. Med. J.* **2**:866–869.

Boveri, T., 1902, Uber mehrpolige Mitosen als mittel zur analyse des Zellkerns, *Verh. Phys. Med. Ges.* **35**:67–88.

Brandt, L., Levan, G., Mitelman, F., Olsson, I., and Sjögren, U., 1974, Trisomy G-21 in adult myelomonocytic leukaemia. An abnormality common to granulocytic and monocytic cells, *Scand. J. Haematol.* **12**:117–122.

Brandt, L., Mitelman, F., Beckman, G., Laurell, H., and Nordenson, I., 1977, Different composition of the eosinophilic bone marrow pool in reactive eosinophilia and eosinophilic leukaemia, *Acta Med. Scand.* **201**:177–180.

Brauer, M. J., and Dameshek, W., 1967, Hypoplastic anemia and myeloblastic leukemia following chloramphenicol therapy. Report of three cases, *N. Engl. J. Med.* **277**:1003–1005.

Brill, A. B., Tomonaga, M., and Heyssel, R. M., 1962, Leukemia in man following exposure to ionizing radiation: Summary of findings in Hiroshima and Nagasaki, and comparison with other human experience, *Ann. Intern. Med.* **56**:590–609.

Brink, A. J., and Weber, H. W., 1963, Fibroplastic parietal endocarditis with eosinophilia, *Am. J. Med.* **34**:52–70.

Brouet, J. C., Flandrin, G., and Seligmann, M., 1973, Indication of the thymus-derived nature of the proliferating cells in six patients with Sezary's syndrome, *N. Engl. J. Med.* **289**:341–344.

Buckton, K. E., Harnden, D. G., Baikie, A. G., and Woods, G. E., 1961, Mongolism and leukaemia in the same sibship, *Lancet* **1**:171–172.

Canellos, G. P., and Whang-Peng, J., 1972, Philadelphia-chromosome-positive preleukaemic state, *Lancet* **2**:1227–1229.

Canellos, G. P., DeVita, V. T., Whang-Peng, J., and Carbone, P. P., 1971, Hematologic and cytogenetic remission of blastic transformation of chronic granulocytic leukemia, *Blood* **38**:671–679.

Canellos, G. P., DeVita, V. T., Arseneau, J. C., and Johnson, R. C., 1974, Carcinogenesis by cancer chemotherapeutic agents: Second malignancies complicating Hodgkin's disease in remission, *Recent Results Cancer Res.* **49**:108–114.

Canellos, G. P., DeVita, V. T., Arseneau, J. C., Whang-Peng, J., and Johnson, R. E. C., 1975, Second malignancies complicating Hodgkin's disease in remission, *Lancet* **1**:947–949.

Cardini, G., Clemente, R., and Bersi, M., 1968, Su di un corredo cromosomico particolare in un caso di leucemia acuta mieloblastica comparsa in un soggetto portatore di un mosaico XY/XO, *Arch. Sci. Med.* **125**:433–438.

Caspersson, T., Farber, S., Foley, G. E., Kudynowski, J., Modest, E. J., Simonsson, E., Wagh, U., and Zech, L., 1968, Chemical differentiation along metaphase chromosomes, *Exp. Cell Res.* **49**:219–222.

Castoldi, G., Yam, L. T., Mitus, W. J., and Crosby, W. H., 1968, Chromosomal studies in erythroleukemia and chronic erythremic myelosis, *Blood* **31**:202–215.

Catovsky, D., and Galtor, D. A. G., 1971, Myelomonocytic leukaemia, supervening on chronic lymphocytic leukaemia, *Lancet* **1**:478–479.

Chusid, M. J., Dale, D. C., West, B. C., and Wolff, S. M., 1975, The hypereosinophilic syndrome: Analysis of fourteen cases with review of the literature, *Medicine* **54**:1–27.

Clarkson, B. D., Dowling, M. D., Gee, T. S., Cunningham, I., Hopfan, S., Knapper, W. H., Vaartaja, T., and Haghbin, M., 1974, Radical therapy for chronic granulocytic leukemia (CGL), in 15th Congress of the International Society of Hematologists, Jerusalem, p. 136 (Abstract).

Cleaver, J. E., 1968, Defective repair replication of DNA in xeroderma pigmentosum, *Nature* **218**:652–656.

Cohen, M. M., and Shaw, M. W., 1964, Effects of mitomycin C on human chromosomes, *J. Cell Biol.* **23**:386–395.

Cohen, T., and Creger, W. P., 1967, Acute myeloid leukemia following seven years of aplastic anemia induced by chloramphenicol, *Am. J. Med.* **43**:762–770.

Conen, P. E., and Erkman, B., 1966, Combined mongolism and leukemia—Report of 8 cases with chromosome studies, *Am. J. Dis. Child.* **112**:429–443.

Court Brown, W. M., 1964, Chromosomal abnormality and chronic lymphatic leukaemia, *Lancet* **1**:986.

Court Brown, W. M., and Doll, R., 1965, Mortality from cancer and other causes after radiotherapy for ankylosing spondylitis, *Br. Med. J.* **2**:1327–1332.

Court Brown, W. M., and Tough, I. M., 1963, Cytogenetic studies in chronic myeloid leukemia, *Adv. Cancer Res.* **7**:351–381.

Court Brown, W. M., Jacobs, P. A., Buckton, K. E., Tough, I. M., Kuenssberg, E. V., and Knox, J. D. E., 1966, *Chromosome Studies on Adults*, Cambridge Univ. Press, London.

Cowdell, R. H., Phizackerley, P. J. R., and Pyke, D. A., 1955, Constitutional anemia (Fanconi's syndrome) and leukemia in two brothers, *Blood* **10**:788–801.

Cox, D., Yuncken, C., and Spriggs, A. I., 1965, Minute chromatin bodies in malignant tumors of childhood, *Lancet* **2**:55–58.

Crossen, P. E., Fitzgerald, P. H., Menzies, R. C., and Brehaut, L. A., 1969, Case reports: Chromosomal abnormality, megaloblastosis, and arrested DNA synthesis in erythroleukaemia, *J. Med. Genet.* **6**:95–104.

Crossen, P. E., Mellor, J. E., Finley, A. G., Ravich, R. B. M., Vincent, P. C., and Gunz, F. W., 1971, The Sezary syndrome. Cytogenetic studies and identification of the Sezary cell as an abnormal lymphocyte, *Am. J. Med.* **50**:24–34.

Dallapiccola, B., and Malacarne, P., 1971, Case report. Di Guglielmo syndrome in a t(DqDq) heterozygote, *J. Med. Genet.* **8**:209–214.

Davidson, W. M., and Knight, L. A., 1973, Acquired trisomy 9, *Lancet* **1**:1510.

DeGrouchy, J., De Nava, C., Zittoun, R., and Bousser, J., 1966, Analyses chromosomiques dans l'anémie sidéroblastique idiopathique asquise, *Nouv. Rev. Fr. Hematol.* **6**:367–387.

de la Chapelle, A., Ericksson, A. W., Kirgarinta, M., and Knutar, F., 1971, Glutathione reductase activity in haematological disorders associated with C trisomy, *Eur. J. Clin. Invest.* **1**:366 (Abstract).

de la Chapelle, A., Vuopio, P., and Icén, A., 1976, Trisomy 8 in the bone marrow associated with high red cell glutathione reductase activity, *Blood* **47**:815–826.

Denver Committee, 1960, A proposed system of nomenclature of human mitotic chromosomes, *Lancet* **1**:1063–1064.

Dewald, G., Spurbeck, J. L., and Vitek, H. A., 1974, Chromosomes in a patient with the Sezary syndrome, *Mayo Clin. Proc.* **49**:553–557.

Diamond, H. D., Craver, L. F., Woodward, H. Q., and Parks, G. H., 1950, Radioactive phosphorus: I. In treatment of lymphatic leukemia, *Cancer* **3**:779–788.

Djernes, B. W., Soukup, S. W., Bove, K. E., and Wong, K. Y., 1976, Congenital leukemia associated with mosaic trisomy 9, *J. Pediatr.* **88**:596–597.

Dosik, H., Hsu, L., Todaro, G., Lee, S., Hirschhorn, K., Selirio, E., and Alter, A., 1970, Leukemia in Fanconi's anemia: Cytogenetic and tumor virus susceptibility studies, *Blood* **36**:341–352.

Dougan, L., Scott, I. D., and Woodliff, H. J., 1966, A pair of twins, one of whom has chronic granulocytic leukaemia, *J. Med. Genet.* **3**:217–219.

Ducos, J., and Colombies, P., 1968, Chromosomes in chronic lymphocytic leukaemia, *Lancet* **1**:1038.

Dutrillaux, B., 1973, Nouveau système de marquage chromosomique: Les Bandes T, *Chromosoma* **41**:395–402.

Dutrillaux, B., and Lejeune, J., 1971, Cytogenetique humaine- sur une nouvelle technique d'analyse du caryotype humain, *C.R. Acad. Sci. Paris* **272**:2638–2640.

Duvall, C. P., Carbone, P. P., Bell, W. R., Whang, J., Tjio, J. H., and Perry, S., 1967, Chronic myelocytic leukemia with two Philadelphia chromosomes and prominent peripheral lymphadenopathy, *Blood* **28**:642–666.

Dyment, P. G., Melnyk, J., and Brubaker, C. A., 1968, A cytogenetic study of acute erythroleukemia in children, *Blood* **32**:997–1002.

Eberle, P., Hunstein, W., and Perings, E., 1968, Chromosomes in patients treated with Imuran, *Humangenetik* **6**:69–73.

Ederer, F., Miller, R. W., and Scotto, J., 1965, U.S. childhood cancer mortality patterns. 1950–1959. Etiologic implications, *JAMA* **192**:593–596.

Engel, E., 1965, X-rays and Philadelphia chromosome, *Lancet* **2**:291–292.

Engel, E., and McKee, L. C., 1966, Double Ph[1] chromosomes in leukaemia, *Lancet* **1**:337.

Engel, E., McGee, B. J., Hartmann, R. C., and Engel-De Montomollin, M., 1965, Two leukemic peripheral blood stemlines during acute transformation of chronic myelogenous leukemia in a D/D translocation carrier, *Cytogenetics* **4**:157–170.

Engel, E., McKee, L. C., and Bunting, K. W., 1967, Chromosomes 17–18 in leukaemias, *Lancet* **2**:42–43.

Engel, E., McGee, B. J., Flexner, J. M., Russel, M. T., and Myers, B. J., 1974, Philadelphia chromosome (Ph[1]) translocation in an apparently Ph[1] negative, minus G22, case of chronic myeloid leukemia, *N. Engl. J. Med.* **291**:154.

Engel, E., McKee, L., Flexner, J., and McGee, B., 1975, 17 long arm isochromosome. A common anomaly in malignant blood disorders, *Ann. Genet.* **18**:56–60.

Engel, E., McGee, B. J., Myers, B. J., Flexner, J. M., and Krantz, S. B., 1977, Chromosome banding patterns of 49 cases of chronic myelocytic leukemia, *N. Engl. J. Med.* **296**:1295.

Engel, W., Merker, H., Schneider, G., and Wolf, U., 1968, Clonal occurrence of a chromosome Dq− in myelosclerosis with myeloid metaplasia, *Humangenetik* **6**:335–337.

Ezdinli, E. S., Sokal, J. E., Aungst, C. W., Kim, U., and Sandberg, A. A., 1969, Myeloid leukemia in Hodgkin's disease: Chromosomal abnormalities, *Ann. Intern. Med.* **71**:1097–1104.

Faber, M., 1973, Follow-up of Danish thorotrast cases, in Proceedings of the Third International Meeting of the Toxicity of Thorotrast, Riso Report n294, pp. 137–147.

Fanconi, G., 1927, Familiäre infantile perniziosaartige anämie (perniziöses Blutbild und Konstitution), *Jahrb. Kinderheilkd.* **117**:257–280.

Fialkow, P. J., Thomas, E. D., Bryant, J. I., and Neiman, P. E., 1971, Leukaemic transformation of engrafted human marrow cells *in vivo*, *Lancet* **1**:251–255.

Fitzgerald, P. H., 1976, Evidence that chromosome band 22q12 is concerned with cell proliferation in chronic myeloid leukaemia, *Hum. Genet.* **33**:269–274.

Fitzgerald, P. H., and Adams, A., 1965, Chromosome studies in chronic lymphocytic leukemia and lymphosarcoma, *J. Natl. Cancer Inst.* **34**:827–839.

Fitzgerald, P. H., and Hamer, J. W., 1976, Karyotype and survival in human acute leukemia, *J. Natl. Cancer Inst.* **56**:459–462.

Fitzgerald, P. H., Adams, A., and Gunz, W. G., 1963a, Chronic granulocytic leukemia and the Philadelphia chromosome, *Blood* **21**:183–196.

Fitzgerald, P. H., Crossen, P. E., and Hamer, J. W., 1963b, Abnormal karyotypic clones in human acute leukemia: Their nature and clinical significance, *Cancer* **31**:1069–1077.

Fitzgerald, P. H., Crossen, P. E., Adams, A. C., Sharman, C. V., and Gunz, F. W., 1966, Chromosome studies in familial leukaemia, *J. Med. Genet.* **3**:96–100.

Fitzgerald, P. H., Pickering, A. F., and Eiby, J. R., 1971, Clonal origin of the Philadelphia chromosome and chronic myeloid leukaemia: Evidence from a sex chromosome mosaic, *Br. J. Haematol.* **21**:473–480.

Fitzgerald, P. H., Rastrick, J. M., and Hamer, J. W., 1973, Acute plasma cell leukaemia following chronic lymphatic leukaemia: Transformation or two separate diseases? *Br. J. Haematol.* **25**:171–177.

Forman, E. N., Padre-Mendoza, T., Smith, P. S., Barker, B. E., and Farmer, P., 1977, Ph[1]-positive childhood leukemias: Spectrum of lymphoid-myeloid expressions, *Blood* **49**:549–558.

Forrester, R. H., and Louro, J. M., 1966, Philadelphia chromosome abnormality in agnogenic myeloid metaplasia, *Ann. Intern. Med.* **64**:622–627.

Fraumeni, J. F., 1968, Constitutional disorders of man predisposing to leukemia and lymphoma, *in Comparative Morphology of Hematopoietic Neoplasms* (C. H. Lingeman and F. M. Garner, eds.), pp. 221–232, U.S. Govt. Printing Office, Washington, D.C.

Fraumeni, J. F., 1969, Clinical epidemiology of leukemia, *Semin. Hematol.* **6**:250–260.

Fraumeni, J. F., and Miller, R. W., 1967, Epidemiology of human leukemia. Recent observations, *J. Natl. Cancer Inst.* **38**:593–605.

Fraumeni, J. F., Vogel, C. L., and DeVita, V. T., 1969, Familial chronic lymphocytic leukemia, *Ann. Intern. Med.* **71**:279–284.

Freireich, E. J., Whang, J., Tjio, J. H., Levin, R. H., Brittin, G. M., and Frei, E., III, 1964, Refractory anemia, granulocytic hyperplasia of bone marrow, and a missing chromosome in marrow cells. A new clinical syndrome? *Clin. Res.* **12**:284 (Abstract).

Frick, P. G., 1969, Primary thrombocythaemia. Clinical, hematological and chromosomal studies of 13 patients, *Helv. Med. Acta* **35**:20–29.

Gahrton, G., Lindsten, J., and Zech, L., 1974a, Clonal origin of the Philadelphia chromosome from either the paternal or the maternal chromosome number 22, *Blood* **43**:837–840.

Gahrton, G., Lindsten, J., and Zech, L., 1974b, The Philadelphia chromosome and chronic myelocytic leukemia (CML)—Still a complex relationship? *Acta Med. Scand.* **196**:353–354.

Garson, O. M., and Milligan, W. J., 1974, Acute leukaemia associated with an abnormal genotype, *Scand. J. Haematol.* **12**:256–265.

Gavosto, F., Pileri, A., and Pegoraro, L., 1965, X-rays and Philadelphia chromosome, *Lancet* **1**:1336–1337.

German, J. L., 1962, DNA synthesis in human chromosomes, *Trans. N.Y. Acad. Sci.* **24**:395–407.

German, J., 1974, Bloom's syndrome. II. The prototype of human genetic disorders predisposing to chromosome instability and cancer, *in Chromosomes and Cancer* (J. German, Ed.), pp. 601–617, Wiley, New York.

Gilman, P. A., Jackson, D. P., and Guild, H. G., 1970, Congenital agranulocytosis: Prolonged survival and terminal leukemia, *Blood* **36**:576–585.

Gmyrek, D., Witkowski, R., Syllm-Rapoport, I., and Jacobasch, G., 1968, Chromosome aberrations and abnormalities of red-cell metabolism in a case of Fanconi's anaemia before and after developing leukaemia, *Ger. Med. Mon.* **13**:105–111.

Goh, K., 1966, Smaller G chromosome in irradiated man, *Lancet* **1**:659–660.

Goh, K., 1968a, Chromosomes in chronic lymphocytic leukaemia, *Lancet* **2**:104.

Goh, K., 1968b, Smaller G(Gp−) and t(Gp−;Dp+) chromosomes. A familial study with one member having acute leukemia, *Am. J. Dis. Child.* **115**:732–738.

Goh, K., 1968c, Large abnormal acrocentric chromosome associated with human malignancies. Possible mechanism of establishing clone of cells, *Arch. Intern. Med.* **122**:241–248.

Goh, K., 1975, Cytogenetic evidence of *in vivo* leukaemic transformation of engrafted marrow cells, *Lancet* **1**:1338–1339.

Goh, K.O., and Swisher, S. N., 1963, Chromosomal studies in patients with chronic myelocytic leukemia and myeloid metaplasia, *Clin. Res.* **11**:194.

Goh, K., and Swisher, S. N., 1965, Identical twins and chronic myelocytic leukemia, *Arch. Intern. Med.* **115**:475–478.

Goh, K., Swisher, S. N., and Rosenberg, C. A., 1965, Cytogenetic studies in eosinophilic leukemia. The relationship of eosinophilic leukemia and chronic myelocytic leukemia, *Ann. Intern. Med.* **62**:80–86.

Golde, D. W., Brugaleta, C., Sparkes, R. S., and Cline, M. J., 1977, The Philadelphia chromosome in human macrophages, *Blood* **49**:367–370.

Golomb, H. M., Vardeman, J., and Rowley, J. D., 1976, Acute nonlymphocytic leukemia in adults: Correlation with Q banded chromosomes, *Blood* **48**:9–21.

Gomez, G., Hossfeld, D. K., and Sobal, J. E., 1975, Removal of abnormal clone of leukaemic cells by splenectomy, *Br. Med. J.* **2**:421–423.

Grebe, S. F., 1954, Beitrag zur Frage der Thorotrast-spätschädigung, *Strahlentherapie* **94**:311–319.

Gruenwald, H., Kiossoglou, K. W., Mitus, W. J., and Dameshek, W., 1965, Philadelphia chromosome in eosinophilic leukemia, *Am. J. Med.* **39**:1003–1010.

Gunz, F. W., Fitzgerald, P. H., and Adams, A., 1962, An abnormal chromosome in chronic lymphocytic leukaemia, *Br. Med. J.* **2**:1097–1099.

Gunz, F. W., Fitzgerald, P. H., Crossen, P. E., Mackenzie, I. S., Powles, C. P., and

Jensen, G. R., 1966, Multiple cases of leukemia in a sibship, *Blood* **27**:482–489.

Hampel, K. E., Kober, B., Rösch, D., Gerhartz, H., and Meinig, K. H., 1966, The action of cytostatic agents on the chromosomes of human leukocytes *in vitro*, *Blood* **27**:816–823.

Hampel, K. E., Löhr, G. W., Blume, K. G., and Rüdiger, H. W., 1969, Spontane und Chloramphenicolinduzierte chromosomen-mutationen und biochemische befunde bei zwei fällen mit glutathionreduktasemangel (NAD(P)H: Glutathione oxidoreductase, E.C.1.6.4.2), *Humangenetik* **7**:305–313.

Hardisty, R. M., Speed, D. E., and Till, M., 1964, Granulocytic leukaemia in childhood, *Br. J. Haematol.* **10**:551–566.

Hardy, W. R., and Anderson, R. E., 1968, The hypereosinophilic syndromes, *Ann. Intern. Med.* **68**:1220–1228.

Hart, J. S., Trujillo, J. M., Freireich, E. J., George, S. L., and Frei, E., III, 1971, Cytogenetic studies and their clinical correlates in adults with acute leukemia, *Ann. Intern. Med.* **75**:353–360.

Hayata, I., and Sasaki, M., 1976, A case of Ph[1]-positive chronic myelocytic leukemia associated with complex translocations, *Proc. Jap. Acad.* **52**:29–32.

Hayata, I., Sakurai, M., Kakati, S., and Sandberg, A. A., 1975, Chromosomes and causation of human cancer and leukemia. XVI. Banding studies of chronic myelocytic leukemia, including five unusual Ph[1] translocations, *Cancer* **36**:1177–1191.

Hayhoe, F. G. J., 1968, Clinical and cytological recognition and differentiation of the leukemia, in Proceedings, International Conference on Leukemia–Lymphoma, 1967, p. 307.

Heath, C. W., 1966, Cytogenetic observation in vitamin $B_{12}$ and folate deficiency, *Blood* **27**:800–815.

Heath, C. W., Bennett, J. M., Whang-Peng, J., Berry, E. W., and Wiernik, P. H., 1969, Cytogenetic findings in erythroleukemia, *Blood* **33**:453–467.

Hecht, F., and McCaw, B. K., 1977, Chromosome instability syndromes, *in Genetics of Human Cancer* (J. J. Mulvihill, R. W. Miller, and J. F. Fraumeni, eds.), pp. 105–123, Raven Press, New York.

Heni, F., and Siebner, H., 1964, Chromosomal abnormality and chronic lymphocytic leukaemia, *Lancet* **1**:1109.

Hennekeuser, H. H., Citoler, P., Niemczyk, H., and Gropp, A., 1970, Klinische, histologische und cytogenetische befunde bei patienten mit thorotrastschaden, *Klin. Wochenschr.* **48**:895–906.

Heston, W. E., 1976, The genetic aspects of human cancer, *Adv. Cancer Res.* **23**:1–21.

Hill, R. D., 1976, Familial cancer on a Scottish island, *Br. Med. J.* **2**:401–402.

Hilton, H. B., Lewis, I. C., and Trowell, H. R., 1970, C group trisomy in identical twins with acute leukemia, *Blood* **35**:222–226.

Hinkes, E., Crandall, B. F., Weber, F., and Craddock, C. G., 1973, Acute leukemia with C-G chromosome translocation, *Blood* **41**:259–263.

Holden, D., and Lichtman, H., 1969, Paroxysmal nocturnal hemoglobinuria with acute leukemia, *Blood* **33**:283–286.

Holden, J. D., Garcia, F. U., Samuels, M., Dupin, C., Stallworth, B., and Anderson,

E., 1971, Myelofibrosis with C monosomy of marrow elements in a child, *Am. J. Clin. Pathol.* **55**:573–579.

Hoppin, E. C., and Lewis, J. P., 1975, Polycythemia rubra vera progressing to Ph[1]-positive chronic myelogenous leukemia, *Ann. Intern. Med.* **83**:820–823.

Horland, A. A., Wolman, S. R., Distenfeld, A., and Cohen, T., 1976, Another variant translocation in chronic myelogenous leukemia, *N. Engl. J. Med.* **294**:164–165.

Hossfeld, D. K., 1975, Additional chromosomal indication for the unicellular origin of chronic myelocytic leukemia, *Z. Krebsforsch.* **83**:269–273.

Hossfeld, D. K., and Schmidt, C. G., 1973, Chromosomal data suggesting a primary role of the spleen in the pathogenesis of chronic myelocytic leukemia (CML) and blastic phase of CML, *in Chemotherapy of Cancer Dissemination and Metastasis* (S. Garattini and G. Franchi, eds.), pp. 223–234, Raven Press, New York.

Hossfeld, D. K., and Wendehorst, E., 1974, Ph[1]-negative chronic myelocytic leukemia with a missing Y chromosome, *Acta Haematol.* **52**:232–237.

Hossfeld, D. K., Han, T., Holdsworth, R. N., and Sandberg, A. A., 1971, Chromosomes and causation of human cancer and leukemia. VII. The significance of the Ph[1] in conditions other than CML, *Cancer* **27**:186–192.

Hossfeld, D. K., Schmidt, C. G., and Sandberg, A. A., 1972, Die "F"-chromosomenanomalie in Erkrankungen der erythropoetischen Systems, *Verh. Dtsch. Ges. Inn Med.* **78**:126–129.

Hossfeld, D. K., Tormey, D., and Ellison, R. R., 1975, Ph[1] positive megakaryoblastic leukemia, *Cancer* **36**:576–581.

Hsu, L. Y., Alter, A., and Hirschhorn, K., 1974, Trisomy 8 in bone marrow cells of patients with PV and myelogenous leukemia, *Clin. Genet.* **6**:258.

Humbert, J. R., Hathaway, W. E., Robinson, A., Peakman, D. C., and Githens, J. H., 1971, Pre-leukaemia in children with a missing bone marrow C chromosome and a myeloproliferative disorder, *Br. J. Haematol.* **21**:705–716.

Hungerford, D. A., and Nowell, P. C., 1962, Chromosome studies in human leukemia. III. Acute granulocytic leukemia, *J. Natl. Cancer Inst.* **29**:545–565.

Inoue, S., Ravindranath, Y., and Zuelzer, W. W., 1975, Cytogenetic analysis of erythroleukaemia in two children—Evidence of nonmalignant nature of erythron, *Scand. J. Haematol.* **14**:129–139.

Irwin, S., and Egozcue, J., 1967, Chromosomal abnormalities in leukocytes from LDS-25 users, *Science* **157**:313–314.

Ishihara, T., Kohno, S.-I., and Kumatori, T., 1974, Ph[1] translocation involving chromosomes 21 and 22, *Br. J. Cancer* **29**:340–342.

Jackson, J. R., and Higgins, L. C., Jr., 1967, Group C monosomy in myelofibrosis with myeloid metaplasia, *Arch. Intern. Med.* **119**:403–406.

Jacobs, N. F., Neu, R. L., and Gardner, L. I., 1969, Phleomycin-induced mitotic inhibition and chromosomal abnormalities in cultured human leucocytes, *Mutat. Res.* **7**:251–253.

Jacobs, P. J., Brunton, M., and Brown, W. M. C., 1964, Cytogenetic studies in leukocytes on the general population: Subjects of ages 65 years and more, *Ann. Hum. Genet.* **27**:353–365.

Jenkins, D. P., and Hartmann, R. C., 1969, Paroxysmal nocturnal hemoglobinuria terminating in acute myeloblastic leukemia, *Blood* **33**:274–282.

Jonasson, J., Gahrton, G., Lindsten, J., Simonsson-Lindemalm, C., and Zech, L., 1974, Trisomy 8 in acute myeloblastic leukemia and sideroachrestic anemia, *Blood* **43**:557–563.

Juberg, R. C., and Jones, B., 1970, The Christchurch chromosome (Gp−), *N. Engl. J. Med.* **282**:292–297.

Kaffe, S., Hsu, L. Y. F., and Hirschhorn, K., 1974, Acquired trisomies 12 and 7, *Lancet* **1**:261–262.

Kamada, N., and Uchino, H., 1967, Double Ph[1] chromosomes in leukaemia, *Lancet* **1**:1107.

Kamada, N., and Uchino, H., 1976, Preleukemic states in atomic bomb survivors in Japan, *Blood Cells* **2**:57–65.

Kamiyama, R., Shibata, T., and Mori, W., 1973, Two autopsy cases of atypical myeloproliferative disorder with group C monosomy occurring in siblings, *Acta Pathol. Jap.* **23**:815–835.

Kaneko, Y., and Sakurai, M., 1977, 15/17 translocation in acute promyelocytic leukaemia, *Lancet* **1**:961.

Kauer, G. L., and Engle, R. L., 1964, Eosinophilic leukaemia with Ph[1]-positive cells, *Lancet* **2**:1340.

Kaufmann, U., Löffler, H., Foerster, W., Desaga, J. F., and Koch, F., 1974, Fehlendes Chromosom nr. 7 in der präleukämischen Phase einer Myeloblastenleukose bei einem Kind, *Blut* **29**:50–61.

Kemp, N. H., Stafford, J. L., and Tanner, R., 1964, Chromosome studies during early and terminal chronic myeloid leukaemia, *Br. Med. J.* **1**:1010–1018.

Khan, M. H., 1972a, Heteromorphic pair of metacentric chromosomes with fused arms and the Philadelphia chromosome in a case of acute myeloid leukemia, *Acta Haematol.* **48**:312–319.

Khan, M. H., 1972b, C trisomy in bone marrow cells in a case of preleukaemic acute myelogenous leukaemia. Remarks on the karyotypic analysis and chemotherapy, *Humangenetik* **16**:323–327.

Khan, M. H., and Martin, H., 1970, Chromosomal aberrations in a case of erythroleukaemia, *Blut* **21**:29–34.

Kihlman, B. A., Nichols, W. W., and Levan, A., 1963, The effect of deoxyadenosine and cytosine arabinoside on the chromosomes of human leukocytes *in vitro*, *Hereditas* **50**:139–143.

Kiossoglou, K. A., Mitus, W. J., and Dameshek, W., 1965a, Chromosomal aberrations in acute leukemia, *Blood* **26**:610–641.

Kiossoglou, K. A., Mitus, W. J., and Dameshek, W., 1965b, Two Ph[1] chromosomes in acute granulocytic leukaemia, *Lancet* **2**:665–668.

Kiossoglou, K. A., Mitus, W. J., and Dameshek, W., 1966a, Double Ph[1] chromosomes in leukaemia, *Lancet* **2**:590–591.

Kiossoglou, K. A., Mitus, W. J., and Dameshek, W., 1966b, Cytogenetic studies in the chronic myeloproliferative syndrome, *Blood* **28**:241–251.

Kohn, G., Manny, N., Eldor, A., and Cohen, M. M., 1975, *De novo* appearance of the Ph[1] chromosome in a previously monosomic bone marrow (45,XX,−6): Conversion of a myeloproliferative disorder to acute myelogenous leukemia, *Blood* **45**:653–657.

Koulischer, L., Fruhlin, J., and Henry, J., 1967, Observations cytogénétiques dans la maladie de vaquez, *Eur. J. Cancer* **3**:193–201.

Knight, L. A., Davidson, W. M., and Cuddigan, B. J., 1974, Acquired trisomy 9, *Lancet* **1**:688.

Krauss, S., Sokal, J. E., and Sandberg, A. A., 1964, Comparison of Philadelphia chromosome-positive and -negative patients with chronic myelocytic leukemia, *Ann. Intern. Med.* **61**:625–635.

Krogh Jensen, M., 1967, Chromosome studies in acute leukaemia. III. Chromosome constitution of bone marrow cells in 30 cases, *Acta Med. Scand.* **182**:629–644.

Krogh Jensen, M., and Killmann, S., 1971, Additional evidence for chromosome abnormalities in the erythroid precursors in acute leukaemia, *Acta Med. Scand.* **189**:97–100.

Kroll, W., and Schlesinger, K., 1970, Chromosome studies in an infant with acute erythremic myelosis, *Blood* **35**:282–285.

Krompotic, E., Lewis, J. P., and Donnelly, W. J., 1968, Chromosome aberration in two patients with chronic granulocytic leukemia undergoing acute transformation, *Am. J. Clin. Pathol.* **49**:161–170.

Lampert, F., Phebus, C. K., Huhn, D., Meyer, G., and Greifenegger, M., 1972, Leukemic xanthomatosis with a missing no. 9 chromosome, *Z. Kinderheilkd.* **112**:251–260.

Lashof, J. C., and Stewart, A., 1965, Oxford survey of childhood cancers. Progress report III. Leukemia and Down's syndrome, *Mon. Bull. Minist. Health (London)* **24**:136–143.

Lawler, S. D., Millard, R. E., and Kay, H. E. M., 1970, Further cytogenetical investigations in polycythaemia vera, *Eur. J. Cancer* **6**:223–233.

Lawler, S. D., Secker Walker, L. M., Summersgill, B. M., Reeves, B. R., Lewis, J., Kay, H. E. M., and Hardisty, R. M., 1975, Chromosome banding studies in acute leukaemia at diagnosis, *Scand. J. Haematol.* **15**:312–320.

Lawrence, J. H., Low-Beer, B. V. A., and Carpender, J. W., 1949, Chronic lymphatic leukemia: A study of 100 patients treated with radioactive phosphorus, *JAMA* **140**:585–588.

Levan, A., Manolov, G., and Clifford, P., 1968, Chromosomes of a human neuroblastoma: A new case with accessory minute chromosomes, *J. Natl. Cancer Inst.* **41**:1377–1387.

Lewis, F. J. W., Poulding, R. H., and Eastham, R. D., 1963, Acute leukaemia in an XO/XXX mosaic, *Lancet* **2**:306.

Lisker, R., Cobo de Gutierrez, A., and Velazquez-Ferrari, M., 1973, Longitudinal bone marrow chromosome studies in potential leukemic myeloid disorders, *Cancer* **31**:509–515.

Littlefield, L. G., 1976, Personal communication to Rowley, J. D., and Potter, D., Chromosomal banding patterns in acute nonlymphocytic leukemia, *Blood* **47**:705–721.

Lobb, D. S., Reeves, B. R., and Lawler, S. D., 1972, Identification of isochromosome 17 in myeloid leukaemia, *Lancet* **1**:849–850.

Lortholary, P., Boiron, M., Ripault, J., Levacher, A., Mielot, T., and Bernard, J., 1966, Trois observations de transformation. Aiguë d'hémopathies lymphocytaires chroniques, *Nouv. Rev. Fr. Hematol.* **6**:637–655.

Lubs, H. A., Jr., Salmon, J. H., and Flanigan, S., 1966, Studies of a glial tumor with multiple minute chromosomes, *Cancer* **19**:591–599.

Lundh, B., Mitelman, F., Nilsson, P. G., Stenstam, M., and Söderström, N., 1975, Chromosome abnormalities identified by banding technique in a patient with acute myeloid leukaemia complicating Hodgkin's disease, *Scand. J. Haematol.* **14**:303–307.

Lundmark, K. M., Thilén, A., and Vahlquist, B., 1967, Familial leukaemia— Three cases of acute leukaemia in four siblings, *Acta Paediatr. Scand. Suppl.* **172**:200–205.

Lutzner, M. A., Emerit, I., Durepaire, R., Flandrin, G., Grupper, C., and Prunieras, M., 1973, Cytogenetic, cytophotometric and ultrastructural study of large cerebriform cells of the Sezary syndrome and description of a small-cell variant, *J. Natl. Cancer Inst.* **50**:1145–1162.

Mabry, J., Gralnick, H., and Carbone, P. P., 1976, Fourteen-year remission of acute leukemia in a patient exposed to Thorotrast, *Cancer* **38**:306–309.

MacDiarmid, W. D., 1965, Chromosomal changes following treatment of polycythemia with radioactive phosphorus, *Q. J. Med. New Ser.* **XXXIV(133)**:133–143.

Macdougall, L. G., Brown, J. A., Cohen, M. M., and Judisch, J. M., 1974, C-monosomy myeloproliferative syndrome: A case of 7-monosomy, *J. Pediatr.* **84**:256–259.

MacMahon, B., 1962, Prenatal X-ray exposure and childhood cancer, *J. Natl. Cancer Inst.* **28**:1173–1191.

MacMahon, B., and Levy, M. A., 1964, Prenatal origin of childhood leukemia; evidence from twins, *N. Engl. J. Med.* **270**:1082–1085.

Mallarme, J., 1949, Les débuts hématologiques des leucoses malignes, *Sang* **20**:429–433.

Mamunes, P., Lapidus, P. H., Abbott, J. A., and Roath, S., 1961, Acute leukaemia and Klinefelter's syndrome, *Lancet* **2**:26–27.

Mandel, E. M., Shabtai, F., Gafter, U., Klein, B., Halbrecht, I., and Djaldetti, M., 1977, Ph[1]-positive acute lymphocytic leukemia with chromosome 7 abnormalities, *Blood* **49**:281–287.

Martineau, M., 1966, A similar marker chromosome in testicular tumours, *Lancet* **1**:839–842.

Mastrangelo, R., Zuelzer, W. W., and Thompson, R. I., 1967, The significance of the Ph[1] chromosome in acute myeloblastic leukemia: Serial cytogenetic studies in a critical case, *Pediatrics* **40**:834–841.

Matsaniotis, N., Kiossoglou, K. A., Karpouzas, J., and Anastasia-Vlachou, K., 1966, Chromosomes in Kostmann's disease, *Lancet* **2**:104.

Matsunaga, M., Sadamori, N., Tomonaga, Y., Tagawa, M., and Ichimaru, M., 1976, Chronic myelogenous leukemia with an unusual karyotype: 46,XY,t(17q+;22q−), *N. Engl. J. Med.* **295**:1537.

McCaffrey, R., Harrison, T. A., Parkman, R., and Baltimore, D., 1975, Terminal deoxynucleotidyl transferase activity in human leukemic cells and normal human thymocytes, *N. Engl. J. Med.* **292**:775–780.

McCaw, B. K., Hecht, F., Harnden, D. G., and Teplitz, R. L., 1975, Somatic rearrangement of chromosome 14 in human lymphocytes, *Proc. Natl. Acad. Sci. U.S.A.* **72**:2071–2075.

McClure, P. D., Manning, M. T., and Conen, P. E., 1965, Chronic erythroleukemia with chromosome mosaicism. Report of a case in a 5-year old boy, *Arch. Intern. Med.* **115**:697–703.

Millard, R. E., Lawler, S. D., Kay, H. E. M., and Cameron, C. B., 1968, Further observations on patients with chromosomal abnormality associated with polycythaemia vera, *Br. J. Haematol.* **14**:363–374.

Miller, O. J., Breg, W. R., Schmickel, R. D., and Tretter, W., 1961, A family with an XXXXY male, a leukaemic male and two 21-trisomic mongoloid females, *Lancet* **2**:78–79.

Miller, R. W., 1964, Radiation, chromosomes and viruses in the etiology of leukemia. Evidence from epidemiologic research, *N. Engl. J. Med.* **271**:30–36.

Miller, R. W., 1966, Relation between cancer and congenital defects in man, *N. Engl. J. Med.* **275**:87–93.

Miller, R. W., 1967, Persons with exceptionally high risk of leukemia, *Cancer Res.* **27**:2420–2423.

Miller, R. W., 1970, Neoplasms and Down's syndrome, *Ann. N.Y. Acad. Sci.* **171**:637–644.

Miller, R. W., 1975, Leukemia in survivors of Wilms' tumor, *J. Pediatr.* **87**:505–506.

Mitelman, F., Brandt, L., and Nilsson, P. G., 1974, Cytogenetic evidence for splenic origin of blastic transformation in chronic myeloid leukaemia, *Scand. J. Haematol.* **13**:87–92.

Mitelman, F., Panani, A., and Brandt, L., 1975, Isochromosome 17 in a case of eosinophilic leukaemia. An abnormality common to eosinophilic and neutrophilic cells, *Scand. J. Haematol.* **14**:308–312.

Mitelman, F., Nilsson, P. G., Levan, G., and Brandt, L., 1976, Nonrandom chromosome changes in acute myeloid leukemia. Chromosome banding examination of 30 cases at diagnosis, *Int. J. Cancer* **18**:31–38.

Mitus, J., Coleman, N., and Kiossoglou, A., 1969, Abnormal (marker) chromosomes in two patients with acute myelofibrosis, *Arch. Intern. Med.* **123**:192–197.

Moake, J. L., Lebos, H., and Warren, R. J., 1974, Chromosomal abnormalities in a patient with adolescent myelofibrosis, *Acta Haematol.* **52**:173–179.

Modan, B., 1975, Interrelationship between polycythaemia vera, leukaemia and myeloid metaplasia, *Clin. Haematol.* **4**:427–439.

Modan, B., and Lilienfeld, A. M., 1965, Polycythaemia vera and leukemia—The role of radiation treatment. A study of 1222 patients, *Medicine* **44**:305–344.

Modan, B., Padeh, B., Kallner, H., Akstein, E., Meytes, D., Czerniak, P., Ramot, B., Pinkhas, J., and Modan, M., 1970, Chromosomal aberrations in polycythemia vera, *Blood* **35**:28–38.

Moore, M. A. S., Ekert, H., Fitzgerald, M. G., and Carmichael, A., 1974, Evidence for the clonal origin of chronic myeloid leukemia from a sex chromosome mosaic, *Blood* **43**:15–22.

Moorhead, P. S., Nowell, P. C., Mellman, W. J., Battips, D. M., and Hungerford, D. A., 1960, Chromosome preparations of leukocytes cultured from human peripheral blood, *Exp. Cell Res.* **20**:613–616.

Najfeld, V., 1976, Isochromosome 17 in a case of chronic erythroleukaemia, *Scand. J. Haematol.* **17**:101–104.

Nasjleti, C. E., and Spencer, H. H., 1966, Chromosome damage and polyploidization induced in human peripheral leukocytes *in vivo* and *in vitro* with nitrogen mustard, 6-mercaptopurine and A-649, *Cancer Res.* **26**:2437–2443.

Nasjleti, C. E., and Spencer, H. H., 1967, Chromosome polyploidization in human leukocyte cultures treated with streptonigrin and cyclophosphamide, *Cancer* **20**:31–35.

Newman, A. J., and Gross, S., 1967, Turner's syndrome and congenital erythroid hyperplasia, *Lancet* **1**:449.

Nicoara, S., Butoianu, E., and Brosteanu, R., 1967, Specificity of the Ph[1] chromosome, *Lancet* **2**:1312–1313.

Nowell, P. C., 1965, Prognostic value of marrow chromosome studies in human "preleukemia," *Arch. Pathol.* **80**:205–208.

Nowell, P. C., 1971, Marrow chromosome studies in "preleukemia." Further correlation with clinical course, *Cancer* **28**:513–518.

Nowell, P. C., and Hungerford, D. A., 1960, A minute chromosome in human chronic granulocytic leukemia, *Science* **132**:1497.

Nowell, P. C., and Hungerford, D. A., 1961, Chromosome studies in human leukemia. II. Chronic granulocytic leukemia, *J. Natl. Cancer Inst.* **27**:1013–1035.

Nowell, P. C., and Hungerford, D. A., 1962, Chromosome studies in human leukemia. IV. Myeloproliferative syndrome and other atypical myeloid disorders, *J. Natl. Cancer Inst.* **29**:911–919.

Nowell, P. C., Jensen, J., and Gardner, F., 1975, Two complex translocations in chronic granulocytic leukemia involving chromosomes 22, 9 and a third chromosome, *Humangenetik* **30**:13–21.

Nowell, P., Jensen, J., Gardner, F., Murphy, S., Chaganti, R. S. K., and German, J., 1976, Chromosome studies in "preleukemia" III. Myelofibrosis, *Cancer* **38**:1873–1881.

Obara, Y., Makino, S., and Sasaki, M., 1969, A chromosome survey in 50 cases of human hematopoietic disorders, *Proc. Jap. Acad.* **45**:495–500.

Odeberg, B., 1965, Eosinophilic leukemia and disseminated eosinophilic collagen disease—A distinct entity?, *Acta Med. Scand.* **177**:129–144.

Ohama, K., and Kadotani, T., 1970, Cytologic effects of bleomycin on cultured human leucocytes, *Jap. J. Hum. Genet.* **14**:293–297.

Okada, M., Miyazaki, T., and Kumota, K., 1977, 15/17 translocation in acute promyelocytic leukaemia, *Lancet* **1**:961.

Osgood, E. E., 1964, Contrasting incidence of acute monocytic and granulocytic leukemias in P[32] treated patients with polycythemia vera and chronic lymphocytic leukemia, *J. Lab. Clin. Med.* **64**:560–573.

Osgood, E. E., and Seaman, A. J., 1952, Treatment of chronic leukemias. Results of therapy by titrated, regularly spaced total body radioactive phosphorus or roentgen irradiation, *JAMA* **150**:1372–1379.

Oshimura, M., and Sandberg, A. A., 1976, Chromosomal 6q− anomaly in acute lymphoblastic leukaemia, *Lancet* **2**:1405–1406.

Oshimura, M., Hayata, I., Kakati, S., and Sandberg, A. A., 1976, Chromosomes and causation of human cancer and leukemia. XVII. Banding studies in acute myeloblastic leukemia (AML), *Cancer* **38**:748–761.

Ostertag, W., and Kersten, W., 1965, The action of proflavin and actinomycin D in causing chromatid breakage in human cells, *Exp. Cell Res.* **39**:296–301.

Pan, S. F., 1976, Personal communications to Rowley, J. D., and Potter, D., Chromosomal banding patterns in acute nonlymphocytic leukemia, *Blood* **47**:705–721.

Paris Conference (1971), 1972, Standardization in human cytogenetics, *Birth Defects, Orig. Art. Ser.* **8**:7.

Parrington, J. M., Delhanty, J. D. A., and Baden, H. P., 1971, Unscheduled DNA synthesis, U.V.-induced chromosome aberrations and $SV_{40}$ transformation in cultured cells from xeroderma pigmentosum, *Ann. Hum. Genet.* **35**:149–160.

Petit, P., Alexander, M., and Fondu, P., 1973, Monosomy 7 in erythroleukaemia, *Lancet* **2**:1326–1327.

Philip, P. E., 1975a, Trisomy 11 in acute phase of chronic myeloid leukemia, *Acta Haematol.* **54**:188–191.

Philip, P., 1975b, Trisomy 8 in acute myeloid leukaemia, *Scand. J. Haematol.* **14**:140–147.

Pierre, R. V., 1975, Cytogenetic studies in preleukemia: Studies before and after transition to acute leukemia in 17 subjects, *Blood Cells* **1**:163–170.

Pierre, R. V., and Hoagland, H. C., 1971, 45, X cell lines in adult men: Loss of Y chromosome, a normal aging phenomenon? *Mayo Clin. Proc.* **46**:52–55.

Pierre, R. V., Hoagland, H. C., and Linman, J. W., 1971, Microchromosomes in human preleukemia and leukemia, *Cancer* **27**:160–175.

Potter, A. M., Sharp, J. C., Brown, M. J., and Sokol, R. J., 1975, Structural rearrangements associated with the Ph[1] chromosome in chronic granulocytic leukaemia, *Humangenetik* **29**:223–228.

Pravtcheva, D., and Manolov, G., 1975, Genesis of the Philadelphia chromosome: Possible points of breakage in chromosome No. 22, *Hereditas* **79**:301–303.

Pravtcheva, D., Andreeva, P., and Tsaneva, R., 1976, A new translocation in chronic myelogenous leukemia, *Hum. Genet.* **32**:229–232.

Prigogina, E. L., Stravrovskaja, A. A., Kakpakova, E. S., Streljuchina, N. V., Zakharov, A. F., Lelikova, G. P., Chudina, A. P., and Pogosianz, E. E., 1970, Congenital chromosome abnormalities and leukaemia, *Lancet* **2**:524.

Propp, S., and Lizzi, F. A., 1970, Philadelphia chromosome in acute lymphocytic leukemia, *Blood* **36**:353–360.

Pruzanski, W., Platts, M. E., and Ogryzlo, M. A., 1969, Leukemic form of immunocytic dyscrasia (plasma cell leukemia), *Am. J. Med.* **47**:60–74.

Randall, D. L., Reiquam, C. W., Githens, J. H., and Robinson, A., 1965, Familial myeloproliferative disease, *Am. J. Dis. Child.* **110**:479–490.

Rastrick, J. M., Fitzgerald, P. H., and Gunz, F. W., 1968, Direct evidence for presence of Ph[1] chromosome in erythroid cells, *Br. Med. J.* **1**:96–98.

Rausen, A. R., Kim, H. J., Burstein, Y., Rand, S., McCaffrey, R. M., and Kung, P. C., 1977, Philadelphia chromosome in acute lymphatic leukaemia of childhood, *Lancet* **1**:432.

Reeves, B. R., Lobb, D. S., and Lawler, S. D., 1972, Identity of the abnormal F-group chromosome associated with polycythaemia vera, *Humangenetik* **14**:159–161.

Reisman, L. E., and Trujillo, J. M., 1963, Chronic granulocytic leukemia of childhood, *J. Pediatr.* **62**:710–723.

Reisman, L. E., Mitani, M., and Zuelzer, W. W., 1964a, Chromosome studies in leukemia. I. Evidence for the origin of leukemic stem lines from aneuploid mutants, *N. Engl. J. Med.* **270**:591–597.

Reisman, L. E., Zuelzer, W. W., and Thompson, R. I., 1964b, Further observation on the role of aneuploidy in acute leukemia, *Cancer Res.* **24**:1448–1455.

Riccardi, V. M., 1976, Trisomy 8 mosaicism in the skin of a patient with leukemia, *Birth Defects, Orig. Art. Ser.* **12**:187.

Ricci, N., Dallapiccola, B., and Preto, G., 1970, Familial transmission of a Gq− (Ph¹-like) chromosome, *Ann. Genet.* **13**:263–264.

Richmond, J. Y., and Kaufmann, B. N., 1969, Studies on busulfan (Myleran) treated leukocyte cultures, *Exp. Cell Res.* **54**:377–380.

Ross, J. D., Moloney, W. C., and Desforges, J. P., 1963, Ineffective regulation of granulopoiesis masquerading as congenital leukemia in a mongoloid child, *J. Pediatr.* **63**:1–10.

Rowley, J. D., 1973a, Deletions of chromosome 7 in haematological disorders, *Lancet* **2**:1385–1386.

Rowley, J. D., 1973b, Acquired trisomy 9, *Lancet* **2**:390.

Rowley, J. D., 1973c, A new consistent chromosomal abnormality in chronic myelogenous leukaemia identified by quinacrine fluorescence and Giemsa staining, *Nature* **243**:290–293.

Rowley, J. D., 1974, Absence of the 9q+ chromosome in Ph¹ negative chronic myelogenous leukaemia, *J. Med. Genet.* **11**:166–170.

Rowley, J. D., 1975, Nonrandom chromosomal abnormalities in hematologic disorders of man (quinacrine fluorescence/trisomy 8/leukemia), *Proc. Natl. Acad. Sci. U.S.A.* **72**:152–156.

Rowley, J. D., 1976a, Chromosomes in malignancies, in Fifth International Congress on Human Genetics, Mexico City, Excerpta Medica Foundation Series 397 (Abstract).

Rowley, J. D., 1976b, The role of cytogenetics in hematology, *Blood* **48**:1–7.

Rowley, J. D., 1976c, 5q− acute myelogenous leukemia: Reply, *Blood* **48**:626.

Rowley, J. D., and Blaisdell, R. K., 1966, Karyotype of treated thrombocythaemia, *Lancet* **2**:104–105.

Rowley, J. D., and Potter, D., 1976, Chromosomal banding patterns in acute non-lymphocytic leukemia, *Blood* **47**:705–721.

Rowley, J. D., Blaisdell, R. K., and Jacobson, L. O., 1966, Chromosome studies in preleukemia. I. Aneuploidy of group C chromosomes in three patients, *Blood* **27**:782–799.

Rowley, J. D., Golomb, H. M., and Dougherty, C., 1977, 15/17 translocation, a consistent chromosomal change in acute promyelocytic leukaemia, *Lancet* **1**:549–550.

Rozynkowa, D., and Marczak, T., 1970, Chromosomes in chronic lymphatic leukaemia: A survey of seven cases, *Genet. Pol.* **11**:415–421.

Rutten, F. J., Hustinx, T. W. J., Scheres, M. J. C., and Wagener, D. J. T., 1974, Trisomy-9 in the bone marrow of a patient with acute myelomonoblastic leukaemia, *Br. J. Haematol.* **26**:391–394.

Saffhill, R., Dexter, T. M., Muldal, S., Testa, N. G., Morris Jones, P., and Joseph,

A., 1976, Terminal deoxynucleotidyl transferase in a case of Ph[1] positive infant chronic myelogenous leukaemia, *Br. J. Cancer* **33**:664–667.

Sakurai, M., 1970a, Chromosome studies in hematological disorders. II. Chromosome findings in acute leukemia, *Acta Hematol. Jap.* **33**:116–126.

Sakurai, M., 1970b, Chromosome studies in hematological disorders. III. Chromosome findings in "preleukemia" and related diseases, *Acta Hematol. Jap.* **33**:127–136.

Sakurai, M., and Sandberg, A. A., 1976a, Chromosomes and causation of human cancer and leukemia. XI. Correlation of karyotypes with clinical features of acute myeloblastic leukemia, *Cancer* **37**:285–299.

Sakurai, M., and Sandberg, A. A., 1976b, Chromosomes and causation of human cancer and leukemia. XIII. An evaluation of karyotypic findings in erythroleukemia, *Cancer* **37**:790–804.

Sakurai, M., and Sandberg, A. A., 1976c, The chromosomes and causation of human cancer and leukemia. XVIII. The missing Y in acute myeloblastic leukemia (AML) and Ph[1]-positive chronic myelocytic leukemia (CML), *Cancer* **38**:762–769.

Sakurai, M., Oshimura, M., Kakati, S., and Sandberg, A. A., 1974, 8–21 translocation and missing sex chromosomes in acute leukaemia, *Lancet* **2**:227–228.

Sandberg, A. A., and Sakurai, M., 1973, The missing Y chromosome and human leukaemia, *Lancet* **1**:375.

Sandberg, A. A., Ishihara, T., Crosswhite, L. H., and Hauschka, T. S., 1962, Comparison of chromosome constitution in chronic myelocytic leukemia and other myeloproliferative disorders, *Blood* **20**:393–423.

Sandberg, A. A., Ishihara, T., and Crosswhite, L. H., 1964, Group C trisomy in myeloid metaplasia with possible leukemia, *Blood* **24**:716–725.

Sandberg, A. A., Takagi, N., Sofuni, T., and Crosswhite, L. H., 1968, Chromosomes and causation of human cancer and leukemia. V. Karyotypic aspects of acute leukemia, *Cancer* **22**:1268–1282.

Sandberg, A. A., Hossfeld, D. K., Ezdinli, E. Z., and Crosswhite, L. H., 1971, Chromosomes and causation of human cancer and leukemia. VI. Blastic phase, cellular origin, and the Ph[1] in CML, *Cancer* **27**:176–185.

Schade, H., Schoeller, L., and Schultze, K. W., 1962, D-Trisomié (Pätau-syndrom) mit kongenitaler myeloischer Leukämie, *Med. Welt* **50**:2690–2692.

Schmidt, R., Dar, H., Santorineou, M., and Sekine, I., 1975, Ph[1] chromosome and loss and reappearance of the Y chromosome in acute lymphocytic leukaemia, *Lancet* **1**:1145.

Schroeder, T. M., and Kurth, R., 1971, Spontaneous chromosomal breakage and high incidence of leukemia in inherited disease, *Blood* **37**:96–112.

Schunk, G. J., and Lehman, W. L., 1954, Mongolism and the congenital leukemia, *JAMA* **155**:250–251.

Seabright, M., 1971, A rapid banding technique for human chromosomes, *Lancet* **2**:971–972.

Secker-Walker, L. M., and Hardy, J. D., 1976, Philadelphia chromosome in acute leukemia, Case report, *Cancer* **38**:1619–1624.

Secker-Walker, L. M., Summersgill, B. M., Swansbury, G. J., Lawler, S. D., Chessells, J. M., and Hardisty, R. M., 1976, Philadelphia positive blast crisis masquerading as acute lymphoblastic leukaemia in children, *Lancet* **2**:1045.

Seif, G. S. F., and Spriggs, A. I., 1967, Chromosome changes in Hodgkin's disease, *J. Natl. Cancer Inst.* **39**:557–570.

Sézary, A., and Bouvrain, Y., 1938, Erythrodermie avec presénce de cellules monstrueuses dans le derme et le sang circulant, *Bull. Soc. Fr. Dermatol. Syphiligr.* **45**:254–260.

Sharp, J. C., Potter, A. M., and Guyer, R. J., 1973, Chromosome changes in congenital lymphoblastic leukaemia, *Lancet* **2**:1448.

Shatkin, A. J., Reich, E., Franklin, R. M., and Tatum, E. L., 1962, Effect of mitomycin C on mammalian cells in culture, *Biochim. Biophys. Acta* **55**:277–289.

Shaw, M. W., 1962, Familial mongolism, *Cytogenetics* **1**:141–179.

Shaw, M. W., 1970, Human chromosome damage by chemical agents, *Annu. Rev. Med.* **21**:409–432.

Shiffman, N. J., Stecker, E., Conen, P. E., and Gardner, H. A., 1974, Males with chronic myeloid leukemia and the 45,XO,Ph[1] chromosome pattern, *Can. Med. Assoc. J.* **110**:1151–1154.

Shiraishi, Y., Hayata, I., Sakurai, M., and Sandberg, A. A., 1975, Chromosomes and causation of human cancer and leukemia. XII. Banding analysis of abnormal chromosomes in polycythemia vera, *Cancer* **36**:199–202.

Sieber, S. M., and Adamson, R. H., 1975, The clastogenic, mutagenic, teratogenic and carcinogenic effects of various antineoplastic agents, *in Pharmacological Basis of Cancer Chemotherapy, Twenty-Seventh Annual Symposium of the Fundamental Cancer Research, Houston, 1974*, pp. 401–468. Williams & Wilkins, Baltimore.

Siegal, F. P., Voss, R., Al-Mondhiry, H., Polliack, A., Hansen, J. A., Siegal, M., and Good, R. A., 1976, Association of a chromosomal abnormality with lymphocytes having both T and B markers in a patient with lymphoproliferative disease, *Am. J. Med.* **60**:157–166.

Silver, H. K., Blair, W. C., and Kempe, C. H., 1952, Fanconi's syndrome: Multiple congenital anomalies with hypoplastic anaemia, *Am. J. Dis. Child.* **83**:14–25.

Sokal, G., Michaux, J. L., van den Berghe, H., Cordier, A., Rodhain, J., Ferrant, A., Moriau, M., De Bruyere, M., and Sonnet, J., 1975, A new hematologic syndrome with a distinct karyotype: The 5q– chromosome, *Blood* **46**:519–533.

Sonta, S., and Sandberg, A. A., 1977, A new complex Ph[1] translocation involving three chromosomes: Brief communication, *J. Natl. Cancer Inst.* **58**:1583–1585.

Spiers, A. S. D., and Baikie, A. G., 1968, Cytogenetic studies in the malignant lymphomas and related neoplasms. Results in twenty-seven cases, *Cancer* **22**:193–217.

Spitzer, G., and Garson, O. M., 1973, Lymphoblastic leukemia with marked eosinophilia. A report of two cases, *Blood* **42**:377–384.

Spriggs, A. I., Boddington, M. M., and Clarke, C. M., 1962, Chromosomes of human cancer cells, *Br. Med. J.* **2**:1431–1435.

Spriggs, A. I., Holt, J. M., and Bedford, J., 1976, Duplication of part of the long arm of chromosome 1 in marrow cells of treated case of myelomatosis, *Blood* **48**:595–599.

Stevenson, A. C., and Patel, C. R., 1973, Effects of chlorambucil on human chromosomes, *Mutat. Res.* **18**:333–351.

Stevenson, A. C., San Roman, C., and Patel, C. R., 1973, Effects of amylobarbitone on the frequency of chromosomal aberrations in human lymphocytes determined by chlorambucil and melphalan *in vitro, Mutat. Res.* **19**:225–229.

Teasdale, J. M., Worth, A. J., and Corey, M. J., 1970, A missing group C chromosome in the bone marrow cells of three children with myeloproliferative disease, *Cancer* **25**:1468–1477.

Thomas, E. D., Bryant, J. I., Buckner, C. D., Clift, R. A., Fefer, A., Johnson, F. L., Neiman, P., Ramberg, R. E., and Storb, R., 1972, Leukaemic transformation of engrafted human marrow cells *in vivo, Lancet* **1**:1310–1313.

Tjio, J. H., and Whang, J., 1962, Chromosome preparations of bone marrow cells without prior *in vitro* culture or *in vivo* colchicine administration, *Stain Technol.* **37**:17–20.

Todd, A. S., Wood, S. M., Robertson, J., and Brown, R. A. G., 1969, A case of leukaemia showing mixed myeloid-lymphoid characteristics and an unusual chromosome pattern, *J. Clin. Pathol.* **22**:743 (Abstract).

Tough, I. M., Court Brown, W. M., Baikie, A. G., Buckton, K. E., Harnden, D. G., Jacobs, P. A., King, M. J., and McBride, J. A., 1961, Cytogenetic studies in chronic myeloid leukaemia and acute leukaemia associated with mongolism, *Lancet* **1**:411–417.

Trübestein, G. K., and Citoler, P., 1973, Drei Falle von Thorotrast-spätschäden, *Med. Klin.* **68**:1442–1447.

Trujillo, J. M., Cork, A., Drewinko, B., Hart, J. S., and Freireich, E. J., 1971, Case report: Tetraploid leukemia, *Blood* **38**:632–637.

Tso, S. C., and Chan, T. K., 1973, Paroxysmal nocturnal haemoglobinuria and chronic myeloid leukaemia in the same patient, *Scand. J. Haematol.* **10**:384–389.

Tsuchimoto, T., Ishii, Y., Uchino, H., and Inoue, S., 1970, Paroxysmal nocturnal haemoglobinuria with chromosome abnormalities: Possible preleukaemia, *Lancet* **1**:617–618.

Tsuchimoto, T., Bühler, E. M., Stalder, G. R., Mayr, A. C., and Obrecht, J. P., 1974, Deletion of chromosome 7 in polycythaemia vera, *Lancet* **1**:566.

van Biervliet, J. P., van Hemel, J., Geurts, K., Punt, K., and De Boer-Van Wering, E., 1975, Philadelphia chromosome in acute lymphocytic leukaemia, *Lancet* **2**:617.

van den Berghe, H., 1976, Personal communications to Rowley, J. D., and Potter, D., Chromosomal banding patterns in acute nonlymphocytic leukemia, *Blood* **47**:705–721.

van den Berghe, H., Fryns, J. P., and Verresen, H., 1972, Congenital leukaemia with 46,XX,t(Bq+,Cq−) cells, *J. Med. Genet.* **9**:468–470.

van den Berghe, H., Cassiman, J. J., and David, G., 1974, Distinct haematological disorder with deletion of long arm of No. 5 chromosome, *Nature* **251**:437–438.

Van De Sande, J. H., Lin, C. C., and Jorgenson, K. F., 1977, Reverse banding on chromosomes produced by a guanosine-cytosine specific DNA binding antibiotic: Olivomycin, *Science* **195**:400–402.

Van Slyck, E. J., Weiss, L., and Dully, M., 1970, Chromosomal evidence for the secondary role of fibroblastic proliferation in acute myelofibrosis, *Blood* **36**:729–735.

vanZyl, J., and Wissmüller, H. F., 1974, The clastogenic effect of azathioprine on human chromosomes *in vitro*, *Humangenetik* **21**:153–165.

Vass, L., and Sellyei, M., 1973, The missing Y chromosome and human leukaemia, *Lancet* **1**:550–551.

Verhest, A., and van Schoubroeck, F., 1973, Philadelphia-chromosome-positive preleukaemic state, *Lancet* **2**:1386.

Verhest, A., Van Schoubroeck, F., Wittek, M., Naets, J. P., and Denolin-Reubens, R., 1976, Specificity of the 5q− chromosome in a distinct type of refractory anemia, *J. Natl. Cancer Inst.* **56**:1053–1054.

Vig, B. K., 1971, Chromosome aberrations induced in human leukocytes by the antileukemic antibiotic adriamycin, *Cancer Res.* **31**:32–38.

Vigliani, E. C., and Forni, A., 1976, Benzene and leukemia, *Environ. Res.* **11**:122–127.

Visfeldt, J., 1971, Primary polycythaemia 2. Types of chromosome aberrations in 21 clones found in bone marrow samples from 50 patients, *Acta Pathol. Microbiol. Scand., Sect. A* **79**:513–523.

Visfeldt, J., Jensen, G., and Hippe, E., 1975, On Thorotrast leucaemia. Evolution of clone of bone marrow cells with radiation-induced chromosome aberrations, *Acta Pathol. Microbiol. Scand., Sect. A* **83**:373–378.

Voorhees, J. J., Janzen, M. K., Harrell, E. R., and Chakrabarti, S. G., 1969, Cytogenetic evaluation of methotrexate-treated psoriatic patients, *Arch. Dermatol.* **100**:269–274.

Wagner, H. P., Tönz, O., and v. Greyerz-Gloor, R. D., 1968, Congenital lymphoid leukaemia. Case report with chromosomal studies, *Helv. Paediatr. Acta* **23**:591–610.

Wald, N., Borges, W. H., Li, C. C., Turner, J. H., and Harnois, M. C., 1961, Leukaemia associated with mongolism, *Lancet* **1**:1228.

Weiner, L., 1965, A family with high incidence leukemia and unique Ph¹ chromosome findings, *Blood* **26**:871 (abstract).

Wertelecki, W., and Shapiro, J. R., 1970, 45,XO Turner's syndrome and leukaemia, *Lancet* **1**:789–790.

Westin, J., 1976, Chromosome abnormalities after chlorambucil therapy of polycythaemia vera, *Scand. J. Haematol.* **17**:197–204.

Westin, J., Wahlström, J., and Swolin, B., 1976, Chromosome studies in untreated polycythaemia vera, *Scand. J. Haematol.* **17**:183–196.

Whang, J., Frei, E., Tjio, J. H., Carbone, P. P., and Brecher, G., 1963, The distribution of the Philadelphia chromosome in patients with chronic myelogenous leukemia, *Blood* **22**:664–673.

Whang-Peng, J., Canellos, G. P., Carbone, P. P., and Tjio, J. H., 1968, Clinical implications of cytogenetic variants in chronic myelocytic leukemia (CML), *Blood* **32**:755–766.

Whang-Peng, J., Leventhal, B. G., Adamson, J. W., and Perry, S., 1969, The effect of daunomycin on human cells *in vivo* and *in vitro*, *Cancer* **23**:113–121.

Whang-Peng, J., Henderson, E. S., Knutsen, T., Freireich, E. J., and Gart, J. J., 1970, Cytogenetic studies in acute myelocytic leukemia with special emphasis on the occurrence of Ph¹ chromosome, *Blood* **36**:448–457.

Whang-Peng, J., Perry, S., Knutsen, T. A., and Gart, J. J., 1971, Cell cycle characteristics, maturation, and phagocytosis *in vitro* of blast cells from patients with chronic myelocytic leukemia, *Blood* **38**:153–161.

Whang-Peng, J., Knutsen, T. A., and Lee, E. C., 1973, Dicentric Ph[1] chromosome, *J. Natl. Cancer Inst.* **51**:2009–2012.

Whang-Peng, J., Lee, E. C., and Knutsen, T. A., 1974a, Genesis of the Ph[1] chromosome, *J. Natl. Cancer Inst.* **52**:1035.

Whang-Peng, J., Gralnick, H. R., Johnson, R. E., Lee, E. C., and Lear, A., 1974b, Chronic granulocytic leukemia (CGL) during the course of chronic lymphocytic leukemia (CLL): Correlation of blood, marrow, and spleen morphology and cytogenetics, *Blood* **43**:333–339.

Whang-Peng, J., Knutsen, T., Ziegler, J., and Leventhal, B., 1976a, Cytogenetic studies in acute lymphocytic leukemia: Special emphasis in long-term survival, *Med. Ped. Oncol.* **2**:333–351.

Whang-Peng, J., Lutzner, M., Edelson, R., and Knutsen, T., 1976b, Cytogenetic studies and clinical implications in patients with Sézary syndrome, *Cancer* **38**:861–867.

Whang-Peng, J., Knutsen, T., Lee, E. C., and Leventhal, B., 1976c, Acquired XO/XY clones in bone marrow of a patient with paroxysmal nocturnal hemoglobinuria (PNH), *Blood* **47**:611–619.

Whang-Peng, J., Broder, S., Lee, E., and Young, R. C., 1976d, Unusual clonal evolution in a case of chronic myelogenous leukemia, *Acta Haematol.* **56**:345–354.

Whang-Peng, J., Gralnick, H. R., Knutsen, T., Brereton, H., Chang, P., Schechter, G. P., and Lessin, L., 1977, Small F chromosome in myelo- and lymphoproliferative diseases, *Leukemia Res.* **1**:19–30.

Whang-Peng, J., Lee, E., Knutsen, T., Chang, P., and Nienhuis, A., Cytogenetic studies in patients with myelofibrosis and myeloid metaplasia, *Leukemia Res.*, in press.

Woodliff, H. J., Chipper, L., and Gallon, W., 1975, Cytogenetic studies in myelofibrosis. Experience in Western Australia, 1963–1970, *Med. J. Aust.* **1**:1075–1078.

Wurster-Hill, D. H., McIntyre, O. R., Cornwell, G. G., III, and Maurer, L. H., 1973, Marker-chromosome 14 in multiple myeloma and plasma-cell leukaemia, *Lancet* **2**:1031.

Wurster-Hill, D., Whang-Peng, J., McIntyre, O. R., Hsu, L. Y. F., Hirschhorn, K., Modan, B., Pisciotta, A. V., Pierre, R., Balcerzak, S. P., Weinfeld, A., and Murphy, S., 1976, Cytogenetic studies in polycythemia vera, *Semin. Hematol.* **13**:13–32.

Yamada, K., and Furnsawa, S., 1976, Preferential involvement of chromosomes no. 8 and no. 21 in acute leukemia and preleukemia, *Blood* **47**:679–686.

Zech, L., Gahrton, C., Killander, D., Franzen, S., and Haglund, U., 1976, Specific chromosomal aberrations in polycythemia vera, *Blood* **48**:687–696.

Zuelzer, W. W., Thompson, R. I., and Mastrangelo, R., 1968, Evidence for a genetic factor related to leukemogenesis and congenital anomalies: Chromosomal aberrations in pedigree of an infant with partial D trisomy and leukemia, *J. Pediatr.* **72**:367–376.

Zussman, W. V., Khan, A., and Shayesteh, P., 1967, Congenital leukemia. Report of a case with chromosome abnormalities, *Cancer* **20**:1227–1233.

# Leukemia Antigens

## Brigid G. Leventhal and Michael Weiner

## 12.1. Introduction

Tumor-specific antigens appear to exist in animal systems and these antigens can be exploited as targets for immunoprophylaxis and immunotherapy in these model systems. The majority of antigens which have been recently detected on the surface of leukemia cells in man appear, however, to be shared with normal human cells. For example, antigens have been described by several authors (Humphrey and Lankford, 1976; Brown and Greaves, 1974, Borella *et al.*, 1977) which appear to be shared with normal T-lymphocytes and thymocytes. Other antigens shared with B-lymphocytes have also been described (Billing *et al.*, 1977; Fu *et al.*, 1975). Nuclear antigens that appear to be proliferation-associated are reported (Klein *et al.*, 1974; Steiner *et al.*, 1975; Russell and Pope, 1976). Tumor cell products such as monoclonal immunoglobulins in chronic lymphocytic leukemia (Preud'homme and Seligmann, 1972) may also serve as antigenic markers. Some antisera raised to viral antigens react with leukemia cells as well. Finally, some of the sophisticated studies by Metzgar and Mohanakumar (1978) with antisera raised in nonhuman primates, by Greaves *et al.* (1975) with antisera raised in rabbits after the normal antigens on the immunizing leukemia cells have been coated with antisera, or by Baker and Taub (1973) in mice rendered tolerant to remission cells prior to immunization suggest that antigens are present on

---

BRIGID G. LEVENTHAL and MICHAEL WEINER  •  The Oncology Center, Johns Hopkins Hospital, Baltimore, Maryland.

human leukemia cells which have not yet been detected on normal cells. In this chapter we will discuss some of the antigens that are shared with normal cells since they may be considered tumor-associated antigens, as well as the possible tumor-specific antigens which are still being characterized.

## 12.2. T Cell Antigens

The ability to form spontaneous rosettes with sheep erythrocytes (E-rosettes) is a function of the majority of circulating thymus-derived (T) lymphocytes in man. Many workers have now described E-rosette-forming lymphatic leukemia cells, and in a recent review (Humphrey and Lankford, 1976) this type of leukemia was estimated to represent 15–25% of childhood cases.

### 12.2.1. Serologic Studies

Antisera have been raised against thymocytes (Kersey *et al.*, 1973), E-rosette positive ALL (Borella *et al.*, 1977), or lymphosarcoma (Metzgar and Mohanakumar, 1978) as well as T cell tissue culture cell lines (Kaplan *et al.*, 1976) and human brain (Brown and Greaves, 1974) which appear to detect antigens present on thymocytes that are shared with E+ leukemia and lymphoma cells. Thus there appears to be no question that the E+ ALL blasts express T cell antigens while leukemic-associated antigens that are detected in sera active against E− leukemic cells may not be present at all on the E+ cells or are buried in the cell membrane under other cell surface antigens (Greaves *et al.*, 1975; Borella *et al.*, 1977).

An antigen common to human thymocytes and acute leukemia cells has been described in an extract of thymic cells, and has been termed HThyL. Rabbit antisera to this antigen reacted with circulating antigen in sera from four patients with untreated E-rosette positive ALL and one patient with previously treated AML. This antigen was not present in 21 patients with E-rosette negative ALL nor seven other patients with AML. The antigen disappeared from the circulation as the percentage of blast cells in the peripheral blood decreased with treatment (Chechik and Gelfand, 1977).

### 12.2.2. Cellular Reactivity

E-rosette-forming lymphoblasts have been studied for their capacity to stimulate in mixed leukocyte culture, and in two separate studies (Tsukimoto *et al.*, 1976; Leventhal *et al.*, 1977) have been shown to lack the capacity to stimulate even allogeneic donors. This is a property which they share with normal human T cells (Lohrmann *et al.*, 1974) and with T cell tissue culture cell lines (Han and Minowada, 1973). This characteristic, however, makes it difficult to evaluate the antigens on their surface by the study of cellular reactivity *in vitro*.

Skin tests with purified membrane antigens from patients with acute lymphatic leukemia have shown positive reactions in ALL patients whose leukemia cells were not classified as E+ or E−. Using similar extraction procedures antigen which appears to be identical has been identified from early human fetal thymus cells. ALL and AML antigens did not cross-react in allogeneic skin tests of both types of leukemia in this study. The clinical significance of these observations awaits clarification (Hollinshead and Herberman, 1975).

It will be of great interest to further subdivide the T lymphoblasts by their functional characteristics. Leukemia cells with *in vitro* suppressor activity have been described (Broder *et al.*, 1978). In addition, T lymphoblasts may react with sera raised against T cell differentiation antigens (Evans *et al.*, 1977). Lymphoblasts with T cell characteristics connote an extremely poor prognosis. The poor response of this group of patients to conventional antileukemia therapy makes their identification essential so that experimental therapy can be employed early in the course of their disease.

## 12.3. B Cell Antigens

Recently, typing sera have been developed which detect new specificities not previously detected serologically (Wernet *et al.*, 1975; Mann *et al.*, 1975; van Rood *et al.*, 1975; Winchester *et al.*, 1975) and which are clearly different from the three previously described SD loci, LA, AJ, and FOUR. These sera appear to react with normal B-lymphocytes rather than with T-lymphocytes. There is speculation that these antisera may be reacting to antigens similar to the Ia antigens in the mouse (Bach and van Rood, 1976). In addition, these "anti-B" sera have recently been reported to react with acute and chronic leukemia cells both of the lymphocytic and the myelogenous variety (Billing *et al.*, 1976b, 1977; Fu *et al.*, 1975). This result was not surprising for chronic lymphatic leukemia since this has been known for some time to be a malignancy of B cell origin which, in general, produces a monoclonal immunoglobulin (Preud'homme and Seligmann, 1972; Seligmann *et al.*, 1973) although an occasional case of polyclonal immunoglobulin production has been reported (Seligmann *et al.*, 1973); however, the other malignancies are not thought to be of B cell origin.

Rabbit antisera raised against B cell lymphoma tissue culture cell lines had been shown to be generally reactive to acute leukemia cells in both cytotoxic (Mann *et al.*, 1975; Billing *et al.*, 1977) and lymphocyte-dependent (Durantez *et al.*, 1975) antibody assay systems. These sera were originally tested against normal human leukocytes and found to be non-reactive. However, the normal peripheral blood in man usually contains less than 20% B lymphocytes and it may well be that reactivity against this small percentage of cells was considered background reactivity. Now that techniques are available for B cell enrichment at least one of these sera (Billing *et al.*, 1977) has been reported to be reactive with normal human B cells.

When the Fab fragment of this antiserum was used to block reactivity of human anti-B cell sera, however, it was found to show a generalized reactivity with all leukemia cells while the human anti-B cell sera reacted in a more specific pattern with the cells (Billing *et al.*, 1977). These and studies showing that anti-B cell sera are generally inhibitory in mixed leukocyte culture suggest that the rabbit antisera were reacting with a common portion of the Ia-like molecules on the surface of the leukemia cells rather than the alloantigenic determinant (Cresswell and Geier, 1975; Winchester *et al.*, 1976).

It is of interest that when human anti-B sera were used to "type" leukemic blast cells, one of the specificities detected on normal human lymphocytes was absent from the leukemic cells. Comparative typing of patients in remission has not been performed to allow the complete evaluation of these data (Billing *et al.*, 1976a).

It has been known for some time that a person would react in *in vitro* mixed leukocyte culture (MLC) to a tissue culture cell line started from his own cells. These cell lines are usually of B cell origin (Green and Sell, 1970; Ling, 1973). Reactivity to T cell lines can be elicited either not at all (Han and Minowada, 1973; Royston *et al.*, 1974) or only when extremely high concentrations of stimulating cells are used (Callewaert *et al.*, 1975). In addition, Opelz *et al.* (1975) have stated that if normal B and T cells are separated, a response of autologous T cells to autologous B cells can be seen in the MLC. The concordance of these observations has placed in doubt the interpretation of the positive MLC reaction of patients to autologous leukemic cells which has been seen by a number of authors (Powles *et al.*, 1971; Gutterman *et al.*, 1972; Leventhal *et al.*, 1972; Viza *et al.*, 1969; Fridman and Kourilsky, 1969) as an indication of the presence of leukemia-associated antigens on the surface of these cells and has forced people to wonder whether this autologous reactivity might represent a response only to the "B cell antigens" on the surface of the leukemia cells.

## 12.4. Proliferation and Fetal Antigens

In 1974 Klein and co-workers reported that sera from 73% of AML patients reacted with the nuclei of fixed myeloblasts when tested by anticomplement immunofluorescence whereas only 10–30% of patients with other leukemias and only occasional normal controls were positive. This reactivity was tentatively designated LANA, for leukemia-associated nuclear antigen, and was clearly distinct from the EBNA or EB virus-associated nuclear antigens which could be detected in nuclei from Burkitt lymphoma cell lines. Further studies by Steiner *et al.* (1975) showed that this antibody was reactive against PHA-stimulated blast cells and T-derived tissue culture cell lines but not against normal lymphocytes. These authors feel therefore that this antigen represents a proliferation-associated antigen. Russell and Pope (1976) confirmed these results and showed that in general nuclear antigen was detected in cell populations reported to have increased levels of DNA synthesis including those from patients with infectious mononucleosis or lymphoproliferative neoplasms as well as leukemia. However, the percentage of antigen positive cells (e.g., 11–70% in AML) in smears in their study was generally higher than the percentage of cells reported by others to be actively synthesizing DNA (0.2–11% in AML) (Clarkson *et al.*, 1965). Reactive sera therefore seemed to be detecting a nuclear component in cells capable of proliferating or possibly cells with a recent history of proliferation. It remains to be determined whether the nuclear antigen in cell lines, normal PHA-transformed blasts, and leukemic cells is identical and why antibodies to it are produced more commonly in myeloblastic leukemias than in other proliferative diseases. This may perhaps be a reflection of the general hyperreactivity of the humoral system that has been seen by several workers in acute myelogenous leukemia (Leventhal *et al.*, 1978).

Harris *et al.* (1971) have suggested the presence of fetal antigen on human leukemic cells as determined by immunological criteria. Bentwich *et al.* (1972) have found that antigens on the surface of CLL cells were shared with newborn lymphocytes but not normal adult lymphoid cells. Granatek *et al.* (1976) immunized BALB/c male mice with human peripheral leukemic blasts and found that these immunizations effectively reduced the later formation of syngeneic fetal liver but not bone marrow hematopoietic colonies in the spleen when these mice were lethally irradiated and challenged intravenously. They felt that this demonstrated the existence of fetal antigen on the immunizing cells. Fetal antigen was detected in 6/6 lymphocytic leukemic patients and 4/8 myelocytic leukemia patients and was correlated with low levels of sialic acid. A rabbit antiserum to BALB/c 15-day fetal liver cells labeled only 0–2% of normal donor peripheral leukocytes in indirect immunofluorescence but reacted with 10–21% of leukemic peripheral blasts and 44% of cells in one relapse bone marrow. These data suggest that there was cross-reactivity of murine and human fetal antigens and that the antigens are expressed on the surface of the leukemia cells.

## 12.5. Leukemia-Associated Antigens

Now that it has been demonstrated that a number of antigens originally thought to be leukemia associated or leukemia specific are shared with normal tissue components, it is time to ask whether there is evidence that leukemia-associated antigens exist which cannot currently be explained away as other than leukemia antigens. Autoantibodies to acute leukemia have been described by several authors and the subject has recently been reviewed (Metzgar and Mohanakumar, 1978). The difficulty with most of these studies has been the inability to prove conclusively the leukemia specificity of the autoantibodies by rigorously controlling for the other antigenic specificities now known to exist on these cells.

However, a few carefully performed experiments deserve mention in this category. Recent studies by Baker and Taub (1973) (see also Baker *et al.*, 1974) describe the production of potent murine antisera against human acute myeloblastic leukemia cell antigens in animals previously rendered tolerant to remission peripheral blood cells from the blast cell donor. Tolerance was achieved by injection of remission lymphocytes from the patient whose leukemia cells were later used as immunogens followed by large doses of cyclophosphamide. The mouse antisera to AML and ALL cells reacted by direct testing with both AML and ALL blasts although after absorption a differential cytotoxic effect could be noted. This differential cytotoxicity of myeloblasts and lymphoblasts cannot be readily explained by our current knowledge of human Ia-like antigen distribution.

Greaves and co-workers (1975) raised antisera to acute lymphoblastic leukemia cells in rabbits by injecting ALL cells coated *in vitro* with rabbit antibodies directed against normal lymphocyte antigens. The resultant antisera were absorbed with various normal tissues. Reactive cells were found in 14/19 ALL patients at presentation. Three of the five nonreactive cases were T cell leukemias. There was weak reactivity against a proportion of cases with AML but this reactivity of myeloid leukemic cells could be abolished by absorption with leukemic myeloblasts, leaving ALL reactivity intact. These sera were not reactive with cells from six patients with CLL, thus again making it unlikely that reactivity to Ia-like antigens could explain all of the reactivity seen in these sera.

Metzgar and Mohanakumar (1978) have recently reviewed their work in immunizing nonhuman primates with leukemia cells. In their studies (Metzgar *et al.*, 1972) cytotoxic antisera raised in monkeys against leukemic peripheral blood cells from individual patients with CLL, AML, and CML were able, after appropriate absorptions, to detect antigens specific for either lymphocytic leukemia or certain myeloid leukemia cells. That is, absorption of chimpanzee antiserum to CLL cells with AML or CML cells did not alter its reactivity with CLL test cells and, similarly, absorption of monkey antiserum to AML with cells from any CLL donor or with cells from certain CML donors did not affect the cytotoxic activity for AML target cells. These data again would be difficult to explain if only a common antigen is being detected on all leukemia cells. The current state of the serologic detection of leukemia-associated antigens would seem then to suggest, not surprisingly, that antisera raised in species which are genetically widely distant from man are likely to detect common antigens in all leukemia cells. If these normal, perhaps stronger, antigens are covered up with antisera, or if the animal is rendered tolerant to these antigens, then specific reactivity to leukemia antigens *per se* may be detected. Antisera raised in genetically closer species such as the nonhuman primates are currently detecting antigenic patterns which may also be leukemia associated. The studies of cellular reactivity to leukemia antigens, although of great interest, do not permit as precise a characterization of the antigens involved since they are currently performed, in general, with whole cells or crude extracts. This subject has recently been reviewed (Leventhal *et al.*, 1978). Studies with more purified antigens as these become available will be of great interest.

## 12.6. Viral Antigens

There are three groups of viruses that have been implicated as oncogenic agents in animals: DNA herpes viruses, type B RNA mammary tumor viruses and type C RNA viruses (Levine, 1976). However, only the type C RNA viruses have been associated with leukemia antigens.

The type C RNA virus-induced tumors have three major groups of antigens: (1) viral antigens as virus components themselves; (2) virus-associated antigens as viral genome-coded antigens; (3) tumor-specific antigens as cellular genome-coded antigens acquired by malignant transformation. The RNA tumor viruses can incorporate viral genetic material into the genome of the host cell with or without subsequent virus production and with or without cell transformation.

Six to seven proteins with a variable spectrum of antigenic determinants have been identified in mammalian viruses and are to be considered major components (Aoki and Sibal, 1976). In the type C RNA viral system there are two antigens which make up the virion particle. One is the primary virion envelope antigen gp 70/71, a glycoprotein with a molecular weight of approximately 70,000 daltons. The other is the major internal core protein, p 30, with an approximate molecular weight of 30,000 daltons (Ikeda *et al.*, 1974; Kennel *et al.*, 1973). Immunofluorescent and virus neutralization tests have shown that these determinants are located in the cytoplasm and probably on the cell surface, as well as on the viral envelope (Ikeda *et al.*, 1974). The discovery of antigens on the cell surface secondary to oncogenic virus infection is important for three reasons: (1) their location on the surface makes them potential targets for host immune defenses; (2) they may serve as markers for the presence of the viral genome; (3) they may be responsible for changes in membrane properties which lead to altered behavior of transformed cells. Glycoprotein 70/71 is a virus gene product expressed on the surface of transformed cells, and antisera directed against gp 70/71 have virus neutralizing activity. Cell surface determinants resembling gp 70/71 have been identified in leukemic and nonmalignant lymphocytes in the murine system and in normal and neoplastic human cells. Hollis *et al.* (1974) have shown that in the murine system antibodies to internal core (p 30) and envelope (gp 70/71) components of type C viruses are present in the sera and antigen–antibody complexes are present in the renal glomeruli. Likewise, antibodies to determinants of p 30 occur in sera or in renal eluates of not only mice but patients with cancer (Charman *et al.*, 1974). Antisera to gp 70/71 and p 30 are cytotoxic for some animal cells which express these antigens on their surface (Grant *et al.*, 1974).

Fink *et al.* in 1964 demonstrated that cross-reactivity existed between leukemia cells and a laboratory strain of RNA leukemia virus. Fink and her group also demonstrated that some patients with acute leukemia possess antibodies that have neutralizing activity against Rauscher leukemia virus (RLV) (Fink *et al.*, 1965). In another study the same investigators isolated an antibody in the sera of patients with erythroleukemia to the RLV envelope antigen (Fink and Cowles, 1965). Biochemical studies have continued to suggest that this cross-reactivity exists (Hehlmann *et al.*, 1972). Ioannides *et al.* (1968) demonstrated immunologically that human leukemia imprints from bone marrow, liver, kidney, and spleen reacted with fluorescein-tagged monkey antisera prepared against murine RLV.

Metzgar and his colleagues (1975) demonstrated that antigenic relationships exist between mouse Friend leukemia virus (FLV) and cells from human patients with myeloid leukemia. These authors prepared rabbit antisera to structural components and membrane antigens of the virus and noted cytotoxic reactions with human myeloblasts. In addition, the FLV antigens absorbed the cytotoxic antibody activity of nonhuman

primate antisera to human myeloid leukemia cells. These antigenic relationships between RNA tumor viruses and human leukemia-associated
antigens exist in other systems as well as the FLV–myeloid leukemia
reactions. For example, cross-reactivity was observed between goat antisera to feline leukemia virus (FeLV) and gibbon ape leukemia virus
(GALV) and human cells from patients with CLL and ALL (Metzgar *et al.*,
1975). Metzgar *et al.* (1975) subsequently showed that it was antisera
prepared against the virion molecular determinants of gp 70/71 and p 30
from the FLV that reacted with the cells from patients with AML and
CML. The data are not conclusive that human AML or CML is caused by
an RNA oncogenic virus. However, it does show that at least two membrane antigens on myeloid leukemia cells cross-react with the well-established gp 70/71 and p 30 components of FLV (Metzgar *et al.*, 1976).

Shew and Todaro (1975) used a radioimmunoassay to detect antigens
related to the major structural protein, p 30, of the type C RNA viruses.
These authors demonstrated that peripheral blood leukocytes from five
patients with acute leukemia possessed antigens related to the p 30
proteins of the woolly monkey simian sarcoma type C virus (SSAV) and
the GALV. This finding suggests that viruses of this group known to be
infectious and tumorigenic in other primate species may be associated
with acute leukemia in man.

Molecular biological data concerning the relationship between RNA
tumor viruses and human leukemia exist. RNA tumor viruses apparently
replicate through a DNA intermediate provirus which requires a polymerase enzyme, "reverse transcriptase" (Temin and Minutzi, 1970). Similar RNA–DNA polymerase activity appears to be present in a cytoplasmic
particulate fraction from fresh peripheral blood white blood cells in
patients with acute leukemia (Gallo *et al.*, 1970). With human AML cells
this polymerase was shown by immunologic studies to be specifically
related to reverse transcriptase from two known oncogenic primate type C
viruses, the SSAV and the GALV (Gallagher *et al.*, 1974). In addition,
nucleic acids associated with the "reverse transcriptase" have some nucleotide sequences that are similar to those of some RNA tumor viruses (Miller
*et al.*, 1974). Gallagher and Gallo (1975) in a recent report demonstrated
the sustained release of typical budding type C virus from a patient with
AML whose peripheral blood white cells were maintained in culture.
Consequently, the reverse transcriptase from AML patients may be of
viral origin and it thus seems conceivable that in some patients with
leukemia a complete virus particle could be assembled.

It is possible to prepare xenoantisera to tumor-specific antigens and
to use the antisera for passive immunization. There are reports in animal
systems that vaccination with formalin-killed virus induces the production
of antibodies, including neutralizing antibodies (Fink *et al.*, 1969). Hersh

*et al.* (1974a,b) immunized 20 patients who had a malignancy with an antigen extracted from RLV-infected Balb/c cells. Two-thirds of the patients developed cell-mediated immunity as assessed by *in vitro* blastogenic lymphocyte response and by delayed hypersensitivity reactions to the immunizing antigen. The same 20 patients were then immunized with 100 $\mu$g of formalin-killed RLV every 2 weeks for a total of 8 weeks. Ten of the 20 patients developed a significant IgG antibody response as measured by radioimmunoprecipitation. The responses were heightened in those patients with malignant melanoma who were receiving BCG immunotherapy in addition to chemotherapy. However, patients not receiving BCG as well as patients with acute leukemia had an increase in their antibody titers although less vigorous than those receiving immunotherapy. In addition, an excellent correlation existed between the cellular and humoral immune responses (Hersh *et al.*, 1974a,b).

In conclusion, immunologic and molecular biochemical data exist to confirm a relationship between type C RNA tumor viruses and human leukemia. However, at the present state of the art, it is not possible to determine precisely what role viruses play in the antigenicity of leukemia cells.

## 12.7. Conclusions

There are numerous antigens in addition to the genetically determined transplantation antigens on the surface of the leukemia cell. A number of these antigens are shared with normal tissue components. These include T cell antigens, B cell antigens, proliferation-associated antigens, and fetal antigens. In addition possible antigens shared with viral components have been detected in these cells. When all of this reactivity is taken into account it appears that there are still some sera detecting specificities which must be called at present leukemia-associated antigens. Whether or not the antigens detected on the surface of the leukemia cell are shared with normal tissue components there are at least four potentially useful applications of the study of these antigens. In the first place, they may serve as sensitive diagnostic tools. In one study, for example, a xenoantiserum raised against a B cell tissue culture cell line was reacting in a cytotoxicity assay with cells in the peripheral blood which were probably leukemic, even though they could not be morphologically distinguished as such (Halterman *et al.*, 1972). The ability to make a more precise diagnosis of residual tumor than that possible with morphology alone is certainly a potentially useful tool in determining such clinical parameters as the necessary duration of drug therapy. In the second place, these antigens could serve as possible useful targets for immunotherapeutic attack. Unfortunately, the data here are more disappointing.

Antibodies that are directly cytotoxic to leukemia cells *in vitro* have been described in the serum of normal individuals. When the serum from one of these individuals was transfused, a fall in peripheral blast count ensued (Bias *et al.*, 1972). However, when more extensive studies with high titer antileukocyte serum was performed (Djerassi, 1968), a fall in peripheral blast count was seen but there was no effect on the bone marrow. Immunization of late stage leukemia patients with lymphoma tissue culture cells resulted in the production of antibody that was cytotoxic to autologous leukemia *in vitro* but no prolongation of remission duration (Sacks *et al.*, 1975). Cytophilic antibodies which allow attachment of immunologically naive macrophages have been described (Mitchell *et al.*, 1973) in the serum of 25 patients. These antibodies recognized not only the patient's own tumor cells but also second-party cells of the same histological type. The possible role of macrophages in tumor control is an intriguing one and should be investigated further. Studies that are underway to attempt to generate cytotoxic lymphocytes *in vitro* and reinfuse them into leukemic patients are interesting but technically demanding, and as yet have no immediate clinical application (Zarling *et al.*, 1976; Zarling and Bach, 1977). Thus at the moment no antigen has been identified which is a useful target for an immunotherapeutic maneuver.

A third reason for studying leukemia antigens is to increase our understanding of the basic biology of the tumor cell itself and the factors which may have led to the malignant transformation. The sharing of reactivity with viral antigens in some leukemia cells, for example, suggests that a virus may play a role in the etiology of some cases of human leukemia.

A final reason for studying the antigenic nature of the leukemic cell is to increase our understanding of the basic biology of the normal cell, since often the malignancy is thought to represent a clonal proliferation of a single cell type. This is the most complicated application of all since, by their nature, malignant cells undergo disordered growth and are not necessarily subject to the same growth controls as normal cells. In fact there are numerous confusing reports of cells which share markers in a way which would be unexpected in normal cells. For example, CLL cells have been described with receptors for both E and EAC rosettes (Toben and Smith, 1977). These same cells may lack Fc receptors or show functionally abnormal Fc receptors (Gale *et al.*, 1975). Another example of multiple marker expression is the presence of terminal deoxynucleotidyl transferase (an enzyme supposedly related to immature T-lymphocytes) on cells from some patients with chronic myelogenous leukemia in blast crisis (McCaffrey *et al.*, 1975). These examples of malignant cells showing markers which in mature cell lines would belong to more than one cell type, are usually interpreted as showing that the malignancy in question is a proliferation of a more immature or "pluripotent" stem cell and the mature cell which it resembles morphologically.

Our understanding of leukemia-associated antigens and markers will increase rapidly over the next several years as our knowledge in the related areas of immunobiology and myelopoiesis expands.

ACKNOWLEDGMENT

This work was supported in part by Grant NIH–NCI CA 06973-14.

## References

Aoki, T., and Sibol, R., 1976, C-type virus-associated antigens and their relevance to human leukemia control, *Cancer Res.* **36**:591.

Bach, F. H., and van Rood, J. J., 1976, The major histocompatibility complex—Genetics and biology, *N. Engl. J. Med.* **295**:806, 872, 927.

Baker, M. A., and Taub, R. N., 1973, Production of antiserum in mice to human leukemia-associated antigens, *Nature New Biol.* **241**:94.

Baker, M. A., Ramachandar, K., and Taub, R. N., 1974, Specificity of heteroantisera to human acute leukemia associated antigens, *J. Clin. Invest.* **54**:1273.

Bentwich, Z., Weiss, D. W., Sultizeanu, D., Kedar, E., Iazk, G., Cohen, I., and Eyal, O., 1972, Antigenic changes on the surface of lymphocytes from patients with chronic lymphocytic leukemia, *Cancer Res.* **32**:1375.

Bias, W. B., Santos, G. W., Burke, P. H., Mullins, G. N., and Humphrey, R. L., 1972, Cytotoxic antibody in normal human serums reactive with tumor cells from acute lymphocytic leukemia, *Science* **178**:304.

Billing, R., and Terasaki, P. I., 1974, Human leukemia antigen I. Production and characterization of antisera, *J. Natl. Cancer Inst.* **53**:1635.

Billing, R. J., Terasaki, P. I., Honig, R., and Peterson, P., 1976a, The absence of B cell antigen B 2 from leukemia cells and lymphoblastoid cell lines, *Lancet* **i**:1365.

Billing, R., Rafizadeh, B., Drew, I., Hartman, G., Gale, R., and Terasaki, P., 1976b, Human B lymphocyte antigens expressed by lymphocytic and myelocytic leukemia cells, *J. Exp. Med.* **144**:157.

Billing, R., Ting, A., and Terasaki, P. I., 1977, Human B lymphocyte antigens expressed by lymphocytic and myelocytic leukemia cells II. Detection by human anti B cell alloantisera, *J. Natl. Cancer Inst.* **58**:198.

Borella, L., Sen, L., and Casper, J. T., 1977, Acute lymphoblastic leukemia (ALL) antigens detected with antisera to E rosette forming and non E rosette forming ALL blasts, *J. Immunol.* **118**:309.

Broder, S., Poplack, D., Whang-Peng, J., Durm, M., Goldman, C., Muul, L., and Waldmann, T. A., 1978, Characterization of a suppressor cell leukemia: Evidence for the requirement of two T cells in the development of human suppressor effector cells, *N. Engl. J. Med.* **298**:66.

Brown, G., and Greaves, M. F., 1974, Antibodies and lymphocytes from multi-transfused donors, *Eur. J. Immunol.* **4**:302.

Callewaert, D. M., Kaplan, J., Peterson, W. D., Jr., and Lightbody, J. J., 1975, Stimulation in the mixed leukocyte culture and generation of effector cells in cell mediated lympholysis by a human T lymphoblast cell line, *Cell. Immunol.* **19**:276.

Charman, H. P., Kim, N., White, M., and Gilden, R. V., 1974, Failure to detect antibodies cross reactive with mouse leukemia virus group specific antigen in human sera, *J. Natl. Cancer Inst.* **52**:1409.

Chechik, B. E., and Gelfand, E. W., 1977, Leukaemia associated antigen in serum of patients with acute lymphoblastic leukemia, *Lancet* **i**:166.

Clarkson, B., Ohkita, T., Ota, K., and O'Connor, A., 1965, Studies of cellular proliferation in acute leukemia, *J. Clin. Invest.* **44**:1036.

Cresswell, P., and Geier, S. S., 1975, Antisera to human B lymphocyte membrane glycoproteins block stimulation in mixed lymphocyte culture, *Nature* **257**:147.

Djerassi, I., 1968, Transfusion of lymphocyte antibodies and lymphocytes from multitransfused donors, *Clin. Pediatr.* **7**:272.

Durantez, P., Zighelboim, J., Thieme, T., and Fahey, J. L., 1975, Antigens shared by leukemic blast cell and lymphoblastoid cell lines detected by lymphocyte dependent antibody, *Cancer Res.* **35**:2693.

Evans, R. L., Breard, J. M., Lazarus, H., Schlossman, S. F., and Chess, L., 1977, Detection, isolation and functional characterization of 2 different human T cell subclasses bearing unique differentiation antigens, *J. Exp. Med.* **145**:221.

Fink, M. A., and Cowles, C. A., 1965, Immunodiffusion: Detection of a murine leukemia virus (Rauscher), *Science* **150**:1723.

Fink, M. A., Malmgrew, R. A., Rauscher, F. J., Orr, H. C., and Karow, M., 1964, Application of immunofluorescence to the study of human leukemia, *J. Natl. Cancer Inst.* **33**:581.

Fink, M. A., Karow, M., and Rauscher, F. J., 1965, Further observations on the immunofluorescence of cells in human leukemia, *CA* **25**:1317.

Fink, M. A., Cohen, M. H., and Sibal, L. R., 1969, The role of cell-associated and circulating antibody in resistance to infection with murine leukemia virus and transplantation of malignant cells in a syngeneis system, Immunity and tolerance in oncogenesis, Proceedings of IV Perugia Quadrennial International Conference on Cancer, pp. 211–219.

Fridman, W. H., and Kourilsky, F. M., 1969, Stimulation of lymphocytes by autologous leukaemia, *Nature* **224**:277.

Fu, S. M., Winchester, R. J., and Kunkel, H. G., 1975, The occurrence of the HL-B alloantigens on the cells of unclassified acute lymphoblastic leukemias, *J. Exp. Med.* **142**:1334.

Gale, R. P., Zighleboim, J., Ossorio, R. C., and Fahey, J. L., 1975, A comparison of human lymphoid cells in antibody-dependent cellular cytotoxicity (ADCC), *Clin. Immunol. Immunopathol.* **3**:377.

Gallagher, R. E., and Gallo, R. C., 1975, Type C RNA tumor virus isolated from cultured human AML cells, *Science* **187**:350.

Gallagher, R., Todaro, G., Smith, R., Levenplow, D., and Gallo, R. C., 1974, Relationship between RNA-directed DNA polymerase (reverse transcriptase) from human acute leukemic blood cells and primate type-C viruses, *Proc. Natl. Acad. Sci. U.S.A.* **71**:1309.

Gallo, R. C., Yang, S. S., and Ting, R. C., 1970, RNA-dependent DAN polymerase of human acute leukemic cells, *Nature* **228**:927.

Granatek, C. H., Hanna, M. G., Jr., Hersh, E. M., Gutterman, J. U., Mavligit, G. M., and Candler, E. L., 1976, Fetal antigens in human leukemia, *Cancer Res.* **36**:3464.

Grant, J. P., Bignev, D. D., Fischenger, P. J., and Bolognese, D. D., 1974, Expression of murine leukemia virus structural antigens on the surface of chemically induced murine sarcomas, *Proc. Natl. Acad. Sci. U.S.A.* **71**:5037.

Greaves, M. F., Brown, G., Rapson, N. T., and Lister, T. A., 1975, Antisera to acute lymphoblastic leukemia cells, *Clin. Immunol.* **4**:67.

Green, S. S., and Sell, K. W., 1970, Mixed leukocyte stimulation of normal peripheral leukocytes by autologous lymphoblastoid cells, *Science* **170**:989.

Gutterman, J. U., Hersh, E. M., McCredie, K. B., Bodey, G. P., Rodriquez, V., and Freireich, E. J., 1972, Lymphocyte blastogenesis to human leukemia cells and their relationship to serum factors, immunocompetence, and prognosis, *Cancer Res.* **32**:2524.

Halterman, R. H., Leventhal, B. G., and Mann, D. L., 1972, A leukemia-associated antigen: Its relationship to clinical status, *N. Engl. J. Med.* **287**:1272.

Han, T., and Minowada, J., 1973, A unique "leukaemic" T lymphoid cell line: Absence of stimulating effect in mixed lymphocyte reaction, *Clin. Exp. Immunol.* **15**:535.

Harris, R., Viza, D., Todd, R., Phillips, J., Sugar, R., Jennison, R. F., Marriott, G., and Gleeson, M. H., 1971, Detection of human leukemia-associated antigens and leukaemic serum and normal embryos, *Nature* **233**:556.

Hehlmann, R., Kufe, D., and Spiegelman, S., 1972, RNA in human leukemic cells related to the RNA of a mouse leukemia virus, *Proc. Natl. Acad. Sci. U.S.A.* **69**:435.

Hersh, E. M., Hanna, M. G., Gutterman, J. U., Mavligit, G., Yarconic, M., and Gschwind, C. R., 1974a, Human immune response to active immunization with Rauscher leukemia virus II. Humoral immunity, *J. Natl. Cancer Inst.* **53**:327.

Hersh, E. M., Gutterman, J. U., Mavligit, G., Gschwind, C. R., Friereich, E. S., Levine, P. H., and Plata, E. J., 1974b, Human immune response to active immunization with Rauscher leukemia virus I. Cell mediated and cell associated immunity, *J. Natl. Cancer Inst.* **53**:317.

Hollinshead, A. C., and Herberman, R. B., 1975, Identification and characterization: Cell membrane antigens associated with the blast phase of human adult leukemia. Comparative Leukemia Research, 1973, *in Leukemogenesis*, Bibl. Haematol. No. 40 (Y. Ito and R. M. Dutcher, eds), pp. 339–348, Univ. Tokyo Press, Tokyo/Karger, Basel.

Hollis, V. W., Aoki, T., Banera, O., Oldstone, M. B. A., and Dixon, F. J., 1974, Detection of naturally occurring Ab's to RNA-dependent DNA polymerase of murine leukemia virus in kidney eluates of AKR mice, *J. Virol.* **13**:448.

Humphrey, G. B., and Lankford, J., 1976, Acute leukemia: The use of surface markers at classification, *Semin. Oncol.* **3**:243.

Ikeda, H., Pincus, T., Yoshiki, T., Shand, M., August, J. T., Boyse, E. A., and Mellas, R. C., 1974, Biological expression of antigenic determinants of murine leukemia virus proteins gp 69/71 and p 30, *J. Virol.* **14**:1274.

Ioannides, A. K., Rosner, R., Brenneo, M., and Lee, S. L., 1968, Immunofluorescent studies of human leukemic cells with antiserum to murine leukemic virus (Rauscher strain), *Blood* **31**:381.

Kaplan, J. T., Tilton, J., and Peterson, W. D., Jr., 1976, Identification of T cell lymphoma tumor antigens on human T cell lines, *Am. J. Hematol.* **1**:219.

Kennel, S. J., DelVillano, B. C., Levy, R. L., and Lerner, R. A., 1973, Properties of an oncornavirus glycoprotein: Evidence for its presence on the surface of virions and infected cells, *Virology* **55**:464.

Kersey, J. H., Sabad, A., Peczalska, K., Hallgren, H. M., Juins, E. J., and Nesbit, M. E., 1973, Acute lymphoblast leukemia cells with T (thymus derived) lymphocyte markers, *Science* **182**:1355.

Klein, G., Steiner, M., Weiner, F., and Klein, E., 1974, *Proc. Natl. Acad. Sci. U.S.A.* **71**:685.

Leventhal, B. G., Halterman, R. H., Rosenberg, E. B., and Herberman, R. B., 1972, Immune reactivity of leukemia patients to autologous blast cells, *Cancer Res.* **32**:1820.

Leventhal, B. G., Leung, E., Johnson, G., and Poplack, D. G., 1977, E rosette forming lymphoblasts fail to stimulate allogeneic cells in mixed leukoycte culture (MLC), *Cancer Immunol. Immunother.* **2**:21.

Leventhal, B. G., Yarbro, G. S., and Mirro, J., Jr., 1978, Immune reactivity to tumor antigens in leukemia and lymphoma, *Semin. Hematol.*, **15**:157.

Levine, P. H., 1976, Approaches to unmorphologic control of virus-associated tumors in man: Introductory remarks, *Cancer Res.* **36**:565.

Ling, N. R., 1973, Immune surveillance of lymphoid tissue. A biological role for the mixed lymphocyte reaction, *Immunol. Commun.* **2(2)**:119.

Lohrmann, H. P., Novikovs, L., and Graw, R. G., Jr., 1974, Stimulatory capacity of human T and B lymphocytes in the mixed leukocyte culture, *Nature* **250**:144.

Mann, D. L., Rogentine, G. N., Halterman, R. H., and Leventhal, B. G., 1971, Detection of an acute leukemia associated antigen, *Science* **174**:1136.

Mann, D. L., Abelson, L., Harris, S., and Amos, D. B., 1975, Detection of antigens specific for B lymphoid cultured cell lines with human alloantisera, *J. Exp. Med.* **142**:84.

McCaffrey, R., Harrison, T. A., and Parkman, R., 1975, Terminal deoxynucleotidyl transferase activity in human leukemic cells and in normal human thymocytes, *N. Engl. J. Med.* **292**:775.

Metzgar, R. S., and Mohanakumar, T., 1978, Tumor-associated antigens of human leukemia cells, *Semin. Hematol.*, **15**:139.

Metzgar, R. S., Mohanakumar, T., and Miller, D. S., 1972, Antigens specific for human lymphocytic and myeloid leukemia cells: Detection by nonhuman primate antiserum, *Science* **178**:986.

Metzgar, R. S., Mohanakumar, T., and Bolognesi, D. P., 1975, Antigenic relationships between murine, feline, and primate RNA tumor viruses and membrane antigens of human leukemic cells. Comparative Leukemia Research, 1975, Bibl. Haematol. #43, pp. 549–554.

Metzgar, R. S., Mohanakumar, T., and Bolognesi, D. P., 1976, Relationships between membrane Ag of human leukemia cells and oncogenic RNA virus structural components, *J. Exp. Med.* **143**:47.

Miller, N., Saxinger, W., Reitz, M., Gallagher, A., Wu, R., Gallo, R., and Gillespie, D., 1974, Systematics of RNA tumor viruses and virus-like particles of human origin, *Proc. Natl. Acad. Sci. U.S.A.* **71**:3177.

Mitchell, M. S., Mokyr, M. B., Aspens, G. T., and McIntosh, S., 1973, Cytophilis antibodies in man, *Ann. Intern. Med.* **79**:333.

Opelz, G., Kiuchi, M., Takasugi, M., and Terasaki, P. I., 1975, Autologous stimulation of human lymphocyte subpopulations, *J. Exp. Med.* **142**:1327.

Powles, R. L., Balchin, L. A., Faurley, G. H., and Alexander, P., 1971, Recognition of leukaemia cells as foreign before and after autoimmunization, *Br. Med. J.* **i**:486.

Preud'homme, J. L., and Seligmann, M., 1972, Surface bound immunoglobulins as a cell marker in human lymphoproliferative disease, *Blood* **40**:777.

Royston, I., Graze, P. R., and Pitts, R. B., 1974, Failure of cultured human T cell lymphoid lines to stimulate in mixed leukocyte culture, *J. Natl. Cancer Inst.* **53**:361.

Russell, A. R., and Pope, J. H., 1976, Reactivity of antibody in acute myeloid leukaemia with proliferation-associated nuclear antigens, *Clin. Exp. Immunol.* **23**:83.

Sacks, K., Olweny, C., Mann, D., Simon, R., Johnson, G., Poplack, D., and Leventhal, B. G., 1975, A clinical trial of chemotherapy and RAJI immunotherapy in advanced acute lymphatic leukemia, *Cancer Res.* **35**:3715.

Seligmann, M., Preud'homme, J. L., and Brouet, J. C., 1973, B and T cell markers in human proliferative blood diseases and primary immunodeficiencies with special reference to membrane bound immunoglobulins, *Transplant. Rev.* **16**:85.

Shew, C. J., and Todaro, G. J., 1975, Primate type-C virus p 30 Ag in cells from humans with acute leukemia, *Science* **187**:855.

Steiner, M., Klein, E., and Klein, G., 1975, Antinuclear reactivity of sera in patients with leukemia and other neoplastic diseases, *Clin. Immunol. Immunopathol.* **4**:374.

Temin, H. M., and Minutzi, S., 1970, RNA-dependent DNA polymerase in Rous sarcoma, *Nature* **226**:1211.

Toben, H. R., and Smith, R. G., 1977, T lymphocytes bearing complement receptors in a patient with chronic lymphocytic leukaemia, *Clin. Exp. Immunol.* **27**:292.

Tsukimoto, I., Wong, K. Y., and Lampkin, B. C., 1976, Surface markers and prognostic factors in acute lymphoblastic leukemia, *N. Engl. J. Med.* **294**:245.

van Rood, J. J., van Leeuwen, A., Keuning, J. J., and van Oud Alblas, A. B., 1975, The serological recognition of the human MLC determinants using a modified cytotoxicity technique, *Tissue Antigens* **5**:73.

Viza, D. C., Bernard Degani, O., Bernard, C., and Harris, R., 1969, Leukaemia antigens, *Lancet* **ii**:493.

Wernet, P., Winchester, R., Kunkel, H. G., Wernet, D., Giphart, M., van Leeuwen, A., and van Rood, J. J., 1975, Serological detection and partial characterization of human MLC determinants with special reference to B cell specificity, *Transplant. Proc.* **7** (Suppl. 1):193.

Winchester, R. J., Fu, S. M., Wernet, P., Junkel, H. G., Dupont, B., and Jersild, C., 1975, Recognition by pregnancy serums of non-HL-A alloantigens selectively expressed on B lymphocytes, *J. Exp. Med.* **141**:924.

Winchester, R. J., Wang, C. Y., Halper, J., and Hoffman, T., 1976, Studies with B cell allo and hetero antisera: Parallel activity and special properties, *Scand. J. Immunol.* **5**:745.

Zarling, J., and Bach, F. H., 1977, Assessment of common target antigens on EBV transformed lymphocytes and fresh human acute leukemia cells, *Proc. Am. Assoc. Cancer Res. Am. Soc. Clin. Oncol.* **18**:249.

Zarling, J. M., Raich, P. C., McKeough, M., and Bach, F. H., 1976, Generation of cytotoxic lymphocytes *in vitro* against autologous human leukaemia cells, *Nature,* **262**:691.

# Recent Advances in the Treatment of Malignant Lymphomas: Hodgkin's Disease

George P. Canellos, Arthur T. Skarin, and Robert L. Goodman

## 13.1. Introduction

No area of investigation in oncology has advanced more rapidly than the pathogenesis and treatment of the malignant lymphomas. The introduction of new immunologic methods has allowed for the characterization of the malignant cell. Such techniques have clearly defined that the majority of cases with Burkitt's lymphoma, nodular lymphoma, and other types described as follicular center cell in origin (Lukes) are derived from B-lymphocytes. The pathologic classification of non-Hodgkin's lymphomas polarized among a number of different classifications, whereas there is more widespread agreement and universality as to the appropriate classi-

GEORGE P. CANELLOS, ARTHUR T. SKARIN, and ROBERT L. GOODMAN •
Sidney Farber Cancer Institute; Harvard Medical School, Boston, Massachusetts.

fication of Hodgkin's disease. There is general agreement among more workers that a systematic staging of Hodgkin's disease is appropriate since therapy can be altered according to the anatomic extent of involvement. This is probably not true for non-Hodgkin's lymphomas. These conclusions are all based on the results of extensive clinical investigations in the last 5 years. The treatment of these disorders is abetted by the fact that a variety of antineoplastic agents and irradiation are efficacious in their treatment. The optimal treatment for these diseases changes with the development of new drug programs as well as the continuous assessment of the long-term results of therapy applied as recently as 5 years ago. It would appear that chemotherapy is to be included earlier in the course of the illness and even in patients who appear to have localized disease. What is optimal today will not be the case tomorrow as we enter yet another generation of therapeutic trials. Yet, chemotherapy is offered to decrease the potential for relapse following radiation therapy and since an expanding number of patients are being cured of disseminated disease with chemotherapy alone, the long-term effects on normal tissue comprise an area of new concern. The authors assume herein that the readers are conversant with terminology of the pathologic subgroups and the generally accepted staging classification applied to the malignant lymphomas.


## 13.2. Hodgkin's Disease

### 13.2.1. Immunologic Aspects

It has been well documented that patients with active Hodgkin's disease have abnormalities of immunologic function characterized by a decrease in delayed hypersensitivity responses as well as impaired lymphocyte reactivity to specific mitogens. Although anergy to a battery of skin test antigens is uncommon, its incidence increases with the stage of disease. In the more advanced stages patients appear to be able to respond to mumps antigen and dinitrochlorbenzene (DNCB), although they may be anergic to other antigens and markedly lymphopenic (Young *et al.*, 1972). Pretreatment skin testing tends to return toward a normal pattern in patients who attain long-term remissions off of all therapy (Chang *et al.*, 1975). *In vitro* lymphocyte transformation (blastogenesis) to mitogenic substances is impaired to an extent which is proportional to the extent of the disease (Hersh and Oppenheim, 1965; Han and Sokal, 1970; Jackson *et al.*, 1970; Corder *et al.*, 1972). As with delayed hypersensitivity, lymphocyte transformation returns to normal in remission. Recently, a more quantitative phytohemagglutinin dose-dependent assay was shown to be capable of demonstrating defects in patients with asymptomatic localized disease, a group which often has normal lymphocyte transformation

(Levy and Kaplan, 1974). Over a range of concentration, normals have a higher stimulation ratio than all patients with Hodgkin's disease regardless of stage. Lymphocytes from patients incubated without mitogen often demonstrate a high spontaneous transformation as measured by the incorporation of thymidine (Matchett *et al.*, 1973). In addition splenic lymphocytes from such patients may demonstrate response to phytohemagglutinin (PHA) even when the peripheral lymphocyte response is reduced (Matchett *et al.*, 1973).

It has long been postulated that the immunologic defect in Hodgkin's disease (HD) involves abnormalities in the number and function of thymus-derived lymphocytes since they are associated with cell-mediated immunity and are more likely to transform with mitogens (Holm *et al.*, 1976). The immunologic abnormalities just described suggest the postulate that the total T-lymphocyte percentages are generally not reduced except in far advanced cases with lymphopenia. The number of B-lymphocytes is generally not altered. Further quantification of lymphocyte subpopulations suggests a reduction in T cells when sheep erythrocyte rosettes or response to PHA are used to quantitate T cells. However, when *in vitro* cytotoxicity with specific anti-T cell serum is used, the numbers appear to be in the normal range, suggesting altered surface properties of the T-lymphocyte in HD (Bobrove *et al.*, 1975). The defective binding of sheep red cells to HD lymphocytes was demonstrated to be due to a specific interaction of the cells with sera from HD patients. Preincubation of HD lymphocytes with tissue culture media containing fetal calf serum restored their ability to bind sheep red cells. The addition of HD serum suppressed this restoration but only in HD lymphocytes (Fuks *et al.*, 1976). Although PHA responsiveness has been the standard assay of T-lymphocyte abnormalities in HD, its specificity has been further questioned by the demonstration that mixed lymphocyte reactions are normal in the face of PHA response impairment, indicating that PHA and MLC may be measuring different functional T cell subpopulations (Lang *et al.*, 1972; Graze *et al.*, 1976). In addition to the suggestion that HD patients have a serum factor which interferes with their own T cell function, elevated serum levels of chemotactic factor inactivator have been demonstrated in HD. This may contribute to a defect in inflammatory cell mobilization (Ward and Berenberg, 1974). The high spontaneous transformation rate and increased levels of nonspecific reactants in addition to constitutional symptoms suggest a generalized host reaction to the disease and perhaps to a specific HD antigen. *In vitro* studies of immunoglobulin synthesis in normal splenic lymphocytes from patients with HD further suggest a humoral response to some antigenic component of HD (Longmire *et al.*, 1973). An antigen has been demonstrated in supernatant of cultured tumor cells derived from splenic tumors (Long *et al.*, 1977a). The antigen was demonstrated only in tissue culture proliferative cells and not from noncultured tumors. Cells from these long-term monolayer cultures are capable of continuous growth, have aneuploid karyotypes, and produce tumors in nude mice (Zamecnik and Long, 1977; Long *et al.*, 1977a). Cell suspensions from these cultured tumors were devoid of surface immunoglobulin, and did not form rosettes with sheep red cells, nor react with antithymocyte serum (Long *et al.*, 1977b). The demonstration of increased quantities of the third component of complement in the plasma of HD patients indirectly suggests the presence of immune complexes (Amlot *et al.*, 1976). In addition these nonspecific abnormalities appear to correlate with constitutional symptoms. Although the significance of this is unclear, there have been rare patients with HD described who had the nephrotic syndrome which disappeared with remission of the disease (Plager and Stutzman, 1971; Sherman *et al.*, 1972; Lokich *et al.*, 1973). It has been described by some as a "lipoid nephrosis" rather than an immune complex type of glomerulonephritis.

### 13.2.2. Staging

The pathologic staging of HD has resulted in the most precise definition of prospects and patterns of dissemination for patients with apparent localized disease and in the various histologic subgroups (Kadin *et al.*, 1971). The necessity and role of extensive pathologic staging including exploratory laparotomy and splenectomy is based on the known pattern of dissemination of the disease through contiguous lymph node areas including the spleen. Whether splenic HD connotes hematogenous dissemination or is a contiguous "lymph node" is unclear and the subject of controversy (Aisenberg and Qazi, 1974). Regardless, in the final analysis, the value of pathologic staging must be in treatment planning for the patient. It is clear that the abdominal involvement undetected by the usual noninvasive techniques occurs in about 26% of asymptomatic patients and 42% of symptomatic patients with disease confined to supradiaphragmatic areas (Table I). The spleen is the most common site of involvement (Kadin *et al.*, 1971; Aisenberg and Qazi, 1974; Gamble *et al.*, 1975; Sutcliffe, 1976; O'Connell *et al.*, 1974; Beretta *et al.*, 1976; Hellman, 1974). Bipedal lymphography has been shown to be accurate in 80–90% of cases. The demonstration of disease below the diaphragm may influence the treatment plan since some may offer only a mantle field of radiation, and others might consider extending the field or total nodal irradiation regardless of the findings (Johnson *et al.*, 1977). The recent demonstration that asymptomatic patients with disease below the diaphragm have a 30–60% 5-year disease-free survival with radiation has prompted the addition of adjuvant chemotherapy to such patients (Pros-

**Table I.**  Results of Staging Laparotomy in Hodgkin's Disease Presenting with Localized Supradiaphragmatic Involvement

| Institution | Positive abdominal disease/total | | Reference |
| --- | --- | --- | --- |
| | Asymptomatic I/IIA | Symptomatic I/IIB | |
| NCI—Baltimore Cancer Research Center | 15/54 | — | O'Connell *et al.*, 1975 |
| NCI, Milan | 9/40 | — | Beretta *et al.*, 1976 |
| M. D. Anderson Hospital | 3/108 | 14/30 | Gamble *et al.*, 1975 |
| Massachusetts General Hospital, Boston | 12/50 | 16/34 | Aisenberg and Qazi, 1974 |
| Joint Center for Radiation Therapy, Harvard | 5/33 | 7/10 | Hellman, 1974 |
| Saint Bartholomew's Hospital, London | 15/45 | 2/5 | Sutcliffe, 1976 |
| Stanford | 5/36 | 3/24 | Kadin *et al.*, 1971 |
| Totals | 95/366 (26%) | 42/103 (42%) | |

nitz *et al.*, 1976; O'Connell *et al.*, 1975; Levi and Wiernik, 1977; Desser *et al.*, 1977; Rosenberg and Kaplan, 1975). Thus, the findings at laparotomy may identify those patients to receive combination chemotherapy in addition to radiation therapy. In more advanced disease the need for laparotomy is to be questioned. Most patients with advanced IIIA or IIIB disease may be equally well treated with chemotherapy. The use of laparotomy to identify liver involvement is also in question. In the combined laparotomy series (Kadin *et al.*, 1971; Aisenberg and Qazi, 1974; Gamble *et al.*, 1975; Sutcliffe, 1976; O'Connell *et al.*, 1974; Beretta *et al.*, 1976; Hellman, 1974) only 2/231 stage IA/IIA patients had liver involvement with 6/53 in I/IIB disease (Table II). Of note is the fact that only 9/104 IIIA cases had liver disease. The Stanford series had 1/63 asymptomatic patients with liver involvement in a setting where liver function studies were generally inaccurate predictors (Kadin *et al.*, 1971). Liver involvement is most likely to occur in the presence of positive retroperitoneal lymph node involvement and splenomegaly and in this setting laparoscopy may be as useful in making the diagnosis (DeVita *et al.*, 1971). In fact the Milan group prospectively compared the utility of laparoscopy prior to laparotomy. Seven of 121 patients had positive livers and 5/7 were diagnosed at laparoscopy. The remaining two were seen in symptomatic patients (Beretta *et al.*, 1976). Bone marrow biopsy in asymptomatic patients with localized disease certainly, and in most other stages probably, is a fruitless

**Table II.** Liver Involvement by Hodgkin's Disease at Staging Laparotomy[a]

| Institution | Stage (positive/total patients) | | | Reference |
|---|---|---|---|---|
| | I/IIA | I/IIB | IIIA | |
| NCI—Baltimore Cancer Research Center | 0/54 | — | 2/32 | O'Connell *et al.*, 1975 |
| M. D. Anderson Hospital | 0/49 | 1/4 | — | Gamble *et al.*, 1975 |
| Massachusetts General Hospital, Boston | 1/50 | 2/34 | 4/16 | Aisenberg and Qazi, 1974 |
| Joint Center for Radiation Therapy, Harvard | 1/45 | 1/5 | 3/18 | Hellman, 1974 |
| Saint Bartholomew's Hospital, London | 0/33 | 2/10 | 0/38 | Sutcliffe, 1976 |
| Totals | 2/231 | 8/54 | 9/104 | |

[a]At Stanford (Kadin *et al.*, 1971) only 1/63 stage A and 8/54 stage B patients had liver involvement. At NCI, Milan (Beretta *et al.*, 1976) only 2/80 I/IIA/B and 3/23 IIIA/B patients had liver involvement.

effort. Bone marrow involvement is usually a late manifestation and rarely detected in initial staging. Only 8/319 patients had positive bone marrow biopsies at initial evaluation and then only in clinical stage III patients (Kadin *et al.*, 1971; Sutcliffe, 1976; Beretta *et al.*, 1976).

Thus, with bone marrow and liver almost never involved and with most centers offering extended field irradiation for disease localized above the diaphragm, the risks and morbidity of a laparotomy have to be weighed against the benefits. The need for laparotomy will vary with the situation. In nodular sclerosing HD the value of laparotomy is seriously questioned by the demonstration of 90% 10-year survival following extended field irradiation without laparotomy (Johnson *et al.*, 1977). Furthermore, these results appear to be equal to those achieved by extended field irradiation (mantle plus para-aortic fields) in a series of 81 cases of I/IIA patients who had undergone staging laparotomy (Goodman *et al.*, 1976). Thus, in nodular sclerosis sparing the risk of pulmonic and renal irradiation by the removal of the spleen is a debatable point when balanced against the morbidity of laparotomy for clinical stage I/IIA disease. Patients in the clinical stage I/II in the other histologic subgroups and those with constitutional symptoms have a 50–70% disease-free survivorship (Johnson *et al.*, 1977; Kaplan, 1976). The importance of staging in this group is especially focused on those patients who may have abdominal disease (pathologic IIIA or IIIB). Extended field or total nodal irradiation has been disappointing in this group. In order to improve disease-free survival combination chemotherapy (MOPP) has been added to extended field or total nodal irradiation (Prosnitz *et al.*, 1976; O'Connell *et al.*, 1975; Levi and Wiernick, 1977; Desser *et al.*, 1977; Rosenberg and Kaplan, 1975). In all series the addition of chemotherapy has improved the disease-free survival. The impact of added chemotherapy appears to be greatest in those patients who have more extensive abdominal lymph node disease (Levi and Wiernik, 1977; Desser *et al.*, 1977). In fact, chemotherapy appears to add little to total nodal or extended field irradiation in those patients whose abdominal disease is confined to spleen, splenic, or celiac nodes. Thus, if these results are confirmed, laparotomy might better be selected for those patients who will benefit from added chemotherapy. Since most patients with stage IIIB disease do poorly with irradiation alone, they are better treated with either radiation and chemotherapy combined or the latter alone. Thus, the need for laparotomy in this group is minimal. A prospective series of trials are currently underway comparing radiotherapy alone in early stages with radiotherapy plus chemotherapy (Rosenberg and Kaplan, 1975). The results are preliminary but in all instances the disease-free survival is equal to or superior than radiation alone. Thus, the possibility exists for a diminishing need for staging laparotomy as more earlier stage groups will be receiving chemotherapy.

## 13.3. Chemotherapy

Chemotherapy of Hodgkin's disease has evolved in the last 20 years from sequential single drug chemotherapy to the application of combination chemotherapy and even the sequential treatment with multiple drug combinations. As with other lymphomas, Hodgkin's disease is responsive to a large number of antineoplastic agents of differing biochemical mechanism of action. The principal drugs include the alkylating agents, especially cyclophosphamide and nitrogen mustard, the vinca alkaloids vinblastine and vincristine, corticosteroids, procarbazine, bis-chlorethyl-nitrosourea (BCNU), adriamycin, and bleomycin. The most extensively applied combination chemotherapy program is that of MOPP which includes intravenous nitrogen mustard 6 mg/m$^2$ and vincristine 1.4 mg/m$^2$ each on days 1 and 8 of a 28-day cycle. Procarbazine 100 mg/m$^2$ and prednisone 40 mg/m$^2$ are given orally daily for 14 days in a 28-day cycle. There is no therapy given between days 14 and 28. Prednisone is generally included only in the first and fourth cycle of a planned six-cycle course of treatment (DeVita *et al.*, 1970). The principal toxicity of this combination is myelosuppression. With modification of the myelosuppressive agents, nitrogen mustard and procarbazine, the combination can be safely administered in an outpatient setting. A progressive decrease in the dose of myelosuppressive agents usually results in the patient receiving 60–70% of the calculated dose by the sixth cycle of treatment. The doses are generally modified according to the blood count before starting each subsequent course. The acute toxicity includes nausea and vomiting with nitrogen mustard and some neurologic toxicity with the vinca alkaloids. The original treatment plan for advanced Hodgkin's disease was to offer six cycles followed by complete clinical restaging. If no evidence of disease was found including biopsy of suspicious sites, the patient was left off of all therapy in complete remission. Under optimal circumstances of patients in the younger age group with advanced disease who have not been previously treated with cytotoxic agents, MOPP can result in a complete clinical remission in approximately 80% of patients. As a general rule approximately 40% of patients who enter complete remission will eventually sustain a relapse of their disease, usually occurring in a median duration of about 18–20 months (DeVita *et al.*, 1972). Long-term follow-up is now available on a total series of 193 patients previously untreated with cytotoxic agents who had received MOPP chemotherapy from 1965 to the present time. It is noteworthy that a plateau at approximately 3 years is reached in the disease-free survival curve and approximately 70% of patients who enter complete remission are alive at 5 and 10 years. The disease-free survivorship at 5 years is close to 70% (DeVita *et al.*, 1976). With so few relapses it is possible now to describe MOPP chemotherapy as curative in patients with advanced Hodgkin's disease. When the patients are analyzed according to a pattern of metastatic disease, it appeared that most extranodal sites were capable of responding to approximately the same extent. The durability of remissions at the sites was somewhat less for liver involvement, but there appeared to be no significant difference among the various extranodal sites including liver, lung, bone, and bone marrow. There seems to be a higher response rate and better disease-free survivorship for patients less than 50 years of age and for those without B symptoms. In patients achieving a complete response at the end of six cycles, the wisdom of continuing intermittent MOPP chemotherapy indefinitely has been questioned.

A prospective randomized trial in patients who have achieved a complete remission was performed comparing no treatment versus intermittent single agent therapy with BCNU versus intermittent MOPP therapy given as two consecutive cycles of chemotherapy every 3 months for 15 months (Young *et al.*, 1973). No significant difference in overall survival was achieved by continuous MOPP therapy. These results have been confirmed in a larger study performed by the Southwest Cooperative Group (Coltman *et al.*, 1976). In addition to a high overall response rate in patients with advanced symptomatic Hodgkin's disease, it was noteworthy that 22 patients in this series of 193 had stage IIIA or IVA disease. Within this group no patient treated with chemotherapy alone has developed relapse, suggesting that asymptomatic advanced Hodgkin's disease may be equally cured by combination chemotherapy. This evidence is further supported by data from Uganda where early stage asymptomatic patients were treated with MOPP chemotherapy in the absence of radiotherapy facilities. All 24 patients achieved a complete remission (Ziegler *et al.*, 1972). A long-term follow-up demonstrated that the majority of asymptomatic patients are continuously free of disease (Olweny *et al.*, 1974). In a prospective comparative trial the British Lymphoma Group demonstrated that the prednisone included in the MOPP program was essential to maintain the high complete remission rate of 80% versus a complete remission rate of 44% without the prednisone (report from the British National Lymphoma Investigation, 1975). This remains a relatively controversial area since there has been an advocacy for the elimination of prednisone especially in patients who have had high dose radiation to the mantle area to reduce the risk of radiation pneumonitis exacerbated by the withdrawal of steroids (Castellino *et al.*, 1974). A number of other groups have confirmed the high order of activity of MOPP chemotherapy demonstrating complete remission rates in the 66–90% range (Nixon and Aisenberg, 1974; Frei *et al.*, 1973).

A number of modified combinations employing other closely related drugs have been employed successfully. One of the early regimens introduced in the Unted Kingdom employed vinblastine 10 mg intravenously on days 1, 7, and 14 with cycles repeated every 44 days rather than 28 days. The results of this regimen seem to be equivalent to MOPP (Nicholson *et al.*, 1970). Similarly, a more contracted regimen utilizing cyclophosphamide, vinblastine, procarbazine, and prednisone (CVPP) on a 21-day cycle has been administered to Hodgkin's patients with no significant improvement in complete remission rate (Diggs *et al.*, 1977; Bloomfield *et al.*, 1976). Advantages of CVPP appear to be somewhat diminished gastrointestinal and neurotoxicity. Maintenance chemotherapy with the nitrosourea, CCNU, and vinblastine did not appear to confer an advantage. For patients resistant to MOPP the availability of other antineoplastic agents that are not necessarily cross-resistant can be administered in new combination chemotherapy programs. Until these were available the patients who relapsed following a protracted remission period off of therapy could be reinduced, in most cases, with the original MOPP program. However, long-term cure was rarely achieved in patients who had relapsed following a MOPP-induced complete remission. In this circumstance, intermittent MOPP treatment was usually required for the remainder of the patient's life. This is in contrast to patients who have relapsed following radiation therapy where MOPP chemotherapy can still achieve prolonged disease-free survival in the setting of MOPP of secondary treatment (Canellos *et al.*, 1972; Weller *et al.*, 1976). In fact the actuarial survival curve of patients treated with MOPP in relapse following radiotherapy is quite similar to that seen with MOPP alone.

For patients resistant to MOPP a number of new programs have been introduced. These must be interpreted with some caution, however, since clear distinctions must be made between those who are primarily refractory or progressive on MOPP chemotherapy and those patients who have recurred during a period off of MOPP treatment. For MOPP-resistant patients a number of programs are available. These include the combination of the nitrosourea, CCNU, vinblastine, and bleomycin which appeared to be capable of inducing a remission in 85% of patients in one series (Goldman and Dawson, 1975). The majority, however, were only partial remissions. The combination includes CCNU 100 mg/m$^2$ on day 1, vinblastine 6 mg/m$^2$ intravenously on days 1 and 8, and bleomycin 15 mg total dose on days 1 and 8 administered every 4 weeks. A more widely applied alternative to MOPP therapy is the ABVD program which consists of six monthly cycles of adriamycin 25 mg/m$^2$ i.v., bleomycin 10 mg/m$^2$ i.v., and vinblastine 6 mg/m$^2$ i.v. on days 1 and 14. Imidazole carboxamide (DTIC) is administered 150 mg/m$^2$ i.v. over the first 5 days of each cycle. No treatment is given between days 15 and 28 and the cycle is repeated for a total of six treatments (Bonadonna *et al.*, 1975). A considerable amount of nausea and vomiting is associated with this program. However, in a prospective randomized trial it appears to be equally as effective as MOPP and, interestingly, is capable of inducing complete remissions in patients who fail to respond to MOPP treatment. The durability of these second line treatments with ABVD is yet unproved for it would be a great advantage in the management of Hodgkin's patients to have a completely non-cross-resistant combination which is able to salvage patients refractory to MOPP. Whether this in fact will be the case, a longer period of follow-up is required. Experience with this program indicates an approximately 60–70% remission rate in patients resistant to MOPP. A modification of this program known as ABVD has been applied at Memorial Hospital with some success and has recently been combined in an alternating sequence with MOPP chemotherapy (Case *et al.*, 1976, 1977). It is interesting that complete remissions were produced in all previously untreated patients. The results are too preliminary for interpretation, although theoretically, this approach has a great deal of appeal since one is combining two non-cross-resistant combination programs. Whether it is to the advantage of the patient to receive them in alternating cycles rather than one 6-month course followed by another 6-month course is speculative. An outline of the principal combination chemotherapy program regimens in current use is shown in (Table III).

**Table III.** Combination Chemotherapy Programs for Advanced Hodgkin's Disease

| Regimen | Number of patients | Percent complete remissions | References |
|---|---|---|---|
| MOPP | | | |
| Mustargen 6 mg/m² days 1,8 | 193 | 80 | DeVita *et al.*, 1970 |
| Oncovin 1.4 mg/m² days 1,8 | | | |
| Procarbazine 100 mg/m² days 1–14 | | | |
| Prednisone* 40 mg/m² days 1–14 | | | |
| *2/6 cycles q. 28 days | | | |
| MVPP | | | |
| Mustargen 6 mg/m² days 1,8 | 26 | 80 | Nicholson *et al.*, 1970 |
| Vinblastine 10 mg days 1,8,14 | | | |
| Procarbazine 100 mg/m² days 1–14 | | | |
| Prednisolone 40 mg days 1–14 | | | |
| q. 44 days | | | |
| CVB | | | Goldman and |
| CCNU 100 mg/m² day 1 | 39 | 25 (MOPP- | Dawson, 1975 |
| Vinblastine 6 mg/m² days 1,8 | | resistant | |
| Bleomycin 15 mg i.m. days 1,8 | | patients) | |
| q. 28 days | | | |
| CVPP | | | |
| Cyclophosphamide 1.0 g/m² | 50 | 62 | Diggs *et al.*, 1977 |
| Vinblastine 0.1 mg/kg days 1,8 | | | |
| Procarbazine 100 mg/m² days 1–7 | | | |
| Prednisone 40 mg/m² days 1–7 | | | |
| q. 21 days | | | |
| CVPP | | | |
| Cyclophosphamide 300 mg/m² days 1,8 | 38 | 74 | Bloomfield *et al.*, 1976 |
| Vinblastine 10 mg days 1,8,15 | | | |
| Procarbazine 100 mg/m² days 1–15 | | | |
| Prednisone* 40 mg/m² days 1–15 | | | |
| *2/6 cycle q. 42 days | | | |
| ABVD | | | |
| Adriamycin 25 mg/m² days, 1,14 | 20 | 76 | Bonadonna *et al.*, 1975 |
| Bleomycin 10 mg/m² days 1,14 | | | |
| Vinblastine 6 mg/m² days 1, 14 | | | |
| DTIC 150 mg/m² days 1–5 | | | |
| q. 28 days | | | |

Chemotherapy is associated with a number of long-term side effects which should be explained to patients. This includes long-term sterility as a result of the azoospermia induced by cytotoxic agents (Asbjrnsen *et al.*, 1976b; Sherins and Devita, 1973). The germinal tissue is seriously injured by chemotherapy and in most patients infertility may be complete and long lasting. A few patients, however, appear to have a return of spermatogenesis after a period of 2–7 years off of treatment (Sherins and DeVita, 1973). The propensity for antineoplastic agents with or without radiation to cause second neoplasms has attracted a great deal of interest (Rosner and Grunwald, 1975). It seems likely that the combination of radiation therapy and combination chemotherapy does increase the statistical likelihood of second tumors especially acute myeloblastic leukemia (Canellos *et al.*, 1975). The incidence may be greater than otherwise expected, but the long-term survival that is now being achieved in Hodgkin's patients far outweighs the slight statistical chance of increased incidence of acute leukemia. It is interesting that the acute leukemias arising in patients who have been previously treated for Hodgkin's disease have marked cytogenetic abnormalities. One study from NCI demonstrated that hypodiploidy occurred in all three patients with acute myeloblastic leukemia. These long-term side effects, however, are worthy of consideration when embarking on combined modality approaches in early stages of Hodgkin's disease.

## 13.4. Current Approaches to Radiation Therapy in the Management of Hodgkin's Disease

The curative intent of irradiation in the treatment of Hodgkin's disease has evolved from low dose, low energy, small field irradiation to high dose, high energy, wide field irradiation over the last several decades. Historically, low doses of irradiation frequently induced a disappearance of pathologic lymphadenopathy, but was associated with recurrence of disease within the same area. Higher dose, but localized irradiation was associated with a greater likelihood of freedom from failure but the disease tended to develop in contiguous lymph-node-bearing areas (Gilbert and Babaintz, 1931; Peters and Middlemiss, 1958; Easson and Russell, 1963). Similarly, low energy irradiation was associated with excessive doses to normal tissue within the treated field. An evolution in radiotherapy technology, technique, and philosophy has led to enhanced survival in patients with Hodgkin's disease. Nevertheless, there is a lack of uniform agreement as to the most appropriate manner of staging and treating either early or late Hodgkin's disease.

### 13.4.1. Stages IA and IIA

Either total nodal irradiation or extended field irradiation to the mantle (lymph-node-bearing areas above the diaphragm, usually excluding Waldeyer's ring) and para-aortic-splenic pedicle regions is associated with a disease-free survival in excess of 80% and an overall survival in excess of 95% (Johnson *et al.*, 1977; Goodman *et al.*, 1976; Kaplan, 1976). Inclusion of the pelvis within the treated region is associated with a high likelihood of sterility in both males and females, and omission of this field has not been associated with a greater likelihood of failure. It is the approach in some centers to include the pelvis within the treated areas in stages IA and IIA with the so-called unfavorable histologic types of mixed cellularity or lymphocyte depleted. In fact, at least two studies have demonstrated that stage for stage, the histologic types are not associated with a greater likelihood of failure and hence should not modify the regions to be treated (Goodman *et al.*, 1976). Several groups are currently studying less field irradiation alone as an alternative to the more traditional extended fields of irradiation. In this trial there has been a high incidence of failure in adjacent lymph-node-bearing areas, although to date the overall survival has been unchanged (Hutchinson, 1976). The addition of chemotherapy to extended field irradiation for localized disease appears to have increased the disease-free survival in a number of trials (Beretta *et al.*, 1976; Prosnitz *et al.*, 1976; O'Connell *et al.*, 1975). Such studies at this time must be viewed as investigational and longer term data must be analyzed regarding the risks of combined modality treatment in this group of patients in whom radiation therapy alone is associated with an excellent prognosis. The 20–30% relapse rate following radiation therapy alone, however, has prompted the addition of chemotherapy.

### 13.4.2. Stage IIIA

The traditional form of treatment for patients with stage IIIA disease has been total nodal irradiation. However, a number of studies recently have reported disease-free survivals ranging from 25 to 75%. The majority of failures in such patients has been in extranodal sites. Even more so than in stage IA and IIA there is a diversity of opinion as to how to best treat this group of patients. There are advocates of chemotherapy only or chemotherapy with low dose irradiation to sites of previous bulk disease. To the contrary, a recent prospective randomized study between total nodal irradiation alone and chemotherapy alone demonstrated a significantly enhanced disease-free survival with total nodal irradiation (British National Lymphoma Investigation, 1976). Nonetheless, the disease-free survival in such patients with radiation therapy alone was sufficiently low to justify alternative forms of treatment. The use of several cycles of multiagent chemotherapy, to be followed by high dose total nodal irradiation or mantle and para-aortic irradiation, with several additional cycles of multiagent chemotherapy after the completion of the irradiation, has proven effective in stage III disease (Goodman *et al.*, 1977). There are also advocates for the continuation of total nodal irradiation with multi-agent chemotherapy reserved for that group of patients who subsequently develop failure. A critical issue which has yet to be answered is whether patients who are given chemotherapy at the time of failure will have the same salvage incidence as those patients who are given chemotherapy prophylactically. Combination chemotherapy appears to be able to induce long-term remissions in patients who relapse following radiation therapy with a disease-free survival which resembles that of previously untreated patients (Canellos *et al.*, 1972; Weller *et al.*, 1976). It is apparent, however, that the higher incidence of second neoplasms occurs in those patients treated with both modalities but who sustain an intervening period of Hodgkin's disease activity in relapse (Canellos *et al.*, 1975).

Associated with the pelvic portal as in earlier stages of disease there is also a higher incidence of sterility in both sexes even without chemother-apy (Asbjbrnsen *et al.*, 1976a; LeFloch *et al.*, 1976).

### 13.4.3. Stages IB, IIB, and IIIB

There are insufficient data to analyze stage IB patients separately because of the paucity of surgically staged patients of this group; thus, for the purposes of this discussion they are included in stage IIB and IIIB patients. It has become common practice to recommend some combina-tion of either high dose total nodal irradiation or mantle and para-aortic irradiation and combination chemotherapy in patients with surgically staged IIB disease (Rosenberg and Kaplan, 1975). Although excellent disease-free and overall survival rates have been reported, it is neverthe-less statistically difficult to prove the efficacy of this treatment over total nodal irradiation alone. Nonetheless, it is policy at a number of centers to recommend several cycles of multiagent chemotherapy, to be followed by high dose mantle and para-aortic irradiation, to be followed by the completion of the chemotherapy in such patients. Treatment regimens for stage IIIB patients are more controversial. Total nodal irradiation alone is clearly associated with at least a 60% incidence of nodal or extranodal failure and no longer should be considered as the sole form of treatment. Recommended forms of therapy include multiagent chemo-therapy alone, multiagent chemotherapy with low or high dose irradiation to sites of previous bulk disease, or mantle and para-aortic irradiation or total nodal irradiation in combination with multiagent chemotherapy (Prosnitz *et al.*, 1976; Rosenberg and Kaplan, 1975). To date, these three regimens have clearly been associated with a higher disease-free and ultimate survival than total nodal irradiation alone. The most efficacious combination of therapies for this stage, however, must await further study.

## 13.4.4. Radiation Therapy Techniques

Careful attention must be paid to the technical factors of radiation therapy in order to maximize dose to the tumor and minimize dose to the normal structures within the irradiated field. The use of high energy irradiation such as cobalt-60 or linear accelerators is essential. Other technical factors include the use of treatment simulators, individualized divergent blocks to protect underlying lung and heart, careful patient positioning, and monitoring of the dose. Frequent portal films are performed to ensure correct treatment, and close cooperation between the radiation therapist, physicist, dosimetrists, technician, and the workshop facility is essential.

## References

Aisenberg, A. C., and Qazi, R., 1974, Abdominal involvement at the onset of Hodgkin's disease, *Am. J. Med.* **57**:870.

Amlot, P. L., Slaney, J. M., and Williams, B. D., 1976, Circulating immune complexes and symptoms in Hodgkin's disease, *Lancet* **1**:449.

Asbjrnsen, G., Molne, K., Kleep, O., and Aakvaag, A., 1976a, Testicular function after radiotherapy to inverted Y field for malignant lymphoma, *Scand. J. Haematol.* **17**:96.

Asbjrnsen, G., Molne, K., Klepp, O., and Aakvaag, A., 1976b, Testicular function after combination chemotherapy for Hodgkin's disease, *Scand. J. Haematol.* **16**:66.

Beretta, G., Spinelli, P., Rilke, F., Tancini, G., Canetta, R., Gennari, L., and Bonadonna, G., 1976, Sequential laparoscopy and laparotomy combined with bone marrow biopsy in staging Hodgkin's disease, *Cancer Treat. Rep.* **60**: 1231.

Bloomfield, C. D., Weiss, R. B., Fortuny, I., Vosika, G., and Kennedy, B. J., 1976, Combined chemotherapy with cyclophosphamide and prednisone (CVPP) for patients with advanced Hodgkin's disease, *Cancer* **38**:42.

Bobrove, A., Funks, Z., Strober, S., and Kaplan, H. S., 1975, Quantitation of T and B lymphocytes and cellular immune function in Hodgkin's disease, *Cancer* **36**:169.

Bonadonna, G., Zucali, R., Monfardini, S., DeLena, M., and Uslenghi, C., 1975, Combination chemotherapy of Hodgkin's disease with adriamycin, bleomycin, vinblastine, and imidazole carboxamide versus MOPP, *Cancer* **36**:252.

British National Lymphoma Investigation, 1975, Value of prednisone in combination chemotherapy of stage IV Hodgkin's disease, *Br. Med. J.* **3**:413.

British National Lymphoma Investigation, 1976, Initial treatment of stage IIIA Hodgkin's disease, *Lancet* **2**:991.

Canellos, G. P., Young, R. C., and DeVita, V. T., 1972, Combination chemotherapy for advanced Hodgkin's disease in relapse following extensive radiotherapy, *Clin. Pharmacol. Ther.* **13**:750.

Canellos, G. P., DeVita, V. T., Arseneau, J. C., Whang-Peng, J., and Johnson, R.,

1975, Malignancies complicating Hodgkin's disease in remission, *Lancet* **1**:947.

Case, D. C., Young, C. W., Nisce, L., Lee, B. J., III, and Clarkson, B. D., 1976, Eight-drug combination chemotherapy (MOPP and ABVD) and local radiotherapy for advanced Hodgkin's disease, *Cancer Treat. Rep.* **60**:1217.

Case, D. C., Young, C. W., and Lee, B. J., III, 1977, Combination chemotherapy of MOPP-resistant Hodgkin's disease with adriamycin, bleomycin, dacarbazine and vinblastine (ABDV), *Cancer* **39**:1382.

Castellino, R. A., Glatstein, E., Turbow, M. M., Rosenberg, S., and Kaplan, H. S., 1974, Latent radiation injury of lungs or heart activated by steroid withdrawal, *Ann. Intern. Med.* **80**:593.

Chang, T., Stutzman, L., and Sokal, J. E., 1975, Correlation of delayed hypersensitivity responses with chemotherapeutic results in advanced Hodgkin's disease, *Cancer* **36**:950.

Coltman, C. A., Frei, E., III, and Moon, T. E., 1976, MOPP maintenance (MM) unmaintained remission (UMR) for MOPP induced complete remission (CR) of advanced Hodgkin's disease (HD): 7.2 year follow-up, *Proc. AACR/ASCO* **17**:289.

Corder, M. P., Young, R. C., Brown, R. S., and DeVita, V. T., 1972, Phytohemagglutinin-induced lymphocyte transformation: The relationship to prognosis of Hodgkin's disease, *Blood* **39**:595.

Desser, R. K., Golomb, H. M., Ultmann, J. E., Ferguson, D. J., Moran, E. M., Griem, M. L., Vardiman, J., Miller, B., Oetzel, N., Sweet, D., Lester, E. P., Kinzie, J. J., and Blough, R., 1977, Prognostic classification of Hodgkin's disease in pathologic stage III, based on anatomic considerations, *Blood* **49**:883.

DeVita, V. T., Serpick, A. A., and Carbone, P. P., 1970, Combination chemotherapy in the treatment of advanced Hodgkin's disease, *Ann. Intern. Med.* **73**:881.

DeVita, V. T., Bagley, C. M., Goodell, B., O'Kieffe, E. A., and Trujillo, N. P., 1971, Peritoneoscopy in the staging of Hodgkin's disease, *Cancer Res.* **31**:1746.

DeVita, V. T., Canellos, G. P., and Moxley, J. H., III, 1972, A decade of combination chemotherapy of advanced Hodgkin's disease, *Cancer* **30**:1495.

DeVita, V. T., Canellos, G., Hubbard, S., Chabner, B., and Young, R., 1976, Chemotherapy of Hodgkin's disease (HD) with MOPP: A 10 yr. progress report, *Proc. ASCO* **17**:269.

Diggs, C. H., Wiernik, P. H., Levi, J. A., and Kvols, L. K., 1977, Cyclophosphamide, vinblastine, procarbazine and prednisone with CCNU and vinblastine maintenance for advanced Hodgkin's disease, *Cancer* **39**:1949.

Easson, E., and Russel, M., 1963, The cure of Hodgkin's disease, *Br. Med. J.* **1**:1704.

Frei, E., III, Coltman, C. A., Talley, R. W., Wilson, H. E., and Delaney, F. C., 1973, Combination chemotherapy in advanced Hodgkin's disease, *Ann. Intern. Med.* **79**:376.

Fuks, Z., Strober, S., and Kaplan, H. S., 1976, Interaction between serum factors and T lymphocytes in Hodgkin's disease, *N. Engl. J. Med.* **295**:1273.

Gamble, J. F., Fuller, L. M., Martin, R. G., Sullivan, M. P., Jing, B., Butler, J. J., and Shullenberger, C. C., 1975, Influence of staging celiotomy in localized presentations of Hodgkin's disease, *Cancer* **35**:817.

Gilbert, R., and Babaintz, L., 1931, Nôtre méthode de roentgenthérapie de la lymphogranulomatose—Résultats élonges, *Acta Radiol.* **12**:523.

Goldman, U. M., and Dawson, A. A., 1975, Combination therapy for advanced resistant Hodgkin's disease, *Lancet* **2**:1224.

Goodman, R. L., Piro, A. J., and Hellman, S., 1976, Can pelvic irradiation be omitted in patients with pathologic stages IA and IIA Hodgkin's disease? *Cancer* **37**:2834.

Goodman, R. L., Rosenthal, D., Botnick, L., Piro, A., and Hellman, S., 1977, Stage IIIA Hodgkin's disease: Results of treatment with total nodal irradiation, *Proc. ASCO* **18**:348.

Graze, P. R., Perlin, E., and Royston, I., 1976, *In vitro* lymphocyte dysfunction in Hodgkin's disease, *J. Nat. Cancer Inst.* **56**:239.

Han, T., and Sokal, J. E., 1970, Lymphocyte response to phytohemagglutinin in Hodgkin's disease, *Am. J. Med.* **48**:728.

Hellman, S., 1974, Current studies in Hodgkin's disease, *N. Engl. J. Med.* **290**:894.

Hersh, E. M., and Oppenheim, J. J., 1965, Impaired *in vitro* lymphocyte transformation in Hodgkin's disease, *N. Engl. J. Med.* **273**:1006.

Holm, G., Mellstedt, H., Bjorkholm, M., Johansson, B., Killander, D., Sundblad, R., and Soderberg, G., 1976, Lymphocyte abnormalities in untreated patients with Hodgkin's disease, *Cancer* **37**:751.

Hutchinson, G. B., 1976, Survival and complications of radiotherapy following involved and extended field therapy of Hodgkin's disease. Stage I and II: A collaborative study, *Cancer* **38**:288.

Jackson, S. M., Garrett, J. V., and Craig, A. W., 1970, Lymphocyte transformation changes during the clinical course of Hodgkin's disease, *Cancer* **25**:843.

Johnson, R. E., Zimbler, H., Berard, C. W., Herdt, J., and Brereton, H. D., 1977, Radiotherapy results for nodular sclerosing Hodgkin's disease after clinical staging, *Cancer* **39**:1439.

Kadin, M. E., Glatstein, E., and Dorfman, R. F., 1971, Clinicopathologic studies of 117 untreated patients subjected to laparotomy for the staging of Hodgkin's disease, *Cancer* **27**:1277.

Kaplan, H. S., 1976, Hodgkin's disease and other human malignant lymphomas: Advances and prospects—G. H. A. Clowes Memorial Lecture, *Cancer Res.* **36**:3863.

Lang, J. M., Oberling, F., Tongio, M. M., Mayer, S., and Waitz, R., 1972, Mixed lymphocyte reaction as assay for immunological competence of lymphocytes from patients with Hodgkin's disease, *Lancet* **1**:261.

LeFloch, O., Donaldson, S., and Kaplan, H. S., 1976, Pregnancy following oophoropexy and nodal irradiation in women with Hodgkin's disease, *Cancer* **38**:2263.

Levi, J. A., and Wiernik, P. H., 1977, The therapeutic implications of splenic involvement in stage IIIA Hodgkin's disease, *Cancer* **39**:2158.

Levy, R., and Kaplan, H. S., 1974, Impaired lymphocyte function in untreated Hodgkin's disease, *N. Engl. J. Med.* **290**:181.

Lokich, J. J., Galvanek, E. G., and Moloney, W., 1973, Nephrosis of Hodgkin's disease, *Arch. Intern. Med.* **132**:597.

Long, J. C., Aisenberg, A. C., and Zamecnik, P. C., 1977a, Chromatographic and electrophoretic analysis of an antigen in Hodgkin's disease tissue cultures, *J. Nat. Cancer Inst.* **58**:223.

Long, J. C., Zamecnik, P. C., Aisenberg, A. C., and Atkins, L., 1977b, Tissue culture studies in Hodgkin's disease, *J. Exp. Med.* **145**:1484.

Longmire, R. L., McMillan, R., Yelenosky, R., Armstrong, S., Lang, J. E., and Craddock, C. G., 1973, *In vitro* splenic IgG synthesis in Hodgkin's disease, *N Engl. J. Med.* **289**:763.

Matchett, K. M., Huang, A. T., and Kremer, W. B., 1973, Impaired lymphocyte transformation in Hodgkin's disease, *J. Clin. Invest.* **52**:1908.

Nicholson, W. M., Beard, M. E. J., Crowther, D., Stansfeld, A. G., Vartan, C. P., Malpas, J. S., Fairley, G. H., and Scott, R. B., 1970, Combination chemotherapy in generalized Hodgkin's disease, *Br. Med. J.* **3**:7.

Nixon, D. W., and Aisenberg, A. C., 1974, Combination chemotherapy of Hodgkin's disease, *Cancer* **33**:1499.

O'Connell, M. J., Wiernik, P. H., Sklansky, B. D., Greene, W. H., Abt, W. B., Kirschner, R. H., Ramsey, H. E., and Murphy, W. L., 1974, Staging laparotomy in Hodgkin's disease, *Am. J. Med.* **57**:86.

O'Connell, M. J., Wiernik, P. H., Brace, K. C., Byhardt, R. W., and Greene, W. H., 1975, A combined modality approach to the treatment of Hodgkin's disease, *Cancer* **35**:1055.

Olweny, C. L. M., Mbidde, E. K., Nkwocha, J., Magrath, I., and Ziegler, J. L., 1974, Chemotherapy of Hodgkin's disease, *Lancet* **2**:1397.

Peters, M. V., and Middlemiss, K., 1958, Study of Hodgkin's disease treated by irradiation, *Am. J. Roentgenol.* **79**:111.

Plager, J., and Stutzman, L., 1971, Acute nephrotic syndrome as a manifestation of active Hodgkin's disease, *Am. J. Med.* **50**:56.

Prosnitz, L. R., Farber, L. R., Fischer, J. J., Bertino, J. R., and Fischer, D. B., 1976, Long-term remissions with combined modality therapy for advanced Hodgkin's disease, *Cancer* **37**:2826.

Rosenberg, S. A., and Kaplan, H. S., 1975, The management of stages I, II, and III Hodgkin's disease with combined radiotherapy and chemotherapy, *Cancer* **35**:55.

Rosner, F., and Grunwald, H., 1975, Hodgkin's disease and acute leukemia, *Am. J. Med.* **58**:338.

Sherins, R. J., and DeVita, V. T., 1973, Effect of drug treatment for lymphoma on male reproductive capacity, *Ann. Intern. Med.* **79**:216.

Sherman, R. L., Susin, M., Weksler, M. E., and Beckner, E. L., 1972, Lipoid nephrosis in Hodgkin's disease, *Am. J. Med.* **52**:699.

Sutcliffe, S. B. J., 1976, Intensive investigation in management of Hodgkin's disease, *Br. Med. J.* **2**:1343.

Ward, P. A., and Berenberg, J. L., 1974, Defective regulation of inflammatory mediators in Hodgkin's disease, *N. Engl. J. Med.* **290**:76.

Weller, S. A., Glatstein, E., Kaplan, H. S., and Rosenberg, S. A., 1976, Initial relapses in previously treated Hodgkin's disease, *Cancer* **37**:2840.

Young, R. C., Corder, M. P., Haynes, H. A., and DeVita, V. T., 1972, Delayed hypersensitivity in Hodgkin's disease, *Am. J. Med.* **52**:63.

Young, R. C., Canellos, G. P., Chabner, B. A., Schein, P. S., and DeVita, V. T., 1973, Maintenance chemotherapy for advanced Hodgkin's disease in remission, *Lancet* **1**:1339.

Zamecnik, P. C., and Long, J. C., 1977, Growth of cultured cells from patients with Hodgkin's disease and transplantation into nude mice, *Proc. Natl. Acad. Sci. U.S.A.* **74**:754.

Ziegler, J. L., Bluming, A. Z., Fass, L., Magrath, I. T., and Templeton, A. C., 1972, Chemotherapy of childhood Hodgkin's disease in Uganda, *Lancet* **2**:679.

# Recent Advances in the Treatment of Malignant Lymphoma: Non-Hodgkin's Lymphoma

Arthur T. Skarin, George P. Canellos, and Robert L. Goodman

## 14.1. Histopathology

A major advance in the understanding of the non-Hodgkin's lymphomas (NHL) was the replacement of the traditional classification, namely lymphosarcoma and reticulum cell sarcoma, by the classification scheme of Rappaport as originally proposed in 1966, but not widely utilized by clinicians until the early 1970s (Table I). This classification forms the basis for most of the therapeutic trials, and emphasizes the more favorable prognosis of nodular histology (with some exceptions, discussed later) compared to those lymphomas without nodules, i.e., diffuse histology (Jones *et al.*, 1972, 1973a,b; Skarin *et al.*, 1974a; Bonadonna *et al.*, 1976).

ARTHUR T. SKARIN, GEORGE P. CANELLOS, and ROBERT L. GOODMAN. • Sidney Farber Cancer Institute; Harvard Medical School, Boston, Massachusetts.

**Table I.**  Histopathologic Classifications[a]

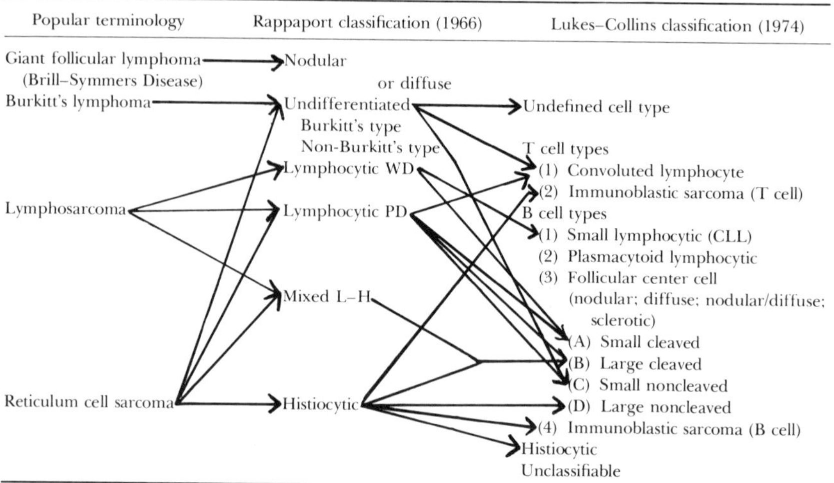



[a] WD, Well differentiated; PD, poorly differentiated; L–H, lymphocytic–histiocytic; T cell, thymus-derived lymphocyte; B cell, bone marrow-derived lymphocyte.

The following is a general review of various histologic subtypes and some recently described clinical–pathologic entities.

Well-differentiated lymphocytic lymphoma, regardless of a nodular or diffuse pattern, carries a better prognosis than the poorly differentiated type (Jones, 1975). While diffuse well-differentiated lymphocytic lymphoma, chronic lymphocytic leukemia, and well-differentiated lymphoproliferative disorders are histologically similar, three distinct clinical entities exist, justifying their separation (Pangalis *et al.*, 1977). Morphologically, poorly differentiated lymphocyte lymphoma (PDLL) can usually be distinguished from acute lymphocytic leukemia by the presence of increased numbers of prolymphocytes in the former disease. However, two clinical–pathologic variants of PDL have recently been reviewed by Nathwani *et al.* (1976), termed convoluted and nonconvoluted lymphoblastic lymphoma (see below).

Diffuse histiocytic lymphoma has a poor prognosis, whether the pattern is diffuse or nodular (Jones, 1975). Undifferentiated or stem cell lymphoma virtually always occurs in a diffuse pattern. In the Rappaport classification Burkitt's lymphoma would be classified as diffuse undifferentiated lymphoma.

Based upon significant differences in survival of histologic subtypes (Jones, 1975), patients can be placed into two groups: favorable prognosis, to include nodular well-differentiated lymphocytic, nodular mixed, nodular poorly differentiated lymphocytic, and diffuse well-differentiated lym-

**Table II.** Median Survival of Histologic Subgroups[a]

| | Median survival (years) | |
| Histologic subgroup | Nodular pattern | Diffuse pattern |
|---|---|---|
| Undifferentiated | — | 0.6 |
| Histiocytic | 3.0 | 1.1 |
| Mixed lymphocytic–histiocytic | 7.5 | 1.5 |
| Poorly differentiated lymphocytic | 7.5 | 1.8 |
| Well-differentiated lymphocytic | >7.5 | >7.5 |

[a]From Jones (1975).

phocytic lymphoma; and unfavorable prognosis histology, to include diffuse poorly differentiated lymphocytic, diffuse histiocytic, diffuse undifferentiated, diffuse mixed, and nodular histiocytic lymphoma (Table II).

The frequency distribution of histologic types of NHL based on the Rappaport classification is presented in Table III. About 45% of patients have nodular histology, with approximately equal numbers of PDL and mixed subtypes. The most common subtype of diffuse histology is histiocytic (24–29%) followed by PDL and mixed types.

**Table III.** Non-Hodgkin's Lymphomas—Percent Distribution of Histologic Types

| | Histology[a] | Stanford[b] (N = 405) | SWOG[c] (N = 420) | Philadelphia[d] (N = 293) | NCI[e] (N = 170) |
|---|---|---|---|---|---|
| Nodular | WDL | 2 | 10 | 1 | 0 |
| | PDL | 17 | 16 | 21 | 29 |
| | M | 18 | 5 | 18 | 15 |
| | H | 7 | 4 | 3 | 4 |
| Subtotal | | 44 | 35 | 44 | 48 |
| Diffuse | WDL | 2 | 11 | 2 | 4 |
| | PDL | 11 | 18 | 15 | 17 |
| | M | 10 | 6 | 10 | 4 |
| | H | 29 | 27 | 26 | 24 |
| | U | 4 | 3 | 3 | 4 |
| Subtotal | | 56 | 65 | 56 | 52 |
| Total | | 100 | 100 | 100 | 100 |

[a]WDL, Well-differentiated lymphocytic; PDL, poorly differentiated lymphocytic; M, mixed lymphocytic–histiocytic; H, histiocytic; U, undifferentiated.
[b]Jones *et al.* (1973a).
[c]McKelvey *et al.* (1976): SWOG, Southwest Oncology Group.
[d]Patchefsky *et al.* (1974).
[e]Chabner *et al.* (1976).

In 1974 Lukes and Collins published a new classification of NHL based on morphological, cytochemical, and immunological membrane marker studies. With use of this system over 70% of histologies are comprised of cleaved and noncleaved follicular center cells of B cell origin, with nodularity occurring only in these types. Lymphomas of "true" histiocytes (and not transformed lymphocytes) are rare. A distinctive clinical–pathologic entity involving large transformed lymphocytes of either B or T cell origin (immunoblastic sarcoma) has been described (Lukes and Collins, 1974). Another clinical–pathologic entity called T cell lymphoma with convoluted lymphocytes, in the past partially confused with acute lymphocytic leukemia or diffuse PDL lymphoma, has been described in detail (Barcos and Lukes, 1975). Patients with this disorder (usually young men) frequently present with massive mediastinal adenopathy and usually develop a leukemic phase which is often refractory to therapy.

Immunoblastic or angioimmunoblastic lymphadenopathy is a recently described lymphoma-like syndrome involving proliferation of lymphocytes and small vessels with resultant generalized adenopathy, hepatosplenomegaly, skin rash, and polyclonal hypergammaglobulinemia (Lukes and Tindle, 1975; Frizzera *et al.*, 1975). Although the disorder appears to be benign microscopically, the clinical course is aggressive with a median survival of 15 months in 18 fatal cases. Of interest, immunoblastic sarcoma has developed in several cases (Lukes and Tindle, 1975). Detailed immunologic and electron microscopic studies in one patient with a leukemic phase revealed plasmacytoid and not lymphocytic features (Fisher *et al.*, 1976).

Two interesting syndromes, the Sezary syndrome and mycosis fungoides, are related to proliferation of thymus-derived lymphocytes, with progressive involvement of skin, lymph nodes, and visceral organs (Lutzner *et al.*, 1975). In Sezary syndrome, a leukemic phase exists with circulation of convoluted lymphocytes (T cells). It has been proposed that both disorders represent variant clinical expressions of the same process, and should be called "cutaneous T-cell lymphoma with or without leukemic phase" (Schein *et al.*, 1976a).

Burkitt's lymphoma, once thought to be restricted to tropical Africa, has become increasingly recognized in the United States and other countries (Ziegler, 1977). The presence of immunologic surface markers has confirmed it to be of B cell origin (Mann *et al.*, 1976). When the disease occurs in temperate climates, abdominal masses are more common and it is seen in older children and young adults. Burkitt's lymphoma, even in the temperate zone, is quite responsive to therapy and long-term cures have been reported in Africa and the United States (Ziegler, 1977). For reasons yet unexplained, elevated titers of antibody to the Epstein–Barr virus have not been seen in the United States studies as compared to the high frequency in Africans (Arseneau *et al.*, 1975; Banks *et al.*, 1975). This may be the only lymphoma that shows a significant response to high dose single alkylating agent chemotherapy (Arseneau *et al.*, 1975), benefits from surgical excision of bulk tumor (Magrath *et al.*, 1974), and is associated with a beneficial host immune response (Arseneau *et al.*, 1975).

The interrelationship between popular terminology and the Lukes and Butler classification and that of Rappaport is indicated by the arrows in Table I. Since the majority of treatment programs are based on the Rappaport classification, and since in one large study (Jones *et al.*, 1977) only 58% of cases had the histologic type confirmed after review by a lymphoma pathology panel, it is imperative that pathologic specimens be carefully evaluated by such a panel or by a regional cancer center. Use of the Lukes and Collins system in planning treatment programs awaits demonstration of reproducibility among various centers and any significant differences in prognosis among the various subgroups. One recent study using B- and T-lymphocyte surface markers suggests that survival of patients whose malignant cells contain B markers was longer than those with no B or T cell markers, or so-called null cells (Bloomfield *et al.*, 1976).

## 14.2. Staging

Considerable data have been accumulated regarding the clinical features and natural history of NHL. Although there is some variation in clinical–pathologic features due to either geographic factors or the type of patient referred to a research center, the following generalities can be made (Jones, 1974, 1975; Jones *et al.*, 1973a). Nodular lymphomas are rare in young adults and children and occur less commonly in patients over the age of 60 years. Women more frequently have nodular lymphoma than men while the reverse is true with diffuse patterns. Adenopathy may be of long-standing duration with nodular histology. Disseminated disease is associated with constitutional symptoms more commonly with diffuse histology (25–30% of cases) than nodular disease (15–20% of cases) but most studies show that symptoms *per se* are not prognostically important. The following areas of involvement are more common with diffuse than nodular histology: localized extralymphatic disease (16 versus 6%); Waldeyer's ring (11 versus 2%); mediastinum (24 versus 18%); skin (15 versus 7%), and gastrointestinal tract (22 versus 7%).

Unlike Hodgkin's disease (HD) the number of occult lesions increases in proportion to the extent of staging procedures (Goffinet *et al.*, 1973; Veronesi *et al.*, 1974; Kim and Dorfman 1974). In a recent NCI study of 170 consecutive untreated patients, sequential staging procedures (short of laparotomy) established stage III or IV disease in 80% of cases (Chabner *et al.*, 1976). Subsequent staging laparotomy revealed disease outside of conventional nodal irradiation fields in 81% (21/26) of patients with a positive lymphangiogram, but in only 18% (3/17) of patients with a negative lymphangiogram. Results of the NCI study showed that patients with nodular histology are almost invariably (94%) stage III and IV, while diffuse histiocytic lymphoma remains localized (stage I or II) in 30%. Unlike HD, it is apparent that staging laparotomy and splenectomy in NHL seldom results in a significant change in management plan. While at the present time no completely satisfactory staging system is available, the four-stage Ann Arbor classification adapted for HD is employed to ensure reasonable comparability among series (Carbone *et al.*, 1971).

## 14.3. Treatment

In the past radiotherapy was used mainly for localized NHL (stages I and II) with chemotherapy reserved for more advanced or disseminated disease (stages III and IV). In the latter category, irradiation is now being employed for residual disease or areas of previous bulk disease, although results of this application await longer follow-up. Similarly, several ongoing studies are evaluating the efficacy of "adjuvant" chemotherapy following radiotherapy for localized disease in poor prognosis histology. Total body irradiation is effective in disseminated disease and is being evaluated as a systemic agent (Chaffey *et al.*, 1975; Canellos *et al.*, 1975). The following is a review of therapy of various stages including approaches to favorable and unfavorable prognosis histology.

### 14.3.1. Early Disease

Medial survival following curative-intent radiotherapy for stages I–$III_E$ is 7.5 years (3.5 years disease-free) in nodular lymphomas compared to 2.6 years (0.9 years disease-free) in diffuse lymphomas (Jones, 1974). The majority of relapses in patients with diffuse histology occur during the first 2 years of follow-up, while nodular types continue to show late relapse, reflecting the favorable natural history of nodular lymphomas (Bonadonna *et al.*, 1976; Jones, 1974). Retreatment of the latter results in further prolongation of survival while most patients with diffuse histology in relapse are generally refractory to further therapy.

Review of recent data from the Harvard Joint Center for Radiation Therapy reveals that while survival of patients with stage I and II disease is impressive and quite comparable (82% at 5 years), relapse-free survival differs (60% for stage I versus 20% for stage II) with sites of failure in nodal as well as extranodal areas (Hellman *et al.*, 1977). Actuarial survival and relapse-free survival appear worse in histiocytic types compared to lymphocytic (and mixed cell) types, and diffuse compared to nodular types. In contrast, another recent radiotherapy study, but involving only 19 patients with pathologic stage I and II diffuse histiocytic lymphoma, revealed a 78% relapse-free survival at 5 years (Bitran *et al.*, 1977).

In an effort to decrease subsequent relapse, two similar controlled adjuvant studies were initiated, employing six cycles of COP following irradiation in pathologic stage I and II patients. In the Bonadonna study (1976), chemotherapy significantly increased the disease-free survival but only in the subgroup with lymphocytic lymphoma. Results from Stanford (Rosenberg and Kaplan, 1975) in patients with unfavorable histology reveal no differences in survival after the addition of COP plus or minus bleomycin after total nodal irradiation. Unfortunately, numbers are small and because of myelosuppression, chemotherapy was started late.

Radiotherapy with curative intent is justified in stage I favorable histology, while in stage I unfavorable histology and stage II (all histologies) regional irradiation followed by adjuvant systemic therapy appears indicated. The most effective combined program remains to be determined.

### 14.3.2. Advanced Disease

Therapy of disseminated NHL (stages III and IV) varies greatly according to the histology, from palliative single drug therapy to intensive combination chemotherapy in advanced stage IV disease. Less aggressive therapy has resulted in satisfactory palliation in the favorable prognosis histologies (defined earlier) which have a protracted natural history. High dose total axial lymphoid radiation therapy for stage III disease has been employed by the Stanford Group (Glatstein *et al.*, 1976) with a 5-year survival of 75% in 51 patients with nodular histology (43% relapse-free). Results were not as good in patients with diffuse histology, with relapse in 83% (14/17 of patients by 5 years. While 50% of relapses in both groups occurred in lymph node areas, extension to nontreated nodal sites (i.e., epitrochlear was frequent in nodular histology with additional benefit from further irradiation.

A systemic modality which is relatively easily administered and tolerated, namely total body irradiation (TBI), has been reintroduced. Recent studies in patients mainly with favorable histology stage III and limited stage IV disease have demonstrated its effectiveness (Chaffey *et al.*, 1975; Hellman *et al.*, 1977). Results in 72 patients at the Harvard Joint Center for Radiation Therapy reveal a 5-year survival of 70%, with a relapse-free survival of 20%. Survival in patients with nodular histology is about twice that in diffuse histology (82 versus 42%) while the majority of both groups relapse. TBI with additional regional XRT was equally effective as CVP chemotherapy in inducing complete remission (55%) in 65 patients with advanced lymphocytic lymphoma in a randomized trial recently reported by Canellos *et al.* (1975). Overall survival at 3 years exceeded 80%, with nodular histology better than diffuse histology. About 50% of patients relapsed but disease was controlled by retreatment with either form of therapy, especially in nodular histology.

### 14.3.2.1. Favorable Histology

Chemotherapy of advanced favorable prognosis histology (mainly nodular) remains controversial. Preliminary results from a prospective trial at Stanford (Portlock *et al.*, 1976) in stage IV disease with favorable histologies, comparing cyclophosphamide, vincristine, and prednisone (CVP), CVP and total lymphoid irradiation, and single alkylating agent therapy, reveal comparable actuarial survival and relapse-free survival at 40 months (approximately 80 and 50%, respectively). Combined modality therapy resulted in increased toxicity compared to minimal morbidity with single agent therapy. Unfortunately, 21 of 63 (33%) patients had progression of disease after therapy. An update of our initial COP study (Skarin *et al.*, 1974a) has revealed a continuous late relapse and death at 7 years in 12 of 13 (92%) patients with favorable histology. The majority of these relapses involved change in histology to a diffuse pattern, mainly histiocytic subtype, with rapidly progressive disease. Results of two BACOP studies (Skarin *et al.*, 1977a; Rodriguez *et al.*, 1977) in advanced favorable histology show impressive results, but longer follow-up is needed to determine possible cures (Fig. 1). Recent data from NCI reveal that achieving a CR with aggressive chemotherapy (C-MOPP) in favorable histology (NM and NPDL) may result in long-term survival (6+ and 9+ years, respectively) compared to partial responders who had a median survival of only 11 and 28 months, respectively (Young *et al.*, 1977). Further documentation of this potentially important data is needed.

### 14.3.2.2. Unfavorable Histology

Combination chemotherapy has been shown to result in higher complete remission (CR) rates in advanced NHL of unfavorable histology than single agent therapy (Bonadonna *et al.*, 1976; Luce *et al.*, 1971). As a consequence, long-term disease-free survival in approximately 40% of patients with diffuse histiocytic lymphoma, which in the past was rapidly fatal in the majority of cases, has recently been reported (DeVita *et al.*, 1975). Results of programs from selected centers are noted in Table IV

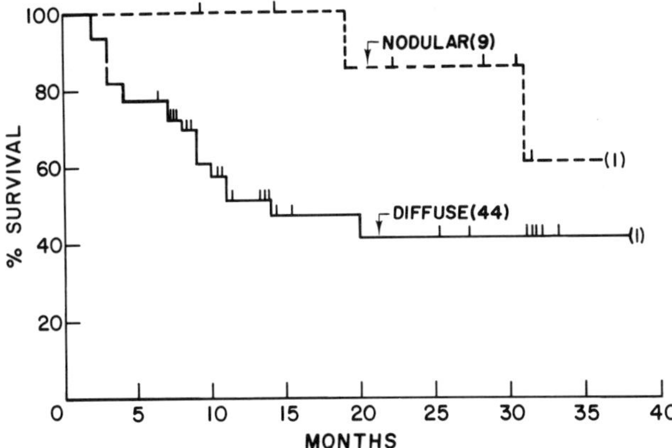



**Fig. 1.** Actuarial survival in advanced non-Hodgkin's lymphoma with nodular histology (9 patients) and diffuse histology (44 patients) from onset of therapy with BACOP—bleomycin, adriamycin, cyclophosphamide, vincristine, and prednisone. (From Skarin *et al.*, 1977. Reproduced by permission of the publisher from *Blood*.)

**Table IV.** Combination Chemotherapy Programs in Advanced Non-Hodgkin's Lymphomas

| Center[a] | Reference | Program[b] | Diffuse No. | Diffuse % CR | Nodular No. | Nodular % CR |
|---|---|---|---|---|---|---|
| SWOG | Luce *et al.*, 1971 | COP | 130 | 27 | 73 | 51 |
| SFCI | Skarin *et al.*, 1974a | COP | 29 | 14 | 13 | 77 |
| NCI | Schein *et al.*, 1974 | COP/C–MOPP' | 43 | 30 | 37 | 62 |
| Chicago | Stein *et al.*, 1975 | COPP' | 11 | 45 | 21 | 70 |
| Stanford | Portlock and Rosenberg, 1976 | COP | 26 | 23 | 32 | 43 |
| ECOG | Lenhard *et al.*, 1976 | COP | 35 | 43 | 7 | 86 |
| SWOG | McKelvey *et al.*, 1976 | AOP | 134 | 60 | 75 | 67 |
| SWOG | McKelvey *et al.*, 1976 | ACOP | 128 | 67 | 73 | 78 |
| SWOG | Luce *et al.*, 1973 | BCOP | 40 | 62 | 8 | 50 |
| SFCI | Skarin *et al.*, 1974b | BACOP | 44 | 66 | 9 | 89 |
| NCI | Schein *et al.*, 1975a | BACOP | 25 | 48[c] | — | — |
| SWOG | Rodriguez *et al.*, 1977 | BACOP | 31 | 67 | 16 | 63 |

[a]SFCI, Sidney Farber Cancer Institute and Peter Bent Brigham Hospital; SWOG, Southwest Oncology Group; NCI, National Cancer Institute; ECOG, Eastern Cooperative Oncology Group.
[b]C, Cyclophosphamide; O, Oncovin (vincristine); P, prednisone; P', procarbazine; A, adriamycin; B, bleomycin.
[c]Diffuse histiocytic only.

(Lenhard *et al.*, 1976; Luce *et al.*, 1973; McKelvey *et al.*, 1976; Portlock and Rosenberg, 1976; Rodriguez *et al.*, 1977; Schein *et al.*, 1974, 1975a,b, 1976b; Skarin *et al.*, 1974a,b, 1977a; Stein *et al.*, 1975). While the exact dose and scheduling of cyclophosphamide, vincristine, and prednisone (CVP or COP) programs vary among the centers, the average CR rate in diffuse histologies is 28% range (14–43%) compared to approximately twice that (57%) in nodular histologies (range 43–86%). With the addition of adriamycin and bleomycin, the CR rate singificantly increases in diffuse histology (range 60–67%) with further increases in nodular types (range 50–89%). While the CR rates with three recently reported five-drug combinations (BACOP) are identical to three- and four-drug combinations (AOP, ACOP, BCOP), long-term disease-free survival may be greater in the BACOP programs (see later).

Complete remission rates of these programs in selected subtypes of diffuse histology are noted in Table V. With COP programs, the average CR appears higher in DPDL versus DH (33 versus 25%) with numbers too small in DM for valid comparison. Response rates with AOP, ACOP, and BCOP are higher than COP (about twice) with no apparent differences in the subtypes. BACOP results in higher CR rates in DPDL (average 78%) than in DH (average 55%).

Most studies have shown that prior chemotherapy significantly lowers the CR rate with combined chemotherapy programs while prior localized XRT may not be an adverse factor. Likewise, the CR rate may vary among centers depending on the extent of restaging procedures. Unlike Hodgkin's disease, patients with NHL are older and frequently have other

**Table V.**   Results of Combination Chemotherapy in Selected Histologic Subtypes[a]

| Center | Program | DPDL | | DH | | DM | |
|---|---|---|---|---|---|---|---|
| | | No. | % CR | No. | % CR | No. | % CR |
| SFCI | COP | 14 | 14 | 12 | 17 | — | — |
| Chicago | COPP' | 4 | 75 | 6 | 17 | | |
| Stanford | COP | 4 | 75 | 13 | 15 | 3 | 0 |
| ECOG | COP | 9 | 33 | 10 | 40 | 5 | 100 |
| NCI | COP/C–MOPP' | 9 | 22 | 26 | 35 | 4 | 0 |
| SWOG | AOP | 38 | 55 | 62 | 66 | 12 | 50 |
| SWOG | ACOP | 38 | 68 | 53 | 68 | 14 | 71 |
| SWOG | BCOP | 12 | 75 | 15 | 60 | — | — |
| SFCI | BACOP[b] | 12 | 80 | 18 | 56 | 6 | 67 |
| NCI | BACOP | — | — | 25 | 58 | — | — |
| SWOG | BACOP | 3 | 67 | 26 | 69 | — | — |

[a]See Tables I and IV for definitions.
[b]Also called B-CHOP.

medical problems, placing them at increased risk for invasive staging procedures such as laparotomy. Nevertheless, pathologic restaging to confirm a complete remission is recommended including rebiopsy of residual or suspicious nodes and repeat baseline studies, especially if previously abnormal.

In a randomized study comparing COP with ABP in 57 evaluable patients (mainly having diffuse histology) with stage IV disease, Monfardini *et al.* (1977) have shown that both programs result in comparable CR rates (50%). Furthermore, crossover for minimal response or relapse after initial remission revealed significant secondary responses in both treatment groups, suggesting that both programs could be used sequentially (or in combination) to improve overall results.

Remission duration varies considerably, depending on histology, stage, drug combination employed, and whether a partial or complete response has been achieved. Partial remissions in unfavorable histology do not favorably affect prognosis, with survival similar to that with no response. A comparison of median CR durations after multiple agent chemotherapy has been prepared by Bonadonna *et al.* (1976).

The BACOP intensive treatment programs (Rodriguez *et al.*, 1977; Skarin *et al.*, 1974b, 1975, 1977a; Schein *et al.*, 1975a, 1976b) were mainly designed to increase the CR rate and duration in unfavorable histology and also to decrease the prospects for relapse which had occurred in earlier three- and four-drug programs between induction cycles during the time of bone marrow recovery. Early results show that the latter has probably been achieved. The projected durations of CR are 14+ months (Skarin *et al.*, 1977a) in excess of 12 months (Schein *et al.*, 1976b) and greater than 2 years (Rodriguez *et al.*, 1977).

The value of maintenance therapy after complete remission has been achieved remains to be resolved. Two COP studies have shown in randomized trials that maintenance chemotherapy prolongs the duration of CR, but survival is probably not affected (Luce *et al.*, 1971; Lenhard *et al.*, 1976). Since nodular lymphomas usually have a progressive relapse rate and death, additional therapy after remission may be required to improve survival. On the contrary, intensive combination chemotherapy for a definite interval may be sufficient for a long relapse-free survival and eventual cure in the unfavorable histologies similar to the results achieved in advanced Hodgkin's disease with MOPP chemotherapy.

Results from several recent studies of patients with advanced diffuse histiocytic lymphoma are of major importance. Prolonged disease-free survival for 26–105 months in 10 patients achieving complete remission with C-MOPP was reported by DeVita *et al.* in 1975 and updated in 1976 (Berard *et al.*, 1976). In another study, 5 of 17 patients with DH achieved disease-free survival for 55–65 months following combined cyclophosphamide, vincristine, methotrexate and leucovorin rescue, and cytosine arabinoside (Berd *et al.*, 1975). Flattening of survival curves in about 40% of patients with DH has been noted with BACOP as used in Boston (Skarin *et al.*, 1977a) (see Fig. 1) and at NCI (Schein *et al.*, 1976b) with a slightly higher projected figure in the Southwest Oncology Group study (Rodriguez *et al.*, 1977).

Early relapse of unfavorable histologies remains a therapeutic challenge (Schein *et al.*, 1975b), especially relapse in the CNS. The latter has been reported to occur in 25–30% of cases (Skarin *et al.*, 1977a; Bunn *et al.*, 1976). Prophylaxis with one dose of intrathecal Ara-C has apparently prevented the latter complication in one recent study (Rodriguez *et al.*, 1977). Studies at the Sidney Farber Cancer Institute using high dose methotrexate with folinic acid rescue in patients failing multiple standard agents reveal a significant although generally brief response (Skarin *et al.*, 1977b). Disease regression occurred in 12 of 20 patients (60%) including four CR (median duration 4.5+ months). Of great interest was response in five of six patients with CNS involvement, with complete resolution of measurable disease in three patients. This regimen, which is nonmyelosuppressive and penetrates the blood–brain barrier, when integrated with other agents, may play a significant role in the chemotherapy of newly diagnosed patients with unfavorable histology NHL.

Whether BACOP, ACOP, C-MOPP, or any other intensive combination chemotherapy program will be the most effective in producing long-term remissions in unfavorable histologies will require longer follow-up and comparison of carefully matched groups of patients with identical prognostic characteristics. Similarly, these programs must be carefully monitored for unusual toxicity as was the case with increased lung toxicity related in part to moderate dose bleomycin in the early phases of two BACOP programs (Skarin *et al.*, 1977a; Schein *et al.*, 1976b). The potential for long-term remissions and eventual cures in diffuse histiocytic lymphoma after combination chemotherapy has been reviewed in a recent editorial (Sweet *et al.*, 1976).

## 14.4. Summary

Considerable progress in the classification, staging, and management of NHL has occurred during the past several years. It is critical that careful pathological review be undertaken to define whether the patient has a favorable histology or unfavorable histology, according to the Rappaport classification. Various immunological studies are currently under investigation in order to identify specific subgroups which might differ prognostically. Extensive pathological staging is recommended, although laparotomy is not generally indicated in the majority of cases. In stage I favorable histology disease, regional irradiation should be employed. All other regional disease, (stage I unfavorable histology, stage II favorable histology or unfavorable histology) may benefit from adjuvant systemic therapy following irradiation. Many therapeutic alternatives are available for patients with greater than stage II disease. Total body irradiation followed by chemotherapy is currently being evaluated in stage III (and some stage IV) patients with favorable histology. Similarly, single agent chemotherapy is effective, although long-term disease control has yet to be proven. For stage III and IV unfavorable histology, various four- and five-drug combination chemotherapy programs are being evaluated. It appears that with intensive treatment (i.e., with C-MOPP and BACOP) long-term disease-free survival may be achieved in 40% of patients with diffuse histiocytic lymphoma.

# References

Arseneau, J. C., Canellos, G. P., Banks, P. M., Berard, C. W., Gralnick, H. R., and DeVita, V. T., Jr., 1975, American Burkitt's lymphoma: A clinicopathologic study of 30 cases, *Am. J. Med.* **58**:314.

Banks, P. M., Arseneau, J. C., Gralnick, H. R., Canellos, G. P., DeVita, V., Jr., and Berard, C. W., 1975, American Burkitt's lymphoma: A clinicopathologic study of 30 cases, *Am. J. Med.* **58**:322.

Barcos, M. P., and Lukes, R. J., 1975, Malignant lymphoma of convoluted lymphocytes: A new entity of possible T-cell type, *Conflicts in Childhood Cancer. An Evaluation of Current Management*, Vol. 4 (L. F. Sinks and J. O. Godden, eds.), pp. 147–178, Alan R. Liss, New York.

Berard, C. W., Gallo, R. C., Jaffe, E. S., Green, I., and DeVita, V., Jr., 1976, Current concepts of leukemia and lymphoma: Etiology pathogenesis, and therapy, *Ann. Intern. Med.* **85**:351.

Berd, D., Cornog, J., DeConti, R. C., Levitt, M., and Bertino, J. R., 1975, Long-term remission in diffuse histiocytic lymphoma treated with combination sequential chemotherapy, *Cancer* **35**:1050.

Bitran, J. D., Kinzie, J., Sweet, D. L., Variakojis, D., Griem, M. L., Golomb, H. M., Miller, J. B., Oetzel, N., and Ultmann, J. E., 1977, Survival of patients with localized histiocytic lymphoma, *Cancer* **39**:342.

Bloomfield, C. D., Kersey, J. H., Brunning, R. D., and Gajl-Peczalska, K. J., 1976, Prognostic significance of lymphocyte surface markers in adult non-Hodgkin's malignant lymphoma, *Lancet* **2**:1330.

Bonadonna, G., Lattuada, A., and Banfi, A., 1976, Recent trends in the treatment of non-Hodgkin's lymphomas, *Eur. J. Cancer* **12**:661.

Bunn, P. A., Jr., Schein, P. S., Banks, P. M., and DeVita, V. T., Jr., 1976, Central nervous system complications in patients with diffuse histiocytic and undifferentiated lymphoma: Leukemia revisited, *Blood* **47**:3.

Canellos, G. P., DeVita, V. T., Young, R. C., Chabner, B. A., Schein, P. S., and Johnson, R. E., 1975, Therapy of advanced lymphocytic lymphoma: A preliminary report of a randomized trial between combination chemotherapy (CVP) and intensive radiotherapy, *Br. J. Cancer* **31**:474.

Carbone, P. P., Kaplan, H. S., Musshoff, K., Smithers, D. W., and Tubiana, M., 1971, Report of the committee on Hodgkin's disease staging classification, *Cancer Res.* **31**:1860.

Chabner, B. A., Johnson, R. E., Young, R. C., Canellos, G. P., Hubbard, S. P., Johnson, S. K., and DeVita, V. T., Jr., 1976, Sequential nonsurgical and surgical staging of non-Hodgkin's lymphoma, *Ann. Intern. Med.* **85**:149.

Chaffey, J. T., Rosenthal, D. S., Pinkus, G., and Hellman, S., 1975, Advanced lymphosarcoma treated by total body irradiation, *Br. J. Cancer* **31**:441.

DeVita, V. T., Chabner, B., Hubbard, S. P., Canellos, G. P., Schein, P., and Young, R. C., 1975, Advanced diffuse histiocytic lymphoma, a potentially curable disease, *Lancet* **1**:248.

Fisher, R. I., Jaffe, E. S., Braylan, R. C., Andersen, J. C., and Tan, H. K., 1976, Immunoblastic lymphadenopathy, *Am. J. Med.* **61**:553.

Frizzera, G., Moran, E. M., and Rappaport, H., 1975, Angioimmunoblastic lymphadenopathy, *Am. J. Med.* **59**:803.

Glatstein, E., Fuks, Z., Goffinet, D. R., and Kaplan, H. S., 1976, Non-Hodgkin's lymphomas of stage III extent, *Cancer* **37**:2806.

Goffinet, D. R., Castellino, R. A., Kim, H., Dorfman, R. F., Fuks, Z., Rosenberg, S. A., Nelsen, T., and Kaplan, H. S., 1973, Staging laparotomies in unselected previously untreated patients with non-Hodgkin's lymphomas, *Cancer* **32**:672.

Hellman, S., Chaffey, J. T., Rosenthal, D. S., Moloney, W. C., Canellos, G. P., and Skarin, A. T., 1977, The place of radiation therapy in the treatment of non-Hodgkin's lymphomas, *Cancer* **39**:843.

Jones, S. E., 1974, Clinical features and course of the non-Hodgkin's lymphomas, *Clin. Haematol.* **1**:131.

Jones, S. E., 1975, Non-Hodgkin's lymphomas, *JAMA* **234**:633.

Jones, S. E., Rosenberg, S. A., Kaplan, H. S., Kadin, M. E., and Dorfman, R. F., 1972, Non-Hodgkin's lymphomas. II. Single agent chemotherapy, *Cancer* **30**:31.

Jones, S. E., Fuks, Z., Bull, M., Kadin, M. E., Dorfman, R. F., Kaplan, H. S., Rosenberg, S. A., and Kim, H., 1973a, Non-Hodgkin's lymphomas. IV. Clinicopathologic correlation in 405 cases, *Cancer* **31**:806.

Jones, S. E., Fukz, Z., Kaplan, H. S., and Rosenberg, S. A., 1973b, Non-Hodgkin's lymphomas. V. Results of radiotherapy, *Cancer* **32**:682.

Jones, S. E., Butler, J. J., Bryne, G. E., Jr., Coltman, C. A., Jr., and Moon, T. E., 1977, Histopathologic review of lymphoma cases from the Southwest Oncology Group, *Cancer* **39**:1071.

Kim, H., and Dorfman, R. F., 1974, Morphological studies of 84 untreated patients subjected to laparotomy for the staging of non-Hodgkin's lymphomas, *Cancer* **33**:657.

Lenhard, R. E., Jr., Prentice, R. L., Owens, A. H., Jr., Bakemeier, R., Horton, J. H., Shnider, B. I., Stolbach, L., Berard, C. W., and Carbone, C. P., 1976, Combination chemotherapy of the malignant lymphomas, *Cancer* **38**:1052.

Luce, J. K., Gamble, J. F., Wilson, H. E., Monto, R. W., Isaacs, B. L., Palmer, R. L., Coltman, C. A., Jr., Hewlett, J. S., Gehan, E. A., and Frei, E., III, 1971, Combined cyclophosphamide, vincristine, prednisone therapy of malignant lymphoma, *Cancer* **28**:306.

Luce, J. K., Delaney, F. C., and Gehan, E. A., 1973, Remission induction chemotherapy of disseminated malignant lymphoma with combination bleomycin, cyclophosphamide, vincristine and prednisone, *Proc. Am. Assoc. Cancer Res.* **14**:66.

Lukes, R. J., and Collins, R. D., 1974, Immunologic characterization of human malignant lymphomas, *Cancer* **34**:1488.

Lukes, R. J., and Tindle, B. H., 1975, Immunoblastic lymphadenopathy—a hyperimmune entity resembling Hodgkin's disease, *N. Engl. J. Med.* **292**:1.

Lutzner, M., Edelson, R., Schein, P., Green, I., Kirkpatrick, C., and Ahmed, A., 1975, Cutaneous T-cell lymphomas: The Sezary syndrome, mycosis fungoides, and related disorders, *Ann. Intern. Med.* **83**:534.

Magrath, I. T., Lwanga, S., Carswell, W., and Harrison, N., 1974, Surgical reduction of tumour bulk in management of abdominal Burkitt's lymphoma, *Br. Med. J.* **1**:308.

Mann, R. B., Jaffe, E. S., Braylan, R. C., Nanba, K., Frank, M. M., Ziegler, J. L., and Berard, C. W., 1976, Nonendemic Burkitt's lymphoma, *N. Engl. J. Med.* **295**:685.

McKelvey, E. M., Gottlieb, J. A., Wilson, H. E., Haut, A., Talley, R. W., Stephens, R., Lane, M., Gamble, J. F., Jones, S. E., Grozea, P. N., Gutterman, J., Coltman, C., Jr., and Moon, T. E., 1976, Hydroxyldaunomycin (adriamycin) combination chemotherapy in malignant lymphoma, *Cancer* **38**:1484.

Monfardini, S., Tancini, G., De Lena, M., Villa, E., Valagussa, P., and Bonadonna, G., 1977, Cyclophosphamide, vincristine and prednisone (CVP) versus adriamycin, bleomycin and prednisone (ABP) in stage IV non-Hodgkin's lymphomas, *Med. Ped. Oncol.* **3**:67.

Nathwani, B. N., Kim, H., and Rappaport, H., 1976, Malignant lymphoma, lymphoblastic, *Cancer* **38**:964.

Pangalis, G. A., Nathwani, B. N., and Rappaport, H., 1977, Malignant lymphoma, well-differentiated lymphocytic, *Cancer* **39**:999.

Patchefsky, A. S., Brodovsky, H. S., Menduke, H., Southard, M., Brooks, J., Nicklas, D., and Hoch, W. S., 1974, Non-Hodgkin's lymphomas: A clinicopathologic study of 293 cases, *Cancer* **34**:1173.

Portlock, C. S., and Rosenberg, S. A., 1976, Combination chemotherapy with cyclophosphamide, vincristine, and prednisone in advanced non-Hodgkin's lymphomas, *Cancer* **37**:1275.

Portlock, C. S., Rosenberg, S. A., Glatstein, E., and Kaplan, H. S., 1976, Treatment of advanced non-Hodgkin's lymphomas with favorable histologies: Preliminary results of a prospective trial, *Blood* **47**:747.

Rappaport, H., 1966, *Tumors of the Hematopoietic System,* p. 91, Armed Forces Institutes of Pathology, Washington, D.C.

Rodriguez, V., Cabanillas, F., Burgess, M. A., McKelvey, E. M., Valdivieso, M., Bodey, G. P., and Freireich, E. J., 1977, Combination chemotherapy ("CHOP-Bleo") in advanced (non-Hodgkin) malignant lymphoma, *Blood* **49**:325.

Rosenberg, S. A., and Kaplan, H. S., 1975, Clinical trials in the non-Hodgkin's lymphoma at Stanford University: Experimental design and preliminary results, *Br. J. Cancer* **31**:456.

Schein, P. S., Chabner, B. A., Canellos, G. P., Young, R. C., Berard, C., and DeVita, V. T., 1974, Potential for prolonged disease-free survival following combination chemotherapy of non-Hodgkin's lymphoma, *Blood* **43**:181.

Schein, P., DeVita, V., Canellos, G., Chabner, B., and Young, R., 1975a, A new combination chemotherapy program for diffuse histiocytic (DHL) and mixed (DML) non-Hodgkin's lymphomas: BACOP, *Proc. Am. Assoc. Cancer Res.* **16**:248.

Schein, P. S., Chabner, B. A., Canellos, G. P., Young, R. C., and DeVita, V. T., Jr., 1975b, Non-Hodgkin's lymphoma: Patterns of relapse from complete remission after combination chemotherapy, *Cancer* **35**:354.

Schein, P. S., MacDonald, J. S., and Edelson, R., 1976a, Cutaneous T-cell lymphoma, *Cancer* **38**:1859.

Schein, P. S., DeVita, V. T., Jr., Hubbard, S., Chabner, B. A., Canellos, G. P., Berard, C., and Young, R. C., 1976b, Bleomycin, adriamycin, cyclophosphamide, vincristine and prednisone (BACOP) combination chemotherapy in the treatment of advanced diffuse histiocytic lymphoma, *Ann. Intern. Med.* **85**:417.

Skarin, A. T., Pinkus, G. S., Myerowitz, R. L., Bishop, Y. M., and Moloney, W. C., 1974a, Combination chemotherapy of advanced lymphocytic lymphoma, *Cancer* **34**:1023.

Skarin, A., Rosenthal, D., Moloney, W., and Frei, E., III, 1974b, Treatment of advanced non-Hodgkin's lymphoma (NHL) with bleomycin (B), adriamycin (A), cyclophosphamide (C), vincristine (O), and prednisone (P) (BACOP), *Proc. Am. Assoc. Cancer Res.* **15**:133.

Skarin, A. T., Frei, E., III, Moloney, W. C., and Gutterman, J. U., 1975, New agents and combination chemotherapy of non-Hodgkin's lymphoma, *Br. J. Cancer* **31**:497.

Skarin, A. T., Rosenthal, D. S., Moloney, W. C., and Frei, E., III, 1977a, Combination chemotherapy of advanced non-Hodgkin's lymphoma with bleomycin, adriamycin, cyclophosphamide, vincristine and prednisone (BACOP), *Blood* **49**:759.

Skarin, A. T., Zuckerman, K. S., Pitman, S. W., Rosenthal, D. S., Moloney, W., Frei, E., III, and Canellos, G. P., 1977b, High dose methotrexate with folinic acid in the treatment of advanced non-Hodgkin's lymphoma including CNS involvement, *Blood,* **50**:1039.

Stein, R. S., Moran, E. M., Dresser, R. K., Miller, J. B., Golomb, H. M., and Ultmann, J. E., 1975, Combination chemotherapy of lymphomas other than Hodgkin's disease, *Ann. Intern. Med.* **81**:601.

Sweet, D. L., Jr., Golomb, H. M., and Ultmann, J. E., 1976, Disseminated malignant lymphoma, histiocytic type: The changing picture, *Ann. Intern. Med.* **85**:521.

Veronesi, U., Musumeci, R., Pizzetti, F., Gennari, L., and Bonadonna, G., 1974, The value of staging laparotomy in non-Hodgkin's lymphomas, *Cancer* **33**:446.

Young, R. C., Anderson, T., Bender, R. A., Norton, L., and DeVita, V. T., 1977, Nodular mixed lymphoma (NML): Another potentially curable non-Hodgkin's lymphoma, *Proc. Am. Assoc. Cancer Res.* **18**:356.

Ziegler, J. L., 1977, Treatment results of 54 American patients with Burkitt's lymphoma are similar to the African experience, *N. Engl. J. Med.* **297**:75.

<h1 style="text-align:right">Index</h1>